CARDIAC RATE AND RHYTHM

DEVELOPMENTS IN CARDIOVASCULAR MEDICINE

VOLUME 17

series ISBN 90-247-2336-1

CARDIAC RATE AND RHYTHM

Physiological, Morphological and Developmental Aspects

Edited by

LENNART N. BOUMAN

and

HABO J. JONGSMA

Department of Physiology
University of Amsterdam

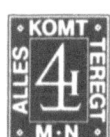

1982

MARTINUS NIJHOFF PUBLISHERS

THE HAGUE / BOSTON / LONDON

Distributors

for the United States and Canada
Kluwer Boston, Inc.
190 Old Derby Street
Hingham, MA 02043
USA

for all other countries
Kluwer Academic Publishers Group
Distribution Center
P.O. Box 322
3300 AH Dordrecht
The Netherlands

Library of Congress Cataloging in Publication Data
Main entry under title:

Cardiac rate and rhythm.

   (Developments in cardiovascular medicine ;
v. 17)
   Includes bibliographical references and index.
   1. Heart beat--Congresses. 2. Sinoatrial node--
Congresses. 3. Pulse--Congresses. I. Bouman,
Lennart Nicolas. II. Jongsma, Habo J. III. Series.
[DNLM: 1. Heart rate--Congresses. 2. Sinoatorial
node--Congresses. W1 DE997VME v. 17 / WG 202
C2693 1980]
QP113.C37   599.01'16   81-22480
ISBN 90-247-2626-3   AACR2

ISBN-13: 978-94-009-7537-8   e-ISBN-13: 978-94-009-7535-4
DOI: 10.1007/978-94-009-7535-4

ACKNOWLEDGEMENT

The editors express their gratitude to all who contributed to the success of the workshop from which these proceedings are the result.

In the first place we want to thank the participants of the workshop for their contribution both in their formal talks and in the ensuing discussions and for the prompt delivery of their manuscripts which are the body of this book.

Secondly our thanks are due to ASTRA Cardiovascular whose generous financial support made this workshop possible; due to their meticulous organization mr. A. van den Elsakker and his co-workers made the workshop a pleasure to attend.

Mrs. Gerie Bouman-Passchier prepared the manuscript for the printer. For this task which implied taming our always resisting laboratory computer she deserves our deepest gratitude.

Finally we want to thank our colleagues in the department of physiology who assisted in the organization of the workshop and the preparation of this volume.

Amsterdam, Spring 1981,

Lennart N. Bouman
Habo J. Jongsma

LIST OF PARTICIPANTS

Allessie, M.A., Dept. of Physiology, Biomedical Center, University of Limburg, Maastricht, The Netherlands

Bleeker, W.K., Dept. of Physiology, Jan Swammerdam Institute, University of Amsterdam, Amsterdam, The Netherlands

Bonke, F.I.M., Dept. of Physiology, Biomedical Center, University of Limburg, Maastricht, The Netherlands

Bouman, L.N., Dept. of Physiology, Jan Swammerdam Institute, University of Amsterdam, Amsterdam, The Netherlands

Brown, H.F., University Laboratory of Physiology, Oxford, United Kingdom

Bukauskas, F.F., Institute for Cardiovascular Research, Kaunas, USSR

Capelle, F.J. van, Dept. of Cardiology and Clinical Physiology, Wilhelmina Gasthuis, The Interuniversity Institute of Cardiology, Amsterdam, The Netherlands

Clapham, D., Dept. of Medicine, Brigham and Women's Hospital, Boston, Massachusetts, U.S.A.

Cranefield, P.F., The Rockefeller University, New York, New York, U.S.A.

DeHaan, R.L., Dept. of Anatomy, Emory University, Atlanta, Georgia, U.S.A.

De Mello, W.C., Dept. of Pharmacology, Medical Sciences Campus, University of Puerto Rico, San Juan, U.S.A.

DiFrancesco, D., Instituto di Fisiologia Generale e Chimica Biologica, University of Milano, Milano, Italy

Ginneken, A.C.G. van, Dept. of Physiology, Jan Swammerdam Institute, University of Amsterdam, Amsterdam, The Netherlands

Gros, D., Laboratoire de Zoologie et Biologie Cellulaire, Universite de Poitiers, Poitiers, France

Irisawa, H., National Institute for Physiological Sciences, Myodaiji, Okazaki, Japan

Jalife, J., Masonic Medical Research Laboratory, Utica, New York, U.S.A.

Janse, M.J., Dept. of Cardiology and Clinical Physiology, Wilhelmina Gasthuis, The Interuniversity Institute of Cardiology, Amsterdam, The Netherlands

Jongsma, H.J., Dept. of Physiology, Jan Swammerdam Institute, University of Amsterdam, Amsterdam, The Netherlands

Karemaker, J.M., Dept. of Physiology, Jan Swammerdam Institute, Unversity of Amsterdam, Amsterdam, The Netherlands

Kimura, J., University Laboratory of Physiology, Oxford, United Kingdom

Kleber, A., Dept. of Physiology, University of Berne, Berne, Switzerland

Kurachi, Y., National Institute for Physiological Sciences, Myodaiji, Okazaki, Japan

Lammers, W., Dept. of Physiology, Biomedical Center, University of Limburg, Maastricht, The Netherlands

Lazdunski, M., Centre de Biochimie C.N.R.S., Universite de Nice, Nice, France

Levy, M.N., Dept. of Investigative Medicine, Mt. Sinai Hospital, Cleveland, Ohio, U.S.A.

Linkens, D.A., Dept. of Control Engineering, University of Sheffield, Sheffield, United Kingdom

Masson-Pevet, M.A., Dept. of Physiology, Jan Swammerdam Institute, University of Amsterdam, Amsterdam, The Netherlands

Meerwijk, W.P.M. van, Dept. of Physiology and Medical Physics, University of Leiden, Leiden, The Netherlands

Moore, E.N., Dept. of Animal Biology, School of Veterinary Medicine, University of Pennsylvania, Philadelphia, Pennsylvania, U.S.A.

Noble, D., University Laboratory of Physiology, Oxford, United Kingdom

Noble, S.J., University Laboratory of Physiology, Oxford, United Kingdom

Op 't Hof, T., Dept. of Physiology, Jan Swammerdam Institute, University of Amsterdam, Amsterdam, The Netherlands

Osterrieder, W., II. Physiologisches Institut, Universitaet des Saarlandes, Homburg/Saar, Germany.

Pappano, A., Dept. of Pharmacology, University of Connecticut Health Center, Farmington, Connecticut, U.S.A.

Pelzer, D., II. Physiologisches Institut, Universitaet des Saarlandes, Homburg/Saar, Germany

Peracchia, C., Dept. of Physiology, University of Rochester, School of Medicine and Dentistry, Rochester, New York, U.S.A.

Renaud, J.F., Centre de Biochimie C.N.R.S., Universite de Nice, Nice, France

Sperelakis, N., Dept. of Physiology, University of Virginia, School of Medicine, Charlottesville, Virginia, U.S.A.

Torre, V., Physiological Laboratory, Cambridge, United Kingdom

Weidmann, S., Dept. of Physiology, University of Berne, Berne, Switzerland

Winfree, A.T., Dept. of Biological Sciences, Lilly Hall of Life Sciences, Purdue

University, West Lafayette, Indiana, U.S.A.

Wojtzcak, J., Dept. of Clinical Physiology, Medical Center of Postgraduate Education, Warsaw, Poland

Ypey, D.L., Dept. of Physiology and Medical Physics, University of Leiden, Leiden, The Netherlands

CONTENTS

XII

SECTION TWO: INTERACTION OF PACEMAKER CELLS

SECTION THREE: ESTABLISHMENT OF CARDIAC RHYTHM

SECTION FOUR: NEURAL CONTROL OF RATE AND RHYTHM

INTRODUCTION

In the denervated state the mammalian heart, both in vivo and in vitro, is excited at very regular intervals, the coefficient of variance of the interbeat intervals not exceeding 2%. The pacemaker that is the source of this regular excitation is localised normally within the sinus node (= sino-atrial node = node of Keith and Flack), a most intriguing small piece of tissue in the caval corner of the right atrium. A small portion of this node containing a group of probably only a few thousands of cells fires spontaneously, that means without any external influence to trigger their activity. The so called pacemaker cells do this by letting their membrane potential fall to the level where an action potential will start which subsequently activates surrounding cells to fire an action potential. The first question which is tackled in this book is which processes underly this spontaneous diastolic depolarization. This is discussed in section I, concerning the fundamental properties of pacemaker cells with special reference to ionic membrane currents. Although views still quite differ about the exact nature of the membrane processes that cause the automatic pacemaker discharge there is agreement that diastolic depolarization is brought about by the interaction of a number of ionic current systems, including both inward and outward going currents.

In the conceptual model that we have in mind nowadays about the basis of the action of the sinus node, the group of several thousands so called leading or dominant pacemaker cells is thought to consist of cells that all fire spontaneously, every cell bringing its membrane potential during diastole down to a level that a propagated action potential can arise. This is as yet merely an assumption, because the intrinsic activity of isolated cells from the dominant pacemaker area is unknown by the lack of an effective isolation procedure. However, even if the assumption would not be correct and only a fraction of the cells in the dominant pacemaker area would exhibit automaticity, it still is likely that the impulse will arise from more than one cell, because the amount of diastolic current that one single cell can generate is too low to excite the adjacent cells if they should have a stable diastolic membrane potential.

Be as that it may, from microelectrode impalements in the sinus node it is
well known that within the group of dominant pacemakers all cells fire together
well in phase with each other. The problem of the coupling of the activity of
the individual pacemaker cells is covered in section II, dealing with the electrical interaction of pacemaker cells. It will appear that via specialized connections between the cells, current can flow from one cell to the other, keeping the
diastolic depolarization of adjacent cells into the same phase. This electrical
interaction seems to be responsible also for another fundamental property of the
cardiac pacemaker, viz. the regularity of its rhythm. From   studies   in   tissue
culture   it   is known that spontaneously beating isolated cardiocytes show a considerable variation in their individual interbeat interval duration.   Only when
the cells grow together forming a multicellular structure the variation in interbeat interval will disappear. The variation in cycle length is likely to be
brought   about   by   the random fluctuations in membrane potential that have been
studied extensively in nerve cells. Membrane noise is a fundamental property of
excitable membranes; it is likely therefore that due to it the intrinsic rhythm
of discharge of a single pacemaker cells should exhibit a certain degree of irregularity.   The interconnection of a multitude of pacemaker cells seems to "level
out" the interference of membrane noise with a regular firing rhythm. The significance of the interaction of pacemaker cells for the establishment of the normal
cardiac rate and rhythm is worked out in a series of papers in section III.   Both
from   experimental   studies   on heart and nerve cells as from model studies using
artificial oscillators it will appear that the degree of coupling between the in-
divual oscillations has a great influence on the rate and the rhythm of the total
system.

In section IV of the book, dealing with the neural control of the cardiac
rate   and   rhythm, we will go into the fundamental processes at the level of the
nerve-muscle interaction in the pacemaker. The membrane action of acetylcholine
has   been elucidated recently: the hyperpolarization and slowing down of the diastolic depolarization, both well known actions of ACh, are caused by an increase
of   the   outward   going   current   of potassium ions by the ACh-induced opening of
specific channels inside the membrane. The existence of an inhibitory effect of
ACh   on   the slow inward current carried by sodium and or calcium ions is however
still controversial.

The same holds true for the membrane activity of catecholamines, of which not yet a comprehensive report can be produced. For both transmitters it has become clear that the responsiveness of cells in different regions of the sinus node to the action of the drug is quite different. This inhomogeneity causes well documented shifts in the site of the pacemaker within the sinus node under the influence of the drug. From a practical point of view it is important that such a drug-induced shift gives an satisfactory explanation for the inhibitory action of acetylcholine on the action of adrenaline.

In the final part of these proceedings, papers on the nervous control in the intact individual are presented. It is a little disconcerting after having understood the complicated mechanisms that turn the irregular rhythm of the isolated cell into the clock-like regularity of the multicellular pacemaker, to find that the intact heart in situ is almost equally irregular as the isolated cardiocyte. But, of course, the basis of this neurogenic irregularity is quite different. It will become clear that a phasic action of the extracardial nerves, and the vagal nerves in particular, can interfere in a complex way with the sinus node in the generation of a constant cycle length.

Summing up the essentials that the workshop has produced we can picture now the events in the cardiac pacemaker in a few lines: In the sinus node, the normal site of the pacemaker of the mammalian heart, there is a small group of cells that will produce an action potential without any external stimulus. A system of membrane currents of different ionic species causes during diastole a fall in membrane potential that will bring those cells gradually into the action potential. Electrical currents flowing through specialized connections between the cells will cause a regular rhythm, of discharge, that takes place in all participating cells at the same moment. Nervous impulses can change the rate of discharge by changing the ionic current flow through the membranes. Unequal distribution of these changes may cause a shifting of the leading pacemakers within the sinus node. The interference of the nervous activity with the rhythmic pacemaker activity may cause irregularities in the cardiac rhythm as they are daily met.

SECTION ONE

FUNDAMENTALS OF PACEMAKER ACTIVITY

PACEMAKER MECHANISMS[*]

Paul F. Cranefield

Our hosts, Drs. Bouman and Jongsma, have asked me to summarize the different mechanisms by which spontaneous activity might arise in a cluster of cells, adding
that, in their view, a cluster of cells must be taken as the model rather than
the single cell to allow for the possible role of reentry as a mechanism for
spontaneous activity. In response to their suggestion, I will point out a few
ways in which a cell or a collection of cells could serve as a pacemaker and consider some ways in which the rate of such a pacemaker might be varied.

To begin, I will repeat the distinctions I made at the Maastricht symposium
(Cranefield, 1978) between automaticity and the mechanisms that can sustain activity once it is initiated. There are at least three kinds of foci of rhythmic
activity that can serve as pacemakers: 1) there are foci that can remain active
and serve as a pacemaker for longer or shorter periods provided they have, in
some manner, become active in the first place but they are not automatic since
they never do become active unless some cell in the focus is excited by an external stimulus or by activity that arises elsewhere and reaches the focus by propagation; 2) a focus may be automatic in the sense that it contains within its
fibers, individually or collectively, a mechanism that will always give rise to
an initial impulse should the focus be or happen to become quiescent but the
rhythmic activity following that initial impulse is sustained by a mechanism
quite different from the mechanism that leads to the first or initiating impulse;
3) a focus may be automatic and both the first and all subsequent impulses may
arise in the same way.

In the first class of pacemakers we may put those examples of circus move-

[*] Supported by a grant from The National Heart Lung and Blood Institute (HL
14899).

ment (Wit and Cranefield, 1978) and triggerable foci (Cranefield, 1977) that never show sustained rhythmic activity until an impulse propagates into the focus from outside. Some potential foci of sustained rhythmic activity of this kind may be quiescent because their fibers are shielded from extrinsic excitation by entry block; the fibers of other may be rhythmically activated by each sinus impulse and thrown into sustained rhythmic activity only when the initiating impulse is premature. Nodal reentry, the WPW syndrome and triggerable activity in the coronary sinus provide specific examples of foci that can become rhythmically active and become the pacemaker of the heart but never do so if the heart is quiescent and never generate an initiating impulse within the focus. In other words such foci are not automatic (Cranefield, 1975, 1977, 1978). Their rhythmic activity is sustained by afterdepolarizations or by circus movement, i.e. by a mechanism different from that which leads to the first impulse in the series.

The second class of foci is that which contains a fiber or fibers that are automatic and can "spontaneously" give rise to an initial impulse which in turn elicits sustained rhythmic activity. Real or hypothetical examples of this could be, e.g., found in foci that contained a fiber or fibers that go from quiescence to activity either by "spontaneous" phase 4 depolarization or by waxing oscillations in membrane potential (see West, 1961; Vassalle, 1965). The first impulse to arise in such a focus may then evoke, in other fibers of the focus, circus movement of excitation or triggering in which the rhythmic activity is sustained by delayed afterdepolarizations or activity sustained by true reflection of the kind discussed later in this chapter.

The third class mentioned above is that in which the first and all subsequent impulses arise "automatically" and by the same mechanism. Every impulse might arise by phase 4 depolarization (Draper and Weidmann, 1951; Trautwein and Zink, 1952) or from waxing oscillations in membrane potential (West, 1961). The situation in which all impulses including the first arise by phase 4 depolarization is that classically associated with "pacemakers" and with the SA node or with rhythmic activity in Purkinje fibers. At the Maastricht symposium (Cranefield, 1978) I questioned whether such foci exist at all, suggesting the possibility that the first impulse in a quiescent fiber, even of the SA node, always arises in a different way from subsequent impulses so that even fibers of the SA node can thus be regarded as triggerable. That does not mean that fibers of the SA node or Purkinje fibers are not automatic, it means only that their ability to pass from quiescence to activity depends on a mechanism that differs, at least in degree, from the mechanism that generates succeeding impulses. Viewed in one way this seems heretical, viewed in another way it is almost a truism since no one would deny that the first action potential in a series sets into motion complex changes in ionic currents that persist into the following diastole and affect subsequent action potentials. I would prefer, at this point to reemphasize the "heretical" aspect, since to me the important notion is that if there are any differences at all between the causes of the first impulse and the causes of subsequent impulses we must look to those differences when we try to figure out how and why rhythmically active foci start or stop. A number of people have claimed to be puzzled by this distinction. Perhaps the replacement of the hand crank by the electric "self-starter" has obscured from view the differences between the way in which the rhythmic activity of an electrically ignited internal combustion engine is initiated and the way in which its rhythmic activity is sustained? And indeed, in these days there must be not only those who have forgotten but those who never even knew that a fully wound pendulum-driven clock will not "spontaneously" start telling time but will begin its sustained rhythmic activity only when an "external stimulus" initiates the first swing of the pendulum. That clock is an interesting example for our purposes since its sustained rhythmic activity can also be interrupted by a single external stimulus that stops the pendulum and, once stopped, it will remain stopped until again "triggered" into activity.

It is possible, therefore, that there is no "Class 3" of rhythmically active foci, since the initiating and sustaining mechanisms may always be different. Nevertheless, in what follows, I will use the term automatic to refer to fibers that move from quiescence to activity "spontaneously", i.e. through intrinsic change that arises within the cell rather than in response to some external stimulus or the arrival of a propagated impulse.

Let me now turn to some examples of pacemakers of a complex kind. Vassalle's studies of rhythmic activity in Purkinje fibers provide a fascinating example of the interaction of different forms of activity with each other and with overdrive suppression (Vassalle et al., 1975; 1977). Under certain conditions such fibers can show both phase 4 depolarization and delayed afterdepolarizations. The addition of epinephrine can increase the rate to the point at which the delayed afterdepolarizations reach threshold, whereupon the fiber is triggered into rapid rhythmic activity sustained by delayed afterdepolarizations. Such activity is usually selflimiting, in part because the increased rate leads to enhanced electrogenic sodium extrusion which generates an outward current capable both of making the maximum diastolic potential more negative and of reducing the amplitude of the delayed afterdepolarizations. When the burst of triggered activity ends, the persistence of the enhanced electrogenic sodium extrusion suppresses the reappearance of the automatic activity which depends on phase 4 depolarization. The return of the latter activity and its gradual increase in rate may again trigger the fiber. The cycle can thus be: quiescence, followed by automatic activity gradually increasing in rate followed by an abrupt increase in rate associated with triggering followed by quiescence and a repeat of the events just described. The response of such a focus to extrinsic overdrive is interesting since overdrive at a moderate rate may suppress the automatic activity and yield post-overdrive suppression whereas overdrive at a higher rate may cause triggering and post-overdrive acceleration.

Activity of the sort seen in Vassalle's experiments can also be seen in the coronary sinus, in which the two forms of activity occur in separate groups of fibers that are close enough together to be regarded, for the sake of discussion, as a single focus. The automatic fibers near the mouth of the sinus can become active when exposed to norepinephrine, and gradually speed up to the rate that triggers fibers within the coronary sinus into rapid rhythmic activity sustained by afterdepolarizations (Wit and Cranefield, 1977; Cranefield, 1977). The resulting burst of triggered activity is eventually suppressed by enhanced electrogenic sodium extrusion (Gadsby, Wit and Cranefield, 1979) which also inhibits the reappearance of activity in the automatic fibers at the mouth of the sinus.

A quite different form of pacemaker can be envisioned in a heart that has two or more foci in which true reflection arises. Some time ago we suggested that the phenomenon of reflection might be important as a cause of re-entry (Wit, Hoffman and Cranefield, 1972). In reflection an impulse arrives at a point in a fiber at which it is delayed: the impulse travels forward slowly and a second impulse is "reflected" to travel back in the direction from which the initiating impulse entered the fiber. Although the underlying cause of reflection might be circus movement of excitation on a microscopic scale it might also result from the fact that the initiating impulse becomes so nearly stationary in the region of slow conduction that the fiber that conveyed it to that region has time to re-

polarize and then be reexcited by the nearly stationary impulse or by electrotonic spread of the rapid upstroke of cells beyond the depressed region (see Cranefield, 1975, p.185). Studies of the giant axon (Ramon and Moore, 1979) have
shown that this latter mechanism can in fact cause "true reflection" in a system
in which, although there is a branch point, there is no syncytium so that there
can be no circus movement. Studies from Moe's laboratory (Antzelevitch et al.,
1980) have offered strong support to the notion that true reflection can cause
reentrant excitation in cardiac fibers. Our further conjecture was that if a
heart contained several foci capable of responding to excitation with true reflection one focus might excite another and so on, producing a form of possibly
irregular but sustained rhythmic activity. That activity would be reentrant but
would not depend on circus movement in the ordinary sense of the word, and would
not arise "spontaneously" but only in response to an initiating impulse.

A large class of mixed causes of sustained rhythmic activity is revealed
when one considers the fact that afterdepolarizations occur remarkably late in
the cycle so that an impulse might return towards a cell that had initiated it at
a moment when the afterdepolarization was nearing its peak and, by electrotonic
interaction, bring a subthreshold afterdepolarization to threshold. This is an
extension of Mines' suggestion (Mines, 1914) that

> "the chief error to be guarded against (in attributing a sequence of
> activity to circus movement of excitation) is that of mistaking a ser-
> ies of automatic beats originating in one point of a ring and travel-
> ling around it in one direction only owing to a complete block close
> to the point of origin of the rhythm on one side of this point."

In our extension of Mines' cautionary remarks we suggested that the impulse
might return to the point of origin and there evoke a "new impulse in some way
other than by continuous conduction" (by, e.g., interaction with an afterdepolarization). As Mayer said (Mayer, 1908) the wave "might be reinforced and sent
forth anew every time it returns to its point of origin." Both foci that show
true reflection and triggerable foci might interact in this way, with or without
the presence of entry block.

At the Maastricht symposium (Cranefield, 1978) I remarked that

"It is not...a verbal quibble to suggest...that at least some of the fibers traditionally regarded as automatic do not derive their automaticity from their familiar phase 4 depolarization, but from some other property such as the ability to show a slow gradual depolarization or oscillatory prepotentials. On the one hand the ionic mechanisms that cause after-potentials and thus permit triggering may be quite different from those that cause oscillatory prepotentials or the very slow and gradual depolarization that leads to the first action potential....On the other hand, we often wish to use drugs to initiate a rhythm or to interrupt a tachycardia. If true automaticity derives from causes different from those which sustain rhythmic activity once it has been triggered, then we must allow for that when we search for drugs that can initiate, modify or terminate rhythmic activity."

In support of the argument expressed in the last sentence of the above remarks let me consider a focus of rhythmic activity in which fibers that show phase 4 depolarization at a high (negative) level of resting potential may also on occasion show an interruption of repolarization leading to rhythmic activity at a low level of resting potential (Fig. 1). Whatever the currents may be that underlie these two forms of rhythmic activity that can be seen in the same single fiber, the activity that occurs at the more negative level is of the sort ordinarily called automatic whereas the activity seen at the more positive level is of the kind ordinarily called triggered because it does not occur unless an initiating action potential triggers it and because it is sustained by delayed afterdepolarizations. Moreover, the two forms of activity are, in fact, differently affected by both arrhythmogenic and anti-arrhythmic agents. The "automatic" activity at the more negative membrane potential is sensitive to catecholamines and beta-blockers and is insensitive to verapamil whereas the rhythmic activity at the more positive membrane potential is sensitive to slow channel blockers. Thus in this, as in many other foci in which multiple mechanisms play a role, the initiating impulse has sensitivities to physiological and pharmacological agents that differ from those of the impulses that sustain rhythmic activity once it has been initiated.

If we accept the existence of two forms of possibly genuine automatic activity, i.e. spontaneous depolarization and waxing oscillations in membrane

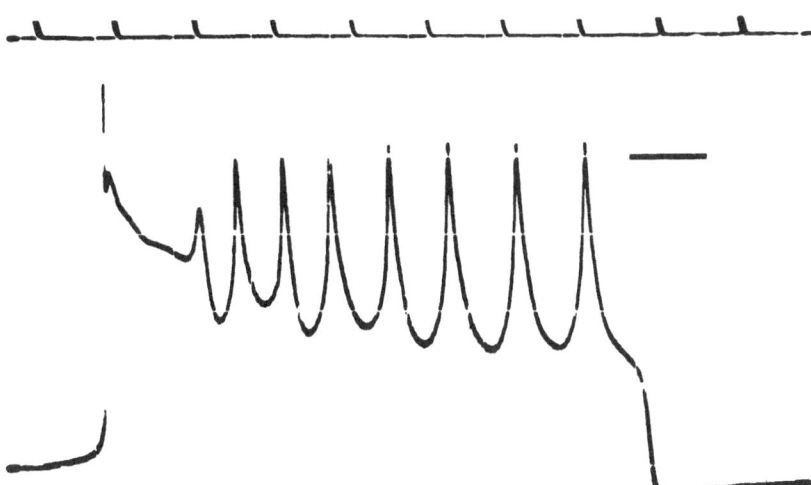

FIGURE 1 *Action potentials recorded from a canine cardiac Purkinje fiber. Spontaneous depolarization occurring at a high negative level of membrane potential evokes a fast upstroke. The repolarization of that upstroke is interrupted by rhythmic activity sustained at a much less negative level of membrane potential. Full repolarization finally carries the membrane back to the original high negative membrane potential and spontaneous depolarization resumes. Calibrations: Time marks occur at 1 s intervals; the point at which the tracing of electrical activity begins corresponds to -81 mV. The short horizontal line to the right corresponds to 0 mV.*

potential, and the existence of some half-dozen ways in which activity can be sustained, namely spontaneous depolarization, waxing oscillations, delayed afterdepolarizations, circus movement, reflection and rhythmic activity at relatively positive levels of resting potential, we are forced to conclude that the number of possible combinations of these mechanisms is rather large. Several such combinations are known to exist and we may surely expect that more will be demonstrated in the future. Recognition of the fact that the mechanism by which the first impulse is initiated may differ from the mechanism by which subsequent activity is sustained may help to explain why certain rhythms respond in complicated ways to physiological and pharmacological agents and to interventions such as overdrive suppression.

In further pursuit of the suggestion made by our hosts that I give some attention to the syncytial properties of the heart I would like to draw your attention to some interesting consequences of the fact that pacemaker fibers are connected to fibers that are not pacemakers. The net inward currents that give rise to phase 4 depolarization, to waxing oscillations and to delayed afterdepolarizations are small and can easily be balanced by small increases in outward current. There has recently been a revival of interest in the well-known phenomenon of electrical "loading" of one part of a cell or syncytium by another part (Joyner et al., 1980) but not too much attention has been paid to the implications of this for pacemaker activity. If a group of cells that has a high resting potential and a high g_K (i.e. a low impedance hyperpolarizing source) is closely connected to a group of cells that can, under appropriate conditions, give rise to spontaneous depolarization, waxing oscillations or delayed afterdepolarizations, the current flowing between the low impedance high resting potential group of cells and the potential pacemaker cells will tend to suppress, in the potentially rhythmically active region, pacemaker activity that depends on small net inward currents. This means that the presence or rate of pacemaker activity could be modulated by changes that act on the "suppressor" region without acting directly on the pacemaker cells. Neural or humoral influences could alter the resting potential or the membrane resistance of the "suppressor" cells in a way that makes them less effective in delivering hyperpolarizing current to the pacemaker cells. Moreover, any increase in internal resistance in the connections between the "suppressor" cells and the pacemaker cells might have the same effect; thus uncoupling of the nexal connections might "release" pacemaker cells and permit them to become rhythmically active whereas better coupling might suppress pacemaker activity. This suggests an explanation for the fact that the true pacemaker cells within the SA node are not connected directly to atrial cells. Atrial cells are cells with a high resting potential and a high g_K and would, were they in direct continuity with SA nodal cells via low resistance pathways, suppress SA nodal activity. The well known relative paucity of nexal junctions within the SA node and the gradual increase both in the density of nexal junctions and cell diameter seen as one moves from true pacemaker cells in the center of the SA node to true atrial cells may be absolutely necessary to permit the functioning of the pacemaker cells.

Similar considerations may explain observations recently made in our laboratory on preparations of the rabbit AV node. When such preparations are reduced in size, by careful dissection, to a bundle about 1 mm long and 0.5 mm in diameter, cells that seem by other criteria to be typical midnodal or N cells become rhythmically active (Wit and Cranefield, unpublished observations). One might suppose that this rhythmic activity results from damage caused by the dissection but the electrical characteristics of the preparation remain constant for many hours. It is possible, therefore, that mid-nodal cells can display phase 4 depolarization but are normally prevented from doing so by the fact that they are connected to cells with a high resting potential that suppress the potential rhythmic activity of the mid-nodal cells. Whether this interpretation is correct or not, it seems certain that we must look at interactions between pacemaker cells and the cells that surround them in the cardiac syncytium not only in terms of propagation but also in terms of variations in the electrical loading of pacemaker cells by cells in their surround.

It is clear then, as our hosts rightly supposed, that pacemaker activity may be altogether more complicated than it seems and certainly cannot be thought about without reference to the fact that pacemaker cells in vivo are part of a syncytium.

REFERENCES

Antzelevitch, C., Jalife, J. and Moe, G.K.: Characteristics of reflection as a mechanism of reentrant arrythmias and its relationship to parasystole. Circulation, 61: 182-191, 1980.

Cranefield, P.F.: The conduction of the cardiac impulse. The slow response and cardiac arrhythmias. Mount Kisco, N.Y., Futura, pp. 185, 1975.

Cranefield, P.F.: Action potentials, afterpotentials and arrhythmias. Circ. Res., 41: 415-423, 1977.

Cranefield, P.F.: Does spontaneous activity arise from phase 4 depolarization or from triggering? In: The Sinus Node. Structure, Function and Clinical Relevance, Bonke, F.I.M., ed., Martinus Nijhoff, The Hague, pp. 348-356, 1978.

Draper, M.H. and Weidmann, S.: Cardiac resting and action potentials recorded with an intracellular electrode. J. Physiol., 115: 74-94, 1951.

Gadsby, D.C., Wit, A.L. and Cranefield, P.F.: Overdrive suppression of trig-

gered atrial tachycardia arising in the canine coronary sinus. (Abstr.)
Amer. J. Cardiol., 43: 374, 1979..

Joyner, R.W., Westerfield, M. and Moore, J.W.: Effects of cellular geometry on
current flow during a propagated action potential. Biophysical J., 31:
183-194, 1980..

Mayer, A.G.: Rhythmical pulsation in Scyphomedusae: II. In: Papers from the
Tortugas Laboratory of the Carnegie Institution of Washington. I: 113-131
(Carnegie Institution of Washington, Publication No. 102, part VII), 1908.

Mines, G.R.: On circulating excitations in heart muscles and their possible relation to tachycardia and fibrillation. Trans. Roy. Soc. Can. Ser. 3,
sec. 4, 8: 43-52, 1914.

Ramon, F. and Moore, J.W.: Propagation of action potentials in squid giant
axons. Repetitive firing at regions of membrane inhomogeneities. J. Gen.
Physiol., 73: 595-603, 1979.

Trautwein, W. and Zink, K.: Ueber Membran und Aktionspotentials einzelner Myokardfasern des Kalt und Warmblueterherzens. Pflueger's Arch., 256: 68-84,
1952.

Vassalle, M.: Cardiac pacemaker potentials at different extra- and intracellular K concentrations. Amer. J. Physiol., 208: 770-775, 1965.

Vassalle, M., Cummins, M., Castro, C. and Stuckey, J.H.: The relationship
between overdrive suppression and overdrive excitation in ventricular pacemakers in dogs. Circ. Res., 38: 367-374, 1975.

Vassalle, M., Knob, R.E., Cummins, M., Lara, G.A., Castro, C. and Stuckey,
J.H.: An analysis of fast idioventricular rhythm in the dog. Circ. Res.,
41: 218-226, 1977.

West, T.C.: Effects of chronotropic influences on subthreshold oscillations in
the sino-atrial node. In: The Specialized Tissues of the Heart, Paes de
Carvalho, A., de Mello, W.C. and Hoffman, B.F., eds., Amsterdam, Elsevier,
pp. 81-94, 1961.

Wit, A.L. and Cranefield, P.F.: Triggered and automatic activity in the canine
coronary sinus. Circ. Res., 41: 435-455, 1977.

Wit, A.L. and Cranefield, P.F.: Reentrant excitation as a cause of cardiac arrhythmias. Amer. J. Physiol., 235: H1-H17, 1978.

Wit, A.L., Hoffman, B.F. and Cranefield, P.F.: Slow conduction and reentry in
the ventricular conduction system. I. Return extrasystole in canine Purk-

inje fibers. Circulation Res., 30: 1-10, 1972.

ON THE ULTRASTRUCTURAL IDENTIFICATION OF PACEMAKER

CELL TYPES WITHIN THE SINUS NODE

Mireille Masson-Pevet, Wim K. Bleeker, Elly Besselsen, Albert J.C. Mackaay, Habo J. Jongsma and Lennart N. Bouman

The heart beat originates within a small group of cells in the sinus node. In the rabbit this site of earliest discharge or leading pacemaker center, is located in the intercaval region, 0.5 - 2 mm away from the medial border of the crista terminalis. It contains typical nodal cells, and is part of a much larger group of cells that all show diastolic depolarization. This latter group of cells, which under standard conditions (see Bleeker et al., 1980) follow the discharge of the leading pacemaker cells and which never reach threshold spontaneously are called transitional cells. From its site of origin the excitation wave propagates through the sinus node preferentially in an oblique cranial direction toward the crista terminalis. In all other directions, the spread of excitation is considerably slower; in the direction of the interatrial septum conduction fails (Fig. 1).

In this zone of conduction block action potentials with double components are recorded (Bleeker et al., 1980). In the present study an answer is sought to the following questions: - Has the electrophysiological differentiation between dominant and following pacemaker cells ultrastructural correlates? - Is there a morphological substrate for the observed conduction block towards the interatrial septum? In a attempt to answer these questions, we will first pay attention to the intracellular structure of the typical nodal cells in the dominant pacemaker center. Thereafter, we will focus our attention on the transitional cells, and more precisely, on the correlation between their electrophysiological and morphological properties.

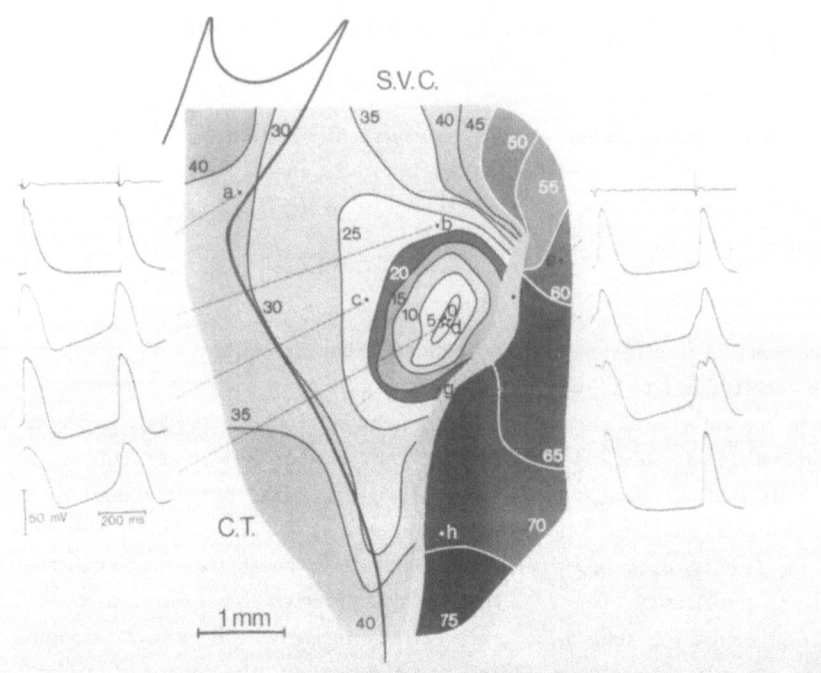

FIGURE 1 *Map of the activation pattern in the nodal region, seen from the endocardial side. The black star indicates the origin of the impulse. The activation times are grouped in classes of 5 ms. The hatched area indicate the zone
with double component action potentials. The action potentials shown were recorded at the sites indicated on the activation map. C.T.= crista terminalis.
SVC = superior vena cava.*

THE DOMINANT PACEMAKER CENTER

Dominant pacemaker cells are defined as cells that show the earliest activation
moment with regard to the activation of the atrium. Bleeker et al. (1980) have
shown that an area, composed of at least 5000 cells, is responsible for initiating pacemaker activity under standard conditions. This area consists of cells of
one type only, the typical nodal cells (Fig. 2).

   Typical nodal cells are also called P cells (James et al., 1966). This term
is very confusing, however, since the term large pale cells or large P cells is
also often used (e.g. Truex, 1976) as a synonym of "intercalated clear cells"

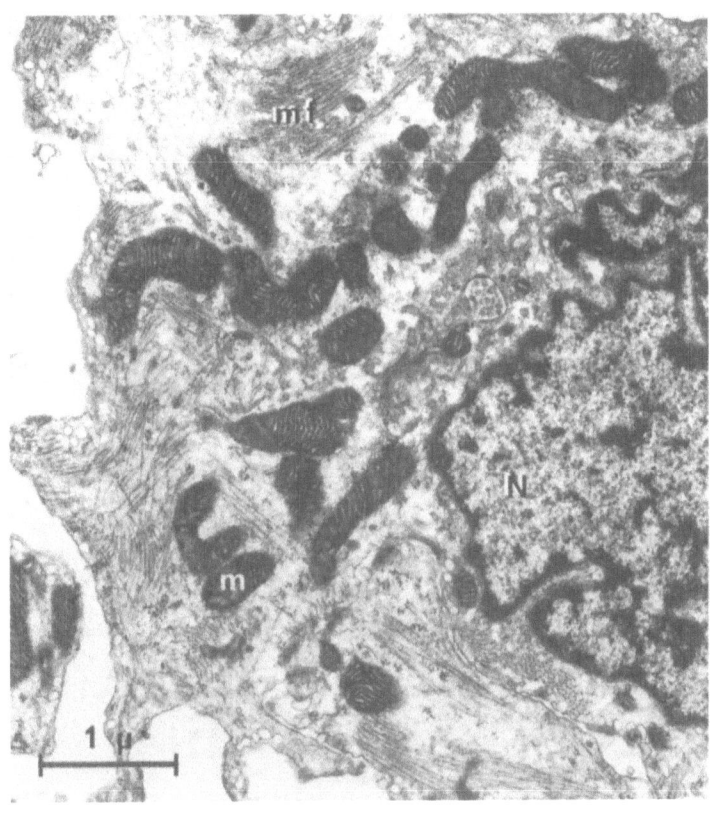

FIGURE 2 *Electronmicrograph of a typical nodal cell. The contractile system (mf) is extremely poorly developed and seems to be distributed at random. N = nucleus.*

(e.g. Viragh and Porte, 1973), which are, according to Tranum-Jensen (1978), artifacts. Typical nodal cells are relatively small cells, roughly spindle-shaped,
about 25 µm long and 5 to 8 µm in diameter, showing a very irregular profile in
cross-section. The smallness of these cells compared to other heart cells, which
results in an increased surface/volume ratio, may be associated with the observed
absence of a T-tubular system (see Table I). Apart from the absence of a
T-tubular system, typical nodal cells are qualitatively similar, however, to the

better-known working myocardial cells. That is to say that with present techniques, exactly the same intracellular and membraneous structures have been found
in both cell types. Quantitatively, however, differences do exist between typical nodal cells and working heart cells, such as atrial cells (Masson-Pevet et
al., 1979a). These differences are summarized in Table I, which shows that about
half of the cell volume in typical nodal cells is free of organized structures as
compared to 10 % in atrial cells. For this reason typical nodal cells have an
"empty" appearance.

TABLE I

SOME CHARACTERISTICS OF THE TYPICAL NODAL CELLS AND OF THE ATRIAL CELLS

	typical nodal cells	atrial cells
size	20 μm / 5-8 μm	80-100 μm / 10 μm
form	irregular	± regular[x]
T system	absent	present[x]
glycogen particles	many	few
arrangement of the	multidirectional	orderly
contractile system	many free myofilaments	parallel myofibrils
myofilaments[*]	15 %	54 %
mitochondria	15 %	23 %
nucleus	13 %	4 %
SR SSV[*]	0.3 %	0.2 %
SR tubules	0.7 %	2.6 %
cytoplasm matrix[+]	± 50 %	± 10 %

[x]Atrial cells in this study were taken from the crista terminalis;
although these cells generally contain a transverse tubular system, it
should be stressed that atrial cells not always contain a T system
(see Forssman and Girardier, 1970).

[*]The percentages given for the myofilaments, mitochondria, nucleus,
subsarcolemmal vesicles (SSV) and sarcoplasmic reticulum tubules (SR
tubules) correspond to the volume fractions occupied by these structures in typical nodal cells and in atrial cells. They have been determined with the point-counting method (Weibel et al., 1966).

[+]The volume density of the cytoplasm matrix is given as 100 % minus
the sum of the relative volumes (in %) of the organized structures,
assuming that the not quanti- fied organized structures occupy between
5 and 10 % of the cell volume.

We will not describe here in detail all structures present in the typical
nodal cells (for more information see Masson-Pevet et al., 1978, 1979a;
Tranum-Jensen, 1978) but we will confine ourselves to a general survey.

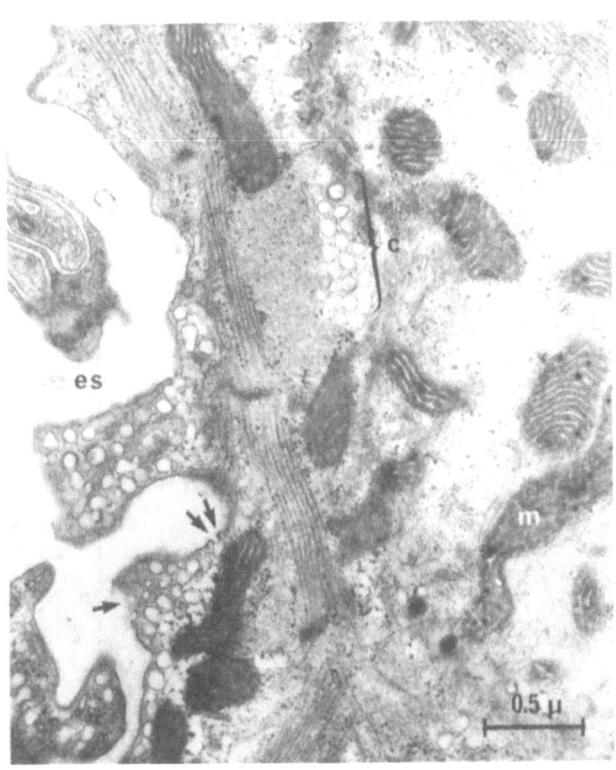

FIGURE 3 *Electronmicrograph of a typical nodal cell showing the presence of a great number of caveolae. The cell has been cut more or less tangentially to its surface. Sometimes it is clear that a caveola communicates with the extracellular space (double arrow). Some caveolae have been cut tangetially at the level of their neck (arrow). c = caveolae, es = extracellular space, ms = mitochondria.*

The cell volume occupied by the organized structures comprises mainly three organelles, present in about equal volume ratio (Table I): myofilaments (15 %), mitochondria (15 %), and nuclei (13 %). It is thus clear that the contractile system, which occupies 54 % of the volume of working heart cells, is only a minor component of typical nodal cells. Contraction seems clearly not to be the primary function of these cells. This point is stressed by the fact that many myofilaments are observed free in the cytoplasm without any obvious orientation (Fig. 2) and not organized into myofibrils with well defined sarcomeres as in working heart cells.

The existence of a longitudinal tubular (SR) system appears to be intimately related with the amount of myofilaments, since the SR tubules to myofilament ratio is equal in nodal and in atrial cells (0.05).

TABLE II

*SOME CHARACTERISTICS OF THE CAVEOLAE IN TYPICAL NODAL CELLS
AND IN ATRIAL CELLS OF THE RABBIT. THESE MEASUREMENTS HAVE
BEEN PERFORMED IN THREE RABBITS*
For details see Masson-Pevet et al., 1980.

	typical nodal cells	atrial cells
number of caveolar openings/ μm^2	21 ± 2	10 ± 1
membrane surface area of one caveola (μm^2)	0.027 ± 0.006	0.026 ± 0.006
increase in membrane surface area (%) due to caveolae	115 ± 3	56 ± 6

The relative volume of the nuclei in leading pacemaker cells is about three times larger than in atrial cells (Table I). If it is assumed that the absolute volume of the nuclei is the same in both cell types, the difference in relative volume occupied by the nuclei is a consequence of a difference in cell volume.

Numerous caveolae are present in the cytoplasm of the heart cells, close to the sarcolemma (Fig. 3). As shown before, these can easily be filled with the extracellular space markers lanthanum and ruthenium red, even after fixation, i.e. after death of the cells (Masson-Pevet et al., 1979b). Caveolae therefore communicate with the extracellular space, as first noted in the frog heart by Lorber and Bertaud (1971).

Caveolae are distributed irregularly. Their density has been determined by counting the number of caveolar openings on replicas of freeze-cleaved specimens. The results are given in Table II. From the measured size of one caveola the increase in membrane surface area due to the presence of these structures has been calculated in nodal and atrial cells. We can see in Table II that the caveolae are very numerous in leading sinus node cells where they increase the membrane surface area by 115 %, as compared with 56 % in atrial cells and 20 and 27 % in ventricular papillary muscle cells (Gabella, 1978; Levin and Page, 1980). The function of the caveolae is still unknown.

It is generally agreed that impulse conduction between heart cells is possible because low resistance pathways (nexuses or gap junctions) exist between cardiac cells.

In the leading center of the sinus node gap junctions (Fig. 4) have been shown to be present (Masson-Pevet et al., 1979b) in low density (about 10 % of the amount found in working myocardium). Due to the small size of sinus node cells, these few gap junctions are sufficient to synchronize the rate of these spontaneously discharging cells, at the same time protecting them from the hyperpolarizing action of the neighbouring atrial cells. The low density of gap junctions between nodal cells is therefore very functional indeed.

THE AREAS OF THE LATENT PACEMAKER CELLS

The largest part of the sinus node consists of latent pacemaker cells, which during diastole depolarize slower than cells in the leading pacemaker centre. Under standard conditions, they serve to conduct the pacemaker impulse toward the atrium and to shield the impulse forming cells from the hyperpolarizing influence of the atrial cells. For certain latent nodal areas, it is demonstrated that they can take over the leading role under special conditions, such as the addition of adrenaline or acetylcholine (Mackaay et al., 1980).

To be able to make a correlation between the electrophysiological and morphological properties of SA nodal cells, we had to chose criteria to qualify these cells. As electrophysiological criterion we chose the shape of the action potential and especially the maximal rate of rise of the action potential. As morphological criteria we assesed the "emptiness" of the cells, the degree of intracellular organization of the cells, and the cellular arrangement. Before we proceed, we will state how we have quantified the "emptiness" of the cells. In a

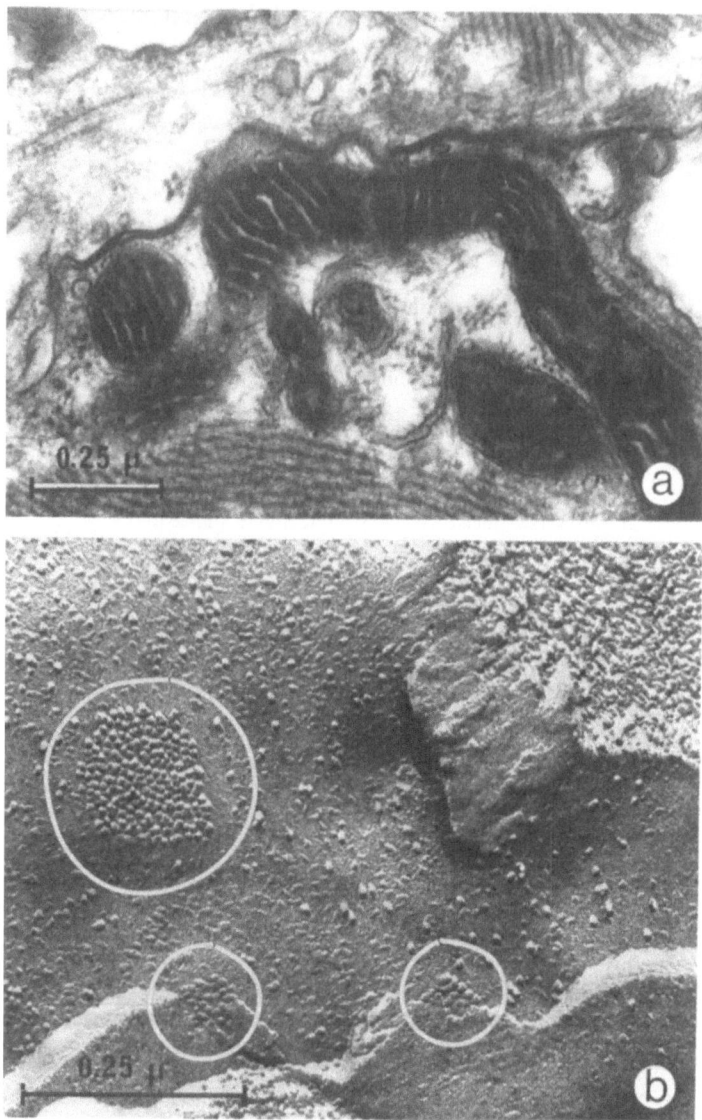

FIGURE 4 a. *Ultrathin section of a gap junction between two sinus node cells.*
b. *Three gap junctions are present on this replica of freeze cleaved sinus node cells. They are seen on PF faces as closely packed partricles.*

heart cell, the intracellular organized structures which occupy most of the cell volume, are: the nucleus, mitochondria, myofilaments and the sarcoplasmic reticulum. In a previous study (Masson-Pevet et al., 1979a) we have estimated the volume densities of the structures for cells from 9 sites in the sinus node and in the atrium. The volume density of the cytoplasm is given as 100 % minus the sum of the relative volume (in %) of the organized structures. We have plotted in Fig. 5, for each site, the volume density of the myofilaments against the volume density of the cytoplasm. The correlation coefficient is - 0.985 (n = 9). It is clear therefore that in typical nodal cells as in transitional and in atrial cells, organized structures others than myofilaments represent a constant percentage of approximately 28, and that if we know the volume fraction of the myofilaments in a cell type, we have a precise idea of the "emptiness" of this cell type.

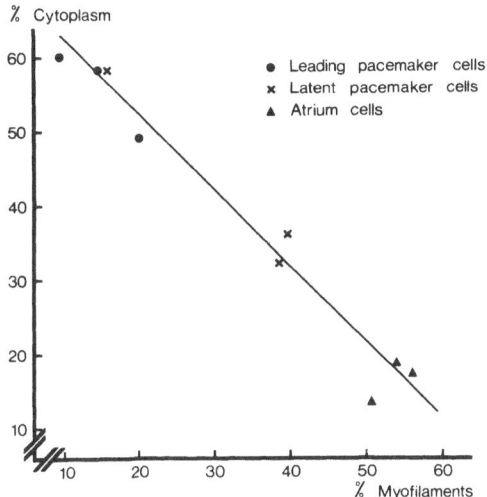

FIGURE 5 *Correlation between the percentages of cell volume occupied by the myofilaments on the one hand and by the cytoplasm on the other hand, for 9 sites situated in the sinus node and in the atrium (For details concerning the methods see Masson-Pevet et al., 1979a).*

For one preparation, we have made an extensive correlative study. The activation pattern of the sinus node of this preparation is given in Fig. 6. It may be seen that the spread of excitation shows a pattern similar to that presented

in Fig. 1. The only difference is that here the hatched area which indicates
the zone in which decremental conduction is observed, is much larger.

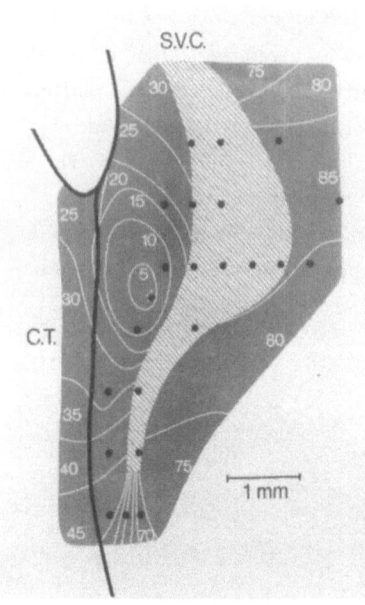 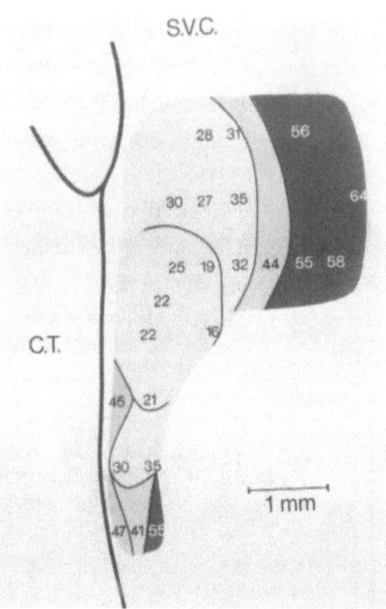

FIGURE 6 *Map of the activation pattern in the nodal region for the preparation
in which we have made an extensive correlative study between electrophysiology
and ultrastructure. The activation times are grouped in classes of 5 ms. The
black dots indicate the sites which have been studied with the E.M., and where
the myofilaments were quantified. As in Fig. 1, the star indicates the origin
of the impulse, and the hatched are the zone of block of conduction. C.T.=
crista terminalis, S.V.C. = superior vena cava.*

FIGURE 7 *Schematic representation of the preparation in which the numbers indicate the volume densities of the myofilaments at the sites where they have been
determined. In the center of the node, the cells contain less than 25 % myofilaments, for all the sites quantified. From the center on, the volume densities
of the myofilaments are grouped in classes of 10%; each class gets its own
shade. (C.T. = crista terminalis, S.V.C. = superior vena cava).*

In Figure 6 are also indicated the sites which have been studied with the electron microscope and where the amount of myofilaments was quantified. Each small
piece of nodal tissue we studied under the electron microscope seemed to be homogeneous with respect to the ultrastructure of the muscle cells. The same is true

for the electrophysiological behaviour, because no difference was found in the
action potentials recorded within the small samples chosen. The volume density
of the myofilaments in the samples studied is given in Fig. 7. It is clear from
this figure that the "emptiest" cells are situated in the center of the node and
that the transition from the center of the node to the working atrial cells is a
gradual one.   The increase in volume density of the myofilaments goes parallel
with an increase degree of intracellular organization of the cells, especially
with regard to the organization of the myofilaments. In Fig. 8, the activation
pattern of the preparation is superimposed on the two-dimensional reconstruction
of the structure, based on the volume density of the myofilaments. It can be
seen that the leading center (star) is situated in the group of the "emptiest"
cells.

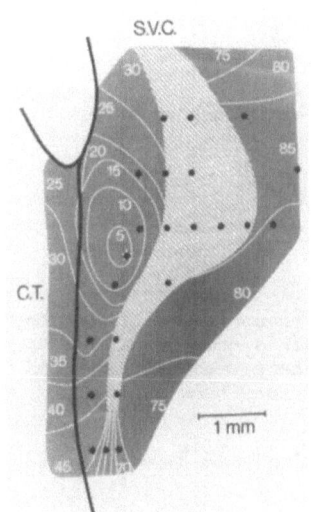 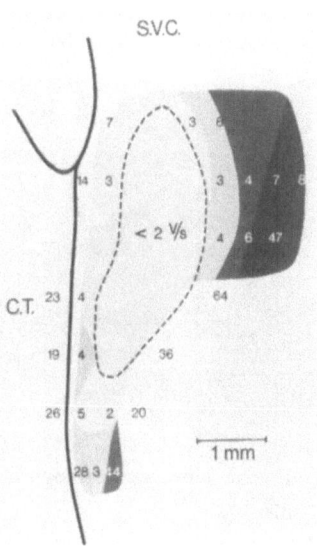

FIGURE 8 *The activation map is projected on the two-dimensional reconstruction
of the structure, based on the volume density of the myofilaments, as visualized
by the different shades of grey (C.T. = crista terminalis, S.V.C. = superior
vena cava).*

FIGURE 9 *The figures which are superimposed on the two-dimensional reconstruction of the structure indicate the maximal rate of rise of the action potentials. Inside the dotted line, all action potentials had a maximal rate of rise
of less than 2 volts per second. (C.T. = crista terminalis, S.V.C. = superior
vena cava).*

In Fig. 9 the cell type and the maximal rate of rise of the action potentials
are correlated.   It is clear that low rates of rise are found in the center of
the node, where the "emptiest" cells are also   present.   A   correlation   between
structure   and function can also be found when the shape of the action potentials
and the cell type are compared.   As an example we present some points in the tail
of   the sinus node, because here very different action potentials can be recorded
at short distances from each other (Fig.   10).

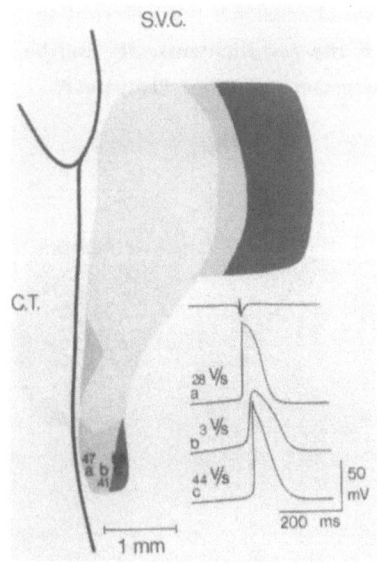

FIGURE 10 *Action potentials recorded   in
the tail of the sinus node at points, a,
b and c, with their maximal rate of
rise. (C.T. = crista terminalis).*

Both the electrophysiological and morphological data obtained   are   sumarized   in
Table III.
For these three sites, located 200 µm apart, we can see that a small   action   potential with a relatively high diastolic depolarization and a low maximum rate of
rise is derived from cells which   contain few randomly oriented myofilaments,
(Fig.   11).   It can be seen on the activation maps presented in Fig. 1 and Fig.
6, that the impulse conduction within the rabbit sinus node has   an   asymmetrical
pattern   and   that in medial direction (toward the interatrial septum) a zone exists in which conduction is decremental.   The activation from encircles the medial   border   of   the node to reach the adjacent atrium.   The septum is activated

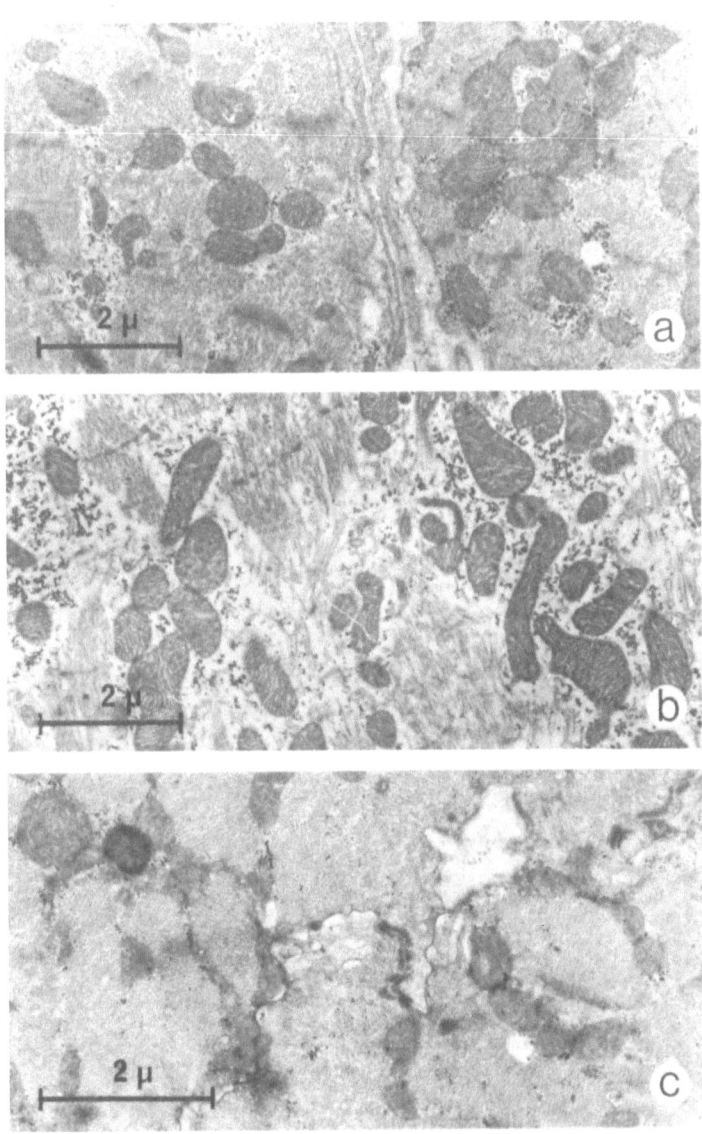

FIGURE 11 *(a-b-c) Electronmicrographs from cells from sites a, b and c, (fig. 10), respectively.*

therefore via a circuitous way instead of via the adjacent septal margin of the
sinus node. The area of conduction block shown in Fig. 1 and 6, is recognized
by the presence of action potentials with double components (Fig. 12). The fine
structure of the zone of decremental conduction was studied extensively in two
hearts. One example is given in Fig. 12. At site a 400 μm from the leading
center, a pacemaker type action potential is recorded whereas site f gives an
atrial type action potential. In between, double component action potentials are
recorded. The percentages of myofilaments present in the cells at each site are
indicated. We can see that the transition between leading center and atrium is a
gradual one. At the nodal side, the cells are similar to those found in the pacemaker region, toward the septum a gradual transition to an atrial cell type is
observed with, as a striking feature, a better organization of the contractile
apparatus. We also observed a transition in tissue architecture: toward the
septum, the cells are more regularly arranged than at the pacemaker side, and
they became oriented approximately parallel to the crista terminalis. It is
clear therefore that in the area of decremental conduction all cell types are
present from the typical nodal type to the atrial type.

TABLE III

ELECTROPHYSIOLOGICAL AND MORPHOLOGICAL DATA OBTAINED FOR THREE
SITES A, B AND C, SITUATED IN THE TAIL OF THE SINUS NODE AS
SHOWN IN FIG. 10

site	dV/dt max (V/s)	amplitude (mv)	diastolic depolarization (mv/s)	myofilaments (%)	cell organization
a	28	80	± 13	47	rather good
b	3	60	± 36	47	bad
c	44	96	± 10	55	good

Nexuses or gap junctions have been found at every site studied in this zone
of decremental conduction. For the preparation shown in Fig. 12, we have counted the number of gap junctions present in micrographs covering an area of 1000
μm^2 per site. This number is given just above the letters a, b.... For sites a,
b and c, only small nexuses have been observed such as those between typical
nodal cells, while at sites d, e and f, longer nexuses were present.

From the results presented it may be concluded that in those areas of the
sinus node where impulse conduction occurs, a correlation can be found between
the cell type present at a given site, and the maximal rate of rise of the action

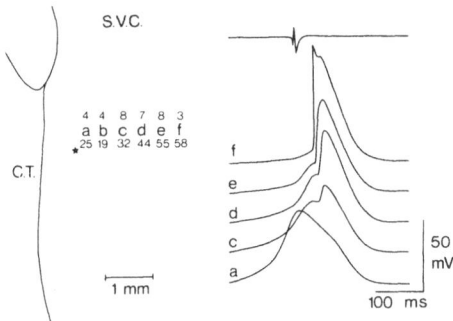

FIGURE 12 Conduction block in the sinus node. The action potentials (on the right side) were recorded at corresponding points a - f of the activation map. The star at the left side indicates the origin of the impulse. The numbers under the letters a - f indicate the volume densities of the myofilaments present at these sites, and the number situated above the letters indicate the number of gap junctions observed on a surface area of 1000 μm^2, also at these sites. (C.T. = crista terminalis, S.V.C. = superior vena cava).

potential or the steepness of the diastolic depolarization. The typical nodal cells, as described in the first part of this article, generate action potentials with a lower rate of rise and a steeper diastolic depolarization than any other cell in the SA node. Consequently, the impulse is initiated in these cells. From this group of cells the impulse is propagated to latent pacemaker cells. With increasing distance from the leading center the gradual decrease in electrophysiological pacemaker properties seems to be correlated with a gradual increase in number and organization of the myofilaments. The existence of a zone of decremental conduction at the septal side of the rabbit sinus node could be explained, neither by the intracellular structure of these cells, nor by the amount of gap junctions between them.

REFERENCES

Bleeker, W.K., Mackaay, A.J.C, Masson-Pevet, M., Bouman, L.N. and Becker, A.E.: Functional and morphological organization of the rabbit sinus node: a correlative study. Circ. Res., 46: 11-22, 1980.

Forssmann, W.G. and Girardier, L.: A study of the T-system in rat heart. J. Cell Biol., 44: 1-19, 1970.

Gabella, G.: Inpocketings of the cell membrane (caveolae) in the rat myocardium. J. Ultrastruct. Res., 65: 135-147, 1978.

James, T.N., Sherf, L., Fine, G. and Morales, A.R.: Comparative ultrastructure of the sinus node in man and dog. Circ., 34: 139-163, 1966.

Levin, K.R. and Page, E.: Quantitative studies on plasmalemmal folds and caveolae of rabbit ventricular myocardial cells. Circ. Res.: 46: 244-255, 1980.

Lorber, V. and Bertaud, W.S.: Cellular surfaces of amphibian atrial muscle. J. Cell. Sci., 9: 427-433, 1971.

Mackaay, A.J.C., Op 't Hof, T., Bleeker, W.K., Jongsma, H.J. and Bouman, L.N.: Interaction of adrenaline and acetylcholine on cardiac pacemaker function. Functional inhomogeneity of the rabbit sinus node. J. Pharm. Exp. Ther., 214: 417-422, 1980.

Masson-Pevet, M., Bleeker, W.K., Mackaay, A.J.C., Bouman, L.N. and Houtkoper, J.M.: Sinus node and atrium cells from the rabbit heart: a quantitative electron microscope description after electrophysiological localization. J. Mol. Cell. Cardiol., 11: 555-568, 1979a.

Masson-Pevet, M., Bleeker, W.K. and Gros, D.: The plasma membrane of leading pacemaker cells in the rabbit sinus node: a qualitative and quantitative ultrastructural analysis. Circ. Res., 45: 621-629, 1979b.

Masson-Pevet, M., Bleeker, W.K., Mackaay, A.J.C., Gros, D. and Bouman, L.N.: Ultrastructural and functional aspects of the rabbit sinoatrial node. In: The Sinus Node. Structure, Function and Clinical Relevance, Bonke, F.I.M., ed., Martinus Nijhoff, The Hague, pp. 195-211, 1978.

Masson-Pevet, M., Gros, D. and Besselsen, E.: The caveolae in rabbit sinus node and atrium. Cell Tissue Res., 208: 183-196, 1980.

Tranum-Jensen, J.: The fine structure of the sinus node. A survey. In: The Sinus Node. Structure, Function and Clinical Relevance, Bonke, F.I.M., ed., Martinus Nijhoff, The Hague, pp. 149-165, 1978.

Truex, R.C.: The sinoatrial node and its connections with the atrial tissue. In: The Conduction System of the Heart, Wellens, H.J.J., Lie, K.I. and Janse, M.J., eds., Stenfert Kroese, B.V., Leiden, pp. 209-227, 1976.

Viragh, S. and Porte, A.: The fine structure of the conducting system of the monkey heart (Macaca mulatta). I. The sinoatrial node and the internodal connections. Zeitschrift fuer Zellforschung, 145: 191-211, 1973.

PACEMAKER MECHANISMS OF RABBIT SINOATRIAL NODE CELLS

Hiroshi Irisawa and Akinori Noma

INTRODUCTION

Since the first voltage clamp experiments in the mammalian sinoatrial (SA) node (Irisawa, 1972), much information on the current systems in this tissue became available. From those studies it appeared that a number of different ionic current systems are involved: 1. the rapid sodium current, i_{Na}, (Noma et al., 1977), 2. the slow inward current, i_s, (Noma et al., 1977; Noma et al., 1980), 3. the potassium current, i_K, (Noma and Irisawa, 1976; DiFrancesco et al., 1979; Yanagihara and Irisawa, 1980), 4. the hyperpolarization-activated current, i_h, (Yanagihara and Irisawa, 1980), and 5. the time-independent background current, i_l of unknown nature. Essentially similar current systems were found in pacemaker cells in the frog heart (Brown et al., 1977). In a simplified model, one might assume that i_s contributes to the upstroke of the action potential, whereas i_K is responsible for the repolarization and the pacemaker potential. However, quantitative insight into the mechanisms of the pacemaker activity is only possible by a reconstruction of the action potential which takes into account all 5 current systems that have been disclosed by the voltage clamp experiments. In Purkinje fibers such a reconstruction has shown that i_{K2} contributes to the pacemaker potential (McAllister et al., 1975), and for the ventricular action potential (Beeler and Reuter, 1977) it was found that the plateau is determined by both i_s and i_K.

A Hodgkin and Huxley type model recently reported by Yanagihara et al. (1980) suggested that i_s is not only important for the upstroke of the action potential but also for the pacemaker depolarization. In this model, however, it was assumed that the fully activated current voltage relation is non-linear while the kinetics of i_s were taken from preliminary data. These aspects were recently examined experimentally (Noma, Kokubun, Kotake and Irisawa, unpublished

observations), and it was confirmed that voltage relationship of the
fully-activated i_s is not lineair, but shows outward-going rectification. Also
it was demonstrated that i_s channels are partially available at a membrane potential positive to -60 mV. The present study extends the previous SA node
model based on new experimental information with respect to i_s.

METHOD

The method of preparing sausage type SA node specimens has been described in detail by Noma and Irisawa (1976a). For the computation of the action potential,
the general form of equations for the time- and voltage-dependent current components has been chosen (Hodgkin and Huxley, 1952; Noble and Tsien, 1968),

$$i = y.\bar{i} \tag{1}$$

where $\bar{i}$ is the product of the driving force and the limiting conductance, the
latter being a function of the membrane potential. The gating variable, y follows the first-order kinetics,

$$dy/dt = \alpha_y(1-y)- \beta_y.y \tag{2}$$

The variable y varies between 0 and 1. α_y and β_y are the rate constants of
opening and closing of the ionic channel. The unit membrane was modeled as a
capacitance of 1 µF (Cm) connected parallel to five different ionic channels.
Mathematically, this equivalent circuit is expressed by the following equation,

$$Cm.\ dE/dt - i_m - (i_s + i_{Na} + i_K + i_h + l_l) \tag{3}$$

where E is the membrane potential and i_m is the total current passing through
the unit membrane. In all calculations i_m was set as zero, thus the action potential being a "membrane action potential". The current components are described by the equations, listed in the appendix section. The differential equa-

tions (2) and (3) were solved by the Runge-Kutta fourth order approximation using a digital computer (Nicolet, Model NIC-80).

GENERAL DESCRIPTION OF THE CURRENT SYSTEMS IN THE SA NODE CELLS

It is well established that the upstroke of the action potential is relatively insensitive to TTX, but sensitive to D 600, verapamil, as well as manganese ion (for review, Brooks and Lu, 1972). These findings strongly suggested a major contribution of i_s to the upstroke of the action potential. This view was confirmed by the results of the recent voltage clamp experiments.

In the nowadays used voltage clamp technique the analysis of the transient inward current is limited by the multicellular nature of the specimens. In many preparations the potential in the periphery can deviates from the command level by several mV within about 5 ms after the onset of the depolarizing pulse, disturbing the analysis of the activation phase of i_s. As a first approximation, we measured i_s as the difference between the currents measured before and after the application of D 600. The amplitude of i_s reached a peak value at a membrane potential of -10 to 0 mV and declined at more positive potentials. The reversal potential was approximately +40 mV. This finding is in good agreement with the observation that i_s is sensitive to both $[Na^+]_o$ and $[Ca^{2+}]_o$.

When the amplitude of the tail current of the fully activated i_s was measured at various potential levels as the difference between the currents, measured before and after the application of D 600, the voltage relation of $\bar{i}_s$ was linear only between 0 to +40 mV, but was almost constant at negative potentials, indicating rectification of i_s channel as has previously been suggested in the frog atrium by DeHemptinne (1978).

The peak amplitude of i_s during depolarizing voltage jumps from a holding potential of -40 mV was reached within 10-20 ms and the time to peak became shorter with increasing depolarization. The voltage relation of the steady state activation variable d_∞ is shown in Fig. 1 (cf. Noma et al., 1980). The time constant of inactivation of i_s, τ_f, is in order of several 10 ms and the voltage dependency is also shown in Fig. 2. At potentials negative to -30 mV the time constant was obtained from the recovery of i_s. The steady state degree of inactivation too was measured from the amplitude of i_s generated by a depolarizing clamp pulse to +10 mV from various potentials and is shown in Fig. 2.

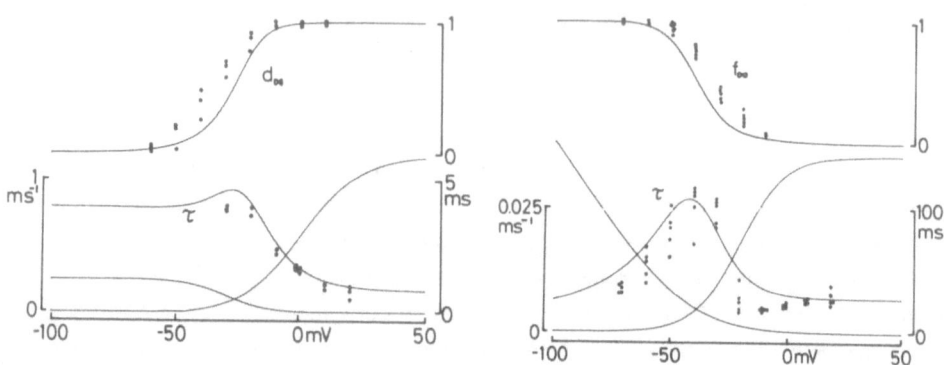

FIGUUR 1 *Steady state activation of i$_s$ and its time constant. Closed circles are the experimentally measured values. The positive slope is the opening rate constant (α), while the negative slope is the closing rate constant (β), in ms^{-1}.*

FIGURE 2 *Steady state inactivation of i$_s$ and its time constant. The closed circles are the experimentally measured values. The positive slope of the rate constant is α and the negative slope is β. The time constant for f was measured by subtracting outward current from the routine voltage clamp record, the resulting inactivation phases reflects τ$_f$.*

The steady state activation curve arises from zero at around -55 mV to saturation at -20 mV. The steady state activation and inactivation curves obtained in the experiments were quite similar to those of i$_s$ in other tissues. However, these two relations gave a large "window current" of i$_s$ in the steady state I-V curve (Fig. 3-A). The discrepancy between these two kinds of experimental data could not simply be attributed to an unknown experimental error. Recently Isenberg and Klockner (1980) obtained similar voltage relations of d$_∞$ and f$_∞$ in single cells. The reconstruction of the experimental I-V curve and the action potential was satisfactory only when the f$_∞$ -curve and d$_∞$ -curve were shifted to the left and right, respectively, as shown in Fig. 3B. Therefore, the kinetics were modified in the present model. With the previous model (Yanagihara et al., 1980), many aspects of the S-A node activity were well simulated by assuming kinetics similar to the present model.

2) i$_{Na}$ Evidence for the presence of i$_{Na}$ in the SA node cells has been suggested by a depressing effect of TTX on the upstroke of the action potential (Kreitner, 1978). In the voltage clamp experiments, a TTX sensitive component

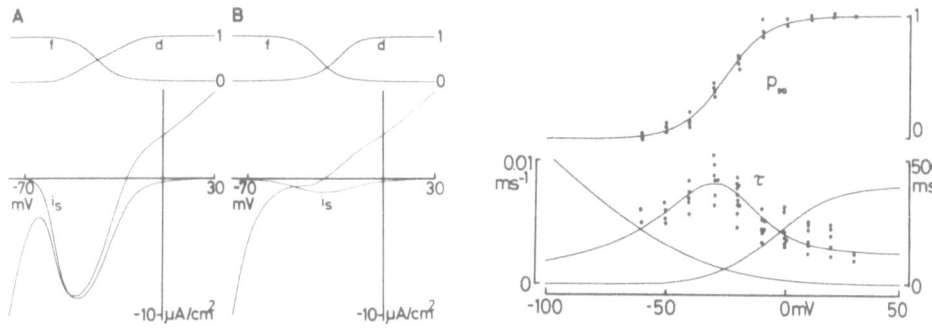

FIGURE 3 *Comparison of the experimentally obtained f- and d-curve against the membrane potential in A and the assumed values of the f- and d-curve in B. When the steady state I-V curve was computed, a marked negative slope at the pacemaker potential range was obtained as shown in A. In the present model, d- and f-curves are shifted so that steady state I-V curve simulates well the experimental curve.*

FIGURE 4 *Steady state activation of i_K, P_∞ and the time constant of i_K. Closed circles are the experimental plots. In the lower panel the positive slope is α, while the negative slope denotes β.*

was recorded in the transient inward current (Noma et al., 1977). In the present study the kinetics used in other cardiac models were adopted (McAllister et al., 1975; Beeler and Reuter, 1977).

3) i_K The kinetics of the outward current has been extensively analysed (Noma and Irisawa, 1976b; DiFrancesco et al., 1979; Yanagihara and Irisawa, 1980). As in other cardiac fibers, the outward current in the S-A node showed slow kinetics. When the membrane potential was held at -40 mV, and various test depolarizing pulses were applied, the outward current was slowly activated after the transient inward current, and on repolarization to the holding potential an outward current tail was observed. The reversal potential of this current was dependent on $[K]_o$ in the same way as a potassium electrode, indicating that the major component of the outward current is carried by K ions (Noma and Irisawa, 1976b). This potassium current, i_K, was most sensitive to Ba; 5 mM Ba^{++} nearly completely blocked the time dependent increase of the outward current. When the time constant of the outward current tail was measured at various potentials, it was approximately 400 ms at -40 mV and decreased with either depolarization or

hyperpolarization (Fig. 4). The steady state activation curve was measured from the amplitude of the i_K tail recorded on repolarization to -40 mV from various amplitude of depolarization or hyperpolarization (Fig. 5).

FIGURE 5 *Reconstructed voltage clamp records using the present model. Numerals on each tracing state the amplitude of the clamp pulses. Current calibration is identical in both upper and lower panel.*

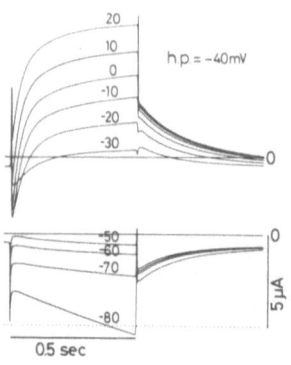

i_K was activated positive to -50 mV and fully saturated at around 0 mV. The fully activated amplitudes of i_k at various membrane potentials were determined from both the amplitude of the tail current and the activation curve (Yanagihara and Irisawa, 1980b). It showed slight inward going rectification without negative slope as i_K in other cardiac fibers.

4) i_h When the membrane was hyperpolarized negative to -60 mV, slowly rising inward current was recorded. Deactivation of i_K can only partially be responsible and only up to 100-200 ms for this current change. The amplitude of the delayed increase became larger with stronger hyperpolarization (Seyama, 1976). On clamping to potentials more negative than E_k (by elevating $[K^+]_o$), the reversal of the i_k tail could clearly be separated from i_h by the different direction of two currents. Thus, another current system which was activated by hyperpolarization was assumed (i_h) (Noma and Irisawa, 1976; Seyama, 1976; Brown et al., 1979), called as i_f by Brown and DiFrancesco (1980) and its kinetics was recently analysed by Yanagihara and Iriwasa (1980a). i_h shows little specificity to any particular ion and its reversal potential was -25 mV. Removal of Cl⁻ as well as low Na reduced the i_h current (Seyama, 1977). This property of i_h was also observed in the AV node cell (Kokubun et al., 1980). i_h began to activate at -50 mV and fully saturated at about -100 mV. The fully activated current-voltage relation showed no rectifying property (Yanagihara an

Irisawa, 1980).

In the range of the pacemaker potential, the activation variable τ_q was between 2 to 3 sec, being smaller at higher and lower membrane potentials. Because of this long time constant, i_h is only of a minor importance for the action potential, but may play a significant role for keeping the maximum diastolic potential 30 mV positive to the potassium equilibrium potential. At present we consider i_h as part of the inward background current.

5) leak current   It was impossible to measure the magnitude of the time-independent leak current directly from the current trace recorded in voltage clamp experiments, because the time-dependent components also contribute to the net current at the onset of the clamp pulse. Therefore, the leakage current was estimated from the difference between the computed total amplitude of the four time-dependent current components and the experimental steady state I-V curve.

RESULTS

RECONSTRUCTION OF THE VOLTAGE CLAMP RECORDS
Since the current components i_s, i_{Na}, i_K and i_l were analysed in different preparations, the relative amplitude of each component has to be determined by simulating the average pattern of the voltage clamp records. First, the amplitude of i_s was determined by adjusting the maximum rate of rise of the action potential to approximately 5 V/s through a membrane capacitance of 1 $\mu F/cm^2$. A family of computed currents during various clamp pulses from the holding potential of -40 mV are shown in Fig. 5 and the I-V curve at 0.5 and 1000 ms as well as the contribution of each current component are shown in Fig. 6.
At the onset of the clamp pulses the model showed sharp spikes, upward on depolarization and downward on hyperpolarization, being due both to instantaneous jump of i_l and the following activation or deactivation of i_s on depolarization or hyperpolarization, respectively. The steady state conductance of i_s at -20 and -30 mV caused inward current tails on repolarization. The outward current decayed exponentially because its second component observed in the experiment

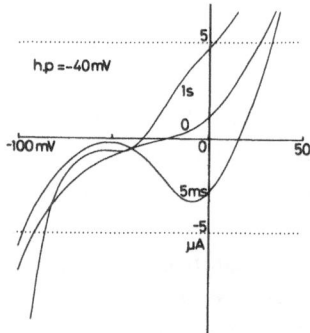
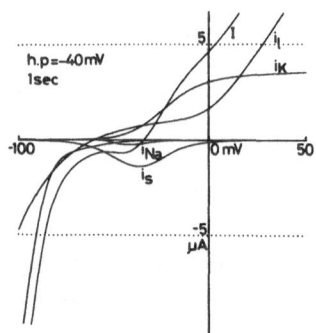

FIGURE 6A *Reconstructed I-V curve. The current-voltage relationship calculated at the holding potential of -40 mV, instantaneously, (0), after 5 ms and at the end of 1s. I is the total membrane current. Dotted horizontal lines indicate 5 and -5 μA.*

FIGURE 6B *Reconstructed current-voltage relationship of individual current systems in a steady state.*

was neglected in the model (DiFrancesco et al., 1979).

Relatively large amplitude of i_l on depolarization and on hyperpolarization (see Fig. 6B) was determined from the difference between the total amplitude of the four time-dependent currents and the experimentally recorded steady state I-V curve. This large amplitude of i_l was suggested by the further experimental observations that the overshoot of the action potential was about 20 mV less positive than the reversal potential of i_s and that the maximum diastolic potential was about 35 mV less negative than E_K. The delayed current systems, i_K and i_h cannot produce such a large current in such a short time because they are slowly activated, and hence i_l has to be large. It is evident in Fig. 6B that the resting potential of about -35 mV is mainly determined by the steady state conductance of i_s and i_k in addition to i_l.

RECONSTRUCTION OF THE PACEMAKER POTENTIAL

In Fig. 7 the computed action potential (lower trace) was compared with the experimental record (upper trace). The maximum diastolic potential in this model was -65.7 mV, and the overshoot is +17.6 mV. The first derivative of the action potential was also illustrated. The model simulated well the pacemaker poten-

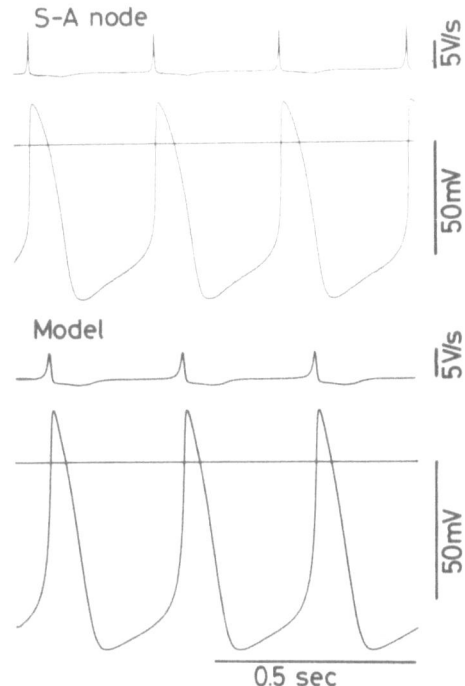

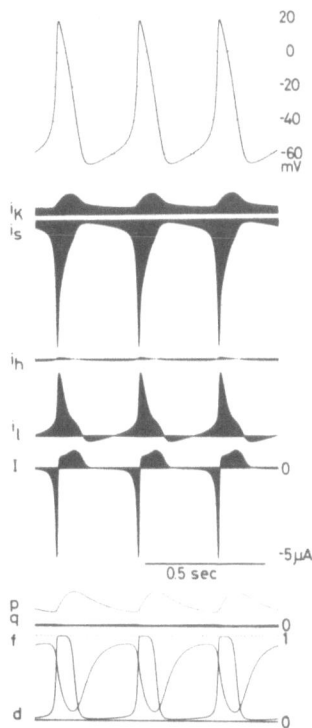

FIGURE 7 *Comparison of experimentally recorded (upper panel) and reconstructed (lower record) SA node action potentials as well as the dV/dt curves.*

FIGURE 8 *Reconstructed SA node action potentials and their composing current systems as well as the kinetic changes during three consecutive cardiac cycles. The two dotted lines indicate -5 μA calibration. During diastolic depolarization, the process of recovery of inactivation and the slight growing, increase of the activation parameter are demonstrated. Concomitant with this change in the inward current parameters, outward current parameter p gradually reduces during pacemaker depolarization. These factors are the major time-dependent factors responsible for the spontaneous depolarization.*

tial and the spontaneous rate. A slight discrepancy between calculations and experiments was noticed which consisted of a relatively short duration of the computed action potential in the positive potential range. The changes of each ionic current during spontaneous activity are shown in Fig. 8. The activation of i_K and the rapid inactivation of i_s repolarized the membrane to the maximum diastolic potential. The following pacemaker depolarization is caused both by gradual decay of i_K and an increase of i_s. Compared to the increase in i_s, the amplitude of reduction in i_K was relatively small. This is explained by the small decrease in p which was counteracted by the increase in i_K, while in the case of i_s, f increased from about 0.1 to 0.9 and d slightly increased during diastole. The i_l significantly changed during cardiac cycle. In the present model i_l accelerated the pacemaker potential negative to -60 mV and decelerated positive to this level. This mechanism may be partially responsible for the two phases of the pacemaker depolarization in the experiment (Fig. 8).

The respective contribution of i_K, i_s, i_h and i_l to the development of the smooth pacemaker depolarization is evident from Fig. 8. Among these current systems i_s appears to be the major contribution to the pacemaker depolarization. This concept was suggested by the experimental finding that the spontaneous activity was resumed when a constant outward current was applied to a SA node cell whose i_K was supressed by application of Ba^{++} (Yanagihara and Irisawa, 1980b). The present model could simulate this experimental finding when i_K was replaced by a constant outward current as shown in Fig. 9. When i_K was deleted, the stimulated spontaneous activity was reduced to small fluctuations around -22 mV. When an external current of 0.25 $\mu A/cm^2$ was applied, the model ensued oscillation which gradually increased in amplitude. As the magnitude of the applied current was increased, a large action potential was initiated with the maximum diastolic potential higher than -60 mV. These simulations clearly indicate that the time dependent characteristics of i_K are not essential for the initiation of the spontaneous action potential in the SA node.

SIMULATION OF SA NODE ACTION POTENTIAL UNDER THE EFFECT OF EPINEPHRINE AND ACETYLCHOLINE

In the Purkinje fiber, epinephrine is known to produce a shift in the kinetics of the potassium current (I_{K2}) by about 24 mV into the depolarization direction. Epinephrine also increases the deactivation rate by a factor 4. These epine-phrine actions produce a positive chronotropic effect in Purkinje fibers as confirmed by the computer simulation (McAllister et al., 1975). Voltage clamp experiments in the SA node disclosed a different ionic mechanism underlying the epinephrine effect. In the rabbit SA node, i_s, i_K and i_h were increased (Brown et al., 1979). The increase of the current was attributed to an increase of

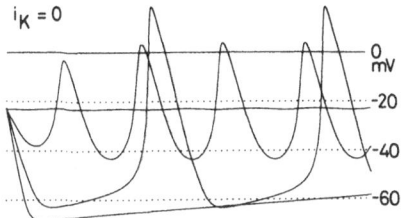
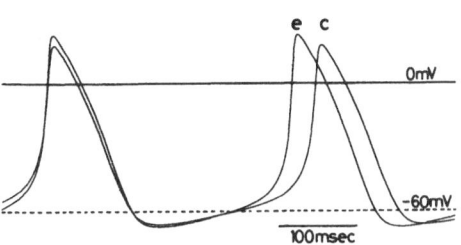

FIGURE 9 *Reconstructed potential tracings under the condition of complete abol-
ition of i_K. The top tracing is the zero line, the second line is the resting
potential level when i_K was abolished to zero; a slight oscillation of the potential was observed. Constant outward current of 0.25 μA, 0.5 μA and 0.75
μA/cm² were applied. As the applied current increased, oscillatory potentials
became greater and finally at 0.5 μA/cm² current full sized action potentials
were observed. At 0.75 μA/cm² membrane became quiescent at least during this
computation.*

FIGURE 10 *Reconstructed action potentials when $\bar{i}_s$, $\bar{i}_K$ and $\bar{i}_h$ were increased
by 30%, 10% and 20%. These conditions well simulated the effect of 5.5 x 10⁻⁷ M
epinephrine in the experiment. c is control and e shows the simulated epinephrine effect.*

the limiting conductances of i_s and i_K, while the kinetics of i_s and i_K remained
constant (Noma et al., 1980). For i_h, changes in both $\bar{i}_h$ and kinetics were
suggested. In the model simulation $\bar{i}_s$, $\bar{i}_K$ and $\bar{i}_h$ were increased by 30%, 10%
and 20%, respectively as observed at 5.5 x 10⁻⁷ M epinephrine in the experiment
(Fig. 10). The heart rate increased by approximately 20% above the control.
The positive chronotropy is quite comparable to the experiment where epinephrine
increased the rate by approximately 17%. The slight increase in the overshoot
is directly due to the increase in i_s and the change in the maximum diastolic
potential is mainly due to the increase of i_K. The relative importance of the
changes in i_s, i_K and i_h for generation of the epinephrine effect was tested by
inducing a change in only one current in the model. The increase of i_s increased the heart rate in almost the same degree as in Fig. 10 without any simultaneous change in i_K or i_h, while the rate was not largely affected by increase
in i_K or by i_h, indicating the major role of i_s for the epinephrine effect.

It is well established that ACh increases the K-conductance by binding to
the muscarinic ACh receptor in the SA node cell. Several characteristics of
this K-current were demonstrated; ACh-induced K-current shows a time- and vol-

tage-dependent change during clamp steps and also shows a miniature fluctuation corresponding to its kinetics, and the ACh-induced hyperpolarization starts approximately 30 ms after an instantaneous application of ACh (Noma and Trautwein, 1978; Noma et al., 1979; Noma et al., 1979; Osterrieder et al., 1980). These characteristics were well explained on the basis of a model proposed by Katz and Miledy. In this model the ACh-receptor complex is assumed to be directly coupled to the specific channel and the channel kinetics are much slower than the binding reaction. The analysis disclosed; 1) a single channel conductance of approximately 4 pS, almost independent of the potential, 2) a channel density of about $1/\mu m^2$, 3) an opening rate constant dependent on ACh concentration, and 4) a closing rate constant dependent on the membrane potential. These kinetics were simulated by equations (5) in appendix. The action potentials in Fig. 11 were calculated by introducing the ACh-induced K current, i_{ACh}, to the SA node model. i_{ACh} increases during the action potential because of increased driving force, but voltage- and time-dependent closing of the channels decreased i_{ACh} and thus i_{ACh} did not reduce the action potential duration as it was the case in the experiment. Unlike i_K the conductance for i_{ACh} gradually increased on repolarization so that the frequency of the cardiac cycle decreased. When the concentration of ACh was further increased, the computed spontaneous activity was ceased.

FIGURE 11 Reconstructed action potential with ACh induced K-current. Heart rate during control was 176.5/s; it was reduced by ACh to 138/s. In the lower panel, the current components due to ACh, i_K and i_s, respectively are illustrated from top to bottom.

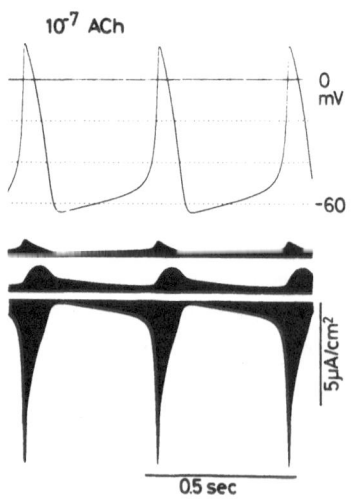

DISCUSSION

The present study demonstrated that the pacemaker depolarization is generated by a gradual deactivation of i_K progressing concomitantly with an increase in i_s on the background of passive changes of i_l. The amplitude of i_h was small during the pacemaker potential compared to i_s and i_K. The increase of i_s during the pacemaker depolarization is caused by a gradual removal of inactivation and a slight increase of the activation variable d. The change of i_K during diastolic depolarization in the SA node was unexpectedly small compared to i_{K2} in the Purkinje fiber. The quantitative difference is mainly due to the difference in the voltage relations of the fully activated amplitude of i_{K2} in the Purkinje fiber and for i_K in the SA node. The negative slope in $\bar{i}_{K2}$ in the range of the pacemaker potential (-80 - -60 mV) was not observed for i_K in the SA node. Furthermore, in the SA node the monotonic increase in $\bar{i}_K$ with diastolic depolarization nearly counterbalanced the decrease of p during diastole, where p decreased only from 0.5 to 0.25. In the Purkinje fiber the kinetic variable s decreases from 1 to 0.5 during the diastolic depolarization (Noble and Tsien, 1968). The participation of i_s to the pacemaker potential critically depends on how much the pacemaker potential range overlaps with that of the d-curve. The experimentally obtained d-curve for i_s shows a threshold potential of about -60 to -50 mV in almost all cardiac fibers examined in the past (for review Carmeliet and Vereecke, 1979). Thus, it is quite natural that i_s contributes to the pacemaker potential in the low membrane potential range (Hauswirth et al., 1961; Beeler and Reuter, 1977.

The amplitude of the slow component of the outward current was found to be up to 20 to 30% of the total amplitude of the outward current tail (DiFrancesco et al., 1979). In the present study this component was neglected and was included in the background current, because of its slow time constant compared to the cardiac cycle.

APPENDIX

SIMULATIONAL EQUATIONS FOR CURRENTS IN THE MAMMALIAN SA NODE CELL

1) $i_s = d.f.\bar{i}_s$

     $\alpha_d = 1.2/(1 + \exp(-E/12))$

     $\beta_d = 0.25/(1 + \exp((E + 30)/8))$

     $\alpha_f = 7 \times 10^{-4}(E + 45)/(\exp((E + 45)/9.5) - 1)$

     $\beta_f = 0.036/(1 + \exp(-(E + 21)/9.5))$

     $\bar{i}_s = 15 (\exp((E - 40)/25) -1)$

2) $i_K = p.\bar{i}_K$

     $\alpha_p = 8 \times 10^{-3}/(1 + \exp(-(E + 4)/13))$

     $\beta_p = 1.7 \times 10^{-4}(E + 40)/(\exp((E + 40)/13.3) - 1)$

     $\bar{i}_K = 0.91 (\exp(0.0277 (E + 90)) - 1)/\exp(0.0277 (E + 40))$

3) $i_h = 0.2 q (E + 25)$

     $\alpha_q = 0.34 \times 10^{-3}(E + 100)/(\exp((E + 100)/4.4) - 1) + 0.0495 \times 10^{-3}$

     $\beta_q = 5 \times 10^{-4}(E + 40)/(1 - \exp(-(E + 40)/6)) + 0.0845 \times 10^{-3}$

4) $i_{Na} = 0.5 m^3. h (E - 40)$

     $\alpha_m = (E + 37)/(1 - \exp(-(E + 37)/10))$

     $\beta_m = 40 \exp(-0.056 (E + 62))$

     $\alpha_h = 1.209 \times 10^{-3} \exp(-(E + 20)/6.534)$

     $\beta_h = 1/(\exp(-(E + 30)/10) + 1)$

5) $i_{ACh} = 0.27 a (E + 90)$

     $\alpha_a = 1.232 \times 10^{-2}/(1 + 4.2 \times 10^{-6}/ACh)$

     $\beta_a = 10^{-2} \exp(0.0133 (E + 40))$

6) $i_1 = 1.2 (1 - \exp(-(E + 60)/25)) + 0.15 (E - 2)/(1 - \exp(-(E - 2)/5))$

The units for the current are: $\mu A/cm^2$, for the rate constants: ms^{-1}, for the membrane potential: mV, for i_{ACh} the concentration of ACh: molar.

REFERENCES

Beeler, G.W., Reuter, H.: Reconstruction of the action potential of ventricular myocardial fibres. J. Physiol. (London), 268: 177-210, 1977.

Brown, H.F., Giles, W. and Noble, S.J.: Membrane currents underlying activity in frog sinus venosus. J. Physiol. (London), 271: 783-816, 1977.

Brown, H.F., DiFrancesco, D. and Noble, S.J.: How does adrenaline accelerate the heart? Nature, 280: 235-236, 1979.

Brown, H.F. and DiFrancesco, D.: Voltage-clamp invevstigations of membrane currents underlying pacemaker activity in rabbit sinoatrial node. J. Physiol., 308: 331-351, 1980.

Carmeliet, E.C. and Vereecke, J.: Electrogenesis of the action potential and automaticity. In: Handbook of Physiology, section 2: The Cardiovascular system, Vol 1: The Heart. Berne, R.M., Sperelakis, N. and Geiger, S.R., eds., Am. Physiol. Soc. Bethesda, Maryland, pp. 269-334, 1979.

De Hemptinne, A.: Identification of ionic currents underlying the repolarization process in the frog auricle. European J. Cardiol., 7: Suppl. 5-15, 1978.

DiFrancesco, D., Noma, A. and Trautwein, W.: Kinetics and magnitude of the time-dependent K current in the rabbit SA node: effect of external potassium. Pfluegers Arch., 381: 271-279, 1979.

Giles, W.R. and Noble, S.J.: Changes in the membrane currents in bullfrog atrium produced by acetylcholine. J. Physiol. (London), 261: 103-123, 1976.

Hauswirth, O., Noble, D. and Tsien, R.W.: The mechanism of oscillatory activity at low membrane potentials in cardiac Purkinje fibres. J. Physiol. (London), 200: 255-265, 1969.

Ikemoto, Y. and Goto, M.: Nature of the negative inotropic effect of acetylcholine on the myocardium: an elucidation on the bullfrog atrium. Proc. Japan Acad., 51: 501-505, 1975.

Irisawa, H.: Comparative physiology of the cardiac pacemaker mechanism. Physiol. Rev., 58: 461-498, 1978.

Irisawa, H. and Yanagihara, K.: The slow inward current of the rabbit sino-atrial nodal cells. In: The Slow Inward Current and Cardiac Arrhythmias, Zipes, D.P. and Bailey, J.C., eds., Martinus Nijhoff, The Hague, pp.

265-284, 1980.

Isenberg, G.: Cardiac Purkinje fibers. $\left[Ca^{2+}\right]_i$ controls steady state potassium conductance. Pfluegers Arch., 371: 71-76, 1977.

Isenberg, G. and Kloeckner, U.: Glycocalyx is not required for slow inward calcium current in isolated rat heart myocyte. Nature, 284: 358-360, 1980.

Kreitner, D.: Effect of polarization and of inhibitors of ionic conductances on the action potentials of nodal and perinodal fibers in rabbit sinoatrial node. In: The Sinus Node. Structure, Function and Clinical Relevance, Bonke, F.I.M., ed., Martinus Nijhoff, The Hague, pp. 270-278, 1978.

McAllister, R.E., Noble, D. and Tsien, W.: Reconstruction of the electrical activity of cardiac Purkinje fibres. J. Physiol. (London), 251: 1-59, 1975.

McDonald, T.F. and Trautwein, W.: The potassium current underlying delayed rectification in cat ventricular muscle. J. Physiol. (London), 274: 217-246, 1978.

Noma, A. and Irisawa, H.: Membrane currents in the rabbit sinoatrial node cell as studied by the double microelectrode method. Pfluegers Arch., 364: 45-52, 1976a.

Noma, A. and Irisawa, H.: A time- and voltage-dependent potassium current in the rabbit sinoatrial node cell. Pfluegers Arch., 366: 251-258, 1976b.

Noma, A., Yanagihara, K. and Irisawa, H.: Inward current of the rabbit sinoatrial node cell. Pfluegers Arch., 372: 43-51, 1977.

Noma, A. and Trautwein, W.: Relaxation of the ACh-induced potassium current in the rabbit sinoatrial node cell. Pflueger Arch., 377: 193-200, 1978.

Noma, A., Osterrieder, W. and Trautwein, W.: The effect of external potassium on the elementary conductance of the ACh-induced potassium channel in the sino-atrial node. Pfluegers Arch., 381: 263-269, 1979a.

Noma, A., Peper, K. and Trautwein, W.: Acetylcholine-induced potassium current fluctuations in the rabbit sino-atrial node. Pfluegers Arch., 381: 255-262, 1979b.

Noma, A., Kotake, H. and Irisawa, H.: Slow inward current and its role mediating chronotropic effect of epinephrine. Pfluegers Arch., 388: 1-9, 1980.

Reuter, H. and Scholz, H.: A study on the ion selectivity and the kinetic properties of the calcium dependent slow inward current in mammalian cardiac muscle. J. Physiol. (London), 264: 17-47, 1977.

Seyama, I.: Characteristics of the rectifying properties of the sinoatrial node cell of the rabbit. J. Physiol. (London), 255: 379-397, 1976.

Yanagihara, K. and Irisawa, H.: Inward current activated during hyperpolarization in the rabbit sinoatrial node cell. Pfluegers Arch., 385: 11-19, 1980a.

Yanagihara, K. and Irisawa, H.: Potassium current during the pacemaker depolarization in rabbit sinoatrial node cell. Pfluegers Arch., 388: 255-260, 1980b.

THE RELATIVE CONTRIBUTIONS OF VARIOUS TIME-DEPENDENT MEMBRANE CURRENTS TO PACEMAKER ACTIVITY IN THE SINO ATRIAL NODE

Hilary Brown, Junko Kimura and Susan Noble

The successful application of the voltage clamp technique to the mammalian sino-atrial node has already given much information about the membrane currents in nodal pacemaking cells. In particular, an apparently new time-dependent current, i_f (or i_h) has been found on voltage clamping SA node cells negative to -50 mV (Brown et al., 1979; Yanagihara and Irisawa, 1980a). It now seems clear that this current, which has been shown to be a developing inward current (DiFrancesco and Ojeda, 1980) is closely related to the current i_{K2} which underlies pacemaking in Purkinje fibres. I_{K2}, whose kinetics were first described by Noble and Tsien (1968) was for many years thought to be an outward current which decays in the pacemaker range and which is carried by potassium ions: hence its name. Recent experiments, using barium to block the background current, i_{K1}, in Purkinje fibres have shown that i_{K2} is in reality a developing inward current which cannot be carried by potassium ions alone (see DiFrancesco, this volume). It problably has the same ionic composition as i_f (i_h) in the SA node and is carried by both sodium and potassium ions (DiFrancesco, 1980; Brown et al., 1980). This being the case, both currents should have the same name, but since no universal agreement has yet been reached as to whether this should be i_f or i_h we here use our original nomenclature i_f.

The discovery of i_f in the SA node brings the number of serious contenders for the title "the pacemaker current" up to three. The term "pacemaker current" is generally understood to mean a time-dependent current whose development or decay controls the rate of the pacemaker depolarization. Time-independent currents may also contribute to a pacemaker depolarization, but in this case it is only their magnitude not their kinetics that control the pacemaker rate.

The three currents in question in the SA node are:

1.   The time-dependent outward current, i_K (also known, particularly in cardiac
tissues other than the SA node, as i_x). This is activated positive to -40 mV so
it develops during an action potential and decays on subsequent repolarization.
It can bring about depolarization only in conjunction with the time-independent
inward background current. This indeed is how pacemaking occurs in depolarized
Purkinje fibres (Hauswirth et al., 1969), in frog atrial trabeculae (Brown
et al., 1976) and in spontaneously beating frog sinus venosus (Brown et al.,
1977) where i_f is present but appears to be activated only at potentials negative to the maximum diastolic potential.

2.   The second time-dependent current present within the voltage range of the
pacemaker depolarization of SA node cells is the slow inward current, i_{si}. This
current is an important (sometimes the sole) component of the action potential
upstroke in SA node cells and fairly substantial claims have recently been made
for its role in controlling the pacemaker depolarization (Yanagihara and Irisawa, 1980b). It certainly always contributes to the last portion of the pacemaker depolarization and may under some circumstances be important earlier in
its time course.

3.   The third and last time-dependent current which may control SA node pacemaking is i_f itself. It appears as a slow change during voltage clamp hyperpolarizations to potentials negative to -50 mV and it has been shown that this
change is the activation of an inward current with a reversal potential at about
-25 mV and an activation range between -50 mV and -120 mV (Yanagihara and Irisawa, 1980a;   DiFrancesco and Ojeda, 1980). Although it is thus by no means
fully activated within the pacemaker range of SA node cells (-70 to -40 mV) and
it also activates rather slowly, taking, for example, seconds to reach steady
state at -60 mV, it generally does start to activate in this voltage range.

      To determine the relative contribution of each of these three   currents   to
SA node pacemaking we have used the very direct method of looking for each of
them in voltage clamp records to see how much is present in the pacing range of
particular SA node cell. Perhaps the most important thing that our observations
show is that the amount of these three membrane currents present in the pacemaker range varies from preparation to preparation.

      Fig. 1 shows records from three SA node preparations prepared as described
elsewhere (Noma and Irisawa, 1976; Brown and DiFrancesco, 1980) and voltage
clamped using two microelectrodes. Action potentials recorded just before the

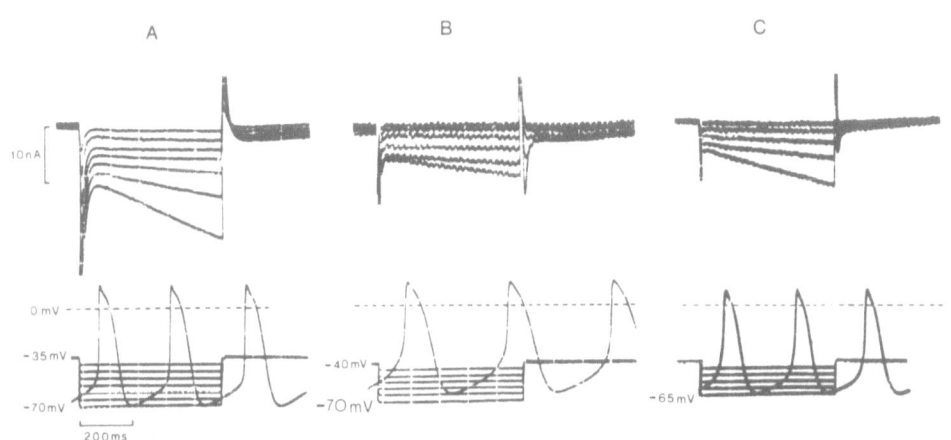

FIGURE 1 *Voltage clamp hyperpolarizations to show the amount of i_f activation in the pacemaker range in three SA node preparations. The pacemaker range has been shown in each case by superimposing the voltage record before clamping on that of clamp hyperpolarizations.*
In A and C there was appreciable i_f activation at the maximum diastolic potential (-70 mV in A and -65 mV in C). In B, the maximum diastolic potential was also -65 mV but here, and similarly at -70 mV, there was very little activation of i_f in this preparation.
Mn^{++} 4 mM and TTX 10^{-6} g/ml present in A and C;
Mn^{++} 2 mM and TTX 5 x 10^{-7} g/ml present in B.

clamp was applied have been superimposed on the voltage record of hyperpolarizing clamp pulses into the pacemaker range. The current records show that the amount of i_f activated within the pacemaker range varies from preparation to preparation: there is a substantial amount in A and C, while in B very little is activated until the preparation is hyperpolarized considerably negative to the maximum diastolic potential. The levels of maximum diastolic potential shown (between -60 mV and -70 mV) are representative of these we find in SA node cells. The most negative maximum diastolic potential we find is -70 mV, with an action potential overshoot of 15 to 20 mV.

To determine the relative amounts of i_K decay and i_f activation which occur over the potential range of the pacemaker depolarization, we first gave hyperpolarizing clamp pulses into the appropriate potential range to see how much i_f was activated (Fig. 2A). Then we preceded each of the same hyperpolarizing

pulses by a depolarizing clamp pulse the magnitude and duration of which was
chosen so that it would activate approxpimately the same amount of i_K as would
be activated by an action potential (Fig. 2B).

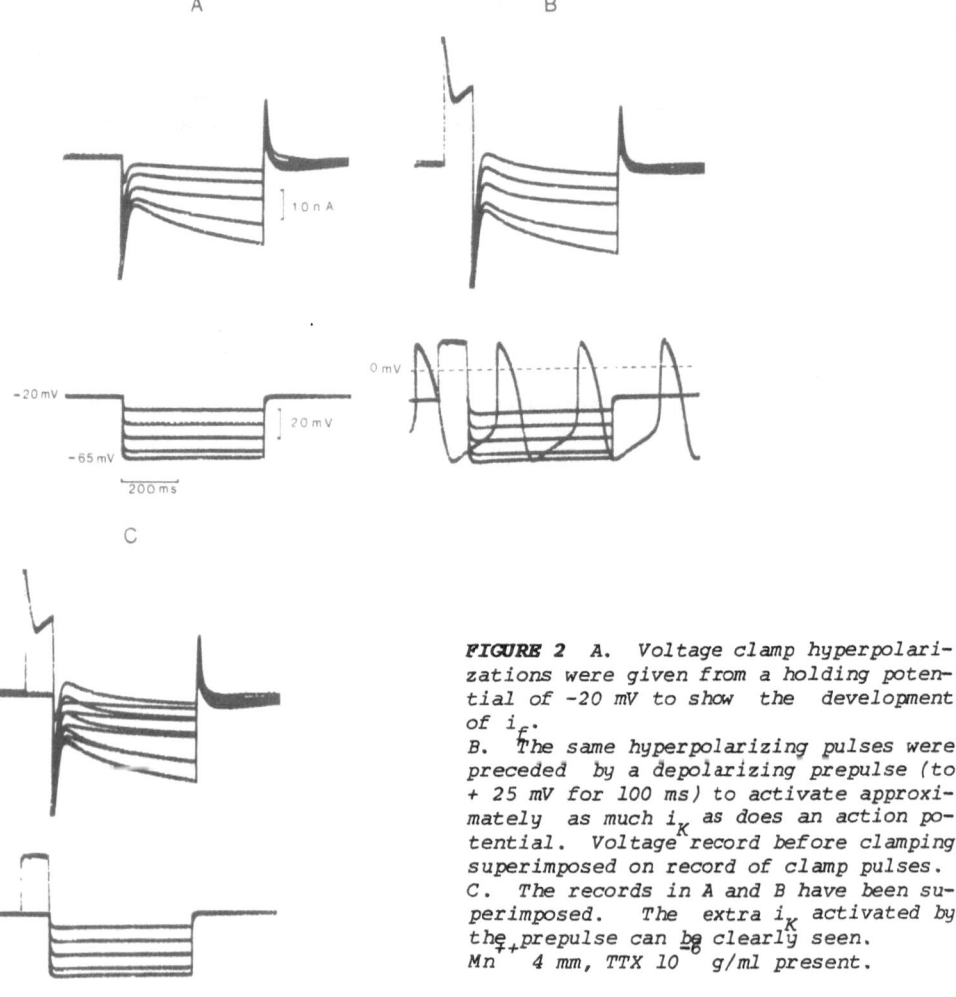

FIGURE 2 A. *Voltage clamp hyperpolari-*
zations were given from a holding poten-
tial of -20 mV to show the development
of i_f.
B. The same hyperpolarizing pulses were
preceded by a depolarizing prepulse (to
+ 25 mV for 100 ms) to activate approxi-
mately as much i_K as does an action po-
tential. Voltage record before clamping
superimposed on record of clamp pulses.
C. The records in A and B have been su-
perimposed. The extra i_K activated by
the prepulse can be clearly seen.
Mn^{++} 4 mm, TTX 10^{-6} g/ml present.

This i_K then decayed during the subsequent hyperpolarization. Superimposing the two sets of current records (i.e. with and without prepulse) demonstrates more clearly the extra i_K activated by the simulated action potential (Fig. 2C).

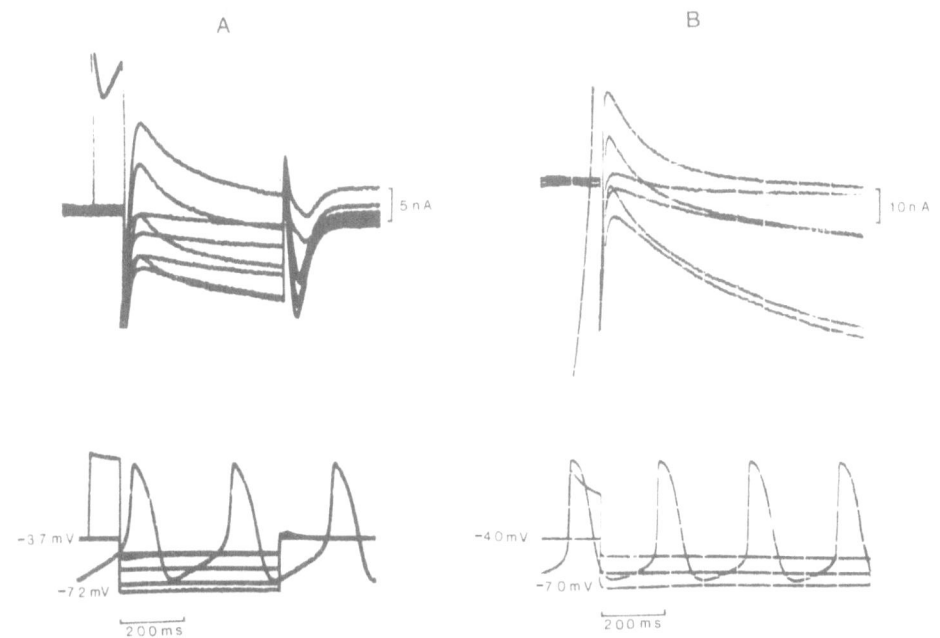

FIGURE 3 *Superimposed records of clamp hyperpolarizations into the pacing range with and without pre-depolarizations in two further preparations, A and B. No manganese present. In A, the prepulse was to +18 mV for 100 ms: in B, to -10 mV for 100 ms but the large amount of i_{si} in this preparation meant that the clamp could not hold the voltage completely constant during the prepulse. Note considerable i_K decay during the hyperpolarizations in both preparations even at levels more negative than the maximum diastolic potential, with appreciable i_f activation at the maximum diastolic level in B, but little in A. TTX 10^{-6} g/ml present in A.*

From Fig. 2C it would appear at first sight that i_K played very little part in controlling the rate of pacemaker depolarization, since during the hyperpolarization to -65 mV, the level of the maximum diastolic potential, the i_K activated by the prepulse decayed so rapidly that the current traces with and without prepulse almost superimpose. This experiment was, however, conducted in manganese (4 mM) which as well as blocking the second inward current, i_{si}, also partially blocks i_K. A better simulation of the real pacemaker situation can be obtained when manganese is not present even though there is then so much i_{si} that it is more difficult to obtain perfectly square voltage clamps.

Fig. 3 shows superimposed clamp hyperpolarizations with and without depolarizing prepulses in two further preparations, both in normal Tyrode solution without manganese. In both preparations the prepulse activated i_K which can be seen decaying during the subsequent hyperpolarizations, even when these were to potentials negative to the maximum diastolic potential. In the preparation shown in Fig. 3A, however, very little i_f was activated by the level of the maximum diastolic potential (-67 mV), whereas in that shown in Fig. 3B, i_f activation as well as i_k decay are evident during the clamp hyperpolarization to the level of the maximum diastolic potential, in this case -64 mV.

Results from experiments such as these must, of course, be interpreted with caution. It is obvious that the depolarizing prepulse can only be an approximation to an action potential and that capacity and other transients mean that the first 50 ms or so of the current records are lost. Nevertheless, results from about 10 preparations do indicate that in some SA node cells sufficient i_f is activated within the pacemaker range to make a significant contribution to pacemaker activity, while in others the decay of i_k is much more significant in controlling the rate of pacemaker depolarization.

In certain SA node cells the ranges of i_K decay and i_f activation appear to be very widely separated. Fig. 4A and B shows the same type of investigation (voltage clamp hyperpolarizations with and without a depolarizing prepulse) as was presented in Fig. 3. As can be seen in Fig. 4A, and more clearly in Fig. 4B where the pre-pulse has activated more i_K, the range of i_K decay and i_f activation did not overlap at all in these cells. The activation range of i_f was very negative (below -90 mV), so that the i_K decay which was present in the pacemaker range must in this case have alone controlled the rate of pacemaker depolarization. Fig. 4C shows the currents recorded in response to similar clamp hyperpolarizations given to the same preparation in the presence of barium and raised external potassium concentration (12 mM). Barium blocks both time-independent and time-dependent potassium currents (see DiFrancesco, this volume). It can be seen that there is a substantial reduction in the

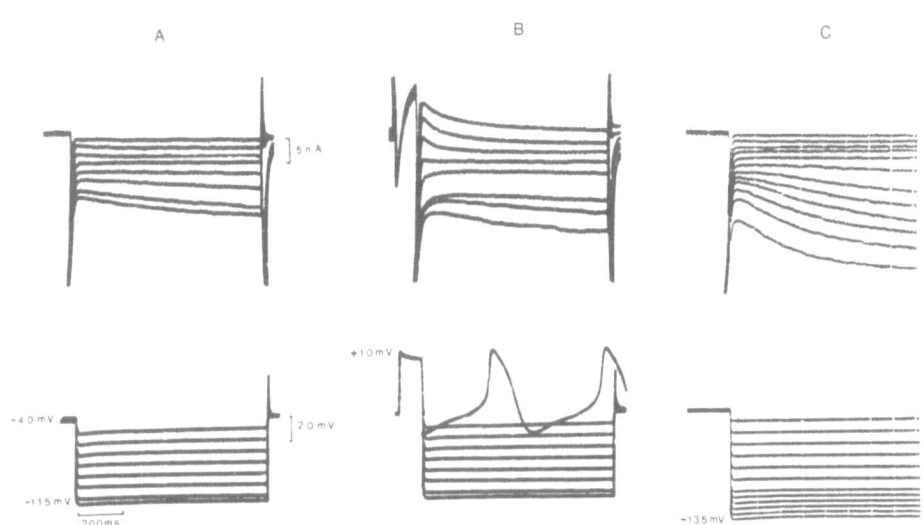

FIGURE 4 A. *Hyperpolarizing clamp pulses from a holding potential of -40 mV show that in this cell i_f is activated only negative to -90 mV. B. A 100 ms prepulse to +10 mV activated considerable i_K which can be seen decaying during the subsequent hyperpolarizations. The reversal of i_K can be seen between -80 and -90 mV. In C, 5 mM barium has reduced the potassium currents present, while raised potassium concentration (now 12 mM instead of 4 mM) has increased i_f which is, however, still in the same very negative voltage range. In B, action potentials recorded before clamping have been superimposed on the record of clamp pulses.*

time-independent current jump at the start of each hyperpolarizing clamp pulse, that no i_f, which might have been masked by depletion, is unmasked in the pacemaker potential range, and that i_f is present in the same very negative voltage range as previously but is now increased in magnitude because external potassium has been raised (see Brown and DiFrancesco, 1980). These findings confirm the suggestion that i_f cannot in any way have controlled the development of the diastolic depolarization in this preparation.

The third time-dependent current in SA node is the slow inward current, i_{si}. To evaluate the part it plays in pacemaking, we have once again tried to use a fairly direct method. By giving a hyperpolarizing clamp pulse to the vol-

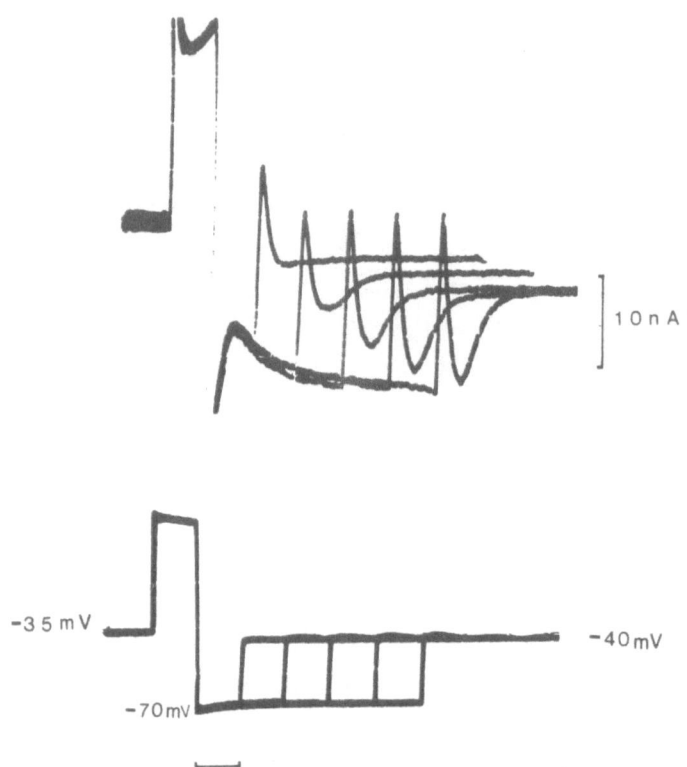

FIGURE 5 *A 100 ms prepulse to +15 mV from the holding potential of -35 mV, was followed by hyperpolarizations of duration between 100 and 50 ms to -70 mV after which the voltage was returned to -40 mV. The amount of i_{si} activated on return to -40 mV can be seen to increase with the duration of the hyperpolarizing pulse. TTX 10^{-6} g/ml present.*

tage level of the maximum diastolic potential for a time comparable to the duration of the pacemaker potential and then pulsing in a positive direction we have determined the threshold of i_{si}, relative to the pacemaker depolarization in a given SA node cell. The question of how long to remain at the maximum diastolic potential is very important as the amount of i_{si} appearing (and therefore, of course, the measured threshold) depends critically on the length of the preceding hyperpolarization.

Fig. 5 shows that as the duration of a hyperpolarizing pulse to -70 mV

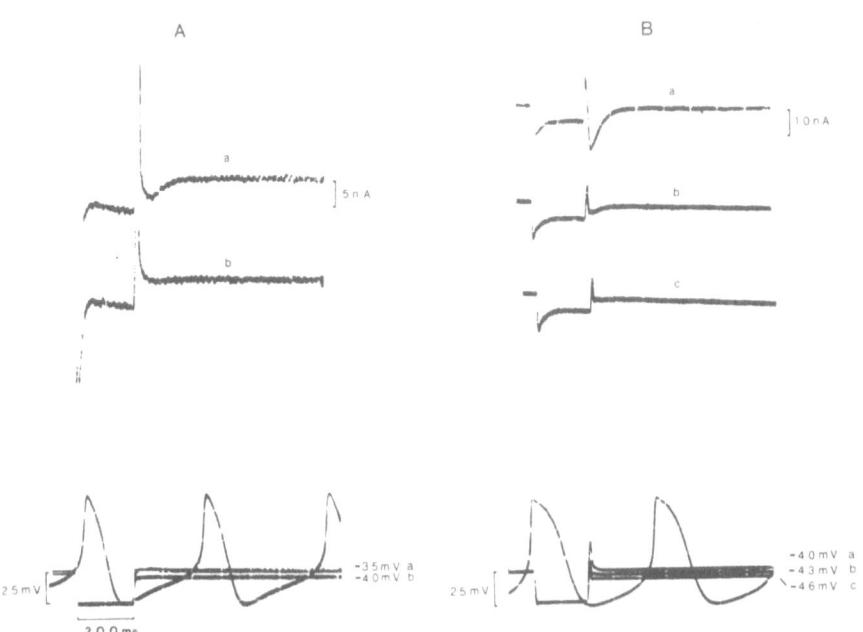

FIGURE 6 *Threshold of slow inward current, i_{si}, in two SA node preparations A and B tested after a 200 ms hyperpolarization to the level of the maximum diastolic potential from a holding potential of -35 mV in A and of -40 mV in B. Action potentials recorded before clamping have been superimposed on the voltage clamp record to show the position of the i_{si} threshold relative to the pacemaker depolarization. Current records shifted for clarity. TTX 10^{-6} g/ml present.*

(the maximum diastolic potential of that cell) is lengthened between 100 and 500 ms, so the amount of slow inward current recorded on pulsing to -40 mV after the pulse increases very markedly. It seems that there is a recovery from inactivation of the i_{si} current system, a process which is known to occur in cardiac membranes and to take place over times up to several seconds (Gettes and Reuter 1974; Noble and Shimoni, 1981). The consequence of this strongly time-dependent recovery from inactivation of the i_{si} system is that the i_{si} threshold appears more and more negative as the hyperpolarization used for the test is prolonged. In view of this we selected short (200 ms) hyperpolarizations to the level of the maximum diastolic potential for the determination of

i_{si} thresholds, as being a reasonable representation of the pacemaker depolarization by a square pulse.

Fig. 6 shows the threshold of i_{si} determined this way in two different preparations. The umclamped voltage record has in each case been superimposed on the record of the clamp pulses to show where detectable i_{si} appears relative to the pacemaker depolarization. As can be seen this is about 150-200 ms after the beginning of the pacemaker depolarization, or put another way, i_{si} contributes at most to the last 1/3 and propably most frequently only to the last 1/4 of the pacemaker depolarization (measured from maximum diastolic potential to "take-off" point). Using the same method we have found that the i_{si} threshold was in about the same place relative to the pacemaker depolarization in 5 preparations.

An even more direct way of looking at the currents involved in pacemaking in SA node is to trigger the voltage clamp circuit from the upstroke of an action potential with a variable delay so that the clamp switches on at different points during the pacemaker depolarization. Thus the currents participating in pacemaking are activated by the preceding action potential and/or the part of the pacemaker depolarization which has elapsed before clamp switch-on. Furthermore, if the level at which the clamp switches on is carefully chosen, capacity artifacts on switching can be avoided. In Fig. 7A the clamp was turned on in this way at the maximum diastolic potential of -60 mV. The current recorded in shown below.

Fig. 7B shows a hyperpolarizing clamp pulse subsequently given to the same potential (-60 mV) from a holding potential of -40 mV. The current record shows the activation of i_f during the first 300 ms at -60 mV. In Fig. 8 have been plotted the total current (open circles) during the first 300 ms after clamp switch on at -60 mV (from Fig. 7A) and (crosses) the amount of i_f activated at the same potential (from Fig. 7B). The decay of i_K (triangles) was obtained by subtracting i_f from the total current.

The information given in Figs. 7 and 8 allows some simple calculations to be made. The rate of rise of the pacemaker depolarization in this preparation was approximately 0.1 V/s. From the capacity transient at the start of the hyperpolarizing pulse in Fig. 7B an estimate of the capacitance of the membrane can be made and comes to 0.05 μF. Using the relationship $c \times dV/dt = -i$, the current flow (i) required through this capacitance (c) to give a rate of rise of

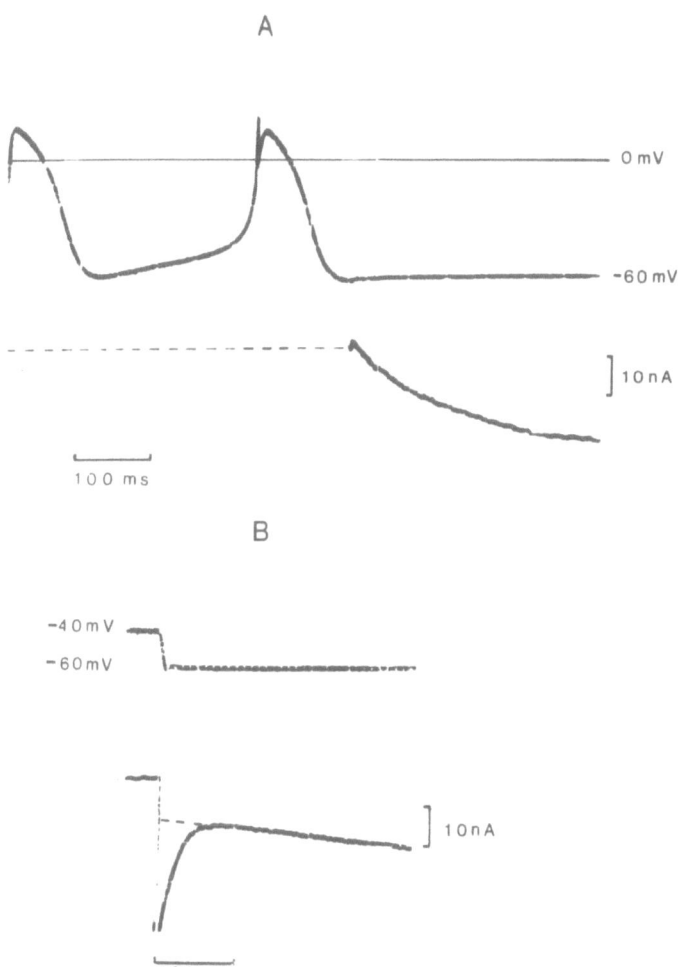

FIGURE 7 A. *Voltage clamp switched on at the maximum diastolic potential (-60 mV). Current trace shows the total current recorded. Dotted line indicates current level at the maximum diastolic potential which since dV/dT is zero must here be zero. The artifact on the voltage line indicates where the delay switch for the clamp circuit was triggered by the upstroke of the action potential.*
B. Voltage clamp hyperpolarization to the same level (-60 mV) as the maximum diastolic potential in A. The current trace shows the i_f activated at this potential during the first 300 ms of the clamp. Dotted line shows extrapolation made to overcome capacitance artifact.

voltage of 0.1 V/s comes to 5 nA. From the graph in Fig. 8, it can be seen
that during the first 50 ms of voltage clamp at -60 mV, a total current of ap-
proximaterly 6 nA is recorded. Hence the current flow during the period of time
(approximately 50 ms) for which the potential at the end of an action potential
is nearly constant: that is while it is at the maximum diastolic potential,
would be sufficient to generate a net inward current of the right magnitude to
achieve a depolarization rate of 0.1 V/s.

FIGURE 8 Plot of the currents recorded in Fig. 7. Open circles: total current change during the first 300 ms of voltage clamp at the maximum diastolic potential (-60 mV) in Fig. 7A. Crosses: i_f activated during the first 300 ms of the clamp hyperpolarization to -60 mV shown in Fig. 7B. Triangles: the change due to i_K decay, obtained by subtracting i_f from total current. All current levels relative to zero current at maximum diastolic potential.

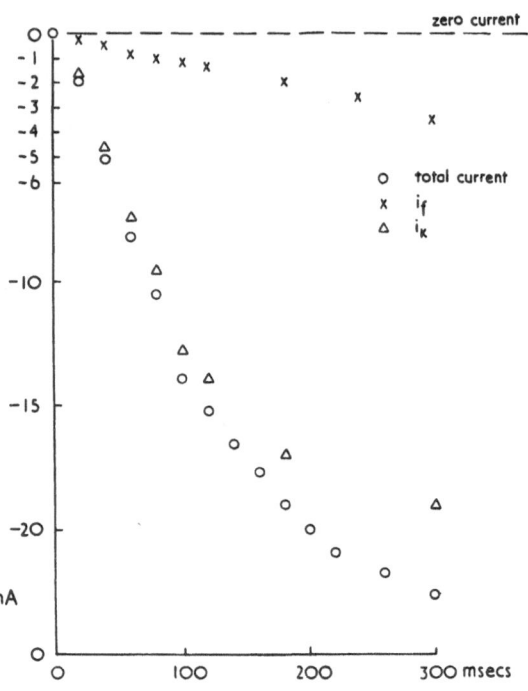

Of the total depolarizing current of 6 nA recorded at the maximum diastolic
potential in the preparation, 1 nA was activating i_f, which leaves over 80%
being provided by deactivating i_K.

Fig. 9 shows the current records obtained when the voltage clamp was
switched on progressively later during the pacemaker depolarization. At first
(Fig. 9C -E) the total amount of current change recorded lessens. In Fig. 9F,
where the pacemaker depolarization was clamped at -47 mV, the slow inward cur-

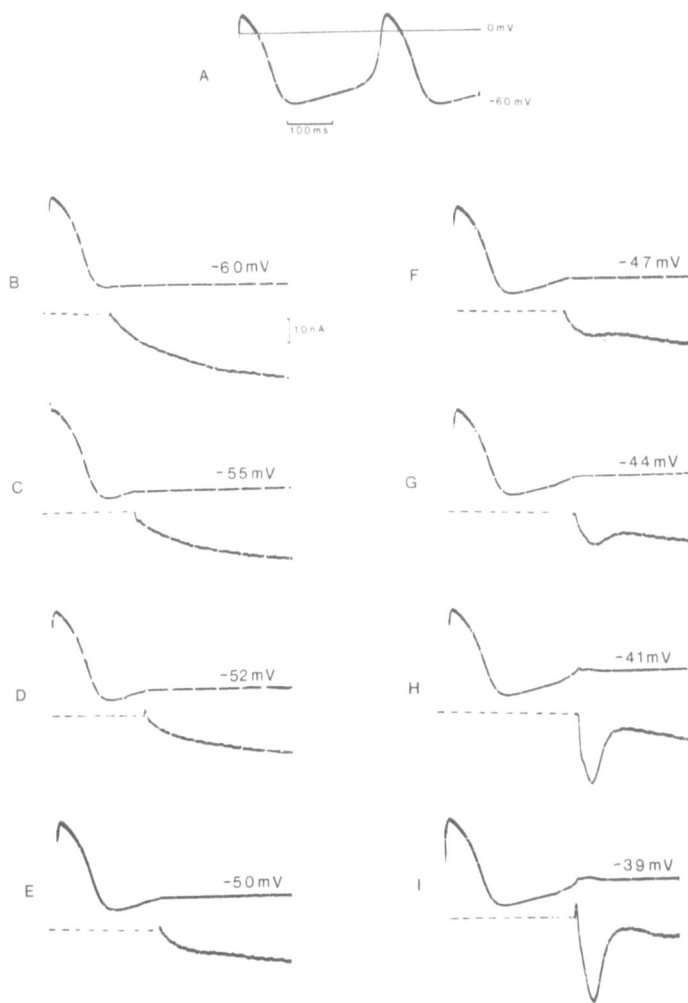

FIGURE 9 *The pacemaker depolarization shown uninterrupted in A was terminated at different points by turning on the voltage clamp with variable delay at the voltage levels indicated (B to I) and the current flowing across the membrane was recorded.*

rent appears for the first time, and in the next three panels (9G - I) it is
seen to be present in increasing amounts. This range of voltages corresponds
well to the region at which the rate of pacemaker depolarization greatly accel-
erates.

It is worth noting that in this work we have not taken into account any effects due to K^+ ion accumulation or depletion in close extracellular spaces.
These effects are very substantial in Purkinje fibres (DiFrancesco and Noble,
1981, this volume). By contrast this problem seems unlikely to be significant
in the SA node. Our own calculations based on the ionic currents we record
(order of 10 nA) and the likely volume of the extracellular space (e.g. 10%)
show that variations of the order of only 0.01 mM are to be expected. Even in a
very restricted space (order of 1%) only a 0.1 mM variation in extracellular potassium concentration is expected. These findings correspond very well to the
range of values of K^+ accumulation measured during repetitive activity in the
rabbit SA node by Kronhaus et al. (1978) using K^+ sensitive electrodes.

The results presented here do not yet form a complete assesment of the relative quantitative contribution on i_K, i_{si} and i_f to sino-atrial node pacemaking since this not only varies between preparations but may also depend on other
conditions that we have not yet investigated systematically. The preparations
used for these experiments, like most SA node preparations successfully clamped
so far, have been taken from near the ring bundle. It should, however, be possible to extend this approach to cells in the centre of the SA node as well as
to cells pacing under the influence of various drugs and transmitters. One
thing that is perhaps already clear is that there is no single pacemaker current
in the SA node but that nodal pacemaking depends upon a balance of membrane currents.

ACKNOWLEDGEMENTS

We should like to thank Dr Denis Noble and Dr Dario DiFrancesco for much helpful
discussion and encouragement, and the Medical Research Council for financial
support.

REFERENCES

Brown, H.F., Clark, A. and Noble S.J.: Identification of the pacemaker current in frog atrium. J. Physiol. (London), 258: 521-545, 1976.

Brown, H.F. and DiFrancesco, D.: Voltage-clamp investigations of membrane currents underlying pacemaker activity in rabbit sino-atrial node. J. Physiol. (London), 308: 331-351, 1980.

Brown, H.F., DiFrancesco, D. and Noble, S.J.: Cardiac pacemaker oscillation and its modulation by autonomic transmitters. J. Exp. Biol., 81: 175-204, 1979.

Brown, H.F., Giles, W. and Noble, S.J.: Membrane currents underlying activity in frog sinus venosus. J. Physiol. (London), 271: 783-816, 1977.

Brown, H.F., Kimura, J. and Noble S.J.: Evidence that the current i_f in sino-atrial node has a potassium component. J. Physiol. (London), 308: 33P, 1980.

DiFrancesco, D.: The pacemaker current "i_{K2}" in Purkinje fibres is carried by sodium and potassium. J. Physiol. (London), 308: 32P, 1980.

DiFrancesco, D.: The current I_{K2} in Purkinje fibres reinterpreted and identified with the current I_f in the SA node. This volume, 1981.

DiFrancesco, D. and Noble, D.: Implications of the reinterpretation of i_{K2} for the modelling of the electrical activity of pacemaker tissues in the heart. This volume, 1981.

DiFrancesco, D. and Ojeda, C.: Properties of the pacemaker current i_f in the sino-atrial node of the rabbit: a comparison with the current I_{K2} in Purkinje fibres. J. Physiol. (London), 308: 353-367, 1980.

Gettes, L.S. and Reuter, H.: Slow recovery from inactivation of inward currents in mammalian myocardium. J. Physiol. (London), 240: 703-724, 1974.

Hauswirth, O., Noble, D. and Tsien, R.W.: The mechanism of oscillatory activity at low membrane potentials in cardiac Purkinje fibres. J. Physiol. (London), 200: 255-265, 1969.

Kronhaus, K.D., Spear, J.F., Moore, E.N. and Kline, R.P.: Sinus node extracellular potassium transients following vagal stimulation. Nature, 275: 322-324, 1978.

Noble, S. and Shimoni, Y.: The calcium and frequency dependence of the slow inward current "staircase" in frog atrium. J. Physiol. (London), 310: 57-75, 1981.

Noble, D. and Tsien, R.W.: The kinetic and rectifier properties of the slow potassium current in cardiac Purkinje fibres. J. Physiol. (London), 195: 185-214, 1968.

Yanagihara, K. and Irisawa, H.: Inward current activated during hyperpolarization in the rabbit sinoatrial node cell. Pfluegers Arch., 385: 11-19, 1980a.

Yanagihara, K. and Irisawa, H.: Potassium current during the pacemaker depolarization in rabbit sinoatrial node cell. Pfluegers Arch., 388: 255-260, 1980b.

THE CURRENT I_{K2} IN PURKINJE FIBRES REINTERPRETED

AND IDENTIFIED WITH THE CURRENT I_F IN THE SA NODE

Dario DiFrancesco

INTRODUCTION

It is well agreed that, because of the problems related to the multicellular nature of cardiac preparations - like voltage non-uniformities in space-clamped preparations - or because of technical limitations, interpretation of voltage-clamp results in cardiac muscle requires a particular caution (Johnson and Lieberman, 1971; McGuigan, 1974; Attwell and Cohen, 1977). Recently, the attention of cardiac electrophysiologists has been concentrating on yet another cause of distortion in the analysis performed under V-clamp conditions, which interferes with the study of current properties, i.e. the phenomenon of accumulation/depletion (Almers, 1972; Noble, 1976; Cohen et al., 1976; Baumgarten and Isenberg, 1977; DiFrancesco et al., 1979; Eisner et al., 1980). It now appears that the distortion induced by accumulation/depletion of potassium ions in close extracellular spaces in the description of any K-dependent current is far more drastic than any distortion induced by non-uniformities. Indeed, evidence given in this paper shows how the presence of strong K-depletion during hyperpolarizations can alter the analysis of the pacemaker current "i_{K2}" so substantially as to make an inward current activating during a hyperpolarization look like an outward current deactivating (DiFrancesco, 1981a).

The observation that K-accumulation/depletion can modify the properties of K-dependent currents as deduced from V-clamp experiments is not, however, the only hint leading to the necessity of a re-evaluation of the properties of "i_{K2}". In the SA node, a "pacemaker" current, i_f, has been found which at least partly underlies the pacemaker depolarization and the acceleratory effect of adrenaline (Brown et al., 1979a,b) in a way similar to that observed for "i_{K2}" in Purkinje fibres (Hauswirth et al., 1968). Furthermore, the two currents have been found to have a similar dependence on Na_b and to be blocked by caesium (DiFrancesco and Ojeda, 1980), which strengthens the hypothesis that the two are identical channels. Despite their similarities, however, the behaviour of i_f in high K solutions and conductance measurements indicate that i_f is not a pure K-current, outward deactivating on hyperpolarization, but is on the contrary an inward current activating on hyperpolarizations below the threshold of -50/-60 mV (DiFrancesco and Ojeda, 1980).

The finding that i_f is an inward current in the pacemaker range, and that the presence of K-accumulation/depletion phenemona intervenes in distorting the analysis of the properties of "i_{K2}", justify the need for a re-investigation of "i_{K2}". Here evidence is presented showing that the pacemaker current in Purkinje fibres is, like i_f in the SA node, an inward current activated on hyperpolarizations in the pacemaker range (DiFrancesco, 1981a). The current reversal observed near E_K is produced by the presence of K-depletion (see also DiFrancesco and Noble, this volume), and is removed by the use of Ba which blocks i_{K1} and thus limits the process of K-depletion taking place during a hyperpolarization. The true reversal potential lies near -30 mV in normal Tyrode, and changes with external potassium (K_b) and sodium (Na_b) as expected if the current were carried by both ions. The fully-activated I/V relations in different potassium and sodium concentrations are linear over a relatively large V-range.

The pacemaker current in Purkinje fibres is here referred to as "i_{K2}", with reference to its former description as a pure K-current (Noble and Tsien, 1968; Peper and Trautwein, 1969), or as "i_f", with reference to its new interpretation as an inward current activated on hyperpolarization in the pacemaker range (DiFrancesco, 1981b). This is not to create confusion, but to distinguish between two quite distinct descriptions. All results described in this paper refer to calf Purkinje fibres V-clamped with the traditional two-microelectrode method.

RESULTS

MEMBRANE CONDUCTANCE MEASUREMENTS IN NORMAL SOLUTION
In principle, following the time course of membrane conductance during a hyperpolarizing V-clamp pulse should enable one to distinguish between an inward current activating and an outward current deactivating (DiFrancesco and Ojeda,
1980). This is only true, however, if the slope conductance of the
fully-activated current is positive at the voltage under consideration, and when
no K-depletion takes place. The membrane conductance can be measured by using
the protocol shown in Fig. 1, where small and short V-pulses are superimposed
on longer pulses during changes of "i_{K2}". If no K-depletion is present, the
total current displacement δi caused by small and short pulses of amplitude δE
is given by

$$\delta i(E,t) = \delta i_b(E) + \delta i_{K2}(E,t) = (di_b/dE)_E \, \delta E + s(E,t)(d\bar{i}_{K2}/dE)_E \, \delta E \qquad (1)$$

where δi_b and δi_{K2} are the contributions of time-independent and time-dependent
components respectively. The current displacement due to "i_{K2}" (δi_{K2}) is proportional to $s(E,t)$, and thus follows the same time-course as the current itself, with the assumption that the pulses used to test the conductance changes
are small and short enough to leave the dependence $s(t)$ unaltered. The ratio
$\delta i(E,t)/\delta E$ represents the time-dependence of the total slope-conductance.
If the hyperpolarization is applied at a potential where $d\bar{i}_{K2}/dE$ is positive,
an outward current deactivating will give rise to a decreasing membrane conductance, while an inward current activating will give rise to an increasing membrane conductance. However, a conductance increase is also expected for an outward current deactivating if, as the case for "i_{K2}" in a certain range, $d\bar{i}_{K2}/dE$
is negative. A further problem arises from the presence of K-depletion. During
a hyperpolarization, by shifting the K-equilibrium potential to more negative
values, K-depletion contributes a conductance decrease due to i_{K1} which overlaps
with the conductance change due to "i_{K2}". The process is further complicated by
the dependence of "i_{K2}" on K_b, and a more detailed analysis of the effects of
K-depletion on the membrane conductance time course requires numerical computation (see DiFrancesco and Noble, this volume).
    In these conditions, conductance measurements during V-clamp hyperpolariza-

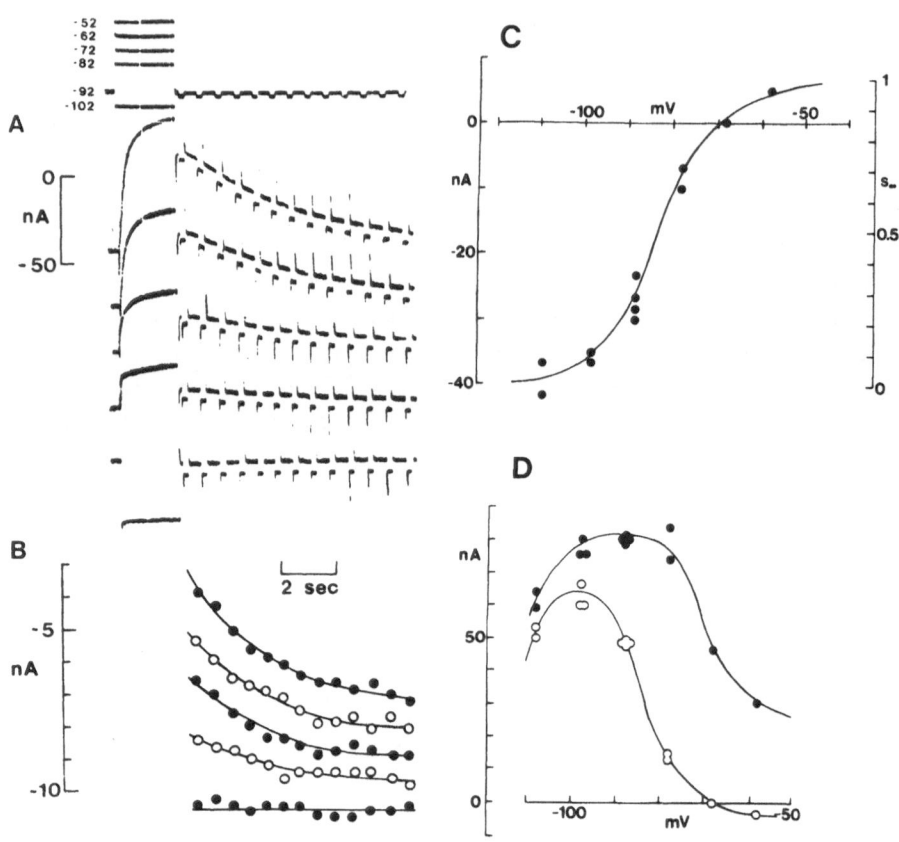

FIGURE 1 *The potential is held at -92 mV and 2 sec pulses are given in the range -52 mV to -102 mV (A). The membrane conductance is measured on returning to the holding potential after every pulse, applying 0.2 sec, 2.5 mV negative pulses at a fixed frequency. The time course of the current displacement δi (B) reveals an increase in membrane conductance on return from each depolarization. Note that at -92 mV the slope of the $i_{K2}(E)$ relation (D) is not negative. Current traces are displaced vertically for clarity. The current scale refers to the pulse to -52 mV. Closed and open circles alternating in the δi(t) curves for clarity. C: activation curve holding the voltage at -68 mV. D: amplitude of time-dependent current changes obtained on pulsing from -68 mV to various potential levels (open circles). These values divided by $s_\infty(E)-s_\infty(-68)$ yield the fully-activated I-V relation i_{K2} (closed circles). The values of $s_\infty(E)$ used in this calculation were the average of several points at the same potential. For details of the construction of activation curve and fully-activated curve see for example DiFrancesco and McNaughton, 1979.*

tions cannot be used to discriminate with certainty between an inward current activating and an outward current deactivating. However, they can be used to check if the Noble and Tsien (1968) model for "i_{K2}" gives a correct interpretation of the experimental data. According to the "outward current" interpretation a conductance decrease is in fact expected during a hyperpolarization at a potential where $d\bar{i}_{K2}/dE$ is positive. As noticed above, the presence of K-depletion should reinforce this decrease. In the experiment of Fig. 1, the potential was held at -92 mV, where according to the fully-activated relation shown in fig. 1D, the slope conductance is positive. 2 sec pulses were given to various potentials and the conductance changes were followed after returning to the holding potential. It can be observed that δi not only increases in magnitude with time for all curves, but is also smaller after larger pre-hyperpolarizations at a fixed time. Thus, in Fig. 1 the increase observed in δi on hyperpolarization is not attributable to the presence of a negative slope conductance in the fully-activated I/V relation for a K-current as described in the conventional way by the Noble and Tsien model. In the same experiment, the membrane conductance time course was followed during a total 82 pulses in the range -68 to -108 mV, and at all voltages where it was followed, the membrane conductance was observed to increase during hyperpolarization, and to decrease during depolarization. Similar results were obtained in two more experiments. These data represent a first indication of the inadequacy of the Noble and Tsien (1968) model to explain conductance measurements.

BLOCKING EFFECT OF LOW CONCENTRATION OF CAESIUM

Caesium has been shown to block at relatively high concentrations (20 mM) i_{K1} and "i_{K2}" in the Purkinje fibre (Isenberg, 1977), as well as i_f in the SA node (DiFrancesco and Ojeda, 1980). On the hypotheses that the block of i_{K1} and "i_{K2}" is the only effect of Cs, its blocking action can be used to discriminate between a time-dependent outward or a time-dependent inward current. According to the "outward current" interpretation in the V-range positive to the "i_{K2}" reversal potential (E_{rev}) both currents are outward, and their reduction would lead to a negative displacement of the current recorded on V-clamp. On the other hand if "i_{K2}" is an inward current activated on hyperpolarization, its block, even if partial, would lead to a positive current shift. To this a further shift due to i_{K1} blocking would add a positive or negative component ac-

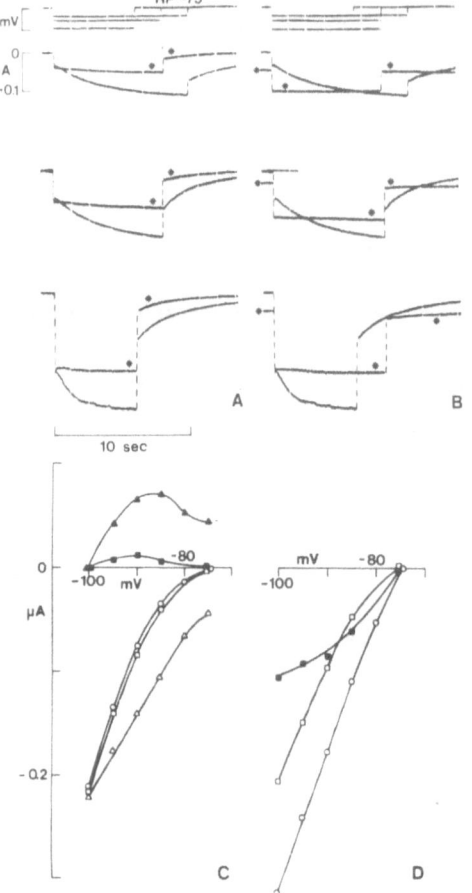

FIGURE 2 *Effect of 1 mM Cs after 3' perfusion (A) and of 5 mM Cs after 3' perfusion (B) during hyperpolarizations in the range -75 to -100 mV. Pulses are of different duration to limit the current through the preparation. Traces in CS are labelled with an asterisk. C: Instantaneous i-V relations in control (○), 1 mM Cs (□), and 5 mM Cs (△). Filled symbols represent the difference between traces in control and 1 mM Cs (■) or 5 mM Cs (▲). D: I-V relations for the pulses in control (○) and 1 mM Cs (□). Filled squares (■) represent the difference between the two curves. In A and B zero current coincides with the holding current in control.*

cording to whether i_{K1} is inward or outward at the voltage analyzed. The records of Fig. 2 show that "i_{K2}" behaves like an inward, rather than an outward current during hyperpolarizations in the range -75 to -100 mV. From a holding potential of -75 mV, hyperpolarizations evoke time-dependent currents which, according to the "i_{K2}" interpretation, occur positive to the reversal potential. Application of 1 mM Cs gives rise to nearly flat records (marked by asterisks), in agreement with the view that at this low concentration Cs already blocks "i_{K2}". When the records are superimposed, it appears that the time-independent component is nearly unchanged at all potentials, and that the current traces have been displaced to the positive direction by Cs, as expected if "i_{K2}" were an inward current. When the Cs concentration is increased up to 5 mM, the background component is also changed (Fig. 2B). The difference curves obtained subtracting the background I/V relation in control solution from those in the two Cs concentrations show inward-going rectification and cross the V-axis near -100 mV. These results (see also DiFrancesco, 1981a) agree with the view that "i_{K2}" is an inward current activated on hyperpolarization, and that is blocked by Cs in low concentrations.

INFLUENCE OF BARIUM ON "I_{K2}" AND ON ITS DEPENDENCE ON EXTERNAL POTASSIUM

The results from conductance measurements and the effect of low Cs concentrations shown above indicate that during a hyperpolarization "i_{K2}" behaves like an activating inward current, rather than a deactivating outward current. How then is it possible that a current reversal is seen on hyperpolarization near E_K? It is important to answer this point, as the existance of a reversal potential near E_K is a central piece of evidence for the view that "i_{K2}" is a pure K-current. A process of K-depletion taking place during large hyperpolarizations has been already found to interfere with the determination of the "i_{K2}" reversal (DiFrancesco et al., 1979). During a hyperpolarization an apparent inward decaying "depletion" component, maily due to a positive shift of i_{K1} along the V-axis caused by K-depletion, overlaps with the time course of "i_{K2}", which is itself distorted by depletion. If the K-depletion is strong enough, during a hyperpolarization even an inward-increasing time-dependent current could be offset by the "depletion" component, the overall result being a nearly flat current trace. Reducing K-depletion, for example by blocking i_{K1}, should be therefore the only way to limit the distortion of the time-course of "i_{K2}". The only known blocker of i_{K1} in Purkinje fibres is Cs (Isenberg, 1977), which however, has the disadventage, seen above, of blocking "i_{K2}" also. The use of Ba is suggested by two considerations: first, Ba is a blocker of the inward-rectifying K-channel in the skeletal muscle (Standen and Stanfield, 1978) as well as in other tissues (Hagiwara et al., 1978); and second, it has little or no effect on the current

FIGURE 3 *Effect of changing K_b in the presence of 5 mM Ba. From a holding potential of -52 mV pulses of various durations and amplitudes are given in 3, 9, 18 and 36 mM K_b. Before application of Ba an "apparent" current reversal was observed at -127 mV (3 mM K_b, not shown), while no current reversal is observed after Ba on hyperpolarizing down to -162 mV. A reversal is not seen even on raising K_b to 36 mM. $MnCl_2$ 8 mM present throughout.*

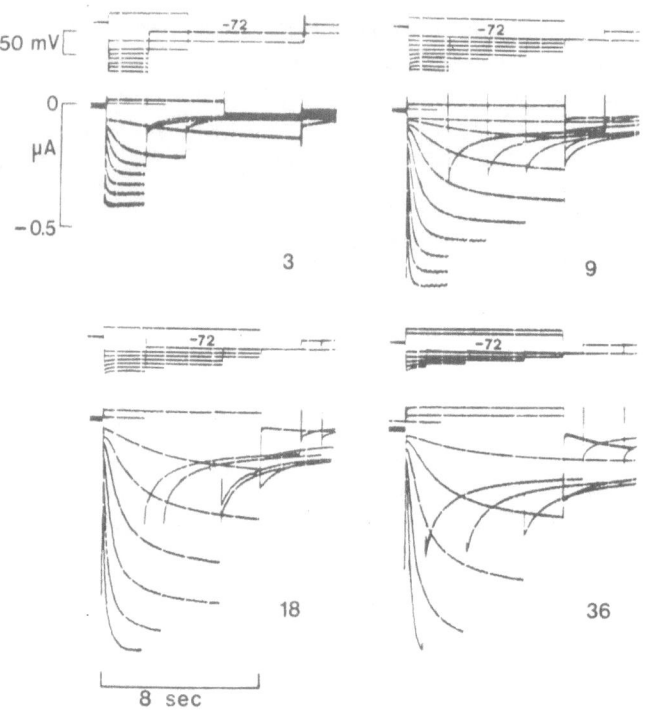

i_f in the SA node (Yanagihara and Irisawa, 1980). Fig. 3 shows the effects of 5 mM Ba on the current time course during hyperpolarizations from a holding potential of -52 mV, and the effect of changing K_b from 3 to 36 mM in the presence of Ba. No current reversal is observed on hyperpolarizing down to -162 mV in normal Tyrode (upper left). In the same fibre, a reversal potential of -127 mV was obtained before application of Ba. A current reversal below -52 mV is not seen even if K_b is increased up to 36 mM. On the contrary, the current increases in the inward direction as K_b is increased. This rules out the possibility that "i_{K2}" is a pure K-current. As expected in the case of a Ba-induced block of i_{K1}, the time-independent component is substantially smaller in Ba than in the control solution (not shown) and varies only a little when K_b is changed, as is more evident in the records of Fig. 4, which are replayed from the same experiment as in Fig. 3 at a higher sweep speed. Subtracting the time-independent current in the control solution from that in 5 mM Ba (3 mM K_b) results in an i_{K1}-type curve displaying inward-going rectification and crossing the V-axis at about -100 mV (see DiFrancesco, 1981a, Fig. 5).

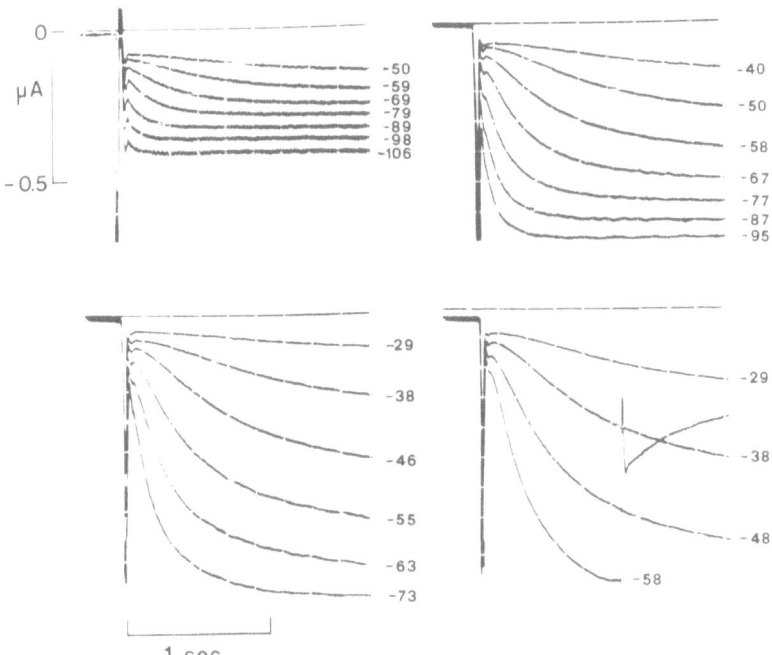

FIGURE 4 *Same traces as in Fig. 3 (only part of the records is shown) replayed from tape at higher sweep speed to illustrate the blocking effect of Ba on i_{K1}. Ba reduces the time-independent component with respect to the control case (not shown) and limits to a small increase the effect of rising K_b on i_{K1}, in contrast with the large effect known to occur in the absence of Ba (Noble, 1965). 3, 9, 18 and 36 mM K_b from left to right, top to bottom. Numbers near each trace represent the corresponding pulse amplitude from the holding potential of -52 mV.*

TIME COURSE OF THE MEMBRANE CONDUCTANCE DURING HYPERPOLARIZATION AFTER BARIUM

When the membrane conductance is measured in Ba-containing solutions (Fig.   5) with   a   protocol   similar   to that shown in Fig.   1, an increase is clearly ob-served at all potentials and potassium concentrations analyzed.   These data con-firm   that   "i_{K2}"   is an inward current activating during a hyperpolarization in the pacemaker range, like i_f in the SA node.

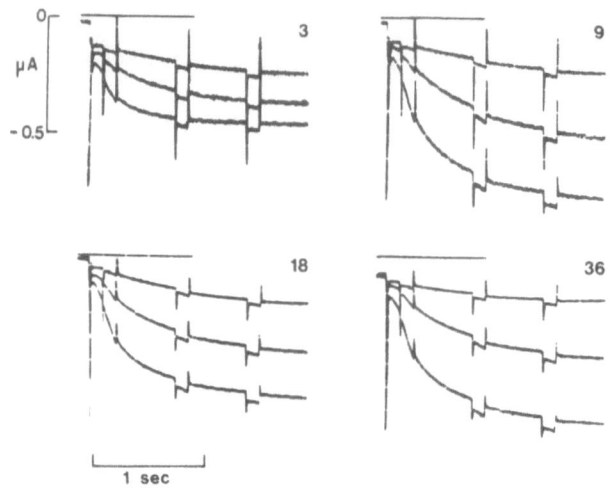

FIGURE 5 *Conductance measurements during hyperpolarizations in Ba 5 mM in 3,   9, 18 and 36 mM K_b, as marked near each panel.   Same experiment as in Fig.   3.   The conductance is measured using a protocol similar to that shown in Fig. 1.   The pulses   used to activate i_f are to -92, -102 and -111 mV at 3 mM K_b, to -82, -92 and -102 mV at 9 mM K_b, to -81, -90 and -98 mV at 18 mM K_b, and to -72, -81 and -90 mV   at   36 mM K_b, from a holding potential of -52 mV.   Test pulse was -5 mV throughout.   The membrane conductance, which is proportional to the current dis-placement   δi   caused by the testing pulse, is seen to increase for all hyperpo-larizations.*

IONIC COMPOSITION OF THE PACEMAKER CURRENT: EFFECT OF EXTERNAL SODIUM

An obvious question arising from the evidence that "i_{K2}" is not a pure K-current concerns   its   ionic composition.   According to the data of Fig.3, a current re-versal is not obtained negative to the holding potential (-52 mV in this case)

FIGURE 6 *Determination of the current reversal potential in Ba (E_f). Following a 100 mV, 0.5 hyperpolarizing pulse from -38 mV to activate i_f, the membrane is depolarized to different levels. Current reversal occurs near -43 mV in 70 mM Na_b (A, see enlarged tails at the bottom) and near -53 mV in 35 mM Na_b (B). Tris-HCL used as a substitute for NaCl in equimolar quantities. K_b is 9 mM. $MnCl_2$ 5 mM and $BaCl_2$ 8 mM present throughout.*

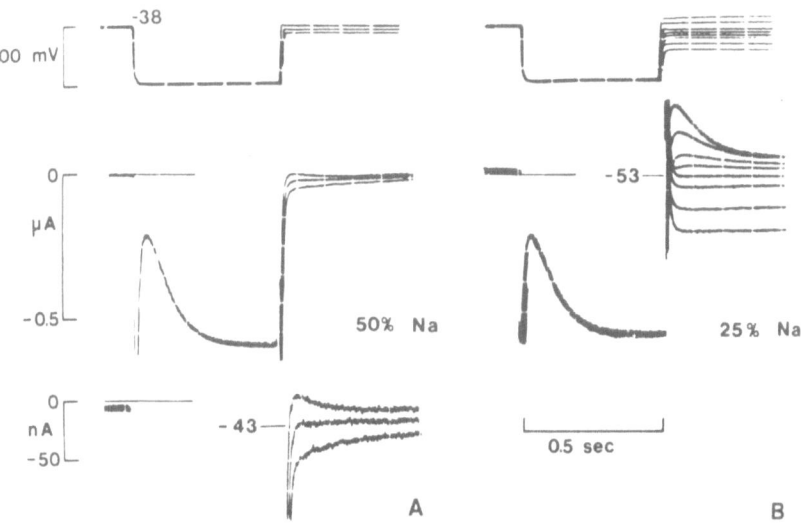

at any K_b. The reversal potential should therefore lie in the region positive to -52 mV. An ion with an equilibrium potential more positive than E_K is therefore required. In view of the known dependence on Na_b of both "i_{K2}" in Purkinje fibres (McAllister and Noble, 1966; DiFrancesco and McNaughton, 1979) and i_f in the SA node (Noma et al., 1977; DiFrancesco and Ojeda, 1980), it is natural to investigate the effects of changing Na_b on the time course of the current in the region positive to E_K. In the experiment of Fig. 6 Na_b was lowered from 140 mM to 70 mM (A) and 35 mM (B), and the potential was stepped to various levels after a hyperpolarization to -138 mV to activate the current. This protocol shows that a current reversal does occur at about -43 mV in 70 mM Na_b (K_b = 9 mM) and that it becomes more negative (about -53 mV) when Na_b is lowered to 35 mM.

The finding that a current reversal dependent on Na_b occurs at potentials much

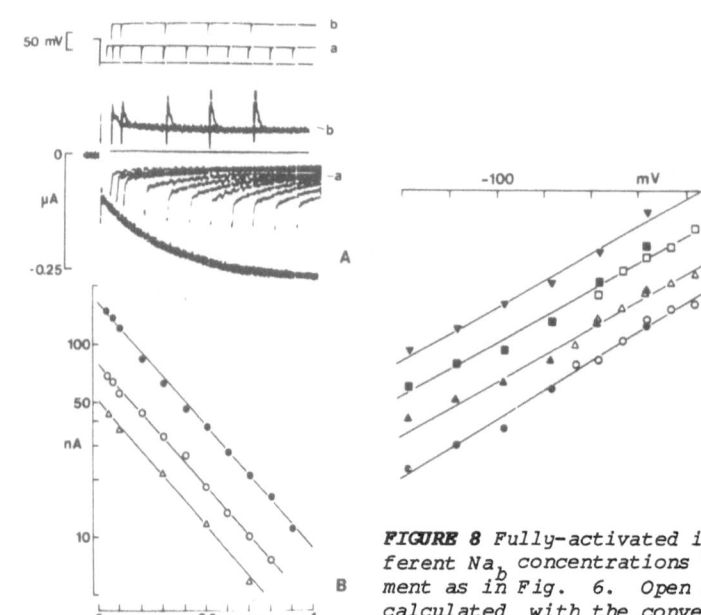

FIGURE 8 Fully-activated $i_f(E)$ relations in different Na_b concentrations $(K_b=9\ mM)$. Same experiment as in Fig. 6. Open symbols refer to values calculated with the conventional two pulse method as in Fig. 1 (see Difrancesco and McNaughton, 1979). Filled symbols refer to values obtained more directly by measuring the sum of the two current changes at a fixed potential obtained after pulsing at the top and the bottom of the activation curve (see DiFrancesco, 1981b, Fig. 1). Na_b varied from 140 (O) to 105 (Δ), 70 (□) and 35 mM (∇). Least squares fitting gave (ranges marked by full lines): 4.8, 4.3, 4.3 and 4.4 nA/mV from 140 to 35 mM.

FIGURE 7 Envelope test at -100 mV in 12 mM K_b. A: from the holding potential of -30 mV the membrane is hyperpolarized to -100 mV for various durations and then stepped to -50 mV, where the current tails are inward deactivating (a), or to 10 mV, where the current is outward (b). B: tail amplitudes at -50 mV (O) and 10 mV (Δ) are plotted against prepulse duration on a semilog scale, together with the current time course during activation at -100 mV (●). Time constants for the least-squares fitting lines are: 347 (●), 346 (O) and 332 ms (Δ). Solutions containing $MnCl_2$ 5 mM and $BaCl_2$ 5 mM. Note the change in τ_f between -50 and 10 mV.

more positive than E_K can be used as an indication that Na crosses the channel only if the time course of the current tails recorded on depolarizations, like those shown in the records of Fig. 6, are proved to reflect i_f deactivation.

This can be checked for example by the use of envelope tests. Identification of the reversal potential in this voltage region, particularly in normal Tyrode solution, is made more difficult by the presence of current components other than i_f in the tails recorded on depolarizations. Separation of i_f from the total current can be simplified, however, by increasing K_b, and this has been done for the envelope test shown in Fig. 7.

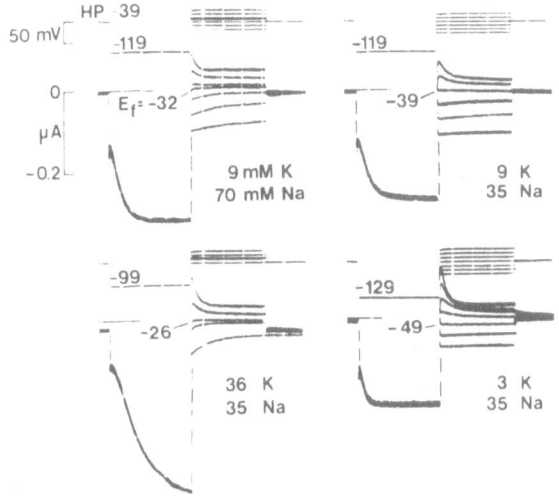

FIGURE 9 *Reversal potential (E_f) measured in solutions with different ionic composition, marked near each panel. E_f values near corresponding records. The protocol used is similar to that shown in Fig. 6. E_f shifts negative when Na_b is lowered (top panels), as in Fig. 6. and also depends on K_b (top right and bottom panels). In the same experiment, values of -34 mV at 35 mM Na_b, 18 mM K_b, and of -19 mV at 140 mM Na_b, 9 mM K_b were obtained for E_f. Pulses duration is 2 sec throughout. $MnCl_2$ 5 mM and $BaCl_2$ 10 mM present in all solutions. Tris-HCl used as a substitute for BaCl. From DiFrancesco, 1980b.*

From the holding potential of -30 mV the voltage is stepped to -100 mV for various durations and then held at -50 mV (a) or +10 mV (b). It is clear from Fig. 7A (b) that the tail amplitude at 10 mV increases with the duration of the hyperpolarization. Plotting on a semilog scale in Fig. 7B the current time course during the pulse to -100 mV and the tail amplitudes as a function of pre-pulse duration for both potentials, shows that the time courses of current

and of tail amplitudes parallel each other, and that therefore the outward decreasing tail observed at +10 mV is i_f deactivating. Similar evidence can be
obtained by plotting activation curves in different Na_b (DiFrancesco, 1981b).
These data confirm the view that Na crosses the i_f channel. Fig. 8 shows the
fully-activated I/V relations for i_f obtained in different sodium concentrations
at K_b = 9 mM. The reversal potential is seen to shift negative when Na_b is
lowered,in accordance with the data of Fig. 6. It is interesting to note that
all the I/V relations display good linearity in a wide V-range and are remarkably parallel. This suggests that changing Na_b does not affect the channel conductance, but only alters the driving force for the current.

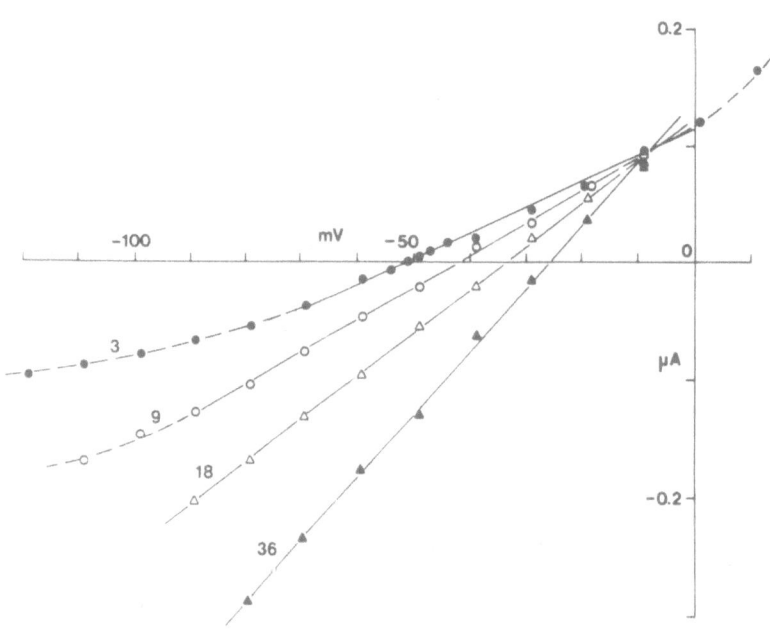

FIGURE 10 Fully-activated $i_f(E)$ relations in 3, 9, 18 and 36 mM K_b (Na_b =
35 mM). Same experiment as in Fig. 9. Slopes of least-squares fitting curves
are (from 3 to 36 mM K_b): 2.2, 2.8, 3.7 and 5.4 nA/mV. Note the increase in
slope conductance with K_b, and the tendency of all curves to meet at about
-10 mV. From DiFrancesco, 1981b.

EFFECT OF EXTERNAL POTASSIUM

The dependence of "i_{K2}" on K_b could be caused by a channel-activation mechanism and/or by the passage of K through the channel. The hypothesis that potassium ions cross the pacemaker channel is favoured by the evidence that the reversal potential is in any case too negative for the current to be carried by Na only (Figs. 6 and 8). In the experiment of Fig. 9 the current reversal was followed first on changing Na_b from 70 to 35 mM (A and B) and then on changing K_b from 9 to 36 and to 3 mM (B,C and D). E_f changes, in agreement with the results shown above, from -32 to -39 mV when Na_b is varied from 70 to 35 mM, and then moves to -26 and -49 mV when K_b is subsequently changed from 9 to 36 and 3 mM, as expected if potassium ions do flow through the channel. The reversal potential can be followed in a variety of different conditions, confirming the observation that both ions contribute to carrying i_f in Purkinje fibres (DiFrancesco, 1981b). In the experiment of Fig. 10 the fully-activated I/V relation has been obtained at different potassium concentrations (Na_b = 35 mM). Together with the expected negative shift of E_f when K_b is lowered, it is worth noting that the slope of the curve decreases with decreasing K_b, in contrast with what is observed in different sodium concentrations (Fig. 8). This suggests that changing K_b not only varies the driving force, but it also affects the channel conductance.

DISCUSSION

The "pacemaker" current in Purkinje fibres was one of the first current systems fully analyzed in the heart. Its outward nature in the pacemaker range of voltages, suggested by Weidmann's (1951) conductance measurements (Dudel and Trautwein, 1958), was confirmed with V-clamp experiments by Vassalle (1966). With the analysis of Noble and Tsien (1968) and Peper and Trautwein (1969), the ionic composition and kinetic properties of "i_{K2}", considered to be a pure K-current outward deactivating on hyperpolarization to below the threshold of about -50 mV, seemed well established. The inward rectification for the fully-activated I/V relation of "i_{K2}" (Noble and Tsien, 1968) did not appear to be a peculiar property, as other K-current systems, like the inward-rectifying channel in the skeletal muscle (Katz, 1949; Hodgkin and Horowitz, 1959) and the i_{K1} channel in the Purkinje fibre itself (Noble, 1965), were known to have similar properties. Nor did it look peculiar that a similar time-dependent system was absent from other parts of the heart (Trautwein, 1973), as natural pacemaker activity is not present in either the atrium or the ventricular muscle.

The reason for investigating the pacemaker mechanism first in the Purkinje fibre, rather in the SA node where pacemaker activity normally originates, was the technical difficulty of V-clamping nodal tissue. These difficulties have been overcome only recently, and the two-microelectrode technique first applied by Noma and Irisawa (1976a) is now being used routinely to yield V-clamp data from the SA node (Brown and DiFrancesco, 1980; Brown et al., this volume). The first V-clamp data reported on rabbit SA node did not seem to provide evidence supporting the existence of a "pacemaker" current similar to "i_{K2}" in the Purkinje fibre (Irisawa, 1978).

Pacemaker activity in the nodal tissue was attributed to the decay of an outward current (i_p in Noma and Irisawa, 1976b), whose characteristics were similar to those of the current i_x in Purkinje fibres (Noble and Tsien, 1969) rather than to those of "i_{K2}". Partly supporting this conclusion was the evidence that in comparison with Purkinje fibres, pacemaker activity had been reported to occur in the SA node in a more depolarized voltage range. More recently, however, it has become evident that action potentials as high as 80 mV can be normally recorded in some regions of the nodal tissue (Brown and DiFrancesco, 1980), and that the pacemaker depolarization can extend in these regions below -50 mV/-60 mV, where little or no i_x-type current is activated (current i_K, DiFrancesco et al., 1979). Furthermore, in the voltage range negative to -50 mV - i.e. in the same range as that in which "i_{K2}" is activated - a new current system, I_f, was found to be important (Brown et al., 1979a,b the problem of the relative magnitude of diffent currents during the pacemaker depolarization in SA node is treated elsewhere in this volume (Brown et al., 1981)). The importance of i_f in determining the pacing rate in SA node was confirmed by the finding that this current partly mediates the acceleratory effect induced by adrenaline as well as that of a temperature increase (Brown and DiFrancesco, 1980). In this i_f shows significant similarity to "i_{K2}". Further investigation of the properties of i_f in the SA node (DiFrancesco and Ojeda, 1980) confirmed the striking similarity between the two current systems, by showing that i_f depends on Na_b and is blocked by Cs like "i_{K2}". Despite this similarity, however, i_f could be shown to be an inward current activated by hyperpolarization in the pacemaker range, in apparent contrast with the seemingly well established properties of "i_{K2}".

The existance of two current systems in two different tissues with very similar properties and the same function, but of different ionic nature, was indeed a surprisingly odd situation, which required clarification. The need to re-investigate the properties of "i_{K2}" was also suggested by a second consideration. The presence of K-accumulation/depletion processes had been noticed in 1956 (Weidmann, 1956), and its importance in interfering with the time course of K-dependent currents in the cardiac muscle had since then been investigated extensively (Maughan, 1973; Kline and Morad, 1976; Noble, 1976; Baumgarten and Isenberg, 1977). DiFrancesco et al. (1979) showed in the Purkinje fibre that a K-depletion process taking place during high hyperpolarizations, such as those used to measure the "i_{K2}" reversal potential (E_{rev}), strongly distorts the current time course and affects the determination of E_{rev} itself. By shifting the K-equilibrium potential to more negative values during a hyperpolarizing V-clamp pulse, the K-depletion process gives rise to an apparently inward-decreasing "depletion" component due to i_{K1}. This component overlaps with "i_{K2}", which is itself modified by the K-depletion, and the whole process results in the appearence of a pseudo-current reversal at a potential where the gated component ("i_{K2}") is still - on the old interpretation - outward deactivating. These results were based on the assumption that "i_{K2}" is a pure K-current, but they apply equally well to a system where the pacemaker current is only partially carried by K (in which case the symbol "i_{K2}" would simply represent the K-component of the current). In other words, the possibility that the K-depletion occurring during V-clamp hyperpolarizations is so strong as to offset an inward activating pacemaker current, and produce a pseudo-current reversal near the expected E_K, could not be excluded.

The conductance measurements in normal Tyrode solution, and the results using low concentrations of Cs shown here (Figs 1 and 2) indicate that "i_{K2}" in Purkinje fibres behaves like an inward current activating on hyperpolarization to below -50/-60 mV, rather than, as in its conventional description, an outward current deactivating on hyperpolarization. It must be noted, however, that there are limits in the interpretation of these results. For example, membrane conductance measurements cannot be interpreted unambiguously. A conductance decrease with time was indeed observed by Vassalle (1966) during V-clamp applied at the MDP of a beating fibre, apparently supporting the hypothesis that the pacemaker depolarization is associated with the decay of an outward current. It is therefore important to establish if a conductance decrease with time during a hyperpolarization is also compatible with the assumption that "i_{K2}" is an inward current. Indeed it is possible to show by computer simulation that even on the "i_f" hypothesis, an apparent current reversal appears on hyperpolarization, when K-depletion is strong enough, and that the apparent reversal potential changes with K_b with an approximately -60 mV/decade slope Nernst dependence (DiFrancesco and Noble, 1980). The degree to which the current time course, and hence the time course of the membrane conductance, is affected by K-depletion is a function of the relative magnitude of i_f versus i_{K1}. Thus, it is not surprising that a conductance decrease can be observed on a hyperpolarization, if the contribution of K-depletion predominates over that of i_f. This problem is dealt with in more detail in an accompanying paper (DiFrancesco and Noble, this volume).

The validity of the "inward current" hypothesis is further verified by the use of barium which by blocking i_{K1} eliminates most of the K-depletion associated with hyperpolarizations, and therefore eliminates the main cause of distortion of "i_{K2}". In Ba-containing solutions no current reversal is seen below -50 mV even in high K_b (Fig. 3), which shows that the current cannot be carried by K only. This result also implies that the apparent reversal potential E_{rev} observed near E_K in normal conditions is an artifact caused by K-depletion. The i_f reversal potential lies in Purkinje fibres near -30 mV in normal Tyrode solution, which is close to the -25 mV found in the SA node (Yanagihara and Irisawa, 1980). E_f changes with Na_b and K_b in a way indicating that both ions contribute to carrying the current (Figs. 6 and 9).

In conclusion, one important consequence of the finding that the pacemaker current (i_f) in the Purkinje fibre is an inward current activated on hyperpolarization, is the identity between the pacemaker channels in Purkinje fibre and SA node. The fact that i_f is partly carried by sodium ions also provides a straightforward explanation for the otherwise unexplained dependence of "i_{K2}" on Na_b (McAllister and Noble, 1966).

The description given in 1968 by Noble and Tsien of the rectifying properties and the cross-over phenomenon for the fully-activated I/V relation of "i_{K2}"
is not applicable any more, as these properties are the result of distortion
from K-accumulation/depletion. The $\bar{i}_f(E)$ relations are linear over a wide voltage range (Figs. 8 and 10), and no cross-over is observed negative to -10 mV.
No regions of negative slope-conductance are detected. Outward going rectification is displayed by $\bar{i}_f(E)$ at low potassium concentrations and at negative potentials, but this could, however, be caused by the residual K-depletion associated with the i_f K-component in the presence of Ba.

It might be interesting to observe that in the records of Figs. 6, 7 and
9, the current time course during the largest depolarizations resembles that
usually attributed to the transient outward current i_{to}. Indeed, the use of envelope tests (Fig. 7) and the comparison between activation curves obtained at
different potentials (DiFrancesco, 1981b, Fig. 7) indicate that the largest
fraction of current observed on depolarizing in the region around 0 mV is i_f deactivating. Even if no experimental evidence on this problem is available at
present, the possibility that some of the current time course commonly atributed
to i_{to} is due to i_f deactivation is worth considering.

ACKNOWLEDGMENTS

I should like to thank Dr Hilary Brown for careful revision of the manuscript,
and the University of Milano and the C.N.R. for financial support. Part of the
data have been obtained with the assistance of D. Janigro.

REFERENCES

Almers, W.: Potassium conductance changes in skeletal muscle and the potassium
concentration in the transverse tubules. J. Physiol. (London), 225:

33-56, 1972.

Attwell, D.   and Cohen, I.:   The voltage clamp of multicellular preparations. Prog. Biophys. Mol. Biol., 31: 201-245, 1977.

Attwell, D., Eisner, D.A. and Cohen, I.: Voltage-clamp and tracer flux data: effects of a restricted extracellular space. Q. Rev. Biophys., 12: 213-261, 1980.

Baumgarten, C.M. and Isenberg, G.: Depletion and accumulation of potassium in the extracellular clefts of cardiac Purkinje fibres during voltage-clamp hyperpolarization and depolarization. Pfluegers Arch., 368: 19-31, 1977.

Brown, H.F. and DiFrancesco, D.: Voltage-clamp investigations of membrane currents underlying pacemaker activity in rabbit sino-atrial node. J. Physiol. (London), 308: 331-351, 1980.

Brown, H.F., DiFrancesco, D. and Noble, S.J.: How does adrenaline accelerate the heart? Nature, 280: 235-236, 1979a.

Brown, H.F., DiFrancesco, D. and Noble, S.J.: Cardiac pacemaker oscillation and its modulation by autonomic transmitters. J. Exp. Biol., 81: 175-204, 1979b.

Brown, H.F., Kimura, J. and Noble, S.J.: The relative contribution of various time-dependent membrane currents to pacemaker activity in the sino-atrial node. This volume, 1981.

Cohen, I., Daut, J. and Noble, D.: The effect of potassium and temperature on the pacemaker current i_{K2} in Purkinje fibres. J. Physiol. (London), 260: 55-74, 1976.

DiFrancesco, D.: The pacemaker current "i_{K2}" in Purkinje fibres is carried by sodium and potassium. J. Physiol. (London), 308: 32P, 1980.

DiFrancesco, D.: A new interpretation of the pacemaker current i_{K2} in Purkinje fibres. J. Physiol. (London), 314: 359-376, 1981a.

DiFrancesco, D: A study of the ionic nature of the pacemaker current in Purkinje fibres. J. Physiol. (London), 314: 377-393, 1981b.

DiFrancesco, D. and McNaughton, P.A.: The effect of calcium on outward membrane currents in the cardiac Purkinje fibre. J. Physiol. (London), 289: 347-373, 1979.

DiFrancesco, D. and Noble D.: Reconstruction of Purkinje fibre currents in sodium-free solution. J. Physiol. (London), 308: 35P, 1980.

DiFrancesco, D. and Noble, D.: Implications of the re-interpretation of i_{K2}

for the modelling of the electrical activity of pacemaker tissues in the heart. This volume, 1981.

DiFrancesco, D., Noma, A. and Trautwein, W.: Kinetics and magnitude of the time-dependent potassium current in the rabbit sino-atrial node. Pfluegers Arch., 381: 271-279, 1979.

DiFrancesco, D., Ohba, M. and Ojeda, C.: Measurement and significance of the reversal potential for the pacemaker current (i_{K2}) in sheep Purkinje fibres. J. Physiol. (London), 297: 135-162, 1979.

DiFrancesco, D. and Ojeda, C.: Properties of the current i_f in the sino-atrial node of the rabbit: a comparison with the current i_{K2} in Purkinje fibres. J. Physiol. (London), 308: 353-367, 1980.

Dudel, J. and Trautwein, W.: Der Mechanismus der automatischen rhythmische Impulsbildung der Herzmuskelfaser. Pfluegers Arch., 267: 553-565, 1958.

Hagiwara, S., Miyazaki, S., Moody, W. and Patlak, J.: Blocking effects of barium and hydrogen ions on the potassium current during anomalous rectification in the starfish egg. J. Physiol. (London), 279: 167-185, 1978.

Hauswirth, O., Noble, D. and Tsien, R.W.: Adrenaline: mechanism of action on the pacemaker potential in cardiac Purkinje fibres. Science, N.Y., 162: 916, 1968.

Hodgkin, A.L. and Horowicz, P.: The influence of potassium and chloride ions on the membrane potentials of single muscle fibres. J. Physiol. (London), 148: 127-160, 1959.

Irisawa, H.: Comparative physiology of the cardiac pacemaker. Physiol. Rev., 58: 461-498, 1978.

Isenberg, G.: Cardiac Purkinje fibres: Caesium as a tool to block inward rectifying potassium currents. Pfluegers Arch., 365: 99-106, 1976.

Johnson, E.A. and Lieberman, M.: Heart: excitation and contraction. Ann. Rev. Physiol., 33: 479-532, 1971.

Katz, B.: Les constantes electriques de la membrane du muscle. Archs. Sci. Physiol., 3: 285-300, 1949.

Kline, R. and Morad, M.: Potassium efflux and accumulation in heart muscle. Evidence from K^+ electrode experiments. Biophys. J., 16: 367-372, 1976.

Maughan, D.N.: Some effect of prolonged depolarization on membrane currents in bullfrog atrial muscle. J. Memb. Biol., 11: 331-352, 1973.

McAllister, R.E. and Noble, D.: The time and voltage dependence of the slow outward current in cardiac Purkinje fibres. J. Physiol. (London), 186: 632-662, 1966.

McGuigan, J.A.S.: Some limitations of the double sucrose gap and its use in a study of the slow outward current in mammalian ventricular muscle. J. Physiol. (London), 240: 775-806, 1974.

Noble, D.: Electrical properties of cardiac muscle attributable to inward-going (anomalous) rectification. J. Cell. Comp. Physiol., 66: 127-136, 1965.

Noble, D. and Tsien, R.W.: The kinetic and rectifier properties of the slow potassium current in cardiac Purkinje fibres. J. Physiol. (London), 195: 185-214, 1968.

Noble, D. and Tsien, R.W.: Outward membrane currents activated in the plateau range of potentials in cardiac Purkinje fibres. J. Physiol. (London), 200: 205-231, 1969.

Noble, S.J.: Potassium accumulation and depletion in frog atrial muscle. J. Physiol. (London), 258: 579-613, 1976.

Noma, A. and Irisawa, H.: Membrane currents in the rabbit sino-atrial node cell as studied by the double microelectrode method. Pfluegers Arch., 364: 45-52, 1976a.

Noma, A. and Irisawa, H.: A time- and voltage-dependent potassium current in the rabbit sino-atrial node cell. Pfluegers Arch., 366: 251-258, 1976b.

Noma, A., Yanagihara K., and Irisawa, H.: Inward current of the rabbit sino-atrial node cell. Pfluegers Arch., 372: 43-51, 1977.

Peper, K. and Trautwein, W.: A note on the pacemaker current in Purkinje fibres. Pfluegers Arch., 309: 356-361, 1969.

Standen, N.B. and Stanfield, P.R.: A potential- and time-dependent blockade of inward rectification in frog skeletal muscle fibres by barium and strontium ions. J. Physiol. (London), 280: 169-181, 1978.

Trautwein, W.: Membrane currents in cardiac muscle fibres. Physiol. Rev., 53: 793-835, 1973.

Vassalle, M.: Analysis of cardiac pacemaker potential using a voltage-clamp technique. Am. J. Physiol., 210: 1335-1341, 1966.

Weidmann, S.: Effect of the current flow on the membrane potential of cardiac muscle. J. Physiol. (London), 115: 227-236, 1951.

Weidmann, S.: Shortening of the cardiac action potential due to a brief injection of KCl following the onset of activity. J. Physiol. (London), 132:

157-163, 1956.

Yanagihara, K. and Irisawa, H.: Inward current activated during hyperpolarization in the rabbit sino-atrial node cell. Pfluegers Arch., 385: 11-19,
1980.

IMPLICATIONS OF THE RE-INTERPRETATION OF i_{K2} FOR THE MODELLING OF THE ELECTRICAL ACTIVITY OF PACEMAKER TISSUES IN THE HEART

Dario DiFrancesco and Denis Noble

INTRODUCTION

Other papers in this volume and elsewhere (Brown et al., 1979; Brown and Di-Francesco, 1980; DiFrancesco and Ojeda, 1980; Yanagihara and Irisawa, 1980) have already described the properties of an inward current, i_f (or i_h), that is slowly activated during hyperpolarization beyond about -50 mV in the SA node. In its time course, its voltage range for activation/deactivation and in its response to adrenaline, this current bears many resemblances to the s-mechanism described by Noble and Tsien (1968) as controlling an outward K^+ current, i_{K2}, in Purkinje fibres (DiFrancesco and Ojeda, 1980). As this resemblance became clear, so also did an obvious puzzle; the s-mechanism is described as activating on depolarization and controls an outward current. This produces the same overall current change as an inward current activated by hyperpolarization; but had nature really developed two systems for producing this current change in the heart by such different means? It seemed rather unlikely.

For some time, therefore, it has been evident that either i_f or i_{K2} might need reinterpretation. Earlier thinking was directed towards finding ways of reinterpreting the "new" current i_f in the SA node (could it not, for example, be an i_{K2} system whose reversal potential was distorted or masked by non-uniform properties of the tissue?) In the event, however, it has been the "old" current, i_{K2}, that has needed reinterpretation. One of us (DiFrancesco, 1981) has described in a previous paper in this volume the compelling experimental reasons for thinking that i_{K2} is in fact the same as the inward current in the SA node and that it is its "reversal potential" E_{rev}, that is misleading.

Our purpose in this paper is to explore the consequences of this reinterpretation for modelling of the electrical properties of pacemaking cells in the heart. The work reported here is part of a development towards constructing a unified model of pacemaker activity that, with only quantitative differences, may be applicable to all the pacemaker regions.

Before we describe the equations we have developed, it is worth recalling the electrical properties that any model must aim to reproduce. These may be divided into specific properties of "i_{K2}" and properties of the pacemaker potential itself.

LIST OF SYMBOLS

t	time	s
E	membrane potential	mV
E_{Na}, E_K	equilibrium potentials for Na$^+$ and K$^+$ ions	mV
K_i, K_c, K_b	internal, cleft and bulk K$^+$ concentrations	mM
F	Faraday's constant	96800 Coul g/ions
V	total cleft volume	μl
D	potassium diffusion constant	$\mu m^2 s^{-1}$
x	distance from fibre centre	μm
P	permeability constant for diffusion between clefts and bulk solution (3 compartment model only)	
C	membrane capacity	μF

Symbols for current (nA), fully-activated current (nA), kinetic variable, rate constants (s^{-1}), time constants (s) reversal potential (mV) respectively are indicated below for the various current components:

i_f, $\bar{I}_f$, y, α_y, β_y, τ_y, E_f "pacemaker" current (new interpretation)

i_{fNa}, $\bar{I}_{fNa}$, y, α_y, β_y, τ_y, E_{Na} sodium component of i_f

i_{fK}, $\bar{I}_{fK}$, y, α_y, β_y, τ_y, E_K potassium component of i_f

i_{K2}, $\bar{I}_{K2}$, s, α_s, β_s, τ_s, E_{rev} "pacemaker" current (old interpretation)

(note: $\alpha_s = \beta_y$, $\beta_s = \alpha_y$, $s = 1 - y$)

i_K (or i_x), $\bar{I}_K$, x, α_x, β_x, τ_x, E_K outward (delayed) current

i_{K1}^o	time-independent K^+ current
i_p	pump current
i_{Na}	fast (sodium) time-dependent current
i_{Ca}	slow (second inward) time-dependent current
i_{inb}	total inward background current
i_{mK}	total potassium current
i	total membrane current
$\beta(E,K_c)$	$= (d\bar{I}_f/dK_c)_{E,K_c}$
$\lambda(E,K_c)$	$= (d(i_{K1} + i_p)/dK_c)_{E,K_c}$

PROPERTIES OF "i_{K2}"

It must be admitted that there is some considerable surprise in the finding that i_{K2} needs reinterpretation for it was so apparently well-established as a highly-specific potassium current. The main experimental findings that gave rise to this view are:

1. On hyperpolarizing Purkinje fibres to different levels of potential, it is found that the total time-dependent current change reverses direction. In Tyrode solutions containing 4 mM K^+ this potential (E_{rev}) occurs in the range -100 to -110 mV (Vassalle, 1966; Noble and Tsien, 1968; Peper and Trautwein, 1969; Cohen et al., 1976a). This reversal is often, (see e.g. Cohen et al., 1976, Fig. 2), though not invariably, a "smooth" process that gives the impression of a single time-dependent mechanism. Even when this is not the case, it could be argued that any diphasic behaviour in the time course near E_{rev} is due to distortion by a process of K^+ depletion in the extracellular spaces (see e.g. DiFrancesco et al., 1979).

2. When the extracellular K^+ concentration is varied in the range 2-12 mM, E_{rev} shifts in the way expected for a K^+ electrode. The slope of the E_{rev} - log K_b relation is often near the expected value (60 mV/decade) for a highly selective

potassium system. This is one of the reasons for which the current was identified as a pure K^+ current. It is, though, worth noting that this interpretation
raised some problems. Although the slope of the Nernst relation (E_{rev} versus
log K_b) is correct, the absolute values of E_{rev} are not. They are invariably
too negative by about 10 mV. Cohen et al., (1976a) interpreted this to mean
that the extracellular cleft K^+ concentration (K_c) was always significantly
lower than the bulk concentration (K_b). This interpretation can be made
self-consistent (Cohen et al., 1979, Appendix) but only at the cost of making
a number of assumptions that are difficult to test experimentally. An alternative explanation is that, when the K^+ depletion that occurs during hyperpolarizations used to determine E_{rev} is taken into account, E_{rev} can be shown to be
more negative than E_K (DiFrancesco et al., 1979).

3. The fully-activated current-voltage relation, $\bar{I}_{K2}$ (see Noble and Tsien,
1968) displays the phenomenon of inward-rectification characteristic of K^+ currents in both skeletal and cardiac muscle. At potentials positive to about -70
mV the slope of the $\bar{I}_{K2}(E)$ relation is negative.

4. Also characteristic of K^+ rectification, the $\bar{I}_{K2}(E)$ curves at different values of K_b cross each other positive to E_K. In this they resemble the properties of i_{K1} (though not of the delayed K^+ rectifier, i_K (or i_x) - see discussion
in Brown et al., 1980).

5. During a hyperpolarizing pulse, the slope conductance, di/dE, is reported as
decreasing (Vassalle, 1966). More recently it has been observed to increase
(DiFrancesco, this volume) with time. Sometimes there is very little net change
in di/dE.

6. The current described as i_{K2} is absent in sodium-free solutions (McAllister
and Noble, 1966).

    At first sight it may seem rather unlikely that all of these properties
should be compatible with an inward current hypothesis. We shall, however, show
that they are indeed compatible with the new interpretation and that, in certain
respects, the new hypothesis provides less complex explanations than the old
one.

PROPERTIES OF THE PACEMAKER POTENTIAL

The relevant properties of the pacemaker potential are:

7. The slope conductance measured on applying small current deflections during the pacemaker depolarization decreases with time (Weidmann, 1951; 1956). This also was an important feature of the "i_{K2}" interpretation and must, clearly, be reproduced by any new model.

8. The pacemaker potential in Purkinje fibres is extremely sensitive to changes in extracellular K^+ concentration (Vassalle, 1965). While this property was not an essential feature of the "i_{K2}" model, it is of great interest to attempt to reproduce it with a new model that incorporates the effects of extracellular K^+ on the ionic currents involved in pacemaker activity.

9. Graded depolarizing and hyperpolarizing pulses have, respectively, strong negative and positive chronotropic effects on the subsequent pacemaker depolarization (Weidmann, 1951). This behaviour was extremely well reproduced by the McAllister, Noble and Tsien (1975) equations, based on the "i_{K2}" hypothesis.

DESCRIPTION OF EQUATIONS

We shall divide the description of the mathematical formulation of the model into two parts: the ionic current equations and the diffusion equations.

IONIC CURRENT EQUATIONS

In formulating the equations for ionic current we have used the McAllister et al. (1975) model where appropriate for all currents except for the new inward current, i_f. For K^+ sensitive currents such as i_{K1} and $i_K(i_x)$ we have also incorporated the modifications designed to reproduce the K^+ dependence introduced by Cohen et al. (1978) for i_{K1} and by Brown et al. (1980) for i_K. Instead of using current density units expressed per unit area of membrane, we have used absolute units of ionic current (in nA) scaled to give total currents similar to those recorded experimentally in a preparation of radius 125 μm and length 2 mm.

(a) THE INWARD CURRENT ACTIVATED ON HYPERPOLARIZATION

This current has so far been referred to either as i_f (Brown et al., 1979) or as i_h (Yanagihara and Irisawa, 1980). We will continue to use the symbol i_f but will use the activation variable, y, (see DiFrancesco, 1981) to avoid confusion with the inactivation variable f in the calcium current equations. Then

$$\frac{dy}{dt} = \alpha_y(E)\ (1 - y) - \beta_y(E)y \tag{1}$$

The equation for $\alpha_y(E)$ was that used by McAllister et al. (1975) for $\beta_s(E)$, while that for $\beta_y(E)$ was $\alpha_s(E)$. This gives an activation curve varying from zero at about -60 mV to 1 at about -90 mV. Clearly, $y(E,t) = 1 - s(E,t)$.

In some preliminary work (DiFrancesco and Noble, 1980) we used a simple linear function for $\bar{I}_f$ with a reversal potential set at 0 mV. Since then, it has become clear that i_f has both sodium and potassium components (DiFrancesco, 1980; 1981). It is not yet clear whether these components are independent, though it is known that a component reversing at E_K exists in completely sodium-free solutions (Hart et al., 1980). A similar result has been obtained for the rabbit SA node (Brown et al., 1980). For simplicity, therefore, we shall represent the components as separate. The sodium component is given by

$$\bar{I}_{fNa} = \bar{g}_{fNa}\ (E - E_{Na}) \tag{2}$$

where E_{Na} was usually set to +40 mV and $\bar{g}_{fNa}$ to 2 μs. To reproduce sodium-free conditions $\bar{g}_{fNa}$ was set to zero.

For the K^+ component we have used two alternative formulations. In the linear case:

$$\bar{I}_{fK} = \bar{g}_{fK}(K)\ (E - E_K) \tag{3}$$

Addition of (2) and (3) gives the total current $\bar{I}_f$:

$$\bar{i}_f = \bar{g}_{fNa} (E - E_{Na}) + \bar{g}_{fK} (Kc) (E - E_K) =$$

$$= (\bar{g}_{fNa} + \bar{g}_{fK}(K_c)) \left(E - \left(\frac{\bar{g}_{fNa}}{\bar{g}_{fNa} + \bar{g}_{fK}(K_c)} E_{Na} + \frac{\bar{g}_{fK}(K_c)}{\bar{g}_{fNa} + \bar{g}_{fK}(K_c)} E_K \right) \right) \qquad (4)$$

The experimental data from DiFrancesco (1981b) can be described in the general form:

$$\bar{i}_f = \bar{g}_f (K_c) (E - E_f) \qquad (5a)$$

where

$$E_f = r_{Na} (K_c) E_{Na} + r_K (K_c) E_K \qquad (5b)$$

The conditions under which the experimental data given by equations (5) can be described by equation (4) are deduced by comparing the two descriptions. In general, the sum of r_{Na} and r_K must be unity at any K_c and a certain relation (as deduced by equation (4)) must exist between the dependence of r_{Na} and r_K on K_c, and the dependence on K_c of the total conductance $\bar{g}_{fNa} + \bar{g}_{fK}$. Within limits the existing experimental data satisfy the above requirements.

We also sometimes used a non linear form for i_{fK}:

$$\bar{i}_{fK} = 2.6 (150 - K_c \exp (-E/25)) \qquad (3a)$$

This equation is based on that for $\bar{i}_K$ (see below). This gives a non-linear relation but the total current in the pacemaker range of potentials then shows more K^+ sensitivity than for most of the linear models. Where appropriate we have checked that our more important results do not depend on the precise formulation used for i_{fK}.

Figure 1 shows the relations generated by one of our linear formulations of i_f for $K_b = 2$ and 10 mM.

(b) THE TIME-INDEPENDENT K^+ CURRENT, i_{K1}

Our first computations were done using the modification of McAllister et al. (1975) equations for i_{K1} and i_{K2} proposed by Cohen et al. (1978). The purpose of this modification was to reproduce the known dependence of potassium current on extracellular potassium. The total time-independent K^+ current is given by

$$i_{K1}(E) = i^o_{K1}(E) + \bar{i}_{K2}(E)$$

where i^o_{K1} refers to the Cohen et al. (1978) function (see DiFrancesco, 1981a). The rationale for adding $\bar{i}_{K2}$ to i^o_{K1} is to ensure that the total value of K^+ current corresponding to the state $y = 0$ (no i_K activated) in the new model corresponds to the state $s = 1$ ($\bar{i}_{K2}$ fully activated in the old model). Clearly though, the component $\bar{i}_{K2}$ is no longer controlled by a gating variable and is therefore indistinguishable from the old i_{K1}. This formulation was satisfactory for many purposes but, in the course of developing the model we have found it desirable to take account of the effects of K^+ depletion and accumulation on the measured i_{K1} relations. We have found that a better reproduction of the steady-state current voltage relations under these circumstances is given by the following equation:

$$i_{K1} = 28 \, \exp(E_K/53) \left\{ \left(\frac{\exp (0.04 (E - E_K)) -1}{\exp (0.08 (E - (E_K + 50)))} \right) + \exp(0.04(E -(E_K + 50))) \right\} +$$

$$+ 0.016 \, (E - (E_K + 80))/(1 - \exp (-0.04 (E - (E_K + 80)))) \qquad (6)$$

This equation is plotted in Figure 1 for K^+ concentrations between 2 and 10 mM. It can be seen that it correctly reproduces the inward-rectification and the "cross-over" phenomenon seen experimentally.

(c) TIME-DEPENDENT (DELAYED) K^+ CURRENT

This component is also known to show inward rectification but with no negative slope conductance (Noble and Tsien, 1969) and no cross-over (DiFrancesco and McNaughton, 1979). Brown et al. (1980) used the equations derived from a rate-theory treatment (Noble, 1972) to give an equation of the form:

FIGURE 1 Top: Current-voltage relations for i_{K1} at various values of K_b
given by equation (6).
Bottom: Example of current-voltage relations for i_f at two values of K_b.
The value of g_{fK} in this example was
given by $(-2007E_K)$. We have also represented g_{fK} in some computations by the
term $\sqrt{K_c} \cdot^{fK}$ Both formulations give linear
$i(E)$ relations with g_{fK} increasing as
K_c is raised, as found experimentally.

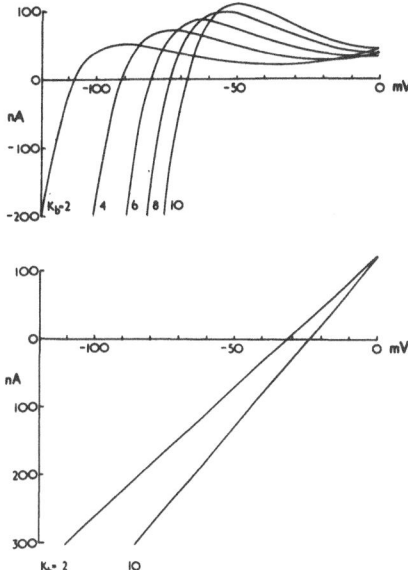

$$\bar{i}_K = 0.67\ (K_i - K_c\ \exp\ (-E/25)) \qquad\qquad (7)$$

where K_i was set to the value 150 mM. Note that we have followed McDonald and
Trautwein (1978), DiFrancesco et al. (1979) in using the symbol i_K for this
current. Noble and Tsien (1969) called it i_x. This notation was chosen to distinguish it from i_{K2} and, since its reversal potential is much less negative
than that for i_{K2}, it was thought to be a less specific channel.   The   new   interpretation of i_{K2} however, means that the real value of E_K without accumulation or depletion (about -90 mV at K_b = 4 mM) may not be as far from the   reversal potential of the delayed K^+ current as previously thought, particularly as
K^+ accumulation during the large depolarizing pulses used to activate i_K may
temporarily shift E_K to values less negative than -90 mV. It is now possible
therefore that i_K (i_x) may be a fairly specific K^+ current.

We shall continue to use McAllister, Noble and Tsien's equations for the activation variable, x, controlling i_K:

$$\frac{dx}{dt} = \alpha_x (1 - x) - \beta_x x \tag{8}$$

$$\alpha_x = 0.08 \exp ((E + 15)/20) \tag{9}$$

$$\beta_x = 0.08 \exp (1 - ((E + 15)/20) \tag{10}$$

(d) INWARD BACKGROUND CURRENT, i_{inb}

As in McAllister et al. (1975) this is represented as a linear function of voltage:

$$i_{inb} = 0.2 (E - 40) \tag{11}$$

(e) THE Na$^+$K$^+$ PUMP CURRENT, i_p

This current was not included in McAllister et al.'s equations (except implicitly as an indistinguishable element of the background current). Since we now wish to develop equations for the variation of extracellular K$^+$ concentration with time it is necessary to include the Na$^+$K$^+$ pump explicitly in the formulation and the current, i_p, that it carries will be represented by the equation

$$i_p = 0.01 K_c VF \tag{12}$$

where V = volume of extracellular space and F is the Farady constant. At $K_b = 4$ mM, and a space of 6.4 %, this gives a pump current of 25 nA. This is less than the maximum pump current estimated by Eisner and Lederer (1980), but, as they also note, the steady state current must be less than the peak current that is activated under optimal conditions.

Strictly speaking, the dependence of i_p on K_c should be non-linear, but this complexity is not yet required in the modelling. It would, though, be relatively easy to incorporate a non-linear relation if needed in future work.

(f) i_{Na} AND i_{Ca}

When required these were represented by the same equations as those used by McAllister et al. (1975). Since, in the present paper, we are concerned only with very slow voltage changes (or with constant voltages) we have simplified the equations by setting the kinetic variables m, h, d and f to their steady state values at each voltage. We intend to remove this restriction in future work.

DIFFUSION EQUATIONS

We shall assume that the extracellular cleft space is uniformly distributed in the preparation. In this case we may use the equation for diffusion in a cylinder to represent the movement of extracellular K^+ ions:

$$\frac{dK_c}{dt} = D\left(\frac{d^2K_c}{dx^2} + \frac{1}{x}\frac{dK_c}{dx}\right) + i_{mK}/FV \qquad (13)$$

where i_{mK} is the net K^+ ion current across the cell membrane. This will, in turn, be represented by the sum of the leak due to passive ionic current carried by K^+ and the active movements due to the Na-K exchange pump:

$$i_{mK} = i_{K1} + i_K + i_{fK} - 2\, i_p \qquad (14)$$

Here i_{fK} is the K^+ component of the inward current activated on hyperpolarization. The K^+ moved by the pump is equal to twice the pump current since we are assuming a 3:2 Na:K exchange. F is the Faraday and V is the extracellular space volume.

Equation (13) was solved numerically by using an inversion procedure for a band matrix of width three (see Fox, 1961). The value of D was chosen to be equal to the free solution value, i.e. 1600 $\mu^2 s^{-1}$, adjusted by a tortuosity factor of 1.6. This assumes that on average a K^+ ion sees a cylinder of 200 μ radius instead of 125 μ, and gives an "effective" value of D of 624 $\mu^2 s^{-1}$. We have checked in our computations that the precise value of D is not in fact very critical.

Various values of V were used to correspond to Purkinje fibres with differ-

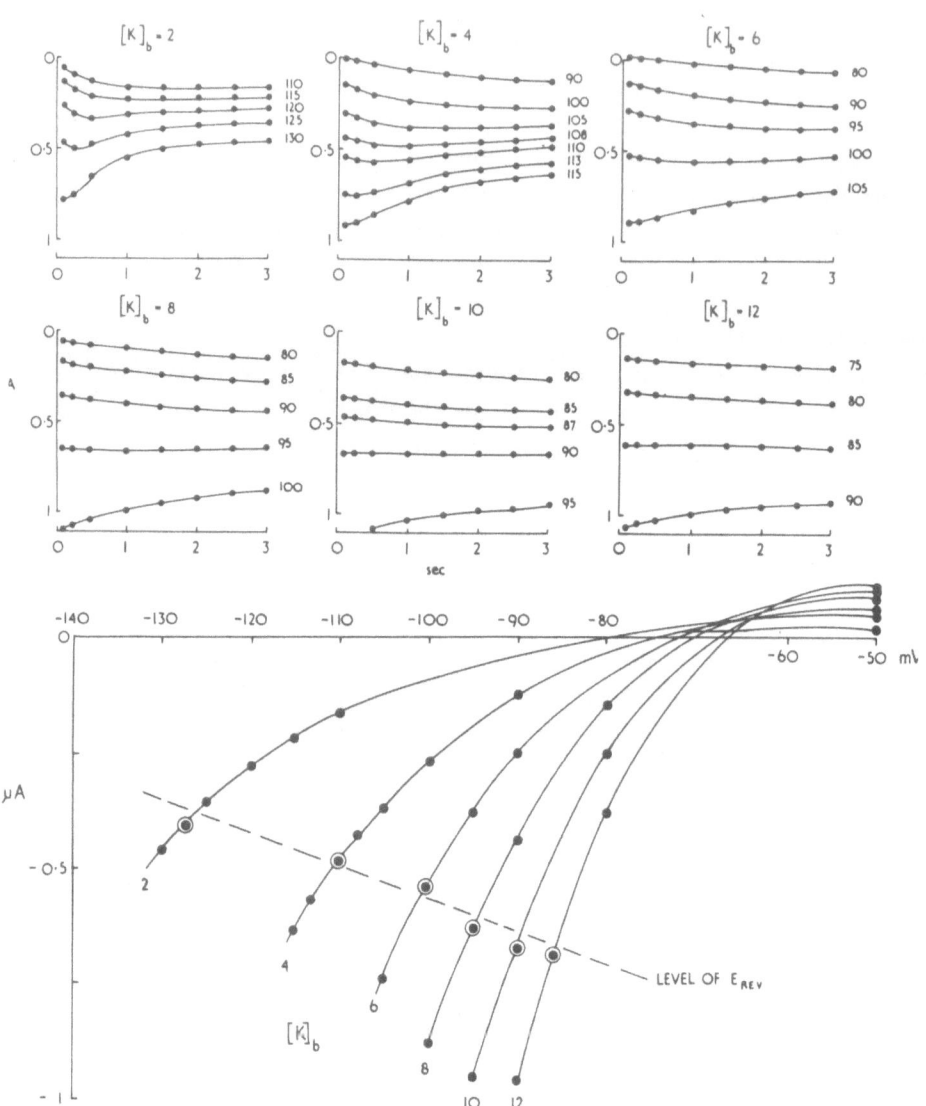

FIGURE 2 *Top: Ionic currents computed on hyperpolarizing to various potentials from -50 mV at various values of K_b. For these computations $\bar{g}_{fK}$ was made proportional to $\sqrt{K_c}$, which gives a good approximation to the K dependence of the total current carried by the i_f channels.*
Bottom: Corresponding steady state current voltage relations. The values for E_{rev} are indicated by ringed symbols.

ent extracellular spaces. For example, canine fibres are known to have a much larger extracellular space (about 30 %) than sheep fibres. In each case we shall indicate the value of V chosen as a percentage of the total fibre volume.

RESULTS AND DISCUSSION

(i) THE APPARENT "REVERSAL POTENTIAL" AND ITS NERNST-LIKE BEHAVIOUR

For these results we computed the total ionic currents in response to hyperpolarizations from -50 mV (where $y_\infty = 0$) to various potentials. The results, for various values of K_b, are shown in Figure 2A. It can be seen that at each value of K_b there is a potential at which the net time-dependent current changes direction. Thus, at $K_b = 4$ mM this potential is about -110 mV. At $K_b = 12$ mM, the reversal occurs at -85 mV. This change of 25 mV is close to the expected change for a Nernst potential (28.6 mV). In Figure 3A we have plotted the results for E_{rev} (●) and compared them with experimental results (□-Noble and Tsien, 1968; △-Peper and Trautwein, 1969; ⍫-Cohen et al., 1976; X - DiFrancesco et al., 1979). We have also plotted the results for resting potentials (▲) obtained by Gadsby and Cranefield, together with the line calculated for E_K from the equation

$$E_K = \frac{RT}{F} \ln \frac{K_b}{140} \tag{15}$$

where 140 mM has been taken as the likely value for K_i. Note that E_K is a good prediction of the resting potential in the range where this varies linearly with log K_b but that, in common with the experimental results, all the values of E_{rev} are significantly more negative than E_K.

Thus, the model reproduces the apparent K^+ specificity of the "reversal potential" very well indeed. Clearly, however, this "reversal" is not a genuine reversal of a single ionic current. We can show this by reproducing DiFrancesco's result using Ba^{++} ions to block i_{K1}. As shown in Fig. 5 (below),

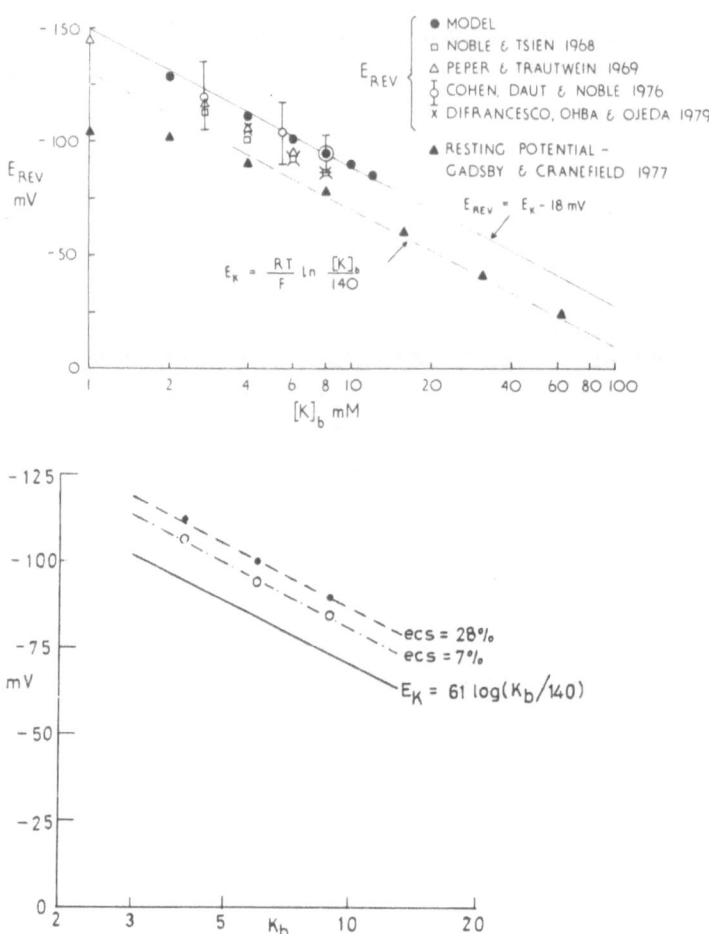

FIGURE 3 Top: ● values of E_{rev} obtained from results shown in Fig.   2.   Also
shown are experimental results of Noble and Tsien (1968) - □, Peper and
Trautwein (1969) - △, Cohen et al., (1976) - ⚵, DiFrancesco et al., (1979) - X,
filled triangles show resting potentials, measured by Gadsby and Cranefield.
The two straight lines are given by $E_K = (RT/F)\ln (K_b/140)$ and $E_{rev} = E_K - 18$
mV.
Bottom: Variation of E_{rev} with K_b for extracellular space volumes of 7 and 28
%. Notice that in both cases a good fit to a 60 mV/decade slope is obtained and
that increasing the space volume by this large factor (x 4) shifts the absolute
values of E_{rev} by only 6 mV. For these computations, equation (3a) was used for
i_{fk}.

once i_{K1} is reduced (in this case to 5 % of its normal value), there is no "reversal potential" at very negative potentials.

Is the apparent K^+ specificity of E_{rev} in the model a fortuitous result or is it expected? First of all, it is not fortuitous. We have found that it does not depend critically on the formulation of the equations for i_f. Thus, DiFrancesco and Noble (1980a) used a simple linear (non K^+ dependent) equation for i_f and obtained a very similar result to that shown here. We have also repeated the computations using a much larger value for V. Increasing V by a factor of 4 to give an extracellular space of about 30 % (which would correspond to the canine Purkinje fibre) shifts the absolute values of E_{rev} by about 6 mV but still gives a nearly linear variation with log K_b with a slope of about 60 mV per decade (DiFrancesco and Noble, 1980b) - see also Figure 3.

The result then is not fortuitous. Is it expected? The answer to this question is that, to a first approximation, the K^+ dependence of E_{rev} reflects the properties of i_{K1} more than of i_f and is not very sensitive to i_f. We can derive this result as follows. The total current change during a hyperpolarization from the holding potential E_H (in this case -50 mV) to E will depend on the changes in $\bar{i}_f$, y, i_{K1}, i_p and K_c. If, for simplicity, we represent the extracellular space by a single compartment we obtain the equations for a 3 compartment model:

$$\Delta i(E) = \bar{i}_f (E, K_c). \ \Delta y + \left(\frac{d(i_{K1} + i_p)}{dK_c}\right)_E \Delta K_c$$

$$= \bar{i}_f (E, K_c). \ \Delta y + \lambda(E) \Delta K_c \tag{16}$$

where $\Delta K_c = K_{c\infty} - K_{co}$ is the change in cleft potassium from its original value K_{co} and $y_\infty - y_0$ is the change in y. Equation (16) can be obtained by integrating equation (24) below on the assumption that $\beta/\lambda < 1$ (equation 26)).

The speed of change in K_c is then given by the continuity equation

$$\frac{dK_c}{dt} = \frac{1}{VF} \left(i_{K1} - 2 i_p + i_{fK} - FP (K_c - K_b) \right)$$

$$= \frac{1}{VF} \left(i_{K1} + i_p - 3 i_p + i_{fK} - FP (K_c - K_b) \right) \tag{17}$$

At potentials near E_{rev}, $i_{K1} + i_p$ is much larger than $-3 i_p$ and i_{fK}. We may therefore simplify (17) to give

$$\frac{dK_c}{dt} = \frac{1}{FV} \left(i_{K1} + i_p - FP (K_c - K_b) \right) \tag{17a}$$

Now, in the steady state, i.e. at $t = \infty$, $dK_c/dt = 0$ and we then have

$$i_{K1} + i_p = FP (K_c - K_b) \tag{18}$$

which simply states that the net K^+ current through the membrane must balance the net K^+ diffusion from the bulk solution. Equation (18) holds for any time t and for a first order approximation may also be written:

$$(i_{K1} + i_p) (E, K_{co}) + \lambda(E) \Delta K_c = FP \Delta K_c - FP(K_b - K_{co})$$

from which

$$\Delta K_c = \frac{(i_{K1} + i_p) (E, K_{co}) - FP (K_b - K_{co})}{FP - \lambda(E)} \tag{19}$$

We now make use of the fact that when the membrane is initially held at a potential (say -50 mV) at which $i_{K1} + i_p$ is small, the initial value of K_c, i.e. K_{co}, will be nearly the same as K_b, so that we may neglect the term $K_b - K_{co}$. We will also assume that over a range of potentials near E_{rev}, the voltage dependence of $i_{K1} + i_p$ is well approximated by a linear function, $i_{K1} + i_p = A(E - E_K)$, where A is a constant. Then (19) becomes

$$\Delta K_c = \frac{A (E - E_K)}{FP - \lambda (E)} \tag{20}$$

Let us now define the "reversal potential" E_{rev} as the potential at which $\Delta i = 0$. (This definition will be exact when the current change near E_{rev} is monotonic, but less so when the time course is diphasic (see DiFrancesco et al., 1979). Then, from (16):

$$\bar{I}_f (E_{rev}, K_c) \Delta y = - \lambda (E_{rev}) \Delta K_c \tag{21}$$

Combining (20) and (21) and rearranging we obtain:

$$E_{rev} = E_K + \frac{\bar{I}_f (E_{rev}, K_c) \Delta y (FP - \lambda(E_{rev}))}{-A \lambda (E_{rev})} \tag{22}$$

E_{rev} will therefore differ from E_k by the value of the expression including $\bar{I}_f$, Δy, P, λ and A. Of these, P, A and Δy may be assumed constant or nearly constant for the relevant voltage range.

Notice that, since $\bar{I}_f$ and λ are always negative, E_{rev} must always be negative to E_k, as observed experimentally. We will now use numerical values for the parameters in equation (22) to see how well it reproduces the computed results. If we consider the case for $K_b = 4$ mM, at which E_{rev} is -105 mV and $E_K = -90$ mV, the values we obtain from the computed results are as follows: $\Delta K_c = -0.8$ mM, $i_{K1} + i_p (t = 0) = -366$, $i_{K1} + i_p (t = \infty) = -140$, $\bar{I}_f = -247$ nA. From these figures we may also compute

FP = 175 nA/mM, $\lambda = -282$ nA/mM, A = 25 nA/mV. Then inserting in (22):

$$E_{rev} = E_K - 16.0 \text{ mV}$$

which, for $E_k = -90$, gives $E_{rev} = -106$ mV. Equation (22) is therefore a very close approximation indeed to the numerical results.

We now ask the question, how constant will be the difference $E_{rev} - E_K$? Clearly for an exact 61 mV/decade slope for E_{rev} plotted against log K_b, the difference needs to be constant. Equally clearly, however, the difference cannot be exactly constant since $\bar{I}_f$ and λ both depend on E and K_b. Of these two, by far the most important variation is in λ, i.e. $d(i_{K1} + i_p)/dK_c$, since, as K_c is increased its influence on $i_{K1} + i_p$ decreases (see Figure 1). By differentiating equation (6) for i_{K1} as a function of E_K we may show that di_{K1}/dE_k is almost constant in the relevant voltage range and, since dE_K/dK_c is proportional to $1/K_c$, λ must vary approximately as $1/K_c$. At 8 mM it will therefore be about half its value at 4 mM. With the same figures for the other parameters this would give a difference $E_{rev} - E_K$ of about -22 mV. This value will in fact overestimate the difference since $\bar{I}_f \Delta y$ decreases, particularly when the value of E_{rev} enters the range of voltages (positive to -90) at which $\Delta y \leftarrow 1$. Nevertheless, it is interesting to note that the deviation from a constant value is in the right direction. Moreover, as expected, a larger hyperpolarizing current is then required to reach E_{rev} at high K_b than at low K_b. This is shown in Figure 2 (bottom) which shows the position of E_{rev} on the steady state current-voltage relations computed at different values of K_b. It is worth comparing these results with those obtained experimentally by Cohen et al. (1976b), for, although these authors made the assumption for theoretical purposes that the current level at E_{rev} is constant, some of their experimental results actually show the same effect as we observe in the numerical model. Thus, in figure 2 of Cohen et al.'s paper, the value of current at E_{rev} becomes significantly more negative when K_b is increased to 8 mM.

In conclusion then:

1. E_{rev} will always be negative to E_K.

2. The difference $E_{rev} - E_K$ changes by only a few mV over the relevant range of K^+ concentrations.

3. Notice also that the difference must depend on Δy. This effect has already been described experimentally by DiFrancesco et al. (1979).

(ii)"INWARD RECTIFICATION" AND "CROSS-OVER"

Noble and Tsien (1968) described $\bar{I}_{K2}$ as a set of current-voltage relations at different values of K_b which show the phenomenon of inward-going rectification and which cross each other when the net current is outward.

The new current $\bar{I}_f$ is opposite in direction to $\bar{I}_{K2}$ in the pacemaker range, and it does not resemble $\bar{I}_{K2}$ even when this difference in direction of current flow is taken into account.

Nevertheless, the new model accounts for the same net current changes as did the old model so, even though $\bar{I}_{K2}$ and $\bar{I}_f$ do not show any simple correspondence, there must be some way of deriving relations between $\bar{I}_{K2}$ and corresponding current terms in the new model. This can be done by taking account of current changes due to i_{K1} as well as those due to i_f.

In the new interpretation the current recorded on hyperpolarizing from the holding potential E_H to a potential E is

$$i(E, K_c, t) = i_f (E, K_c, t) + i_{K1} (E, K_c) + i_p(K_c) + i_{inb}(E) \qquad (23)$$

Differentiating with respect to time gives:

$$\frac{di}{dt} = \bar{I}_f \frac{dy}{dt} + \lambda \frac{dK_c}{dt} + \beta\, y \frac{dK_c}{dt} \qquad (24)$$

where $\bar{I}_f$ is the initial value of this parameter, β is $(d\,\bar{I}_f/dK_c)$ and λ, as before, is $d(i_{K1} + i_p)/dK_c$. We will assume that these parameters are independent of K_c (i.e. they depend on voltage only). Then the total current change during the hyperpolarization can be obtained by integrating (24):

$$\Delta i\,(E) = \int_0^\infty \frac{di}{dt}\, dt = \bar{I}_f\, \Delta y + \lambda\, \Delta K_c + \beta \int_0^\infty y \frac{dK_c}{dt}\, dt \qquad (25)$$

In the APPENDIX we shall give a fuller treatment of this equation. Here we will note that β is usually small compared to λ so that the final term can be neglected in a first approximation. Then

$$\Delta i(E) = \bar{I}_f (E) \Delta y + \lambda (E) \Delta K_c \qquad (26)$$

In the old model the same current change was described as

$$\Delta i(E) = \bar{I}_{K2} (E) \Delta s \qquad (27)$$

Since $\Delta y = -\Delta s$, it is clear that

$$-\bar{I}_{K2}(E) = \bar{I}_f(E) \Delta y + \lambda \Delta K_c/\Delta y \qquad (28)$$

and, in particular, for values of E such that $\Delta y = 1$ (full activation)

$$-\bar{I}_{K2}(E) = \bar{I}_f(E) + \lambda \Delta K_c \qquad (28a)$$

This "dissection" of $\bar{I}_{K2}$ into two components is illustrated in Figure 4A. Notice that the negative slope region of $\bar{I}_{K2}$ is generated by the fact that when ΔK_c is small (positive to -90 mV) $\bar{I}_{K2}$ is simply $-\bar{I}_f$. When ΔK_c is large, $\bar{I}_{K2}$ is dominated by $\Delta(i_{K1} + i_p)$ (i.e. $\lambda \Delta K_c$). We have also shown (in the points indicated by x) the effect of depletion on i_f, which corresponds to the third term in equation (26). It can be seen that the deviation of $\bar{I}_f$ from its value for $\beta = 0$ is indeed quite small, (though this effect can be seen in some of the experimental results (DiFrancesco, 1981b).

In figure 4B we have illustrated the result of increasing the extracellular K^+ concentration. This has two effects:
1. At each potential $\bar{I}_f$ is increased in magnitude (cf. Figure 1).
2. The voltage range at which Δi_{K1} becomes significant is shifted in a positive direction. This is because i_{K1} becomes large and negative at a less negative range of potentials (see Fig. 1).

Clearly the total current will display a "cross-over" at about -85 mV. Thus the "negative slope" and the "cross-over" are necessary consequences of considering as one current alone the superimposition of the inward component i_f and the effects of K^+ depletion on i_{K1} during strong hyperpolarizations, even if neither of these characteristics feature as properties of $\bar{I}_f$.

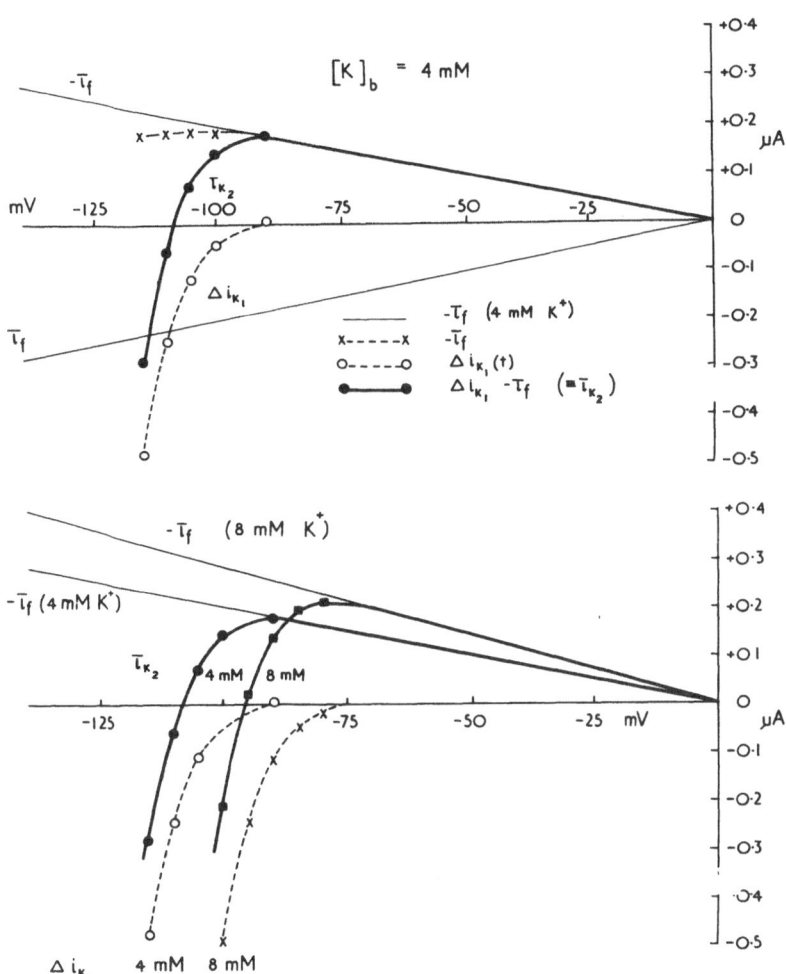

FIGURE 4 Top: *Diagram showing how* $\bar{i}_{K2}$ *is generated by new model as the alge-braic sum of* $-i_f$ *and* $\Delta(i_{K1} + i_p)$. *We have also shown the small effect of de-pletion on* i_f *(xxx). This corresponds to the last term in equation (25) and can for most purposes be neglected.*
Bottom: Effect of increasing K_b. *For strong depolarizations, where* $\bar{i}_f$ *domi-nates the total current,* $\bar{i}_{K2}$ *is increased. At more negative potentials where* $\Delta(i_{K1} + i_p)$ *dominates, the opposite effect occurs. This generates the "cross-over" phenomenon observed experimentally (Noble and Tsien, 1968). In both diagrams the very small values of* Δi_{K1}, *when this term is positive have been neglected.*

(iii) SLOPE CONDUCTANCE MEASUREMENTS

When small voltage steps (δE) are applied the membrane current will change. The current displacement (δi (E, t)) is given by

$$\delta i \ (E, \ t) = \delta (i_{K1} + i_p) + \delta i_f + \delta i_{inb}$$

$$= \left(\frac{d(i_{K1} + i_p)}{dE}\right)_{E,t} \delta E + y(E, \ t)\left(\frac{di_f}{dE}\right) \delta E + \left(\frac{di_{inb}}{dE}\right) \delta E$$

The conductance ($\delta i/\delta E$) measured in this way is given by

$$\frac{\delta i}{\delta E}(E, \ t) = \lambda(E, \ t) + y(E, \ t) \ \beta(E) + g_{inb} \ (E) \tag{29}$$

It is worth noting that in equation (29) the restriction on the dependence of λ on K_c has been removed and λ is considered to be changing even during the relatively small K_c changes occurring during hyperpolarization. As we shall show below, the decrease in λ with time is of crucial importance since, while λ is decreasing, y increases with time. Clearly the net result will depend on the relative magnitudes of these two time-dependent changes in conductance.

In Figure 5 we show the result of applying repetitive 5 mV hyperpolarizations in the numerical model during clamp pulses to various voltages. Notice that at -95, -100 and -105 mV the slope conductance decreases as a function of time. At -95 mV the change in g is about 10 %. At -100 mV it is 23 % and at -105 mV it becomes 33 %. Vassalle (1966) reported approximately a 20 % decrease during a voltage clamp applied at the level of the maximum diastolic potential. Clearly, this result is not inconsistent with the new model.

When i_{K1} is made very small (reduced to 5 %) to reproduce the effect of Ba^{++}, the conductance increases with time, as shown experimentally by DiFrancesco (1981b).

It should be noted that, although the model can reproduce Vassalle's (1966) result, this result is not the only one expected. If i_{K1} is reduced (though not necessarily as much as in the presence of barium), or if a larger extracellular

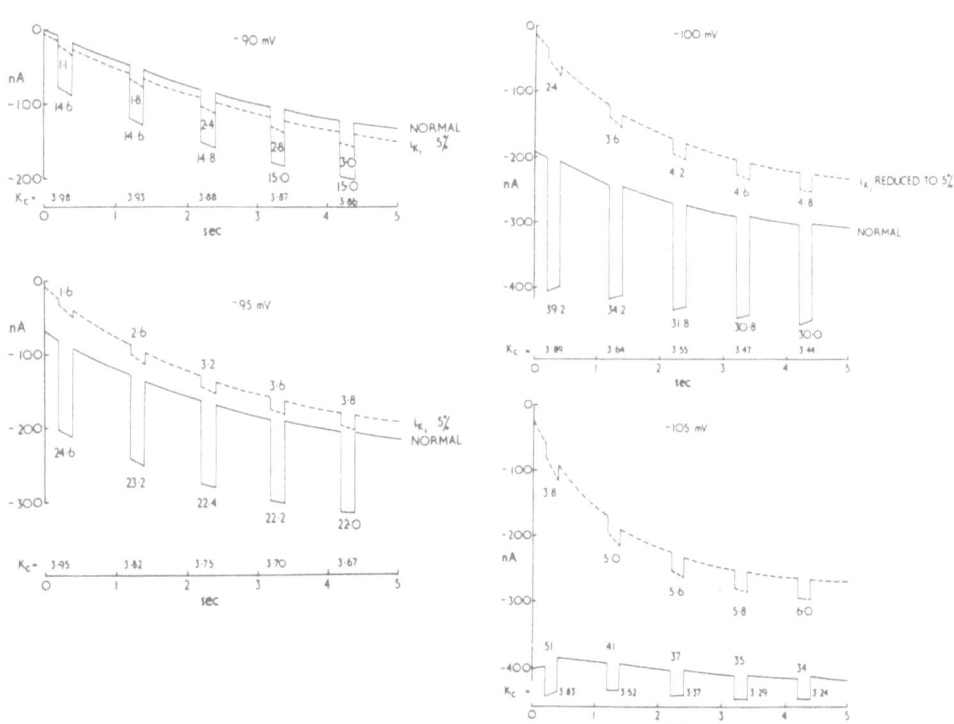

FIGURE 5 *Reconstruction of Vassalle's (1966) slope conductance measurements. For these calculations we set K_b = 4 mM and the extracellular space was 7 %. The membrane was hyperpolarized from -50 mV to the voltages shown. 5 mV test pulses were then applied (1 mV in the case of the pulse in normal solution to -105 mV). The figures on each test pulse are the value of slope conductance in µS. At -90 mV there is almost no net change in g. At all other voltages the slope conductance decreases as a function of time. When i_{K1} is reduced to 5 % of its normal value (to reproduce the effect of barium) large increases in slope conductance occur at each voltage and the net current no longer displays a reversal at -105 mV. The figures at the bottom of each graph show the mean value of the cleft K concentration, K_c, at the time of each test pulse. Notice that the slope in normal solution can be dominated by the properties of i_{K1} (and the effects of changes in K_c on its slope conductance) even though the total current change is dominated by i_f. The reason for this is that, in general for this range of voltages, di_{K1}/dE is much larger than di_f/dE - see figure 1. (Note also that the slope conductance values given here are the mean values obtained by calculating the current jumps at the "on" and "off" of each pulse after correcting for the change in net current with time. This calculation was performed automatically by the computer programme from the formula $\delta i = (i_{t+\delta t} - i_t) - (i_t - i_{t-\delta t})$ where t is the time of onset of the voltage change and δt is the integration step length).*

space is used, or if a function for i_f is chosen for which $d\bar{I}_f/dE$ is larger, the balance can be shifted in favour of the second term in equation (29). We then obtain a small increase in conductance with time even in normal conditions. This is the result reported by DiFrancesco (this volume). It is important to note that while Vassalle's (1966) results are consistent with both old and new models, DiFrancesco's results in both normal and barium solutions cannot be reproduced by the old i_{K2} explanation except in the range of voltages where the negative slope characteristic is found.

(iv) SODIUM-FREE SOLUTIONS

The "sodium-dependence" of "i_{K2}" has always been a puzzle. Since, in the new theory, a major part of i_f is carried by sodium ions it is to be expected that a large change will occur in sodium-free solutions. The existence of a K^+ component in i_f may nevertheless seem to pose a problem. It is therefore important to check on the effect of removing the sodium component alone on the total ionic current. This has been done in the calculations shown in Figure 6. Here we have chosen to use the large extracellular space of 30% to correspond to the situation found in canine Purkinje fibres.

As can be seen, the effect of removing the Na^+ component of i_f is the apparently complete disappearance of "i_{K2}", even though a large K^+ component of i_f is still present. The reason for this result is that the K^+ component of i_f is large and negative only in the range of voltages (negative to about 10 mV from E_K) over which i_{K1} is also large and negative. Hence, as i_f grows on applying stronger hyperpolarizations, so does i_{K1} and this generates sufficient Δi_{K1} to mask i_f. Only when i_{K1} is reduced, by applying Ba^{++}, is it possible to record the K^+ component of i_f in completely sodium-free solutions (Hart et al., 1980). In this connection it is interesting to note that, even in normal Na^+ containing Tyrode solution, results like those in Na-free solution occasionally occur, i.e. there appears to be no "i_{K2}". Exposure of such preparations to Ba^{++} then reveals that i_f is nevertheless present (Hart, Noble and Shimoni, unpublished). It is likely therefore that in such preparations, either the Na component of i_f is already relatively weak or the magnitude of i_{K1} is sufficient to generate a depletion component, i_{K1}, that masks i_f even in normal solutions.

One consequence of the explanation for results in Na^+-free solutions given here is that the time-dependent current change obtained cannot be attributed un-

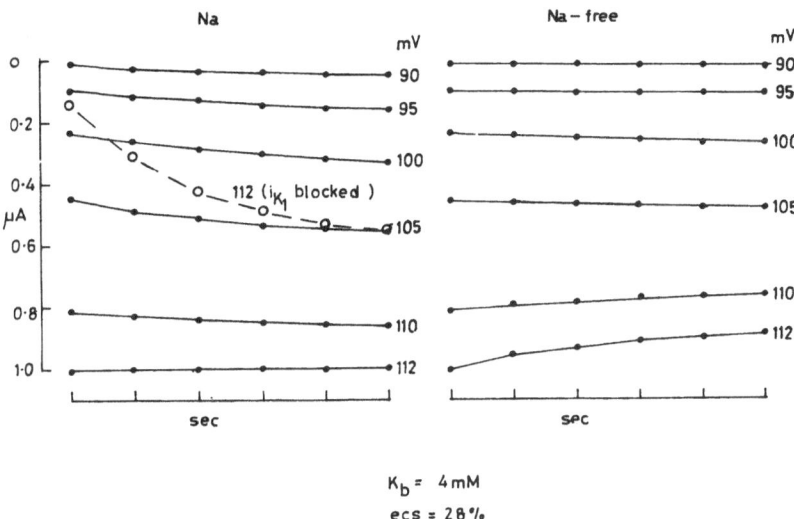

$K_b = 4\,mM$

$ecs = 28\%$

FIGURE 6 *Example of reconstruction of the effect of sodium-free solution on net ionic currents.*
Left: The net ionic current shows a reversal at -112 mV. At this voltage, the change in i_f is shown by the interrupted line (i_{K_1} blocked). The K component of i_f was represented by equation (3a). The extracellular space was set to 28 %. Right: After removing i_{fNa}, the current records are almost flat at potentials between -90 and -105 mV. At -112 mV the current change is now reversed and appears to represent a simple depletion process. In fact, a substantial current change due to i_{fK} is still present.
We have carried out a number of such computations for various formulations of i_f and for various values of K_b (for K_b = 6 mM see DiFrancesco and Noble, 1980b) and extracellular space. The precise quantitative results depend on the equations and conditions used, but in all cases the apparent disappearance of "i_{K2}" in Na-free solutions is well reproduced. The reason is that, at potentials close to E_K, i_{fK} is too small to be evident (it reverses at E_K) and at more negative potentials it is always effectively masked by the effect of depletion on i_{K1}. The result is therefore a necessary one given the known voltage and K^+ dependence of i_{K1} and of i_{fK}.

iquely to K^+ depletion.

(v) THE SLOPE CONDUCTANCE DURING THE PACEMAKER POTENTIAL

Weidmann's (1951) experiment showing that the voltage change produced by applying small current pulses increases during the pacemaker depolarization in Purkinje fibres has been of seminal importance in the study of pacemaker mechanisms.

The simplest interpretation of the result is that a time-dependent decay of, e.g., K^+ conductance is responsible for pacemaker activity. It has, however, also been clear since the discovery of inward-going rectification that the decrease in conductance recorded in Weidmann's experiment might also (or entirely) be a consequence of the depolarization rather than its cause (see Hutter and Noble, 1960). The relation between slope conductance and total ionic conductance is in fact quite complex (Noble and Tsien, 1972) and it has already been shown that the slope conductance change during the plateau of the cardiac action potential may not reflect the total conductance change.

It is clearly very important to check whether the new model can reproduce Weidmann's result in the pacemaker range of potentials. It might be thought that we have already done this in principle in our reconstruction of Vassalle's result (see Figure 5). However, this is by no means the case. Thus, at -90 mV we found that $\delta i/\delta E$ is almost constant. At -85 mV it in fact slightly increased (not shown in figure 5). It is, however, important to note that in these calculations the voltage level at which the conductance is measured is constant (apart from the small voltage step used to make the measurement). No voltage-dependent conductance changes were therefore involved.

To reproduce Weidmann's result we have let the voltage change spontaneously by using the equation:

$$\frac{dE}{dt} = \frac{-\Sigma i_i}{C} \tag{30}$$

where Σi_i was set equal to the sum of all ionic currents calculated at every point in the preparation. The capacitance, C, was set to 0.05 µF, which is a typical value obtained for Purkinje fibre preparations of the size we have assumed. As explained in an earlier part of the paper, the sodium and calcium currents were set equal to their steady state values at each potential. This means that the calculation is restricted for all practical purposes to the slow pacemaker depolarization.

Figure 7 shows one of our results. The initial conditions were chosen to correspond to the end of an action potential: E = -90 mV, y = 0. Since the model was quiescent at this value of K_b, we shifted the y curve in the depolar-

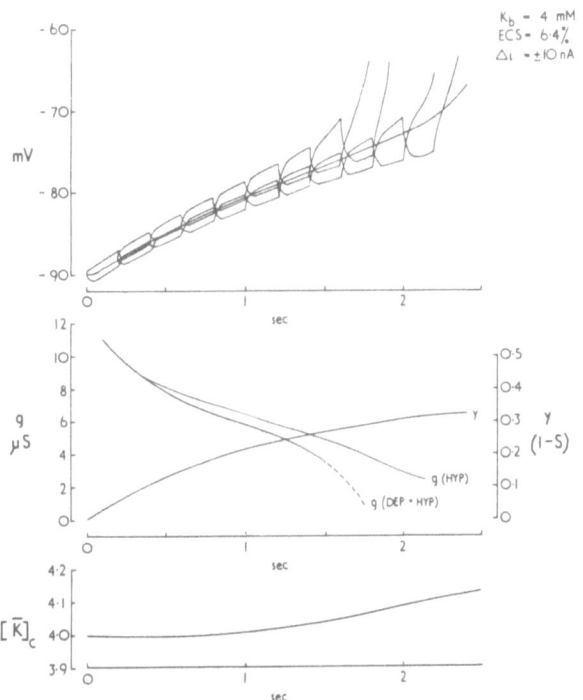

FIGURE 7 *Reconstruction of Weidmann's (1951) measurement of slope conductance during the pacemaker potential in Purkinje fibres.*
Top: pacemaker depolarization with and without ± 10 nA repetitive current pulses. Note that voltage deflection increases with time.
Middle: variation in calculated slope conductance with time and of activation, y, of i_f with time. The slope conductance was calculated either for depolarizing and hyperpolarizing pulses combined (g DEP + HYP) or for hyperpolarizing pulses only (g(HYP)). Note that g varies in the opposite direction to y. The slope conductance is therefore dominated by the voltage-dependent decrease in i_{K1} slope conductance, not by the time-dependent increase in g_f.
Bottom: Variation in mean value of K_c with time. There is a small (0.12 mM) increase in K_c. This would slightly increase g for i_{K1}. It is not therefore responsible for the decrease in g with time. This means that the explanations for Weidmann's g measurements and those of Vassalle (see figure 5) are quite different.

izing direction by 5 mV. This produced the pacemaker potential shown in the diagram. We then repeated the calculation with small (10 nA) repetitive current
pulses added to Σi_i. The slope conductance was calculated either as the mean
value of $\delta i/\delta E$ for both hyperpolarizing and depolarizing pulses or as the value
for hyperpolarizing pulses alone. In both cases a very substantial decrease in
$\delta i/\delta E$ was obtained, as observed by Weidmann.

Note, however, that this result cannot be due to changes in K_c. First of
all, the change in the mean value of K_c was very small (only 0.1 mM). Secondly,
the change in K_c is in the wrong direction: it slightly increases during the
later part of the pacemaker depolarization which by itself would increase the
slope conductance.

The decrease in conductance computed here is in fact produced by the effect
of voltage on i_{K_1}. It is therefore a consequence of the pacemaker depolarization, not its primary cause.

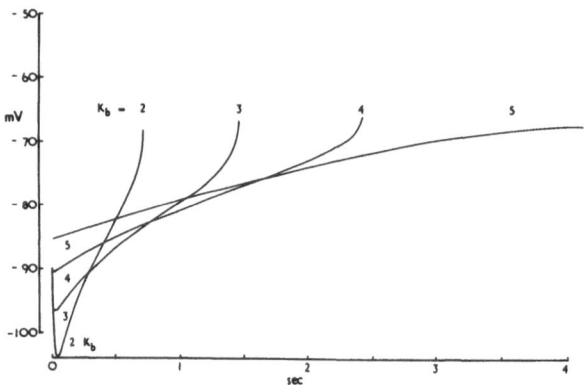

FIGURE 8 *Pacemaker depolarizations computed at various values of K_b between 2
and 5 mM. At 5 mM the "fibre" becomes quiescent. As in Vassalle's (1965) experimental results, the maximum diastolic potential becomes more negative and
the slope of the pacemaker potential greatly increases as K_b is reduced. For
these computations the voltage dependence of y was shifted by 10 mV in a positive direction. Without this shift, the "fibre" is also quiescent at $K_b = 4$ mM.*

(vi) INFLUENCE OF EXTRACELLULAR K⁺ ON PACEMAKER ACTIVITY

In 1965 Vassalle described some important experiments designed to clarify the
extreme sensitivity of pacemaker activity in Purkinje fibres to the level of the

extracellular K^+ concentration. Having constructed a model which, for the first time, takes account of the effects of K^+ on ionic currents and of the extracellular space it seemed possible that we should be able to reproduce Vassalle's results. This is indeed the case, as Figure 8 shows. We computed the pacemaker depolarization in our model for values of K_b = 2, 3, 4, 5, 6 and 8 mM. It can be seen that high K_b suppresses pacemaker activity and that at low K_b the maximum diastolic potential becomes more negative while the slope of the pacemaker depolarization greatly increases. These computations reproduce all the main features of Vassalle's experimental results.

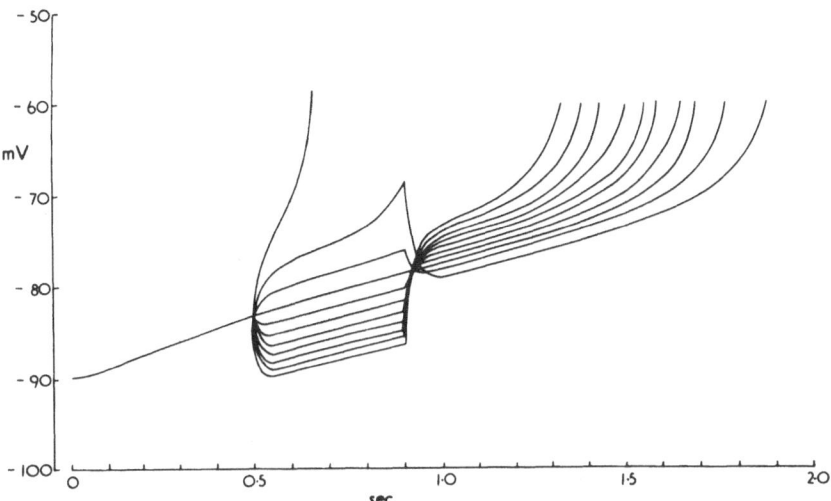

FIGURE 9 *Reconstruction of Weidmann's (1951) experiment showing effect of short hyperpolarizing and depolarizing current pulses applied at about the middle of the pacemaker depolarization. The current used were: depolarizing: 10,   20, and 30 nA.*
hyperpolarizing: 10, 20, 30, 40, 50, 60, 70 nA
Weidmann's result is well reproduced by the new model, just as it was reproduced by McAllister, Noble and Tsien's (1975) equations.

(vii) INFLUENCE OF GRADED CURRENT PULSES

In Figure 9 we show the results of calculations designed to reproduce Weidmann's experiment using positive and negative current pulses of varying amplitude applied at about the middle of the pacemaker depolarization. As in Weidmann's experiment hyperpolarizations are followed by accelerated depolarization and more rapid firing, whereas depolarizations (unless they induce firing themselves) are followed by a less rapid approach to threshold. This result was also well reproduced by the McAllister, Noble and Tsien equations. Clearly, the new interpretation of i_{K2} does not influence this result. The reason is that the result depends only on the fact that the activation curve for the current controlling the rate of depolarization varies steeply in the pacemaker range. A less dramatic result, or even the opposite result, would be obtained if the time-dependent current involved had its activation curve outside the pacemaker range.

CONCLUSIONS

The computations we have described in this paper show that all the major features of the ionic currents in Purkinje fibres that led so apparently conclusively to the "i_{K2}" interpretation receive full and natural explanations with the new "i_f" interpretation. In some respects the new interpretation offers less complex explanations, as, for example, for the behaviour of the ionic current in sodium-free solution (for which the "i_{K2}" hypothesis offered no explanation) and the relatively negative level of E_{rev} (for which the "i_{K2}" hypothesis required more complex explanations - see Cohen et al., 1979; Appendix, and DiFrancesco et al., 1979).

This conclusion is both reassuring and disturbing. It is reassuring inasmuch as it is no longer necessary to suppose that the different pacemaker regions possess fundamentally different ionic current mechanisms. Yet it is also disturbing. For all the standard criteria for a pure K^+ current in the heart had been so fully satisfied that, without the uneasy analogy with the SA node and, even more, the striking and unexpected results of blocking i_{K1} with barium, no-one would have seen any reason to replace i_{K2} with a simple, non-specific linear conductance that carries current in the opposite direction.

Any lessons here for the philosophy of science? Perhaps; and if so, they are fairly obvious: the troughs and peaks are not so very far apart -

*Ara vos prec, per aquela valor

Que vos guida al som de l'escalina:

Sovenhatz vos a temps de ma dolor!

(Dante, Divina Commedia, Purgatorio,

end of song XXVI)

APPENDIX

Equation (25) may be further treated by noting that the integral

$$\int_0^\infty y \frac{dK_c}{dt} \, dt$$

can be obtained as follows.   In general

$$y(E, t) = (y_0 - y_\infty) \exp (-t/\tau_f) + y_\infty$$

or, if $y_0 = 0$

$$y(E, t) = y_\infty(1 - \exp (-t/\tau_f)) \tag{A1}$$

Hence

*Now, preie you, by that power whiche not in vayn

up this high montaigne-staire hath lad you sure,

bethynke you in due sesoun of my payne!

(Translation into archaic English of Dante's Occitan)

$$\int_0^\infty y \, \frac{dK_C}{dt} \, dt = y_\infty \int_0^\infty \frac{dK_C}{dt} \, dt - y_\infty \int_0^\infty \exp(-y/\tau_f) \, \frac{dK_C}{dt} \, dt \qquad (A2)$$

Now,

$$\int_0^\infty e^{-pt} \frac{dK_C}{dt} \, dt$$

is, by definition, the Laplace transform of dK_C/dt and

$$\int_0^\infty e^{-pt} \frac{dK_C}{dt} \, dt = \mathcal{L} \left\{ \frac{dK_C}{dt} \right\} = -K_{CO} + p\bar{K}_C(p)$$

where $\bar{K}_C(p)$ is the Laplace transform of $K_C(t)$.
Therefore

$$\int_0^\infty e^{-t/\tau_f} \frac{dK_C}{dt} \, dt = -K_{CO} + \frac{1}{\tau_f} \bar{K}_C \left(\frac{1}{\tau_f} \right) \qquad (A3)$$

Suppose the decay of K is exponential, then

$$K_C(t) = (K_{CO} - K_{C\infty}) \exp(-t/\tau_K) + K_{C\infty}$$

and

$$\bar{K}_C(p) = \frac{K_{C\infty}}{p} + \frac{K_O - K_{C\infty}}{p + 1/\tau_K}$$

which leads to

$$\int_0^\infty e^{-t/\tau_f} \frac{dK_c}{dt} \, dt = -K_{co} + \frac{1}{\tau_f} \left(\tau_f K_{c\infty} + \frac{K_{co} - K_{c\infty}}{(1/\tau_f + 1/\tau_k)} \right)$$

$$= -K_{co} + K_{c\infty} + (K_{co} - K_{c\infty}) \frac{1/\tau_f}{(1/\tau_f + 1/\tau_k)}$$

$$= \Delta K_c - \Delta K_c \left(\frac{1/\tau_f}{(1/\tau_f + 1/\tau_K)} \right) \tag{A4}$$

So, from (A2)

$$\int_0^\infty y \frac{dK_c}{dt} \, dt = y_\infty \Delta K_c \left(\frac{1/\tau_f}{1/\tau_f + 1/\tau_K} \right) \tag{A5}$$

In the limiting case when $y_\infty = 1$ (i_f fully activated by strong hyperpolarization) and τ_f if short compared to τ_K, this expression simplifies to ΔK_c. For all other cases it will be less than ΔK_c.

ACKNOWLEDGEMENTS

We are grateful to the Medical Research Council and the British Heart Foundation for financial support. We are also indebted to the Wellcome Trust for providing funds to enable one of us (D.D.) to visit Oxford to complete this work.

REFERENCES

Brown, H.F. and DiFrancesco, D.: Voltage clamp investigations of membrane currents underlying pacemaker activity in rabbit sino-atrial node. J. Physiol. (London), 308: 331-351, 1980.

Brown, H.F., DiFrancesco, D., Noble, D. and Noble S.J.: The contribution of potassium accumulation to outward currents in frog atrium. J. Physiol. (London), 306: 127-149, 1980.

Brown, H.F., DiFrancesco, D. and Noble, S.J.: Cardiac pacemaker oscillation and its modulation by autonomic transmitters. J. Exp. Biol., 81: 175-204, 1979.

Brown, H.F., Kimura, J. and Noble, S.J.: Evidence that the current i_f in sino-atrial node has a potassium component. J. Physiol. (London), 308: 33P, 1980.

Cohen, I., Daut, J. and Noble, D.: The effects of potassium and temperature on the pacemaker current, i_{K2}, in Purkinje fibres. J. Physiol. (London), 260: 55-74, 1976a.

Cohen, I., Daut, J. and Noble, D.: An analysis of the actions of low concentrations of ouabain on membrane currents in Purkinje fibres. J. Physiol. (London), 260: 75-103, 1976b.

Cohen, I., Eisner, D. and Noble, D.: The action of adrenaline on pacemaker activity in cardiac Purkinje fibres. J. Physiol. (London), 280: 155-168, 1978.

Cohen, I., Noble, D., Ohba, M. and Ojeda, C.: Actions of salicylate ions on the electrical properties of sheep cardiac Purkinje fibres. J. Physiol. (London), 297: 163-185, 1979.

DiFrancesco, D.: The pacemaker current, i_{K2}, in Purkinje fibres is carried by sodium and potassium. J. Physiol. (London), 308: 32P, 1980.

DiFrancesco, D.: A new interpretation of the pacemaker current in Purkinje fibre. J. Physiol. (London), 314: 359-376, 1981a.

DiFrancesco, D.: A study of the ionic nature of the pacemaker current in Purkinje fibres. J. Physiol. (London), 314: 377-393, 1981b.

DiFrancesco, D.: The current "i_{K2}" in Purkinje fibres reinterpreted and identified with the pacemaker current i_f in the SA node. (this volume), 1981c.

DiFrancesco, D. and McNaughton, P.A.: The effects of calcium on outward membrane currents in the cardiac Purkinje fibre. J. Physiol. (London), 289, 347-373, 1979.

DiFrancesco, D. and Noble, D.: If "i_{K2}" is an inward current, how does it display potassium specificity? J. Physiol. (London), 305: 14-15P, 1980a.

DiFrancesco, D. and Noble, D.: Reconstruction of Purkinje fibre currents in sodium-free solution. J. Physiol. (London), 308: 35P, 1980b.

DiFrancesco, D., Noma, A. and Trautwein, W.: Kinetics and magnitude of the time-dependent K-current in the rabbit SA node: effect of external potassium. Pfluegers Arch., 381: 271-279, 1979.

DiFrancesco, D., Ohba, M. and Ojeda, C.: Measurement and significance of the reversal potential for the pacemaker current (i_{K2}) in sheep Purkinje fibres. J. Physiol. (London), 297: 135-162, 1979.

DiFrancesco, D. and Ojeda, C.: Properties of the pacemaker current i_f in the sinoatrial node of the rabbit compared with those of the current i_{k2} in Purkinje fibres. J. Physiol. (London), 308: 353-367, 1980.

Eisner, D.A. and Lederer, W.J.: Characterisation of the electrogenic sodium pump in cardiac Purkinje fibres. J. Physiol. (London), 303, 441-474, 1980.

Fox, L.: In: Modern Computing Methods, Chapter 12. H.M.S.O. London, 1961.

Gadsby, D.C. and Cranefield, P.F.: Two levels of resting potential in cardiac Purkinje fibres. J. Gen. Physiol., 70: 725-746, 1977.

Hart, G., Noble, D. and Shimoni, Y.: Adrenaline shifts the voltage dependence of the Na^+ and K^+ components of i_f in sheep Purkinje fibres. J. Physiol. (London), 308: 34P, 1980.

Hutter, O.F. and Noble, D.: Rectifying properties of heart muscle. Nature, 188: 495, 1960.

McAllister, R.E. and Noble, D.: The time and voltage dependence of the slow outward current in cardiac Purkinje fibres. J. Physiol. (London), 186: 632-662, 1966.

McAllister, R.E., Noble, D. and Tsien, R.W.: Reconstruction of the electrical activity of cardiac Purkinje fibres. J. Physiol. (London), 251: 1-59, 1975.

McDonald, T.F. and Trautwein, W.: The potassium current underlying delayed rectification in cat ventricular muscle. J. Physiol. (London), 274: 217-246, 1978.

Noble, D.: Conductance mechanisms in excitable cells. Biomembranes 3, Kreuzer, F. and Slegers, J.F.G., eds., Plenum Press, New York, pp. 427-447, 1972.

Noble, D. and Tsien, R.W.: The kinetics and rectifier properties of the slow potassium current in cardiac Purkinje fibres. J. Physiol. (London), 195: 185-214, 1968.

Noble, D. and Tsien, R.W.: Outward membrane currents activated in the plateau range of potentials in cardiac Purkinje fibres. J. Physiol. (London), 200, 205-231, 1969.

Noble, D. and Tsien, R.W.: The repolarization process of heart cells. In: Electrical Phenomena in the Heart, De Mello, W.C., ed., Academic Press, New York, pp. 133-161, 1972.

Peper, K. and Trautwein, W.: A note on the pacemaker current in Purkinje fibres. Pfluegers Arch., 309: 356-361, 1969.

Vassalle, M.: Cardiac pacemaker potentials at different extracellular and intracellular K concentrations. Am. J. Physiol., 208: 770-775, 1965.

Vassalle, M.: Analysis of cardiac pacemaker potential using a "voltage clamp" technique. Am. J. Physiol., 210: 1335-1341, 1966.

Weidmann, S.: Effect of current flow on the membrane potential of cardiac muscle. J. Physiol. (London), 115: 227-236, 1951.

Weidmann, S.: Electrophysiologie der Herzmuskelfaser. Huber, Bern, 1956.

Yanagihara, K. and Irisawa, H.: Inward current activated during hyperpolarization in the rabbit sinoatrial node cell. Pfluegers Arch., 385: 11-19, 1980.

PACEMAKER MECHANISMS IN MYOCARDIAL CELLS DURING

DEVELOPMENT OF EMBRYONIC CHICK HEARTS

Nick Sperelakis

INTRODUCTION

Important changes occur in the heart during embryonic development, including ultrastructural, metabolic, pharmacological, and electrophysiological changes. For example, striking changes occur in the electrical properties of ventricular myocardial cells during embryonic development of chick heart. These electrophysiological changes include changes in automaticity and pacemaker capabilities of the cells. The electrical properties at each stage of development determine many of the functional properties of the heart at that stage. Studies on the electrophysiological properties of embryonic heart cells are useful, not only for elucidating the changes during differentiation, but also may provide clues for understanding the complex electrophysiology of adult hearts. Similarly, cultured heart cells may prove useful as a model system in which to study automaticity of heart cells.

In this article, some of the important facts concerning changes in the properties of the heart during development are reviewed. Most of the data presented are for the chick, although some are for developing mammalian hearts. Some findings on organ-cultured hearts and cultured heart cells are presented for purposes of comparison and illustration of related phenomena. Because the electrical properties may be influenced by morphological, biochemical and pharmacological changes, some relevant changes in these parameters are also mentioned. A brief discussion of the mechanisms underlying automaticity of heart cells is given, and how these vary during development.

The following points are proposed, and they may serve as a guide for the facts, interpretations, and hypotheses to be presented subsequently. (1) All excitable cells, including all heart cells (e.g., nodal, Purkinje and atrial and ventricular myocardial), are capable of automaticity under the right conditions. (2) These conditions include: (a) a low Cl^- conductance (g_{Cl}), (b) a low K^+ permeability (P_K) (e.g., by addition of some agent, like Ba^{++} ion, that decreases P_K and (c) depolarization by some means into the pacemaker voltage range. (3) In cells that possess automaticity, the slope of the pacemaker potential is very sensitive to changes in membrane potential (E_m), application of small hyperpolarizing currents diminishing the slope and small depolarizing currents increasing the slope, thereby altering the frequency of discharge correspondingly. (4) The slope of the pacemaker potential is also very sensitive to temperature and to agents that affect the various ion conductances, such as acetylcholine and norepinephrine. (5) In the early embryonic heart (tubular), all the heart cells exhibit automaticity, including the cells in the presumptive ventricular region; P_K is low and E_m is low. (6) During development, P_K increases, resting E_m increases, and automaticity decreases in the myocardial cells; in some cells, e.g., the presumptive nodal cells, these changes do not occur. (7) The early tubular heart (e.g., days 1.5 - 3 in the embryonic chick) resembles a pulsating blood vessel, and the cells behave electrically like vascular smooth muscle cells, namely they have a low P_K, a low resting potential (e.g., -55 mV), and no (or very few) functional fast Na^+ channels. (During subsequent development, the myocardial cells proceed to further differentiate, including an increase in the density of functional fast Na^+ channels.) (8) Decrease in basal cyclic AMP level, decrease in the cyclic AMP response to beta-adrenergic agonists, and increase in (Na, K) - ATPase activity occur during development, and these changes might affect some of the electrical properties. (9) Differentiation of the heart cells does not normally proceed in vitro during cell culture or organ culture, but can be made to do so under certain conditions. (10) In cell culture of old embryonic heart cells that have adult-like electrical properties, many of the cells rapidly revert back (partially dedifferentiate) towards the young embryonic state; namely, they lose functional fast Na^+ channels, P_K and E_m decrease, and they gain automaticity. (11) Postdrive hyperpolarization and overdrive suppression of automaticity occur in cultured heart cells, and even in those derived from very young embryonic hearts.

INTACT HEARTS DEVELOPING IN SITU

PRECARDIAC AREAS OF THE CHICK BLASTODERM

Explants of the bilateral precardiac areas of the anterior half of the   16-17 hr
(chick) blastoderm develop spontaneous electrical activity after several days in
culture, which include spontaneous action potentials of   about   50 mV   amplitude
(LeDouarin et al., 1966).   In culture, a spontaneously beating tubular heart
develops within a vesicle.   If the precardiac area is treated   with   trypsin   to
facilitate   mechanical separation of the three germ layers, culture of the mesoderm alone gives rise to a solid mass of cells which fire spontaneous action potentials and contract (Renaud, 1973).

The postnodal piece (posterior third of the blastoderm dissected) from   the
19 hr   chick   blastoderm   does not normally give rise to heart tissue in culture.
If, however, the postnodal piece is cultured in the presence of an   RNA-enriched
fraction   obtained   from   adult   chicken hearts, a spontaneously-beating tubular
heart forms within a vesicle (Niu and Deshpande, 1973), and   it   exhibits   spontaneous action potentials (McLean et al., 1978).   Thus, it appears that either
RNA or some other material within the extract can induce cells in the   postnodal
piece,   normally   not destined to form the heart, to take on many of the properties of cardiac myoblasts.

Subsequently in development in situ, the twin   tubular   primordia   formed
bilaterally   from   the   precardiac mesoderm fuse to form a single tubular heart.
This fusion begins from the head end and proceeds posteriorly by   a   zipper-like
process,   such that the first region fused (ventricle) begins contracting first;
the atria are added posteriorly later.   The   tubular   heart   begins   contracting
spontaneously at   30-40 hr   (9-19   somite stage).   Cutting the 2-day heart into
bulbus, ventricle, and sinoatrium regions shows that each region has its characteristic automaticity, the sinoatrium being the fastest.   The velocity of propagation of the peristaltic contraction wave in 3-day hearts is   approximately   1
cm/s (Romanoff, 1960).

The heart rate of the chick embryo increases from about 50 beats/min at day
1.5   to   the   maximal   value   of   about 220 beats/min by day 8 (Romanoff, 1960).
Ignarro and Shideman (1968) observed a rate of about 20/min on day 1, 170/min on
day 4,   and   250/min   on   day 16.   Girard (1973) found the following heart rate
changes during development: 138 (day 3), 191 (day 5), 222 (day 7),   233   (days

10-20); there was a sharp decrease in heart rate at hatching which lasted for several days. Loffelholz and Pappano (1974) measured the SA nodal pacemaker rate of isolated chick embryonic hearts (at 30 $^{\circ}$C) by intracellular microelectrodes and also observed an increase during development, a peak occurring on about days 11-15, and decreasing thereafter until hatching.

The influence of temperature on heart rate decreases markedly during development (Romanoff, 1960). The Q_{10} decreases from about 3.6 on day 3 to about 2.0 on day 18 for the same temperature range (Sperelakis and McLean, 1977).

Innervation reaches the heart on about day 5 (Romanoff, 1960), but does not become functional, with respect to neurotransmitter release and effect, until about 12 for cholinergic nerves (Pappano, 1974), or day 16 for the adrenargic nerves (Enemar et al., 1965).

DEVELOPMENT OF AUTOMATICITY IN MAMMALIAN HEARTS

In mammals, the heart also begins beating early in development, e.g. on embryonic day 8.5 (6-7 somite stage) in rabbit and day 9.5 (stage 16 of Nicholas) in rat (Goss, 1938). The heart beat initially appears in the primitive ventricle or conoventricular region, which is the first region formed. The primordial atrium, and later the sinus venosus, become established caudally, and the rate of beating increases progressively. All cells of the early tubular heart possess automaticity, but there is a cephalocaudal progression of pacemaker dominance, each region of the developing heart having its intrinsic rhythm, as verified by cutting the heart into its various regions. The cells of the sinus venosus exhibit the fastest intrinsic rate. Thus, the cells destined to become part of the ventricle, atrium, or node differ in their degree of inherent automaticity.

The SA node arises from the primitive sinus venosus, and can be morphologically identified in the human fetus at 15.5 weeks (Anderson et al., 1977; Brooks and Lu, 1972). Whether the cells of the sinus node are derived from specialized cells or are simply embryonic cells that have failed to differentiate is controversial (James, 1970). Although the cells of the fetal sinus node appear to be all of one type, the adult node is characterized by two distinct cell groups, P (pacemaker) cells and transitional cells (James, 1970).

DeHaan (1961) has described the histodifferentiation of the AV node for the developing human heart. Early in the 6th week (9-10 mm embryo), the AV node makes its appearance as a cluster of cells in the posterior wall of the AV canal (cf. Bonke, 1977). Shortly thereafter, the AV bundle branches arise. The cells of the AV node and AV bundles contain few myofibrils and numerous glycogen granules, thus resembling early embryonic myocardial cells.

TABLE I

SUMMARY OF DATA OBTAINED FROM E_m VS. LOG $[K]_o$ CURVES AND FROM INPUT RESISTANCE (R_{in}) MEASUREMENTS FOR CHICK EMBRYONIC HEARTS (VENTRICULAR CELLS) AT VARIOUS STAGES OF DEVELOPMENT

Embryonic Age (days)	E_m (mV)	Slope (mV/decade)	Extrapolated $[K]_i$ (mM)	E_K (mV)	P_{Na}/P_K ratio	r_{in} (MΩm)
2	-40	30	125	-100	0.21	13.0
3	-51	40	130	-101	0.17	8.5
4	-57	46	140	-103	0.08	6.5
5-6	-58	50	130	-101	0.08	5.5
7-9	-71	51	145	-104	0.07	5.5
11-13	-80	53	145	-104	0.07	4.7
14-20	-78	52	155	-106	0.05	4.5

Data were taken from Sperelakis and Shigenobu, 1972, and from Sperelakis et al., 1975.
The resting potential (E_m) values are given for a $[K]_o$ of 2.7 mM. The slope is the average at $[K]_o$ levels between 10 and 100 mM. $[K]_i$ was estimated from the extrapolation of fitted curves to zero potential. The P_{Na}/P_K ratios were calculated from the Goldman constant-field equation.
Similar values for slope and $[K]_i$ were obtained by Pappano (1972) for embryonic chick atrium at 4 days, 6 days, and 12 days; the 18-day values were -59 mV/decade and 125 mM $[K]_i$, respectively.

RESTING MEMBRANE PROPERTIES

The transmembrane resting potential (E_m) of the ventricular portion of the chick and rat hearts increases during embryonic development (Bernard, 1976; Boethius and Knutsson, 1970; Couch et al., 1969; McDonald and DeHaan, 1973; Pappano, 1972; Shigenobu and Sperelakis, 1971; Sperelakis and Shigenobu, 1972; Yeh and Hoffman, 1967)(cf. Renaud, 1973). In the case of the embryonic chick heart,

However, it is possible that the low recorded potentials in young hearts are partly an artifact caused by current leakage around the electrode tip due to improper sealing of the microelectrode; this effect would be most prominent in small cells having a high input resistance.

the greatest changes occur between days 2 and 7, and thereafter the increase is
smaller.

INTACT HEARTS

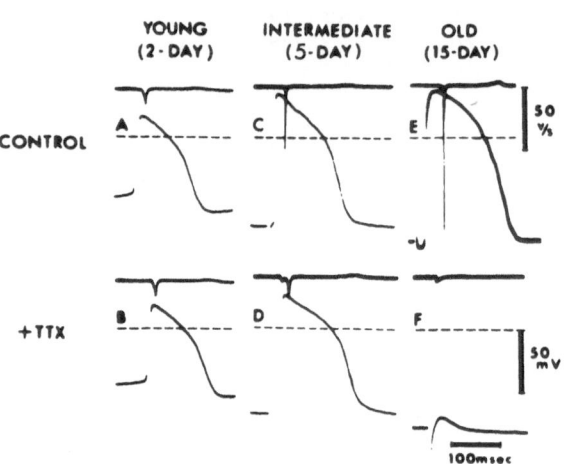

FIGURE 1 *Resting potential (E_m) plotted as a function of $[K]_o$ on a logarithmic
scale for three representative hearts of different ages. $[K]_o$ was elevated by
substitution of K^+ for equimolar amounts of Na^+. Continuous lines give theoretical calculations from the constant-field equation (inset) for P_{Na}/P_K ratios of
0.001, 0.01, 0.05, 0.1 and 0.2. Calculations were made assuming $[K]_i$ and $[Na]_i$
values shown. For a P_{Na}/P_K ratio of 0.001, the curve is linear over the entire
range with a slope of 60 mV/decade, i.e., it closely follows E_K. Symbols give
representative data obtained from embryonic chick hearts at days 3(○), 5(△) and
15 (●). The data for the 3-day heart follow the curve for a P_{Na}/P_K ratio of
0.2, those for the 5-day heart follow the curve for 0.1 , and those for the
15-day heart fall between the curves for 0.01 to 0.05. The estimated intracellular K^+ activities ($[K]_i$) obtained by extrapolation to zero potential are nearly the same for all ages. (Modified from Sperelakis and Shigenobu, 1972.)*

The mean resting potential is about -51 mV on day 3, and is close to -80 mV by
day 12, nearly the final adult value. The large increase in resting E_m during
the first few days is primarily due to an increase in K^+ permeability (P_K) and
not in the K^+ equilibrium potential (E_K). The $[K]_i$ is already high in young em-

bryonic chick hearts.

The relationship between resting potential and external K^+ concentration ($[K]_o$) was determined for embryonic hearts of different ages (Sperelakis and Shigenobu, 1972). Data for 3-day, 5-day, and 15-day old embryonic chick hearts are shown in Figure 2.

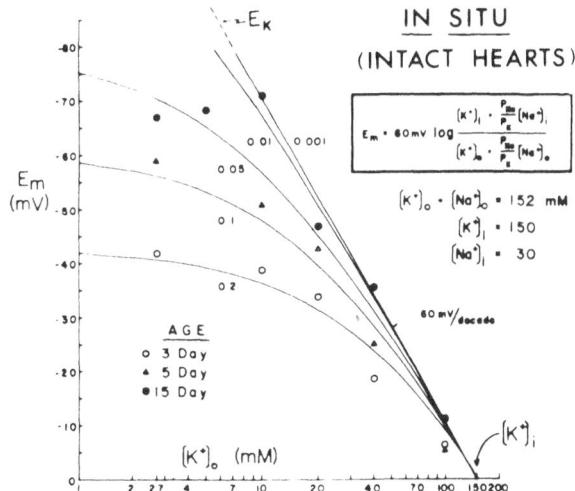

FIGURE 2 *Development of sensitivity to tetrodotoxin (TTX) of intact embryonic chick hearts with increasing embryonic age.*
A-B: Intracellular recordings from a 2-day-old heart before (A) and 20 min after (B) the addition of TTX (20 μg/ml).
C-D: Recordings from a 7-day heart before (C) and 2 min after (D) the addition of TTX (2 μg/ml). Note depression of the rate of rise in D.
E-F: From a 15-day-old heart prior to (E) and 2 min after (F) the addition of TTX (1 μg/ml). The action potentials were abolished and excitability was not restored by strong field stimulation in F. The upper traces give dV/dt; this trace has been shifted relative to the V-t trace to prevent obscuring dV/dt. The horizontal broken line in each panel represents zero potential. dV/dt calibration (in E) and voltage and time calibrations (in F) pertain to all panels. (Modified from Sperelakis and Shigenobu, 1972.)

$[K]_i$ was estimated by extrapolation of the curves to zero potential, and the values varied between 125 mM (for 2-day-old hearts) and 155 mM (for 14-20-day hearts) (Table I). Also plotted in Figure 2 are the theoretical curves (calculated from the Goldman constant-field equation given in the inset and assuming that $[Na]_i$ was 30 mM and $[K]_i$ was 150 mM) for five different ratios of P_{Na}/P_K: 0.001, 0.01, 0.05, 0.1 and 0.2. It can be seen that the data points for the 3-day heart most closely fit the theoretical curve for a P_{Na}/P_K ratio of 0.2; those for the 5-day heart fit a P_{Na}/P_K of 0.1, and those for the 15-day heart fit between the 0.05 and 0.01 curves. These data suggest that the P_{Na}/P_K ratio is very high in young hearts, and that this accounts for the low measured resting potential. Only a small increase in the calculated E_K occurs during development: from about -100 mV on day 2 to -106 mV on days 14-20. Pappano (1972) also reported high values of $[K]_i$ (145 mM) on day 4 for chick atrial cells, and Carmeliet et al. (1976) calculated $[K]_i$ values of 151 mM for chick hearts on days 6-8. (It has been reported that $[K]_i$ may actually decrease during development (Carmeliet et al., 1976; Harsch and Green, 1963; McDonald and DeHaan, 1973).) Thus, in the young hearts, the resting potential is far from E_K due to the high P_{Na}/P_K ratio. In this respect, the myocardial cells in young embryonic hearts resemble SA nodal cells in adult hearts.

In old embryonic chick or adult hearts, the E_m vs log $[K]_o$ curve is nearly linear above 10 mM K^+, with a slope approaching the theoretical 61 mV/decade (from the Nernst equation). The data in Figure 2 and Table 1 show that the slope for hearts 7-20 days old is 51-53 mV/decade, whereas the average slopes (curves continually bend) for 4-day, 3-day and 2-day hearts are 46, 40 and 30 mV/decade, respectively. Pappano (1972) found similar values for $[K]_i$ and slope for embryonic chick atrial cells at various stages of development.

In order to ascertain whether the P_{Na}/P_K ratio is high in the young embryonic chick hearts because of a high P_{Na} or a low P_K, input resistance (r_{in}) was determined from steady-state voltage-current curves. The r_{in} of the cells is high (13 MOhm) in young 2-day-old hearts, and rapidly declines over the next few days, reaching the adult value of about 4.5 MOhm by day 14 (Table 1). If the average cell size and the degree of electrical coupling between the cells remains unchanged, the high r_{in} of young hearts would suggest that membrane resistivity (R_m) is very high, consistent with a low K^+ conductance and P_K. Consistent with this is the finding that the chronaxie, hence the membrane time constant, of young hearts (2-day-old) is about four-fold higher than that of 9-16 day hearts (Shimizu and Tasaki, 1966); if membrane capacitance remains constant, membrane resistivity must be four-fold higher. Thus, the P_{Na}/P_K ratio is high in young hearts probably because P_K is low.

Consistent with this conclusion, Carmeliet and coworkers (1976) reported on the basis of ^{42}K flux measurements, that P_K is about 2-3-fold lower in 6-8 day hearts (13.2×10^{-8} cm/s) than in 18-20 day hearts (27.5×10^{-8} cm/s). (Although they reported that P_K for 3-5 day hearts was high, lack of control for spontaneous beating and action potentials, hence increased K^+ efflux, could cause an erroneously high calculated P_K.) The P_{Na}/P_K ratios were 0.018 for the 19-day hearts and 0.037 for the 7-day hearts. P_{Na} (calculated from P_K and P_{Na}/P_K ratio) did not change during development (about 0.50×10^{-8} cm/s.).

Young hearts are less affected by elevation of $[K]_o$ that are older hearts (DeHaan, 1970; Sperelakis and Shigenobu, 1972), as expected by the much more prominent flattening of the resting potential vs log $[K]_o$ curve (at lower $[K]_o$ levels) in young hearts, i.e., they are depolarized less by a given increment in $[K]_o$ (see Fig. 2). This is true for both inhibition of automaticity of the whole heart, as well as for loss of excitability of the ventricle to electrical stimulation. Automaticity and excitability fail at about 25 mM K^+ in 2-3-day-old hearts, whereas failure occurs at about 15 mM (automaticity) and 20 mM (excitability) in the 14-20 day hearts. Depression of automaticity was evident by 12 mM in hearts of all ages.

The young ventricular cells of the chick heart are not hyperpolarized by acetylcholine (ACh), even though a large hyperpolarization is theoretically possible because the resting potential is much below E_K (Sperelakis and Shigenobu, 1972). In addition, the action potential duration is not shortened by ACh. Therefore, it is likely that ACh does not significantly increase P_K in ventricular cells. In old embryonic hearts also, ACh has little or no effect on shortening the ventricular action potential, whereas the atrial action potential is markedly shortened. Pappano (1972) reported that the atrial cells of young hearts are slightly depolarized by ACh in normal medium, and slightly hyperpolarized in Na-free medium, and he suggested that ACh increases both Na^+ conductance and K^+ conductance in young hearts.

The specific activity of the (Na,K)-ATPase is low in young embryonic chick hearts and rises during development (Sperelakis, 1972). The average value on day 4 is about 35% of that on day 16. Thus, while P_K is increasing during development, and hence the membrane passive leaks, the capability of the Na-K pump is increasing. The pumping capacity of the young hearts, however, must be sufficient to maintain the relatively high $[K]_i$ and low $[Na]_i$ already found in young cells. When the ventricular myocardial cells from 16-days hearts are placed into monolayer cell culture, the specific activity of the (Na,K)-ATPase decreases by more than threefold (Sperelakis and Lee, 1971); this is consistent with the lower K^+ permeability and somewhat lower $[K]_i$ generally observed in these cells.

The $[Na]_i$ in the chick heart does not change greatly during development (Harsch and Green, 1963; McDonald and DeHaan, 1973). For example, Carmeliet et al. (1976) measured $[Na]_i$ values of 16 mM and 15 mM for 7-day and 19-day embryonic chick hearts, respectively. Electrophysiological studies also indicate that the free intracellular Na^+ must not be too high in young hearts, because the Na^+-dependent action potentials already overshoot to +11 mV in day 2 hearts (Sperelakis and Shigenobu, 1972). The overshoot increases rapidly, so that by day 7, it is +28 mV, which is close to the adult value.

TABLE II

INCIDENCE (%) OF PACEMAKER POTENTIALS AND HYPERPOLARIZING AFTERPOTENTIALS IN VENTRICULAR MYOCARDIAL CELLS DURING EMBRYONIC DEVELOPMENT OF CHICK HEARTS

Embryonic Age (days)	Hyperpolarizing Afterpotentials Intact Hearts	Pacemaker Potentials Intact Hearts	Cut Ventricles
2-3	81	80-100	100
4	63	60-100	100
7	38	20-40	100
10	0	0	100
12	0	0	0
17	0	0	0
20	0	0	0
27	0	0	0

Data taken from Sperelakis and McLean (1978) and from Sperelakis and Shigenobu (1972).
Cells which exhibit pacemaker potentials usually also possess hyperpolarizing afterpotentials, but the converse is not always true.

AUTOMATICITY; OVERDRIVE SUPPRESSION

The major requirements for automaticity appear to be a low chloride conductance and a low K^+ conductance (g_K). A low g_K may be considered as enhancing the inductance in series with one type of K^+ channel (the inward-rectifying or anomalous rectification channel having a negative slope conductance region), and tends to cause oscillations in membrane potential. The low g_K also produces some depolarization, moving the resting potential farther from E_K and placing the membrane potential in the region that can support pacemaker oscillations.

Pronounced changes in automaticity of the ventricular cells occur during development, as would be predicted from the changes in P_K. The incidence of hyperpolarizing afterpotentials and pacemaker potentials is very high (80-100%) in the young hearts, and this incidence decreases to 0% in the old embryonic hearts (Table II) (Sperelakis and Shigenobu, 1972). If a portion of the ventricle is cut and isolated to remove drive from the nodal cells, the incidence of pacemaker potentials observed in the impaled cells was 100% for embryos up through day 10, whereas the incidence was 0% in embryos day 12 or older (Table II; Figs. 3,4). Thus, the ventricular myocardial cells possess automaticity capability when they are young, but this capability diminishes as the cells become older.

However, old ventricular cells again become automatic when trypsin-dispersed and placed into monolayer culture. For example, ventricular cells dispersed from 16-day-old chick hearts and cultured as monolayers usually revert back towards the young embryonic state with respect to their electrical properties, including gain of automaticity (Sperelakis, 1967). When the cells are allowed to reaggregate into small spheres, however, they often retain their highly differentiated electrical properties, including lack of automaticity (Jongsma et al., 1975; McLean and Sperelakis, 1976). In some cases, the reaggregates may exhibit automaticity, even though the action potentials are relatively fast-rising and TTX-sensitive. The gain in automaticity of cultured cells appears to reflect a decrease in P_K (Sperelakis, 1967; Sperelakis and Lehmkuhl, 1966). Isolated single ventricular cells in culture often have such a low P_K that they are depolarized too far and do not normally exhibit automaticity or excitability (Pappano and Sperelakis, 1969). However, if these cells are hyperpolarized by the intracellular application of current, then spontaneous action potentials and contractions occur. The retention of automaticity of cultured isolated single heart cells or monolayers suggests that mechanical factors

FIGURE 3 *Electrophysiological recordings from ventricular fragments cut from chick embryonic hearts of various ages.*
A-D: Pacemaker potentials preceded the action potentials in impaled cells within fragments from 3-day (A), 4-day (B), 7-day (C) and 10-day-old (D) hearts. Maximal rate of rise and maximal diastolic potentials in the fragments were the same as in the intact heart. The fragments contracted spontaneously.
E-F: Cut ventricular fragments from hearts 12-day-old and older did not exhibit automaticity. Action potentials with fast rates of rise (equal to those recorded from cells in the intact hearts of the respective ages) were elicited by field stimulation (shock artifacts visible) from fragments of 12-day (E), 17-day (F) and 20-day (G) ventricles. Time calibration in D applies to A-D. (Taken from Sperelakis and McLean, 1978.)

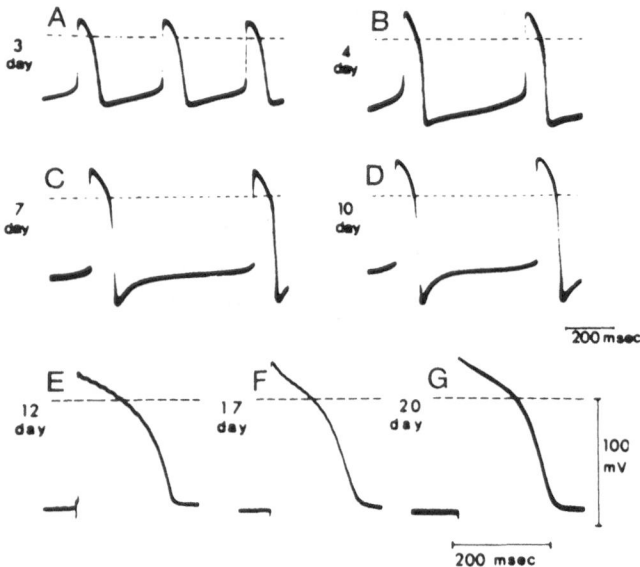

Embryonic Chick Ventricular Fragments

may play little or no role in automaticity.

Pacemaker-like activity also can be produced by the application of small depolarizing currents to adult ventricular myocardial cells (Katzung, 1974, 1975). This indicates that cells with normally high resting potentials retain the ability to generate spontaneous rhythm, and that the ontogenic increase in the resting potential may be an important factor in the absence of automaticity under normal conditions. Membrane resistance increases during diastolic depolarization, and the rhythmic activity is inhibited by inhibitors of slow current, such as verapamil. These findings suggest that automaticity of adult myocardial cells induced by depolarization is similar to that in natural pacemaker (nodal) cells. It has been proposed that the deactivation of the delayed K^+ conductance (g_{x1}) is responsible for the diastolic depolarization in partially depolarized ventricular muscle (Beeler and Reuter, 1977).

An electrogenic Na^+ pump potential has been demonstrated in various tissues of the heart (Page and Storm, 1965; Vassalle, 1970; Glitsch, 1973; McLean et al., 1979; Sperelakis, 1979), and it contributes to the resting potential under normal physiological conditions in Purkinje fibers (Deleze, 1960; Isenberg and Trautwein, 1974), atrial fibers (Glitsch, 1973), sinoatrial nodal cells (Noma and Irisawa, 1975), in cultured embryonic chick (11-day-old) myocardial cells (Lieberman et al., 1977), and in cultured embryonic heart cell reaggregates derived from early (3-day-old) and late (16-day) stages of development (Pelleg et al., 1980). Thus, the ability to carry out electrogenic transport is acquired in early stages of ontogenesis, and this ability is retained in vitro.

When automatic heart cells are driven at a faster rate than their intrinsic rate, upon termination of the drive there is a transient pause followed by a gradual recovery to the predrive firing rate (Lu et al., 1965; Vassalle, 1970). This phenomenon of overdrive suppression of automaticity is usually accompanied by a small hyperpolarization of a few millivolts; the transient hyperpolarization presumably is the cause of the suppression of the automaticity. Vassalle (1970) presented evidence that the hyperpolarization was due to stimulation of an electrogenic Na^+ pump potential, presumably resulting from an increase in $[Na]_i$ and in $[K]_o$ during the drive. Overdrive suppression was observed in intact young 3-day-old hearts (prior to innervation of the heart), and was attributed to the release of an ACh-like substance from within the heart cells (Coraboeuf et al., 1970). It was recently demonstrated by Pelleg et al. (1980) that cultured heart cells (ventricular and atrial) from both young and old embryonic chick heart that are automatic in vitro exhibit the phenomena of postdrive hyperpolarization and overdrive suppression of automaticity. These phenomena were blocked by ouabain but not by atropine, thus supporting the view that stimulation of an electrogenic pump is the underlying me-

FIGURE 4 *Electrophysiological recordings from an intact 6-day-old embryonic chick heart (ventricle) (A) and from a ventricular fragment cut from the apex of the same heart (B).*
A: Ventricular action potentials (maximal rate of rise 70 V/s) recorded in spontaneously-contracting heart in response to conduction of the impulse from the sino-atrial pacemaker; note stable resting potential, i.e., absence of pacemaker potentials.
B: Pacemaker potentials preceded the action potentials in the cells of the cut ventricular fragment, revealing intrinsic automaticity. The cut fragment contracted spontaneously. (Taken from Sperelakis and McLean, 1978.)

Embryonic Chick Ventricular Cells — 6 days In ovo

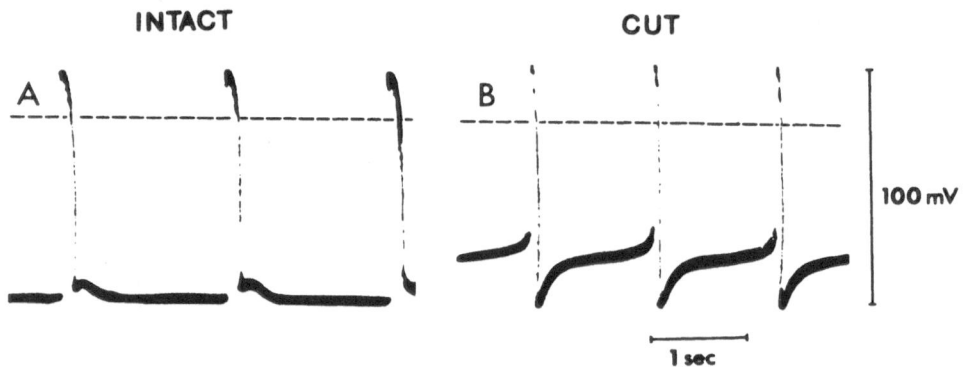

chanism.

ACTION POTENTIALS

The action potentials of the cells of intact chick hearts undergo sequential changes during development in situ (Sperelakis and Shigenobu, 1972; Sperelakis, 1972; Sperelakis et al., 1976). Young 2-3-day-old embryonic chick hearts have action potentials with relatively low rates of rise and which are only little depressed by tetrodotoxin (TTX), a specific blocker of fast Na^+ channels (Shigenobu and Sperelakis, 1971; Sperelakis and Shigenobu, 1972; McDonald et al., 1972; McDonald and Sachs, 1975; DeHaan et al., 1976). During development, there is a progressive increase in maximal rate of rise $(+\dot{V}_{max})$ and overshoot of the action potential, as well as in resting potential

(Fig. 1). The overshoot averaged +11 mV on day 2, and increased progressively to reach the maximal value of about +28 mV by day 8. The duration (at 50% repolarization) was not significantly changed during development, the average value being 110 ms. The time course of the increase in $+\dot{V}_{max}$ was not parallel to the increase in resting E_m, the increase in resting E_m usually preceeding the increase in $+\dot{V}_{max}$. For example, in young hearts, it was not unusual to find a cell with a large resting potential but with a low $+\dot{V}_{max}$.

Young (2-3 days in ovo) myocardial cells possess slowly rising (15-40 V/s) action potentials preceded by pacemaker potentials (Fig. 1A). TTX has either no effect or only little effect on the action potential rate of rise or overshoot (Fig. 1B) (Table III). Hyperpolarizing current pulses do not greatly increase the rate of rise of the action potential, thus indicating that inactivation of fast Na^+ channels at the low resting potential is not a major reason for the low $+\dot{V}_{max}$, but rather a low density of fast channels. Excitability is not lost until the membrane is depolarized to less than -20 mV, also consistent with a preponderance of slow channels. Nathan and DeHaan (1978) also found that TTX-sensitive fast Na^+ conductance channels were absent or nonfunctional in cultured cell reaggregates derived from 3-day-old embryonic chick hearts.

TABLE III

EFFECT OF TETRODOTOXIN (TTX) ON THE ACTION POTENTIAL MAXIMAL RATE OF RISE ($+\dot{V}_{max}$) OF CHICK EMBRYONIC HEARTS (VENTRICULAR MUSCLE) AS A FUNCTION OF DEVELOPMENTAL AGE

Embryonic Age (days)	$+\dot{V}_{max}$ (V/s) Control	+TTX	TTX Sensitivity
2-3	15-40	10-30	Little or none
5-6	50-70	10-30	Partial
8-10	75-90	0	Complete
12-16	90-140	0	Complete
17-21	140-170	0	Complete

*Data taken from Sperelakis and Shigenobu, 1972.

The action potential upstroke in young hearts is generated by Na^+ influx through TTX-insensitive slow Na^+ channels, as indicated by the dependence of the action potential overshoot and rate of rise on $[Na]_o$. The slope of overshoot as a function of $[Na]_o$ approaches the theoretical 61 mV/decade at the lower $[Na]_o$

levels.

Kinetically fast Na^+ channels, which are sensitive to TTX, are substantial in number by day 5. At this time, $+\dot{V}_{max}$ is about 50-70 V/s (Fig. 1C; Table III). During this intermediate stage of development (from about day 5 through day 7), a large number of slow channels still coexist with the fast Na^+ channels. TTX causes a reduction in $+\dot{V}_{max}$ to about 10-20 V/s, but the action potentials and accompanying contractions persist (Fig. 1 D; Table III).

After day 8, the action potentials are completely abolished by TTX (Fig. 1F; Table III). Depolarization to less than -50 mV now abolishes excitability. This indicates that the action potential-generating Na^+ channels now consist predominantly of fast Na^+ channels. The density of fast Na^+ channels continues to increase until about day 18, when the adult maximal rate of rise of about 150 V/s is achieved (Fig. 1E). A large fraction of the slow Na^+ channels appear to have been inactivated, and insufficient numbers remain to support regenerative excitation in the presence of TTX. (In addition, the simultaneous increase in resting potential might render propagation more difficult for any given density of slow channels.) Addition of some positive inotropic agents, such as beta-adrenergic agonists, histamine or methylxanthines, increases the number of slow Ca-Na channels available in the membrane, and leads to the regaining of excitability in cells whose fast Na^+ channels have been voltage inactivated or blocked (Pappano, 1970; Shigenobu and Sperelakis, 1972).

The slow-channel blocking drugs, verapamil and D-600, abolish the action potentials of the young embryonic hearts (Shigenobu et al., 1974). In contrast, Mn^{++} (at 1 mM) does not depress the action potentials of young hearts (although it does block the contractions), indicating a greater specificity for slow Ca^{++} channels (Sperelakis and Shigenobu, 1972). Kasuya et al. (1977) also reported that the slowly-rising action potentials of 3-days-old embryonic chick hearts involved cation channels that were pharmacologically different from those of old embryonic hearts. The contractions of 3-5-day-old embryonic chick hearts are insensitive to TTX, but are sensitive to D-600 (Galper and Catterall, 1978; Ishima, 1978). During subsequent development, the sensitivity to TTX increased and the sensitivity to D-600 decreased in a reciprocal manner.

In summary, young 2-3-day-old embryonic chick hearts have Na-dependent action potentials with relatively low rates of rise and which are only little depressed by TTX. Hyperpolarization does not greatly increase the rate of rise.

Therefore, the density of functional fast Na^+ channels is low. In contrast, the density of slow Na^+ channels is high in the young hearts, and verapamil-type agents block the slow Na^+ channels, whereas Mn^{++} does not. During development, the number of functional fast Na^+ channels increases progressively, reaching the final adult level by about day 18. In contrast, the number of available slow channels, in the absence of positive inotropic agents, decreases during development, falling substantially by day 8. At this time, TTX completely blocks the action potential, indicating that the number of available slow channels is not enough to support regenerative excitability. However, addition of some positive inotropic agents rapidly increases the number of available slow channels, and thus allows regenerative slow action potentials to be generated. During an intermediate stage of development, a sizeable number of functional fast Na^+ channels coexist with the original high density of functional slow channels, so that blockade of the fast Na^+ channels by TTX allows slow action potentials to be generated that resemble those present in young hearts.

BIOCHEMICAL AND ULTRASTRUCTURAL CHANGES

1. Cyclic AMP levels.

Changes in cyclic AMP content occur during embryonic development of the chick heart. The cyclic AMP level is highest in young hearts and it decreases during development, the greatest changes occurring before day 8 (McLean et al., 1975; Renaud et al., 1978). The level decreased gradually thereafter to a plateau level of 9.4 pmoles/mg protein, which is about the adult level, by day 16.

Isoproterenol markedly elevated the cyclic AMP level in the young hearts; this effect was much less in the old hearts. For example, 10^{-6} M isoproterenol elevated the cyclic AMP level of 4-day-old chick hearts from 34 to 119 pmoles/mg protein (peak effect at 3 min) (Renaud et al., 1978). These findings also clearly demonstrate that young hearts prior to innervation have functional beta-adrenergic receptors.

The relationship, if any, between changes in membrane properties and changes in cyclic AMP levels during development of heart remains to be clarified. However, since increase in cyclic AMP level is associated with increase in the number of available slow channels, it is possible that the decrease in number of available slow channels during development of chick heart results from the concomitant drop in cyclic AMP level. This would allow positive inotropic agents, that increase cyclic AMP level, to increase the number of available slow channels transiently back towards the density present in young embryonic hearts. In other words, the decrease in steady-state level of cyclic AMP during development may allow the fraction of slow channels that are available for activation to be modulated by inotropic agents.

2.   Biochemical changes

Glucose uptake is very high in young hearts, and decreases during development. Glucose uptake by hearts 5-days-old and younger seems to be by simple diffusion across the membrane (Guidotti et al., 1966). A carrier-mediated saturable glucose transport system, that can be stimulated by insulin appears on about day 7 (Guidotti et al., 1961). In addition, hexokinase activity increases several fold during development (Seltzer and McDougal, 1975).

Amino acid uptake decreases during development (Elsas et al., 1975). Amino acids are actively transported in 5-day-old embryonic chick hearts, and insulin enhances their rate of transport.

There are also changes in membrane fluidity (microviscosity) during development of chick hearts, the trend being towards an increase in fluidity (Kutchai et al., 1977). The cholesterol/phospholipid ratio of the sarcolemma increases during development, concomitant with an increase in the number of unsaturated fatty acid residues.

Young 2-3-day-old embryonic chick hearts have large pools of glycogen, and their metabolism is mainly by anaerobic glycolysis. The circulation to the chorioallantoic membrane for gas exchange is not established until day 5. Following this event, there is a shift toward aerobic metabolism, accompanied by changes in various enzymes. For example, there is an increase in pyruvate kinase activity (Cardenas et al., 1978; Harris et al., 1977), and lactic dehydrogenase (LDH) shifts from the embryonic M-form isoenzyme (which catalyzes the reduction of pyruvate to lactate) to the adult-like H-form (which facilitates pyruvate oxidation to CO_2 and H_2O) (Fine et al., 1963). (When old embryonic chick myocardial cells are cultured in monolayers, they again synthesize the early embryonic M-LDH (Cahn, 1964).) Enzymes of the pentose shunt pathway, such as glucose-6-P dehydrogenase and 6-P-gluconic dehydrogenase, decrease from day 4 to day 20, whereas enzymes of the Krebs cycle, such as isocitric dehydrogenase and alpha-ketoglutaric dehydrogenase, increase during development (Seltzer and McDougal, 1975).

Consistent with the fact that they have a low rate of aerobic metabolism, being mainly dependent on glycolysis, young hearts are relatively resistant to metabolic interventions. For example, hypoxia does not block the slow action potentials of young embryonic chick hearts (Thyrum, 1973; Vleugels et al., 1976). Similarly, monolayer cultures of chick embryonic heart cells, that have reverted in electrical properties, are relatively insensitive to a variety of metabolic poisons (Sperelakis and Lehmkuhl, 1967).

3. Ultrastructural changes.

Thin myofilaments appear in the tubular heart of the embryonic chick between 18-30 hr, and they begin to collect into groups by 36 hr (Hibbs, 1956). The my- ofibrils in 2-3 day hearts are relatively sparse, short, in various stages of formation, and are not aligned. The sarcomeres are usually incomplete. H zones first become obvious at 8 days, and M lines do not appear untill about day 18. By day 18, the embryonic myocardial cell closely resembles the adult cell, and has a close packing of completed myofibrils with rows of mitochondria in between. The large pools of glycogen and the abundant rough ER tubules observed in the young 2-3-day-old hearts are greatly reduced in amount. Sarcoplasmic re- ticulum (SR) is found in the young hearts, and it increases with development. Subsarcolemmal cisterns, regions in which terminal elements of the SR (continu- ous with the network SR) come in close apposition to the surface sarcolemma, are observed in young hearts (Sperelakis et al., 1974). A transverse (T) tubular system is not present.

CULTURED HEARTS AND HEART CELLS

ORGAN-CULTURED YOUNG EMBRYONIC HEARTS

Culture of embryonic heart in vitro provides a means of analyzing the changes that occur during normal development, and provide a useful model for studying the regulation of membrane differentiation. When young (2-3-day-old) embryonic chick hearts are placed into organ culture for 1-2 weeks, they fail to gain TTX-sensitive fast Na^+ channels and they retain automaticity (Shigenobu and Sperelakis, 1974; Sperelakis and Shigenobu, 1974). The action potentials continue to be slowly-rising and generated by TTX-insensitive slow Na^+ channels, the rates of rise remain slow, and are preceded by pacemaker potentials. Similar findings were obtained when the young hearts were grafted on to the chorioallantoic membrane of host chicks for blood perfusion (Renaud and Sperelakis, 1976). Thus, organ-cultured young hearts do not differentiate further in vitro, but appear to be arrested in the young embryonic state (cf. DeHaan et al., 1976). When such hearts are treated with RNA-enriched fractions obtained from adult chicken hearts, they gain fast Na^+ channels, become completely sensitive to TTX, and lose their automaticity (McLean et al., 1976). That is, young hearts in vitro can be induced to undergo further membrane differentiation.

CULTURED HEART CELLS

Various stages of cardiac electrical differentiation can be simulated in vitro using cell culture techniques, and their study may facilitate elucidation of the mechanisms operating during normal heart development. The electrophysiological properties observed depend to a large extent on the age of the hearts from which the cells are isolated, and on the method of cell culture. Reverted old embryonic cells or non-differentiated young embryonic cells may provide a useful model system for nodal cells of the heart and for study of mechanisms of automaticity.

1. MONOLAYER CULTURES PREPARED FROM OLD EMBRYONIC HEART

When cells are dispersed from old embryonic hearts using trypsin or collagenase and standard monolayer cultures are prepared, the cells are found to possess slowly-rising TTX-insensitive action potentials with pacemaker potentials (Fig. 5 C-D). These action potentials are similar to those recorded from young (2-3-day-old) hearts, rather than the old hearts from which the cells were taken (Fig. 5 A-B) (Sperelakis, 1967; Sperelakis and Lehmkuhl, 1964). It appears that cell separation results in a rapid reversion toward the young embryonic state. This reversion can be partially prevented by separating the cells and culturing them in solutions containing elevated K^+ concentrations (12-60 mM) and ATP (5 mM) (McLean and Sperelakis, 1974). Action potentials recorded from these cells fire from moderately high stable resting potentials of about -60 mV, and they are completely sensitive to TTX; however, $+\dot{V}_{max}$ is still rather slow (Fig

FIGURE 5 *Comparison of electrophysiological properties of the intact old (16-day) embryonic chick heart in situ (A-B) with those of trypsin-dispersed old ventricular myocardial cells in cultures prepared by three different methods (C-H).*
A-B: Intact heart: control action potential (A) was rapidly-rising (150 V/s), had a high stable resting potential (about -80 mV), and was completely abolished by tetrodotoxin (TTX; 0.1 µg/ml) (B).
C-D: Standard reverted monolayers; control action potential was slowly-rising (10 V/s), was preceded by a pacemaker potential, the resting potential was low (about -50 mV) (C), and TTX did not alter the action potential (D).
E-F: Partially reverted cells cultured as monolayers in media containing elevated K⁺ concentration (25 mM); control action potential had a rate of rise of 30 V/s (E), lacked a pacemaker potential, had a moderately high resting potential (~60 mV), and was completely abolished by TTX (F).
G-H: Highly differentiated cells in spherical reaggregate culture; control action potentials were rapidly-rising (150 V/s), the resting potentials were high (~80 mV) (G), and TTX abolished the action potentials (H). (Taken from Sperelakis and McLean, 1976.)

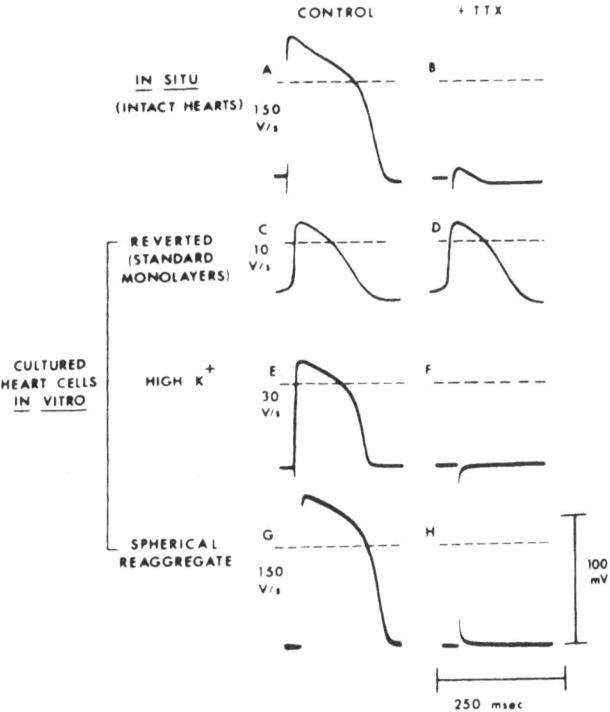

5 E-F).

Shortly after enzymatic separation from the ventricle of old embryonic hearts, many of the myocardial cells in suspension beat spontaneously at independent rhythms (Sperelakis and Lehmkuhl, 1964). This indicates that the normally nonpacemaker ventricular cells rapidly gain automaticity upon cell separation. When the cells are allowed to adhere to the glass for a few days and are subsequently impaled, the resting potentials are low and many cells exhibit pacemaker potentials (Figs. 5 C-D; 6 D-F). The input resistance increases, the average value being close to double (10 MOhm) that of cells in intact hearts. These facts are consistent with a low P_K. A plot of resting potential versus log $[K]_o$ suggests that the extrapolated $[K]_i$ is 90-100 mM in the reverted cells, corresponding to an E_K (at a $[K]_o$ of 4 mM) of -82 mV. This value is considerably greater than the measured resting potential of about -55 mV, hence indicating that the P_{Na}/P_K ratio is high (presumably because P_K is low). Thus, P_K also tends to revert back towards the young embryonic state in cultured monolayers.

In fact, in some isolated single cells in culture, P_K is so low that the cells are depolarized beyond the level that action potentials can be produced (beyond the inactivation potential for the slow channels); therefore, these cells do not contract spontaneously (Pappano and Sperelakis, 1969). However, if impaled with one or two microelectrodes, it is found that the membrane resistance is very high and that spontaneous action potentials and contractions appear upon application of hyperpolarizing current pulses (Fig. 6 J-L). Such cells exhibit a prominent hyperpolarization when $[K]_o$ is raised to 10-15 mM.

Some of the monolayer cells behave as non-pacemaker cells. Application of depolarizing or hyperpolarizing current pulses does not alter the frequency of firing in these cells (Fig. 6 A-B). Sufficient hyperpolarization causes failure of the action potentials, but unlike the true pacemaker cells, small driving junctional potentials that propably represent the interaction with contiguous firing cells) continue at unaltered frequency during the pulse (Fig. 6C). Although hyperpolarizing current pulses increase action potential amplitude (Fig. 6B), $+\dot{V}_{max}$ is increased only a relatively small amount; with depolarizing pulses, spike amplitude decreases (Fig. 6 A), and $+\dot{V}_{max}$ decreases and goes to zero at an E_m of about -20 mV.

In contrast, true pacemaker cells respond to small depolarizing current pulses by an increase in firing rate, and to small hyperpolarizing pulses by a

FIGURE 6 *Effect of polarizing current on nonpacemaker and pacemaker reverted heart cells in monolayer culture.*
A-C: Nonpacemaker cell; frequency of firing unaltered by current pulses of 0.6 (A) and 1.4 nA (B); at 1.5 nA, action potentials were prevented but driving junctional potentials remain at unaltered frequency (C).
D-F: Three pacemaker cells, depolarizing current pulse of 1.2 nA markedly increases rate of firing (D), whereas hyperpolarizing pulses slow the frequency (E, 0.6 nA) or cause cessation of firing (F, 1.2 nA).
G-I: Quiescent cells can be induced to fire during depolarization current pulses (1.4 nA in G and 0.2 nA in H), or at the termination of hyperpolarizing current pulses (I, 2 nA).
J-L: Recordings from an isolated single cell in culture which was quiescent and had a very low resting potential. Hyperpolarizing current pulses of 0.2 and 0.4 nA (J), 0.8 nA (K), and 0.9 nA (L) elicited anodal break responses as well as spontaneous firing during the pulse (J-K); the frequency of firing during the pulse was a function of the degree of hyperpolarization, indicating true pacemaker behavior. (Modified from Sperelakis and Lehmkuhl, 1966 and Pappano and Sperelakis, 1969.)

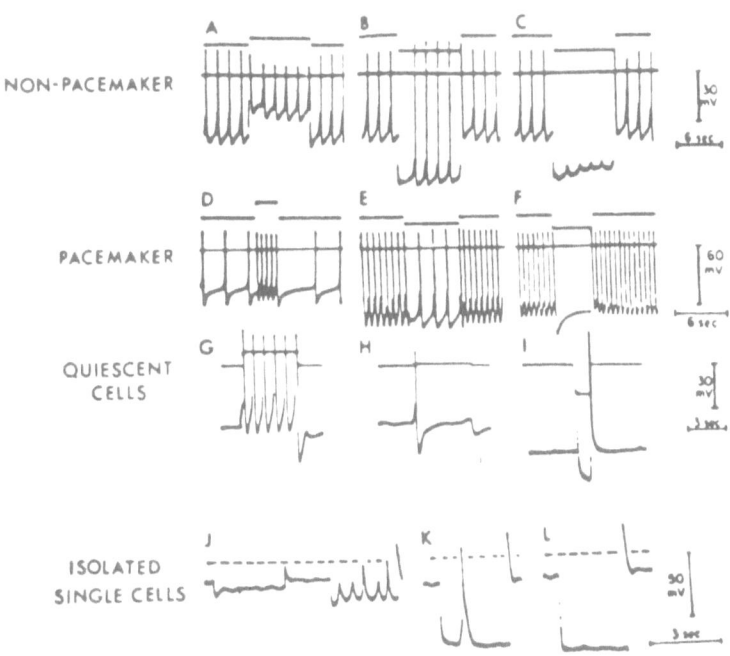

decrease in firing frequency (Fig. 6 D-F). There is an absence of junctional potentials when firing is abolished (Fig. 6 F). The slope of the pacemaker potential is a function of E_m.

Some quiescent cells can be induced to exhibit trains of action potentials during application of long-duration depolarizing pulses (Fig. 6 G-H), and anodal-break excitation can be elicited by brief hyperpolarizing pulses (Fig. 6 I). Some cells possessing automaticity function as latent pacemakers in that they are driven by true pacemaker cells which have greater intrinsic firing rates.

The action of Ba^{++} ion, an agent that greatly depresses P_K (Sperelakis and Lehmkuhl, 1966; Sperelakis et al., 1967), on the induction of automaticity in quiescent cells is illustrated in Fig. 7 A-C. The marked depolarization produced by Ba^{++} is shown in Fig. 7 A-B and D-E. When the cells are excessively depolarized by Ba^{++}, and therefore quiescent, the application of hyperpolarizing current pulses to return E_m close to the resting level allows the spontaneous production of large action potentials during the pulse (Fig. 7 F). The frequency and magnitude of the action potentials so produced is a function of the level to which the membrane has been artificially repolarized.

2. SPHERICAL REAGGREGATE CULTURES

Cells with highly differentiated electrophysiological properties can be obtained following trypsinization (in solutions containing elevated K^+ and ATP) and subsequent reaggregation in vitro to form small spheres (0.05 to 0.4 mm in diameter) (McLean and Sperelakis, 1976). (Reaggregation is achieved either by gyrotation for 24-48 hr or by plating the cells on cellophane to which they adhere poorly.) Action potentials recorded from cells in such reaggregates possess rapid rates of rise (up to 200 V/s) and fire from high stable resting potentials (about -80 mV), and TTX completely abolishes all excitability (Fig. 5 G-H). These action potentials are indistinguishable from those of the intact 16-day ventricle (Fig. 5 A-B). As in the case of the intact old embryonic or adult hearts, positive inotropic agents induce slowly-rising action potentials following blockade of the fast Na^+ channels with TTX (Freer et al., 1976; Josephson et al., 1976; McLean and Sperelakis, 1976; Vogel et al., 1977). However, not all such reaggregates consist of highly differentiated cells, i.e., some contain reverted cells.

FIGURE 7 *Effects of Ba^{++} amd Sr^{++} on reverted heart cells in monolayer culture. In a quiescent cell, Ba_{++} (5 mM) depolarized and induced spontaneous firing: A: Two successive sweeps superimposed at 20 s after addition of Ba^{++} showing onset of depolarization and oscillations. B: After 3 min, the action potentials acquired prolonged plateaus with repetitive discharges on the plateau. C: At 5 min, sustained depolarization occured with repetitive action potentials. In a firing cell (D), Ba^{++} (7 mM) rapidly depolarized and increased membrane resistance (E); repolarizing current pulse (1.2 nA) applied during te sustained depolarization initiated action potentials during the pulse (F). In a quiescent cell (G), 10 mM Sr^{++} produced hyperpolarization and converted the cell to a true pacemaker (H), as evidenced by cessation of firing during applied hyperpolarizing pulses of 4.8 nA. Elevation of Sr^{++} to 19 mM (I) induced sinusoidal-like oscillations with several action potentials superimposed and produced prominent depolarizing afterpotentials; current pulse of 6.0 nA applied. (Modified from Sperelakis and Lehmkuhl, 1966.)*

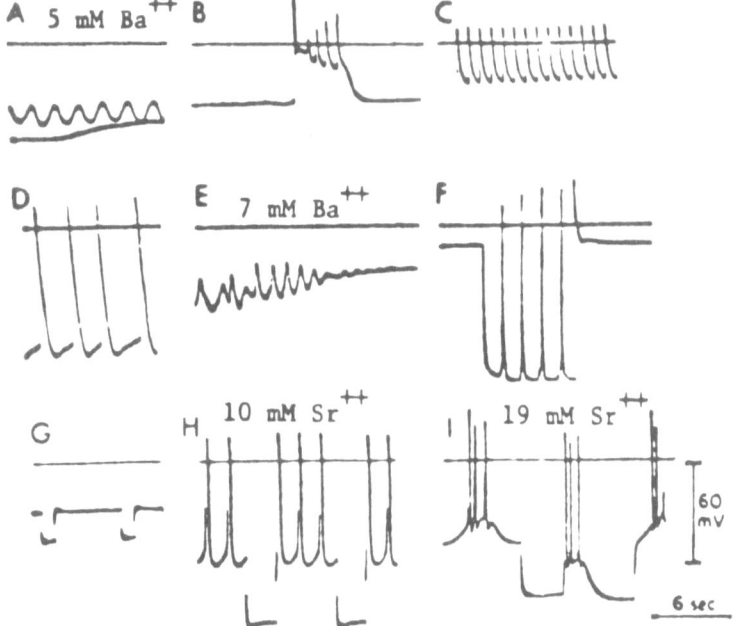

Acetylcholine did not affect the action potential duration of the cultured ventricular cells cultured either as monolayers or as reaggregates (Sperelakis and Lehmkuhl, 1965; McLean and Sperelakis, 1976).

When reaggregates are prepared from young (2-3-day-old) embryonic hearts the cells retain electrical activity characteristic of the young heart, i.e., the cells have low resting potentials, and they fire spontaneous slowly-rising action potentials, which are unaffected by TTX (McLean et al., 1976) (cf. DeHaan et al., 1976). However, as observed with the young organ-cultured hearts, the addition of RNA-enriched extracts induces differentiation, namely the appearance of rapidly-rising (e.g., 100 V/s) TTX-sensitive action potentials which fire from high stable resting potentials (-70 to -80 mV) (McLean et al., 1976, 1977).

Many cells in reverted reaggregates (ventricular cells) were found to be electrically coupled, whereas no evidence of low-resistance connections was obtained in the highly differentiated reaggregates (McLean and Sperelakis, 1980). In reverted reaggregates, automaticity of the entire reaggregate is suppressed by small hyperpolarizing current pulses. These results suggest that the degree of electrotonic interaction among the cells is a function of the state of differentiation.

Shrier and Clay (1980) employed a two-microelectrode voltage clamp technique to investigate the pacemaker current (I_p) from cultured reaggregates prepared from 7, 12, and 17-day-old chick embryo ventricles. The reversal potentials for I_p indicated that it is a pure K^+ current. The intensity of the pacemaker current was markedly reduced by day 17, and this reduction paralleled the decline of spontaneous activity in these preparations. Shrier and Clay (1980) suggested that the diminished magnitude of I_p during development is one factor in the decline of automaticity in ventricular cells, and that an additional factor could be a diminished inward background current (time-independent).

SIMILARITY BETWEEN UNDIFFERENTIATED MYOCARDIAL CELLS AND ADULT NODAL CELLS

In isolated rabbit SA node, electrotonic potentials could not be detected at a recording microelectrode 50-100 μm away from a current-injecting microelectrode, but when the nodal preparation was pared down to a 0.3 mm length, then the point source of current was effective in polarizing the preparation uniformly, suggesting that the cells became electrotonically coupled (Irisawa, 1978). Using this truncated rabbit SA node preparation, Irisawa (1978) characterized the ionic currents by a two-microelectrode voltage clamp method. Depolarizing clamps, from a holding potential of -35 mV, elicited a transient inward current whose threshold was 3-5 mV positive to the holding potential and had a rise time to peak of 10-20 ms. The peak current density was 13 $\mu A/cm^2$, consistent with a rate of rise of 5 V/s for the nodal action potential (assumed specific capacitance of 2.5×10^{-6} F/cm^2). The slow inward current was TTX-insensitive but was reduced by D-600, and disappeared in Na^+-free solution. Li^+ ions could not substitute for Na^+ ions as carrier of the slow current (Goto and Irisawa, 1977). Variations in $[Ca]_o$, although not affecting the $+\dot{V}_{max}$ of the nodal action potential, did increase its amplitude (Noma and Irisawa, 1974). In summary, the nodal action potential is generated by an influx of Na^+ ions, possibly through a selective slow Na^+ channel, similar to that observed in the young embryonic chick heart.

At holding potentials that were greater than -50 mV, an early and more rapid component of inward current was found that was sensitive to TTX (Noma et al., 1977). Although this indicates that the SA nodal cells contain some fast Na^+ channels, these channels probably inactivate during the pacemaker potential, and hence may not play a role in the nodal action potential.

SUMMARY AND CONCLUSIONS

This article summarizes some of the facts and hypotheses dealing with automaticity in embryonic myocardial cells. All cells in the young embryonic tubular hearts possess automaticity, but the degree of automaticity varies among regions of the heart. Automaticity and spontaneous action potential discharge even occurs in the presumptive cardiac areas of the early blastoderm stage. During development, the degree of automaticity diminishes in the myocardial cells, concomitant with an increase in resting potential. The old embryonic and adult ventricular myocardial cells are normally quiescent (non automatic). However, even these differentiated cells can become automatic if depolarized experimentally to levels that support automaticity or partially depolarized under pathological conditions. Although the origin of the SA and AV nodal cells is not fully known, they may arise from special groups of cells in the early embryonic heart that fail to differentiate further, and thus retain their relatively un-differentiated characteristics.

The most important single factor that changes during development and controls the degree of automaticity is P_K. The young tubular hearts (2-3 days old) have a resting potential of about -50 mV, even though $[K]_i$ is nearly as high as the adult value. The low resting potential is caused by a low P_K. The low P_K (coupled with the naturally low P_{Cl} of heart cells) can also account for the high degree of automaticity observed in the myocardial cells of the young embryonic heart. P_K increases rapidly during development, nearly attaining the final adult value by day 12; the resting potential increases to about -80 mV, and automaticity of the ventricular cells is suppressed.

The young heart has a low (Na, K)-ATPase activity, and this enzyme activity increases during development. The basal cyclic AMP level is high in young hearts and decreases during development. The elevation in the cyclic AMP level by isoproterenol is much greater in young 4-day-old heart than in older hearts. Therefore, functional beta-adrenergic receptors are present prior to innervation.

The young 2-3-day-old hearts have slow-rising action potentials (10-40 V/s) which are dependent mainly on $[Na]_o$ and TTX has little or no effect on them; hyperpolarization does not greatly increase $+\dot{V}_{max}$. Thus, fast Na^+ channels are absent or relatively few in number in young hearts, the inward current during the action potential being carried predominantly through slow Na^+ channels. (Young embryonic rat hearts also fire slowly-rising TTX-insensitive action potentials, but the slow channels are predominantly of the slow Ca^{++} type.) The slow Na^+ channels are blocked by verapamil, but not by 1 mM Mn^{++} (Mn^{++} does block the contractions). In some respects, the electrical properties of the young tubular hearts are similar to those of vascular smooth muscle.

There is a progressive increase in $+\dot{V}_{max}$ during development. By day 5, $+\dot{V}_{max}$ is about 50-80 V/s, and TTX reduces $+\dot{V}_{max}$ to 10-20 V/s, i.e., close to the value observed in day 2 hearts. Thus, the TTX-sensitive fast Na^+ channels progressively increase in number until they attain the final adult level by day 18. Between day 5 and day 7, fast Na^+ channels and a high density of slow Na^+ channels coexist. After day 8, TTX usually completely abolishes excitability, suggesting that the number of functional slow channels have decreased sufficiently so as to not support regenerative excitation. But positive inotropic agents that elevate cyclic AMP can increase the number of available slow channels.

Young (day 2-3) embryonic chick hearts placed into organ culture for two weeks do not gain fast Na^+ channels and they retain their automaticity and low resting potential. If, however, such hearts are exposed to an RNA-enriched fraction obtained from adult chicken hearts, they do gain TTX-sensitive fast Na^+ channels, develop greater resting potentials, and lose their automaticity. Trypsin-dispersed myocardial cells obtained from young hearts and placed in cell culture for several weeks also do not proceed with differentiation in vitro, unless exposed to the RNA extract.

Cultured heart cells prepared from old embryonic heart (ventricles) and allowed to form monolayers, rapidly revert back to the young embryonic state. That is, they lose most or all of their fast Na^+ channels, gain slow Na^+ channels, and gain automaticity because of a low P_K. If, however, the cells are allowed to reaggregate into small spheres, they often will regain highly differentiated electrical properties. The cultured heart cells retain their membrane receptors for catecholamines, histamine, angiotensin, and acetylcholine. Overdrive suppression of automaticity, related to stimulation of the electrogenic Na-K pump, can be demonstrated in young and old embryonic myocardial cells in culture.

Thus, ventricular myocardial cells in culture, that have reverted in electrical properties to the young embryonic state, may make a useful model system for nodal cells. Both types of cells have a low resting potential due to a low P_K and exhibit automaticity. Polarizing current pulses affect the frequency of firing in a similar manner, and neurotransmitters and other agents exert similar effects on their rhythmicity. Thus, undifferentiated myocardial cells, either in intact young hearts or in various types of culture, have many properties that are identical to those of nodal cells.

ACKNOWLEDGMENTS

The work of the author summarized and reviewed in this chapter was supported by a grant (HL-18711) from the National Institutes of Health. The author wishes to gratefully acknowledge his colleagues who have participated in this work, including Dr. D. Lehmkuhl, Dr. A.J. Pappano, Dr. K. Shigenobu, Dr. M.J. McLean, Dr. J.-F. Renaud, Dr. J.A. Schneider, Dr. S. Vogel, Dr. L. Belardinelli, Dr. A. Pelleg, and Dr. I. Josephson.

REFERENCES

Anderson, R.H., Yen, H.S., Becker, A.E. and Gosling, J.A.: The development of the sinoatrial node. In: The Sinus Node. Structure, Function and Clinical Relevance, Bonke, F.I.M., ed., Martinus Nijhoff, The Hague, pp. 166-182, 1977.

Beeler, G.W. and Reuter, H.: Reconstruction of the action potential of ventricular myocardial fibres. J. Physiol. (London), 268: 177-210, 1977.

Bernard, C.: Establishment of ionic permeabilities of the myocardial membrane during embryonic development of the rat. In: Developmental and Physiological Correlates of Cardiac Muscle, Lieberman, M. and Sano, T., eds., Raven Press, New York, pp. 169-184, 1976.

Boethius, J. and Knutsson, E.: Resting membrane potential in chick muscle cells during ontogeny. J. Exp. Zool., 174: 281-286, 1970.

Bonke, F.I.M.: A general introduction about the current status of the electrophysiology of the sinus node. In: The Sinus Node. Structure, Function and Clinical Relevance, Bonke, F.I.M., ed., Martinus Nijhoff, The Hague, pp. 225-232, 1977.

Brooks, C.M. and Lu, H.: The Sinoatrial Pacemaker of the Heart, Thomas, C.C., ed., C.C.Thomas, Co., Springfield, 1972.

Cahn, R.D.: Developmental changes in embryonic enzyme patterns: the effect of oxidative substrates on lactic dehydrogenase in beating chick embryonic heart cell cultures. Devel. Biol., 9: 327-346, 1964.

Cardenas, J.M., Bandman, E. and Strohman, R.C.: Hybrid isozymes if pyruvate kinase appear during avian cardiac development. Biochem. and Biophys. Res. Comm., 80: 593-599, 1978.

Carmeliet, E., Horres, C.R., Lieberman, M. and Vereecke, J.S.: Developmental aspects of potassium flux and permeability of the embryonic chick heart. J. Physiol. (London), 254: 673-692, 1976.

Coraboeuf, E., LeDouarin, G. and Obrecht-Coutris, G.: Release of acetylcholine by chick embryo heart before innervation. J. Physiol. (London), 206: 383-395, 1970.

Couch, J.R., West, T.C. and Hoff, H.E.: Development of the action potential of the prenatal rat heart. Circ. Res., 24: 19-31, 1969.

DeHaan, R.L.: Differentiation of the atrio-ventricular conducting system of the heart. Circulation, 24: 458-470, 1961.

DeHaan, R.L.: The potassium-sensitivity of isolated embryonic heart cells increases with development. Devel. Biol., 23: 226-240, 1970.

DeHaan, R.L., McDonald, R.F. and Sachs, H.G.: Development of tetrodoxotin sensitivity of embryonic chick heart cells in vitro. In: Developmental and Physiological Correlates of Cardiac Muscle, Lieberman, M. and Sano T., eds., Raven Press, New York, pp. 158-168, 1976.

Deleze, J.: Possible reasons for drop of resting potential of mammalian heart preparations during hypothermia. Circ. Res., 8: 553-557, 1960.

Elsas, L.J., Wheeler, F.B., Danner, D.J. and DeHaan, R.L.: Amino acid transport by aggregates of cultured chicken heart cells (Effect of insulin), J. Biol. Chem., 250: 9381-9390, 1975.

Enemar, A., Flack, B. and Hakanson, R.: Observations on the appearance of norepinephrine in the sympathetic nervous system of the chick embryo. Devel. Biol., 11: 268-283, 1965.

Fine, I.H., Daplan, N.V. and Kuftinec, D.: Developmental changes of mammalian lactic dehydrogenases. Biochem., 4: 116-124, 1963.

Freer, R.J., Pappano, A.J., Peach, M.J., Bing, K.T., McLean, M.J., Vogel, S. and Sperelakis, N.: Mechanism for the positive inotropic effect of angiotensin II on isolated cardiac muscle. Circ. Res., 39: 178-183, 1976.

Galper, J.B. and Catteral, W.A.: Developmental changes in the sensitivity of embryonic heart cells to tetrodotoxin and D-600. Devel. Biol., 65: 216-227, 1978.

Girard, H.: Arterial pressure in the chick embryo.   Am.   J.   Physiol., 224:
    454-460, 1973.

Glitsch, H.G.: An effect of the electrogenic sodium pump on the membrane poten-
    tial in beating guinea-pig atria. Pfluegers Arch., 334: 169-180, 1973.

Goss, C.M.: The first contractions of the heart in rat embryos.   Anat.   Rec.,
    70: 505-524, 1938.

Goto, J. and Irisawa, H.: Effects of lithium ions on rabbit   sinoatrial   node
    cell. Japan Circ. J., 41: 749, Abst., 1977.

Guidotti, G., Kanemeishi, D. and Foa, P.P.: Chick embryo heart as a tool for
    studying cell permeability and insulin action. Am. J. Physiol., 201:
    863-868, 1961.

Guidotti, G., Loreti, L., Gaja, G. and Foa, P.P.: Glucose uptake in the devel-
    oping chick embryo heart. Amer. J. Physiol., 211: 981-987, 1966.

Harris, W., Days, R., Johnson, C., Finkelstein, I., Stallworth, J. and Hubert,
    C.: Studies on avian heart pyruvate kinase during development. Biochem.
    Biophys. Res. Commun., 75: 1117-1121, 1977.

Harsch, M. and Green, J.W.: Electrolyte analyses of chick embryonic fluids and
    heart tissues. J. Cell. Comp. Physiol., 62: 319-326, 1963.

Hibbs, R.G.: Electron microscopy of developing cardiac muscle in chick embryos.
    Am. J. Anat., 99: 17-52, 1956.

Ignarro, L.J. and Shideman, F.E.: Catechol-o-methyl transferase and monoamine
    oxidase activities in the heart and liver of the embryonic and developing
    chick. J. Pharmacol. Ex. Ther., 159: 29-37, 1968.

Irisawa, H.: Comparative physiology of the cardiac pacemaker mechanism.
    Physiol. Rev., 58: 461-498, 1978.

Isenberg, G. and Trautwein, W.: The effect of dihydroouabain and lithium ions
    on the outward current in cardiac Purkinje fibers: evidence for electro-
    genicity of active transport. Pfluegers Arch., 350: 41-54, 1974.

Ishima, Y.: The effect of tetrodoxotin and sodium substitution on the   action
    potential in the course of development of the embryonic chicken heart.
    Proc. of Jap. Acad., 44: 170-175, 1978.

James, T.N.: Cardiac conduction system: fetal and postnatal development.
    Amer. J. Cardiol., 25: 213-226, 1970.

Jongsma, H.J., Masson-Pevet, M. and DeBruyne, J.: Synchronization of the beat-
    ing frequency of cultured rat heart cells. In: Developmental and Physio-

logical Correlates of Cardiac Muscle, Lieberman, M.   and Sano T., eds.,
Raven Press, New York, pp. 185-196, 1975.

Josephson, I., Renaud, J-F., Vogel, S., McLean, M.   and Sperelakis, N.:
Mechanism of the histamine-induced positive inotropic action in cardiac
muscle. Europ. J. Pharmacol., 35: 393-398, 1967.

Kasuya, Y., Matsuki, N. and Shigenobu, K.: Changes in sensitivity to anoxia of
the cardiac action potential plateau during chick embryonic development.
Devel. Biol., 58: 124-133, 1977.

Katzung, B.G.: Electrically induced automaticity in ventricular myocardium.
Life Sci., 14: 1133-1140, 1974.

Katzung, B.G.: Effects of extracellular calcium and sodium on
depolarization-induced automaticity in guinea pig papillary muscle. Circ.
Res., 37: 118-127, 1975.

Kutchai, H., King, S.L., Martin, M. and Daves, E.D.: Glucose uptake by chicken
embryo hearts at various stages of development. Devel. Biol., 55:
92-102, 1977.

LeDouarin, G., Obrecht, G. and Coraboeuf, E.: Determinations regionales dans
l'air cardiaque presomptive mises en evidence chez l'embryon de poulet par
la methode microelectrophysiologique. J. Embryol. Exp. Morph., 15:
153-167, 1966.

Lieberman, M., Horres, C.R., Aiton, J.F. and Johnson, E.A.: Active transport
and electrogenicity of cardiac muscle in tissue culture. XXVIIth Proc. of
Internat. Cong. of Physiol. Sci. (Paris), 13: 446, 1977.

Loeffelholz, K. and Pappano, A.J.: Ontogenetic changes in the pacemaker activity in chick heart. Life Sci., 14: 1755-1763, 1974.

Lu, H., Lange, G. and Brooks, C.M.: Factors controlling pacemaker action in
cells of the sinoatrial node. Circ. Res., 17: 460-471, 1965.

McDonald, T.F. and DeHaan, R.L.: Ion levels and membrane potential in chick
heart tissue and cultured cells. J. Gen. Physiol., 61: 89-109, 1973.

McDonald, T.F. and Sachs, H.G.: Electrical activity in embryonic heart cell
aggregates (Developmental aspects). Pfluegers Arch., 354: 151-164, 1975.

McDonald, T.F., Sachs, H.G. and DeHaan, R.L.: Development of sensitivity to
tetrodotoxin in beating chick embryo hearts, single cells, and aggregates.
Science, L76: 1248-1250, 1972.

McLean, M.J. and Sperelakis, N.: Rapid loss of sensitivity to tetrodotoxin of chick ventricular myocardial cells after separation from the heart. Exp. Cell Res., 86: 351-364, 1974.

McLean, M.J. and Sperelakis, N.: Differences in degree of electrotonic inter- action between highly differentiated and reverted cultured heart cell reag- gregates. J. Memb. Biol., (in press), 1980.

McLean, M.J. and Sperelakis, N.: Retention of fully differentiated electrophy- siological properties of chick embryonic heart cells in culture. Devel. Biol., 50: 134-142, 1976.

McLean, M.J., Lapsley, R.A., Shigenobu, K., Murad, R. and Sperelakis, N.: High cyclic AMP levels in young chick embryonic hearts. Devel. Biol., 42: 196-201, 1975.

McLean, M.J., Pelleg, A. and Sperelakis, N.: Electrophysiological recordings from spontaneously contracting reaggregates of cultured smooth muscle cells from guinea pig vas deferens. J. Cell Biol., 80: 539-552, 1979.

McLean, M.J., Renaud, J-F. and Sperelakis, N.: Cardiac-like action potentials recorded from spontaneously-contracting structures induced in post-nodal pieces of chick blastoderm exposed to an RNA-enriched fraction from adult heart. Differentiation, 11: 13-17, 1978.

McLean, M.J., Renaud, J-F., Sperelakis, N. and Niu, M.C.: RNA induction of fast Na^+ channels in cultured cardiac myoblasts. Science, 191: 297-299, 1976.

McLean, M.J., Renaud, J-F., Niu, M.C. and Sperelakis, N.: Membrane differenti- ation of cardiac myoblasts induced in vitro by an RNA-enriched fraction from adult heart. Exp. Cell Res.,110: 1-14, 1977.

Nathan, R.D. and DeHaan, R.L.: **In vitro** differentiation of a fast Na^+ con- ductance in embryonic heart cell aggregates. Proc. of Nat'l. Acad. Sci., 75: 2776-2780, 1978.

Niu, M.C. and Deshpande, A.K.: The development of tubular heart in RNA-treated post-nodal pieces of chick blastoderm. J. Embryol. Exp. Morphol., 29: 485-501, 1973.

Noma, A. and Irisawa, H.: The effect of sodium ion on the initial phase of the sinoatrial pacemaker action potentials in rabbits. Japan. J. Physiol., 24: 617-632, 1974.

Noma, A. and Irisawa, H.: Contribution of an electrogenic sodium pump to the membrane potential in rabbit sinoatrial node cells. Pfluegers Arch., 358:

289-301, 1975.

Noma, A., Yanagihara, K. and Irisawa, H.: Inward current of the rabbit sinoatrial node cell. Pfluegers Arch., 372: 43-51, 1977.

Page, E. and Storm, S.R.: Cat heart muscle in vitro. Active transport of
sodium in papillary muscles. J. Gen. Physiol., 48: 957-972, 1965.

Pappano, A.J.: Calcium-dependent action potentials produced by catecholamines
in guinea pig atrial muscle fibers. Circ. Res., 27: 379-390, 1970.

Pappano, A.J.: Sodium-dependent depolarization of non-innervated embryonic
chick heart by acetylcholine. J. Pharmacol. Exp. Ther., 180: 340-350,
1972.

Pappano, A.J.: Development of autonomic neuroeffector transmission in the chick
embryo heart. In: Developmental and Physiological Correlates of Cardiac
Muscle, Lieberman, M. and Sano, T., eds., Raven Press, New York, pp.
235-248, 1976.

Pappano, A.J. and Sperelakis, N.: Low K^+ conductance and low resting potentials of isolated single cultured heart cells. Am. J. Physiol., 217:
1076-1082, 1969.

Pelleg, A., Vogel, S., Belardinelli, L. and Sperelakis, N.: Overdrive suppression of automaticity in cultured chick myocardial cells. Amer. J.
Physiol., 238: H24-H30, 1980.

Renaud, D.: Etude electrophysiologique de la differentiation cardiaque chez
l'embryon de poulet. Thesis Univ. of Nantes, 1973.

Renaud, J-F. and Sperelakis, N.: Electrophysiological properties of chick embryonic hearts grafted and organ cultured in vitro. J. Mol. Cell.
Cardiol., 8: 889-900, 1976.

Renaud, J-F., Sperelakis, N. and LeDouarin, G.: Increase of cyclic AMP levels
induced by isoproterenol in cultured and non-cultured chick embryonic
hearts. J. Mol. Cell. Cardiol., 10: 281-286, 1978.

Romanoff, A.: The Avian Embryo, Structure and Functional Development, Macmillan
Press, New York, 1960.

Seltzer, J.L. and McDougal, D.B.: Enzyme levels in chick embryo heart and
brain from 1 to 21 days of development. Devel. Biol., 42: 95-105, 1975.

Shigenobu, K. and Sperelakis, N.: Development of sensitivity to tetrodotoxin
of chick embryonic hearts with age. J. Mol. Cell. Cardiol., 3:
271-286, 1971.

Shigenobu, K. and Sperelakis, N.: Ca^{++} current channels induced by catecholamines in chick embryonic hearts whose fast Na^+ channels are blocked by tetrodotoxin or elevated K^+. Circ. Res., 31: 932-952, 1972.

Shigenobu, K. and Sperelakis, N.: Failure of development of fast Na^+ channels during organ culture of young embryonic chick hearts. Devel. Biol., 39: 326-330, 1974.

Shigenobu, K., Schneider, J.A. and Sperelakis, N.: Blockade of slow Na^+ and Ca^{++} currents in myocardial cells by verapamil. J. Pharmacol. Exp. Ther., 190: 280-288, 1974.

Shimizu, Y. and Tasaki, K.: Electrical excitability of developing cardiac muscle in chick embryos. Tohuku J. Exp. Med., 88: 49-56, 1966.

Shrier, A. and Clay, J.R.: Low K^+ conductance and low resting potentials of isolated single cultured heart cells. Nature, 283: 670-671, 1980.

Sperelakis, N.: Electrophysiology of cultured chick heart cells. In: Electrophysiology and Ultrastructure of the Heart, Sano, T., Mizuhira, V. and Matsuda, K., eds., Bunkodo Co., Ltd., Tokyo, pp. 81-108, 1967.

Sperelakis, N.: Na^+, K^+-ATPase activity of embryonic chick heart and skeletal muscles as a function of age. Biochim. Biophys. Acta, 266: 230-237, 1972.

Sperelakis, N.: Origin of the cardiac resting potential. In: Handbook of Physiology, the Cardiovascular System, Vol. 1, Berne, R.M. and Sperelakis, N., eds., Am. Physiol. Soc., Bethesda, pp. 187-267, 1979.

Sperelakis, N. and Lee, E.E.: Characterization of (Na^+,K^+)-ATPase isolated from embryonic chick hearts and cultured chick heart cells. Biochim. Biophys. Acta, 233: 562-579, 1971.

Sperelakis, N. and Lehmkuhl, D.: Effect of current on transmembrane potentials in cultured chick heart cells. J. Gen. Physiol., 47: 895-927, 1964.

Sperelakis, N. and Lehmkuhl, D.: Insensitivity of cultured chick heart cells to autonomic agents and tetrodotoxin. Am. J. Physiol., 209: 693-698, 1965.

Sperelakis, N. and Lehmkuhl, D.: Ionic interconversion of pacemaker and nonpacemaker cultured chick heart cells. J. Gen. Physiol., 49: 867-895, 1966.

Sperelakis, N. and Lehmkuhl, D.: Effects of temperature and metabolic poisons on membrane potentials of cultured heart cells. Am. J. Physiol., 213:

719-724, 1967.

Sperelakis, N. and McLean, M.J.: The electrical properties of embryonic chick cardiac cells. In: Fetal and Newborn Cardiovascular Physiology, Vol. 1, Longo, L.D. and Renaud, D.D., eds., Garland Press, New York, pp. 191-236, 1978.

Sperelakis, N. and Shigenobu, K.: Changes in membrane properties of chick embryonic hearts during development. J. Gen. Physiol., 60: 430-453, 1972.

Sperelakis, N. and Shigenobu, K.: Organ-cultured embryonic hearts of various ages. Part I: Electrophysiology, J. Mol. Cell. Cardiol., 6: 449-471, 1974.

Sperelakis, N., Forbes, M. and Rubio, R.: The tubular systems of myocardial cells: ultrastructure and possible function. In: Recent Advances in Studies on Cardiac Structure and Metabolism, Vol. 4, Dhalla, N.S. and Rona, G., eds., University Park Press, Baltimore, pp. 163-194, 1974.

Sperelakis, N., Schneider, M.F. and Harris, E.J.: Decreased K^+ conductance produced by Ba^{++} in frog sartorius fibers. J. Gen. Physiol., 50: 1565-1583, 1967.

Sperelakis, N., Shigenobu, K. and McLean, M.J.: Membrane cation channels - changes in developing hearts, in cell culture and in organ culture. In: Developmental and Physiological Correlates of Cardiac Muscle, Lieberman, M. and Sano, T., eds., Raven Press, New York, pp. 209-234, 1976.

SECTION TWO

INTERACTION OF PACEMAKER CELLS

168

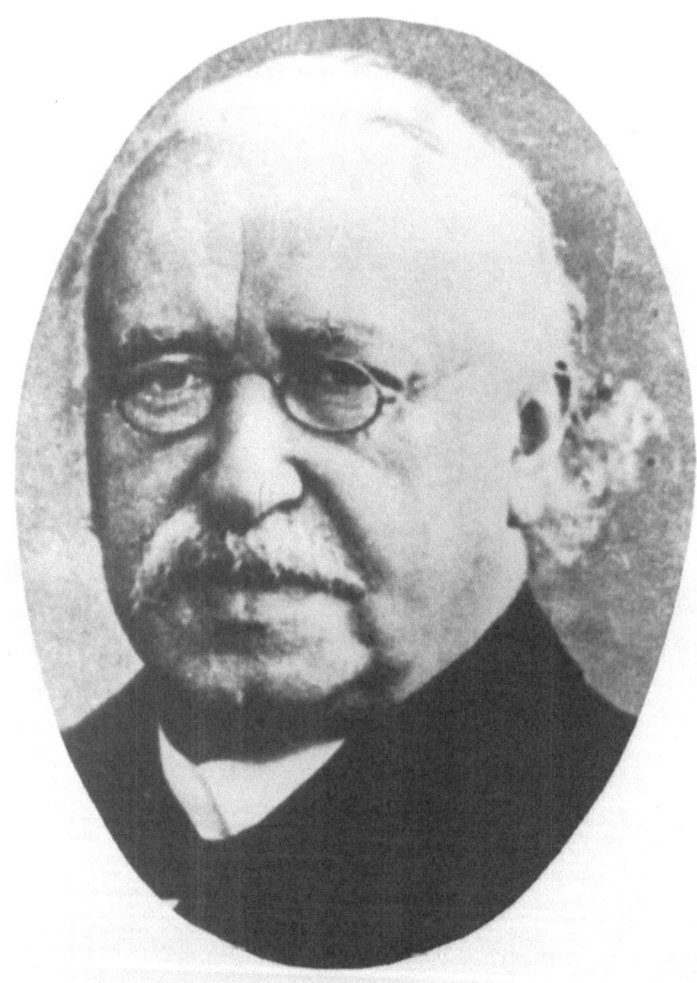

FIGURE 1 *Kingreen Helmut: Theodor Wilhelm Engelmann (1843-1909). Ein bedeu-tender deutscher Physiologe an der Schwelle zum 20. Jahrhundert. Med. Diss. Muenster, 1968.*

CELLULAR COMMUNICATION: INTRODUCTORY REMARKS

Silvio Weidmann

Theodor Wilhelm Engelmann (1843-1910), when working as an assistent to Franciscus Cornelius Donders in Utrecht, published several remarkable articles in "Pfluegers Archiv fuer die gesamte Physiologie des Menschen und der Thiere", got married to Donders' daughter and, in 1897, succeeded du Bois-Reymond to the chair of Physiology in Berlin (Rothschuh, 1953). One of these papers entitled "Ueber die Leitung der Erregung im Herzmuskel" (1875) describes morphological and functional similarities between heart and the ureter (Engelmann, 1869). Thus stimulation of any site would be followed by contraction of all other sites, wherever situated and however thin the connecting bridge. In a paper dated 1877 Engelmann gives a detailed report on the electrical changes following injury under one of two recording electrodes and concludes "Es gilt fuer die Kammermuskulatur dasselbe Gesetz wie fuer andere animale Zellketten (...): die einzelnen Zellen vermoegen sich zwar waehrend des Lebens den Erregungsvorgang durch Contakt mitzutheilen, sterben aber jede fuer sich ab". In a publication dated 1876 Engelman attempted to extend the general validity of his idea to single nerve fibres. His observations, to judge from the illustrations, are beyond question: A damaged nerve fibre, two days after injury, shows a process of decay (Entartungsprocess) which comes to a halt exactly at the nearest node of Ranvier, this being so for the central as well as for the peripheral stump. His comment that only those cells decay which have undergone direct damage is an example of what might happen if one is eager to formulate unifying theories. Having thus paid due respect to Dutch Physiology of the past century let us focus on heart and review work done in the 20th century.

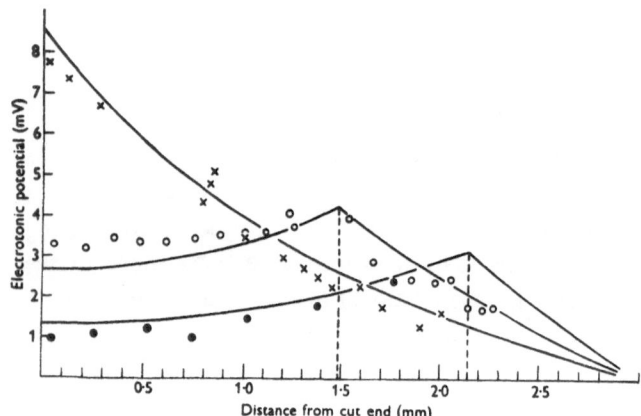

FIGURE 2. Spatial distribution of electrotonic potential within a single ungulate (kid) Purkinje fibre (Purkinje strand). Its diameter was 53 µm and there was no branching between the cut end (left) and a distance of 3.0 mm from the cut end. Forty-four impalements on the same fibre. Subthreshold current pulses were applied through a microelectrode positioned near the cut end (crosses), at a distance of 1.48 mm (open circles) and at a distance of 2.14 mm (closed circles) from the cut end. All 3 curves are fitted by assuming a space constant (λ) of 1.40 mm. Note that curves tend to be flat near the cut end, suggesting that the cable is terminated by a large resistance typical for "healing over" to be complete. From Weidmann (1952).

THE SPATIAL DISTRIBUTION OF ELECTROTONIC POTENTIALS

Cardiac cells are of the order of 100 µm in length and 10 µm in diameter. An answer to the question "high vs. low resistance cell contacts" is obtained from the method of "cable analysis". In a strand of cells, e.g. a Purkinje fibre, subthreshold current steps can be introduced through a first intracellular electrode, and changes of membrane potential can be recorded at various distances from the first by means of a second microelectrode. Plots of electrotonic potentials vs. distance (Fig. 2) indicate that the so-called space constant (λ) of the cable (distance over which the amplitude of the electrotonic potential falls by a factor of e) is of the order of one mm, i.e. many times the length of a single cell. Similar results have been reported for ventricular trabeculae of dog, calf, sheep and frog (Kamiyama and Matsuda, 1966; Weidmann, 1970; Chapman and Fry, 1978), for rabbit crista terminalis (Bonke, 1973a), for rabbit sinoatrial node (Bonke, 1973b; Bukauskas et al., 1977), for rabbit atrioventricular node (De Mello, 1977) and for "artificial cables" from tissue culture cells (Lieberman et al., 1975).

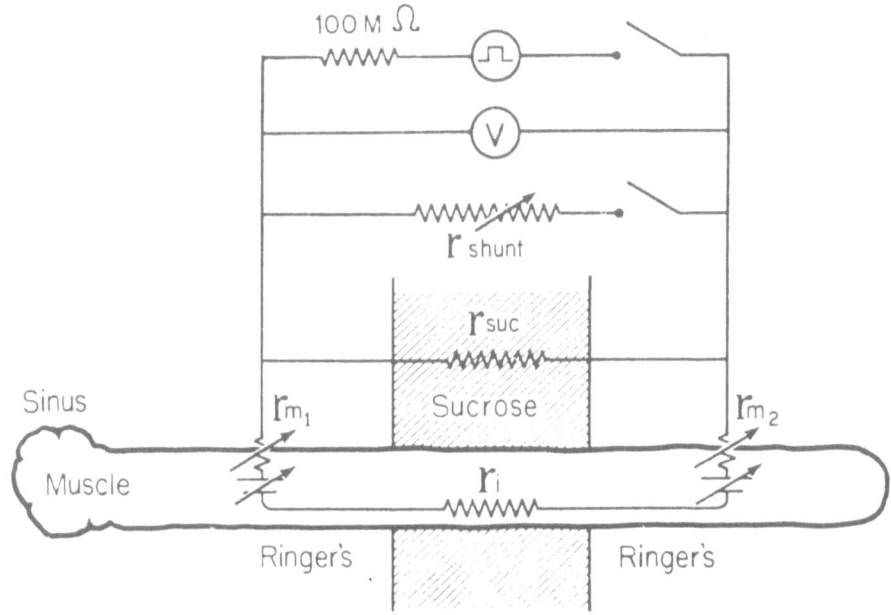

FIGURE 3 *Atrial trabecula of the frog with its central part being washed by ion-free sucrose. There is no conduction of the impulse from left to right in the absence of a shunt resistance. However, when the shunt resistance is decreased below a critical value, the impulse jumps from Ringer pool to Ringer pool. From Barr, Dewey and Berger (1965).*

EXTRA- AND INTRACELLULAR CONDUCTANCE AS A PREREQUISITE FOR IMPULSE PROPAGATION

Impulse propagation by "local circuits" (Hermann, 1879) necessitates a low electrical resistance of both the intracellular and the extracellular pathway. If either of these resistances is artificially increased, propagation in a frog atrial trabecula is blocked (Barr et al., 1965). The extracellular resistance is conveniently increased by exposing part of the trabecula to isotonic sucrose

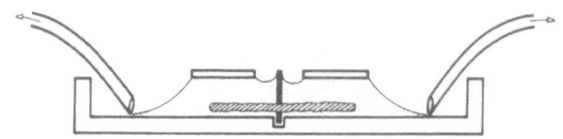

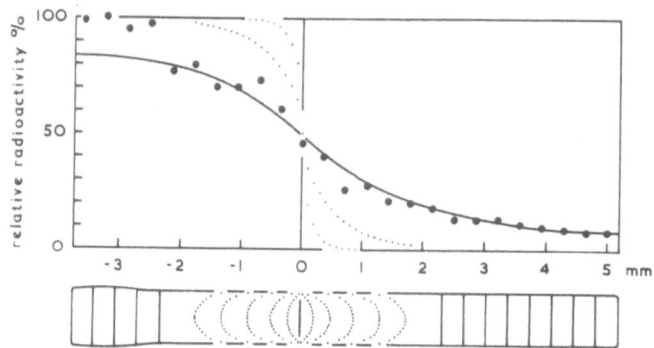

FIGURE 4 *Top: Ventricular trabecula pulled through a tight-fitting hole. Middle: Radioactivity vs. distance from the partition, 6 hrs after the start of the experiment. The continuous line is based on cable equations (appendix by A.L. Hodgkin to Weidmann, 1966) and is drawn to give a reasonable fit. Steady-state diffusion and a space constant of 2 mm are assumed. A thickening of the preparation near the left-hand end (bottom drawing) had been noted and accounts for the relatively high radioactivity in this part of the bundle. Radioactivity is seen to decrease to a finite value near the right-hand end, indicating the presence of a large barrier to the escape of ^{42}K (healing over). The dotted lines in the lowest graph give the expected admixture due to extracellular diffusion of ^{42}K and K, respectively (1/e, 1/10, 1/100, 1/1000 and 1/10000). When averaged over cross sections, the dotted values closer to the diaphragm (middle graph) are obtained for D-longitudinal = D-transverse, those further apart from the diaphragm for D-longitudinal = 10 x D-transverse. From Weidmann, 1966.*

solution (Fig. 3), resulting in conduction block. When the value of a resistor bridging the gap is gradually decreased, propagation is restored in an "all-or-nothing" way. This is in principle the "salt bridge experiment" first performed with the alga Nitella (Osterhout and Hill, 1930).

Hypertonic Ringer solution has been shown to block conduction of the impulse. If the experiment is performed with frog auricle, the effect is reversible. The ultrastructural picture shows wide extracellular clefts, and it must be speculated that the cell-to-cell pathway for current flow has risen above a critical value (Barr et al., 1965).

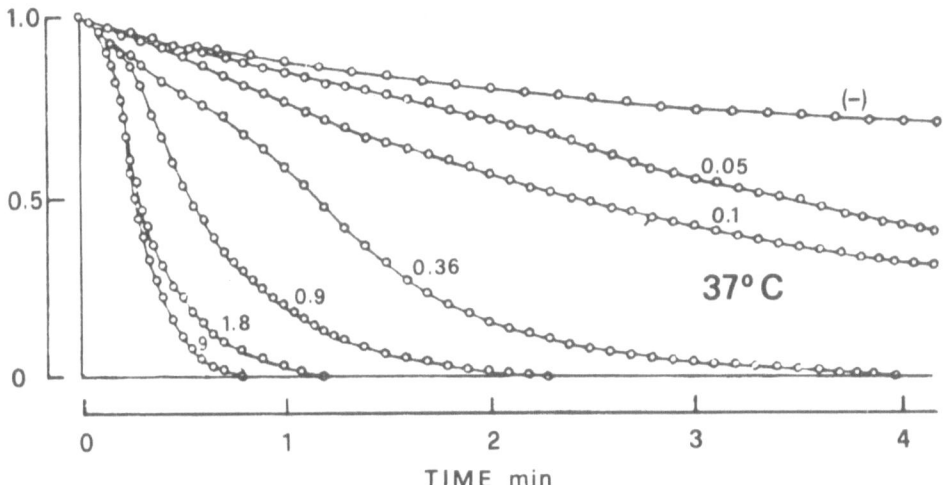

FIGURE 5 *The time course of healing over. A guinea pig's papillary muscle is cut in solutions containing various concentrations of Ca^{2+}, as indicated by the numbers (mM) near the curves. The data have been normalized, zero referring to the potential difference recorded (extracellularly) before cutting, 1.0 to the maximal potential drop observed as a result of cutting. Recovery takes a time of the order of one minute with normal Ca^{2+} but is extremely slow with Ca^{2+} nominally zero (-). From Nishiye, 1977.*

DIFFUSION OF ^{42}K FROM CELL TO CELL

The ion most important as a carrier of electrical charge within the intracellular compartment (K^+) has been shown to diffuse from cell to cell (Weidmann, 1966; Fig. 4). A bundle of fibres, less than 1 mm in diameter and 7-10 mm in length, is placed in a double chamber. One part is superfused with ^{42}K Tyrode solution (charging compartment), the other part continuously washed by non-radioactive Tyrode. At the end of several hours, when steady-state diffusion is reached, the bundle is rinsed with non-radioactive solution and frozen in liquid N_2. Slices of equal length are counted for radioactivity. The spatial distribution of ^{42}K, together with a knowledge of the influx and efflux rate constants, lead to the following results: (i) K^+ permeability of the intercalated disks separating adjoining cells is less than 1/5000 of K^+ permeability of the surface membrane, and (ii) the electrical resistance to the flow of K^+ current is 3 Ohm or less for one cm^2 of disk membrane.

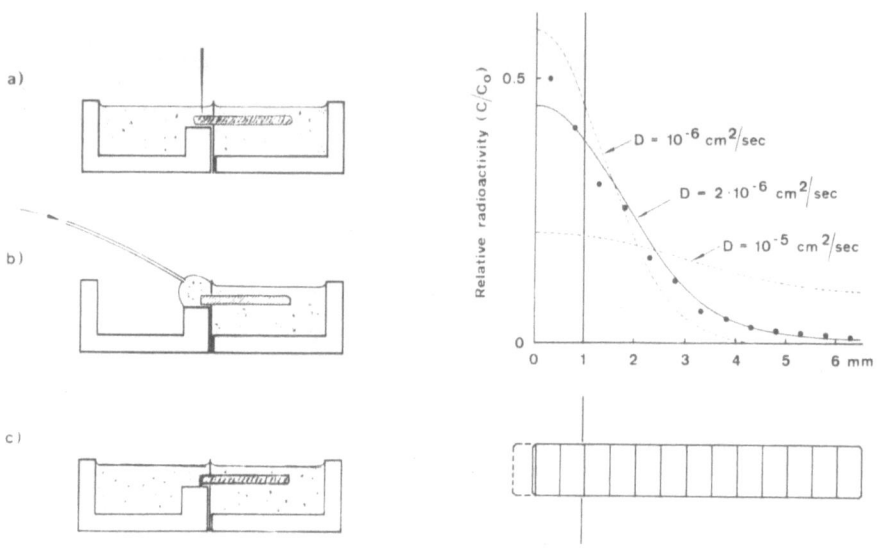

FIGURE 6 The cut-and-seal method. Left: A trabecula, pulled through a tight-fitting hole in a rubber membrane, is cut close to this membrane in Ca^{2+}-free solution. A droplet of Ca^{2+}-free Tyrode containing the tracer is brought into contact with the cut end. Sealing is achieved by circulating tracer-free and Ca^{2+}-containing solution. Right: Radioactivity (^{14}C of tetraethylammonium) plotted against distance. Diffusion in non-steady-state, 2 hrs after sealing. The best fit to the experimental values is obtained on the assumption of a diffusion coefficient of $D = 2 \times 10^{-6}$ cm^2/s. From Weingart, 1974.

DIFFUSION OF TRACER MOLECULES INTRODUCED BY A CUT-END METHOD

If a cardiac preparation is damaged by cutting, there will be a strong tendency for the surviving cells to isolate themselves from the damaged neighbours (Engelmann, 1875). Demarcation can be prevented by washing the preparation with Ca^{2+}-free solution (Déléze, 1970; Nishiye, 1977, Fig. 5). Use has been made of these observations to admix tracers to a Ca^{2+}-free bathing solution and to let them diffuse into the intracellular compartment. Subsequently, the preparation is "sealed" by a Ca^{2+}-containing, tracer-free solution. Longitudinal distribution down the concentration gradient now takes place during several hours. To set an end to tracer diffusion the preparation is frozen in liquid N_2. A block of razor blades, spaced 0.5 mm from one another, is used to obtain slices of equal dimensions. A plot of radioactivity (or fluorescence) vs. distance allows to calculate a diffusion coefficient for the tracer molecule (see Weingart, 1974; Fig. 6). So far, this method had yielded quantitative data for tetraethylammonium$^+$ (M.W. = 130; Weingart, 1974), cyclic AMP$^-$ (M.W. 328; Tsien and Weingart, 1976) and Procion Yellow^{3-} (M.W. = 697; Imanaga, 1974). There is a steep fall of diffusivity with increasing molecular weight by almost 3 orders of magnitude from TEA (M.W. 130) to Procion Yellow (M.W. = 697), and there is reason to assume (Imanaga, 1974) that the tracer Chicago Blue (M.W. about 1000) does not move from cell to cell. The diameter of (aequous?) pores connecting adjoining cells has been estimated at 1-1.5 nm (McNutt and Weinstein, 1973) while the largest molecule to pass, Procion Yellow, is an elongated structure measuring 0.5 x 1.0 x 2.7 nm. The molecular weights of many substances of importance in metabolism are within the range where cell-to-cell diffusion is expected to take place, thus the concept of the heart as a nutritional syncytium.

REFERENCES

Barr, L., Dewey, M.M. and Berger, W.: Propagation of action potentials and the structure of the nexus in cardiac muscle. J. Gen. Physiol., 48:

797-823, 1965.

Bonke, F.I.M.: Passive electrical properties of atrial fibers of the rabbit heart. Pfluegers Arch., 339: 1-15, 1973a.

Bonke, F.I.M.: Electrotonic spread in the sinoatrial node of the rabbit heart. Pfluegers Arch., 339: 17-23, 1973b.

Bukauskas, F.F., Veteikis, R.P., Gutman, A.M. and Mutskus, K.S.: Intercellular coupling in the sinus node of the rabbit heart. Biofizika, 22: 108-112, 1977.

Chapman, R.A. and Fry, C.H.: An analysis of the cable properties of frog ventricular myocardium. J. Physiol. (London), 283: 263-282, 1978.

Délèze, J.: The recovery of resting potential and input resistance in sheep heart injured by knife or laser. J. Physiol. (London), 208: 547-562, 1970.

De Mello, W.C.: Passive electrical properties of the atrioventricular node. Pfluegers Arch., 371: 135-139, 1977.

Engelmann, Th. W.: Zur Physiologie des Ureter. Pfluegers Arch., 2: 243-293, 1869.

Engelmann, Th. W.: Ueber die Leitung der Erregung im Herzmuskel. Pfluegers Arch., 2: 465-480, 1875.

Engelmann, Th. W.: Ueber Degeneration von Nervenfasern. Pfluegers Arch., 13: 474-491, 1876.

Engelmann, Th. W.: Vergleichende Untersuchungen zur Lehre von der Muskel- und Nervenelektricitaet. Pfluegers Arch., 15: 116-148, 1877.

Hermann, L.: Allgemeine Muskelphysiologie. In: Handbuch der Physiologie, Vol. 1, Vogel, Leipzig, 1879.

Imanaga, I.: Cell-to-cell diffusion of Procion Yellow in sheep and calf Purkinje fibers. J. Memb. Biol., 16: 381-388, 1974.

Kamiyama, A. and Matsuda, K.: Electrophysiological properties of the canine ventricular fiber. Jap. J. Physiol., 16: 407-420, 1966.

Lieberman, M., Sawanobori, T., Kootsey, J.M. and Johnson, E.A.: A synthetic strand of cardiac muscle. Its passive electrical properties. J. Gen. Physiol., 65: 527-550, 1975.

McNutt, N.S. and Weinstein, R.S.: Membrane ultrastructure at mammalian intercalated junctions. Progr. Biophys. Mol. Biol., 26: 45-101, 1973.

Nishiye, H.: The mechanism of Ca^{2+} action on the healing-over process in mammalian cardiac muscles: a kinetic analysis. Jap. J. Physiol., 27: 451-466, 1977.

Osterhout, W.J.V. and Hill, S.E.: Salt bridges and negative variations. J. Gen. Physiol., 13: 547-552, 1930.

Rothschuh, K.E.: Geschichte der Physiologie, Springer, Berlin-Goettingen-Heidelberg, 1953.

Tsien, R.W. and Weingart, R.: Inotropic effect of cyclic AMP in calf ventricular muscle studied by a cut end method. J. Physiol. (London), 260: 117-141, 1976.

Weidmann, S.: The electrical constants of Purkinje fibres. J. Physiol. (London), 118: 348-360, 1952.

Weidmann, S.: The diffusion of radiopotassium across intercalated disks of mammalian cardiac muscle. J. Physiol. (London), 187: 323-342, 1966.

Weidmann, S.: Electrical constants of trabecular muscle from mammalian heart. J. Physiol. (London), 210: 1041-1054, 1970.

Weingart, R.: The permeability to tetraethylammonium ions of the surface membrane and the intercalated disks of sheep and calf myocardium. J. Physiol. (London), 240: 741-762, 1974.

ON THE CONTROL OF CELL COMMUNICATION IN HEART

Walmor C. De Mello

There is extensive electrophysiological and electronmicroscopic evidence that heart cells are connected through low resistance channels (see, for instance, De Mello, 1977a).

Ions, such as potassium (Weidmann, 1966) and molecules - fluorescein (mol. wt. 320; Pollack, 1973; De Mello, 1979a), TEA (tetraethylammmonium, mol. wt. 130; see Weingart, 1974), Procion Yellow (mol. wt. 625 - see Imanaga, 1974) and Lucifer Yellow (mol. wt. 476 - De Mello, 1979b) flow from cell-to-cell through intercellular junctions.

The hydrophyllic channels between apposing cardiac cells constitute, therefore, an internal pathway, making feasible the metabolic cooperation and the ionic flow throughout the heart.

The synchronization of the heart beat, for instance, depends greatly on the preservation of high conductance gates between heart cells (DeHaan and Hirakow, 1972). How intercellular communication is controlled? Since intercellular junctions are not permanent structures but can be formed or disrupted according to the physiological needs of the tissue (Keeter et al., 1974), one might think that the spread of electrical current in heart fibres could be modified by variations on the number or permeability of the intercellular channels. No information is available, however, if intercellular junctions can be synthetized or destroyed on adult heart tissues. The permeability of the existing junctions, however, can be modulated.

When Ca ions are injected iontophoretically inside a cardiac Purkinje cell, the electrical coupling is gradually reduced leading to cell decoupling (De Mello, 1975 - see Fig. 1). Concurrently with the fall in cell communication, the input resistance of the injected cell is enhanced (see Fig. 1).

This effect of Ca, which is reversible, indicates that the junctional resistance can be gradually increased by incrementing the free $[Ca^{2+}]_i$. This rise

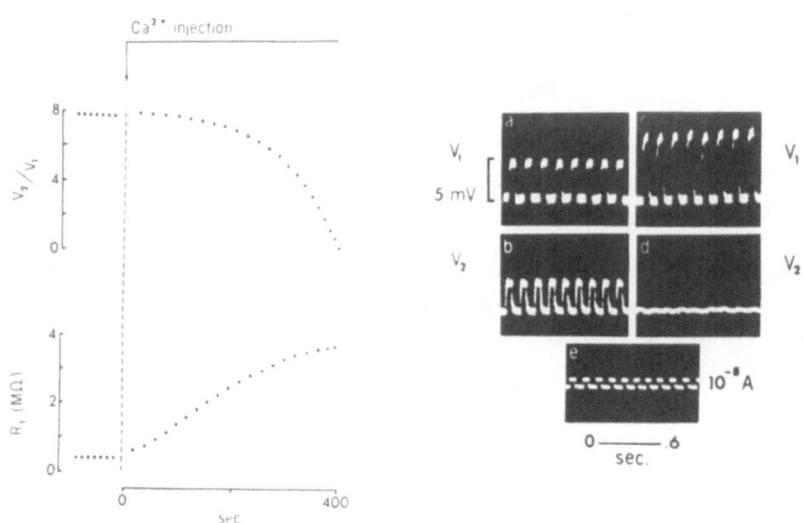

FIGURE 1 *Effect of intracellular Ca injection on the electrical coupling of Purkinje cells.*
At right - typical effect of intracellular Ca injection on the electrical coupling. a) and b) show V_1 and V_2 - control; c) and d) recorded after 410 s of Ca injection showing cell decoupling. e) outward current pulses (60 ms duration, 5 Hz, 10^{-8} A).
At left - influence of intracellular Ca injection on the coupling coefficient (V_2/V_1) and on input resistance (R_1) of Purkinje cells (average from 6 experiments). Temperature - $37^{\circ}C$.

in junctional resistance is probably related to a reduction in diameter or in the number of permeable channels.

The free $\left[Ca^{2+}\right]_i$ required to cause suppression of the electrical coupling is difficult to precise since part of the amount of Ca injected is taken by the sarcoplasmic reticulum, mitochondria or is extruded from the cell. The total amount of Ca injected can be calculated taking the transfer number of Ca as 0.32 (see Gorman and Herman, 1979). This amount is 1.5×10^{-13} moles (S.E. $\pm$ 0.45 - average from 8 experiments). Assuming a cell volume of 0.3×10^{-9} l, the approximate concentration of Ca inside the cell required to suppress the electrical coupling is about 10^{-4} M.

INFLUENCE OF THE INTRACELLULAR SODIUM CONCENTRATION
ON THE ELECTRICAL COUPLING OF HEART CELLS

It is known that the inward movement of Ca through the non-junctional membrane is sensitive to variations in $[Na^+]_i$ and that a small increase in $[NA^+]_i$ results in a substantial rise in free $[Ca^{2+}]_i$ (see Reuter and Seitz, 1968; Glitsch and Reuter, 1970).

In order to investigate the possible role of the Ca/Na transport on the process of cell-to-cell communication, I decided to inject Na ions into the cytosol of a heart cell and search for changes in coupling. Micropipettes filled with NaCl (1 M) were used to inject the ion electrophoretically into the cell.

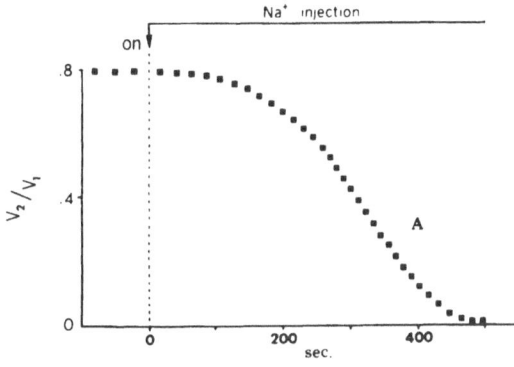

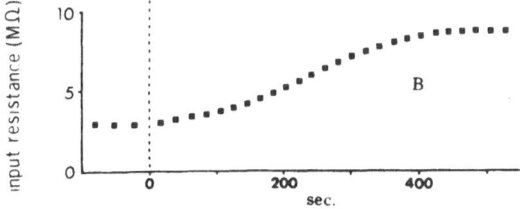

FIGURE 2 *Influence of intra-cellular Na injection on the electrical coupling and input resistance of Purkinje cells (average from 5 experiments).*

As it can be seen in Fig. 2 the increment of $[Na^+]_i$ elicited a decline in the electrical coupling and finally, a total decoupling is achieved (De Mello, 1974, 1976). The determination of the space constant and input resistance made possible to calculate the intracellular longitudinal resistance per unit length (r_a) and the membrane resistance per unit length (r_m). Table I shows that the intracellular Na injection enhanced r_a by 250% while r_m is reduced by 23%. Assuming that the rise in $\left[Na^+\right]_i$ is not altering the myoplasmic resistivity, one can conclude that the ion increased the junctional resistance. The abolishment of the electrical coupling by high $\left[Na^+\right]_i$ is totally reversible (see De Mello, 1976).

TABLE I

*EFFECT OF INTRACELLULAR SODIUM INJECTION ON INPUT RESISTANCE (R_o), SPACE CON-
STANT (λ), MEMBRANE RESISTANCE PER UNIT LENGTH (r_m) AND AXIAL RESISTANCE PER
UNIT LENGTH (r_a)

	R_o (x 10^6 Ω)		λ (mm)		r_m (kΩcm)		r_a (MΩ/cm)	
Fibre	Normal	After Na injection	Normal	After Na injection	Normal	After Na injection	Normal	After Na injection
1	2.5	5	1.3	0.5	650	500	38	200
2	3	4.3	1.4	0.58	840	498	40	140
3	2	6	1.6	0.51	640	600	25	230

*Values of R_o and λ were experimentally determined. Values of r_m and r_a were
calculated by equations $r_m = 2 R_o \lambda$; $r_a = 2 R_o / \lambda$.
+Determination of λ and R_o were made after 250-300 s of sodium injection. From
de Mello, 1976, with permission of Cambridge University Press.

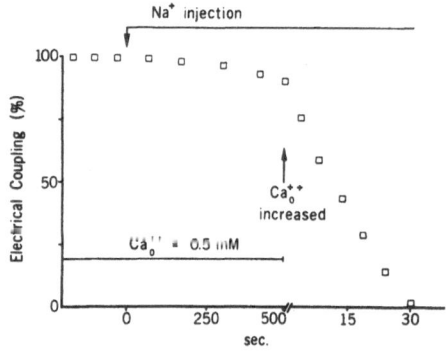

FIGURE 3 Effect of extracellular Ca concentration on the decoupling action of intracellular Na injection (average from 5 experiments). The normal coupling coefficient (V_2/V_1) was taken as 100%. Arrow, at right, indicates increase in $\left[Ca^{2+}\right]_o$. From De Mello, 1976, with permission of Cambridge University Press.

An activation of the Na/Ca exchange seems involved on the decoupling action of $\left[Na^+\right]_i$ because Na injection has a neglegible effect on the electrical coupling if the extracellular Ca concentration is kept low (see Fig. 3). The re-admission of Ca to the extracellular fluid elicit quick decoupling of the injected cell (Fig. 3).

These findings not only support the Ca hypothesis (De Mello, 1975;   Rose and Loewenstein, 1975), but also denote that the maintenance of a low $\left[Na^+\right]_i$ is vital for preservation of cell communication.

Studies performed on Purkinje fibres exposed to ouabain to inhibit the Na pump have shown that the glycoside increases the junctional resistance (De Mello, 1976; Weingart, 1977). More recent observations have shown that the cell-to-cell movement of Lucifer Yellow (mol. wt. 476) is also suppressed by ouabain (De Mello, 1979b;   1980a).

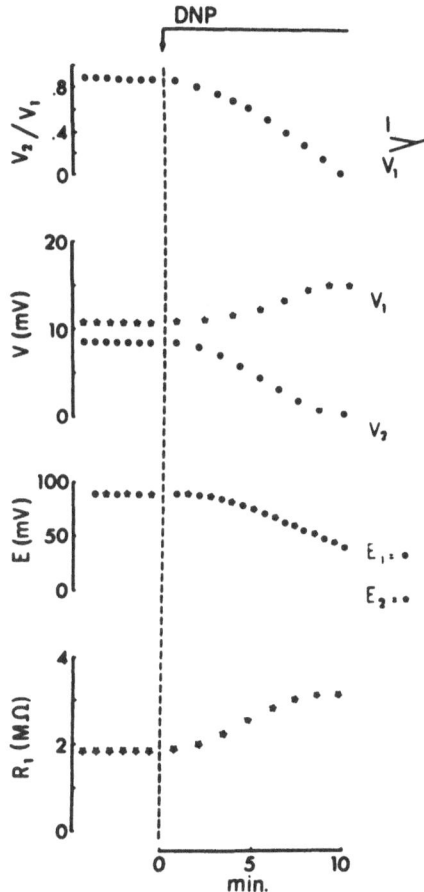

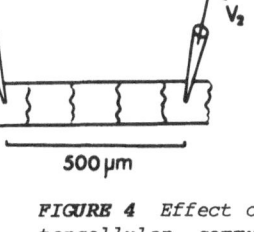

FIGURE 4 *Effect of DNP on intercellular communication in dog   Purkinje   fibre. Time-course of R_1 (input resistance of cell 1), V_1 and V_2 (changes in membrane potential in cells 1 and 2, respectively), E_1 and E_2 (membrane potentials of cells 1 and 2 at zero current taking as outside minus inside potential) and coupling coefficient (V_2/V_1). Arrow indicates start of treatment with DNP (0.5 mM). At right - drawing, that is not to an exact scale, shows experimental procedure used during this experiment and distance between cells 1 and 2. Cells impaled were not located at   the   end   of   strand. Temperature, 37 ^{o}C. From De Mello, (1979a), with permission of Springer-Verlag.*

IS METABOLIC ENERGY NECESSARY FOR THE MAINTENANCE OF INTERCELLULAR COMMUNICATION?

Since the permeability of the intercellular channels is modulated by $\left[Ca^{2+}\right]_i$, the obvious question is - can cell metabolism control or influence intercellular communication by regulating the free $\left[Ca^{2+}\right]_i$?

Recent observations with 2-4-dinitrophenol, an uncoupler of oxydative phosphorylation, show that this compound increases the intracellular longitudinal resistance in Purkinje fibres, suppresses the electrical coupling and the cell-to-cell movement of fluorescein (De Mello, 1979a - see Figs. 4 and 5, and Table II). In myocardial fibres, 2-4-dinitrophenol increases the resting tension markedly (De Mello, 1979a), denoting that the free $\left[Ca^{2+}\right]_i$ is enhanced. This increment in free $\left[Ca^{2+}\right]_i$ seems related to the release of the ion by intracellular stores because contractures are developed by dinitrophenol even in preparations immersed in Ca-free solution.

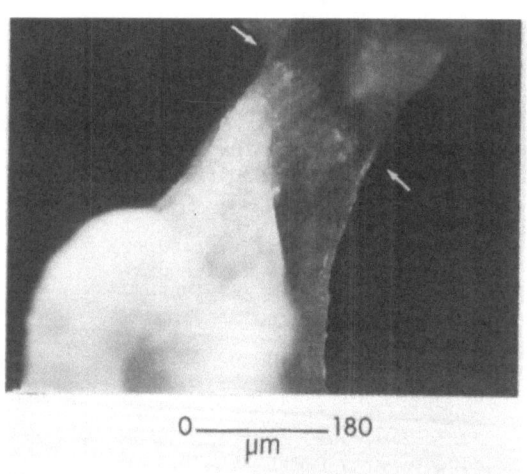

0————180
μm

FIGURE 5 *Lack of longitudinal movement of fluorescein along a strand of Purkinje fibres exposed to DNP (0.5 mM). The distribution of the dye was followed with the cut-end method. Picture taken 1 1/2 hr after removal of the dye from right compartment. Arrows indicate site of partition. Below the arrows, part of right segment loaded with fluorescein. Above the arrows, part of left segment showing absence of the dye. Temperature, 37 °C. From De Mello (1979a), with permission of Springer-Verlag.*

The iontophoretic injection of EDTA into cardiac cells re-establishes the electrical coupling previously abolished by dinitrophenol, supporting the view that a rise in free $[Ca^{2+}]_i$ is, indeed, involved on the decoupling action of the compound (see Fig. 6).

The sequence of events in the effect of dinitrophenol seems to start with a reduction of cell ATP content with ulterior impairment of the active Ca uptake by mitochondria and sarcoplasmic reticulum and consequent rise in free $[Ca^{2+}]_i$.

An inhibition of the Na-pump and the activation of a Na/Ca transport might be also involved on the suppression of cell communication produced by the metabolic inhibitor.

ON THE MECHANISM OF CELL DECOUPLING BY HIGH $[Ca^{2+}]_i$

The intimate mechanism by which Ca increases the junctional resistance is not known. A reasonable assumption is that the diffusion of monovalent cations (such as K^+) or of molecules (such as fluorescein, or Lucifer Yellow) through the intercellular channels might be blocked by the interaction of Ca with negative binding sites, probably located at the cytoplasmic end of the channel.

The presence of negative binding sites seems supported by the finding that La^{3+} is more effective than Ca in suppressing the electrical coupling when injected intracellularly (see Fig. 7 - and De Mello, 1979c).

Sr^{2+} has effects similar to those of Ca (De Mello, 1975), while Mn^{2+} is less effective than Ca^{2+} or La^{3+} in abolishing cell communication (De Mello, 1979c).

EFFECT OF INTRACELLULAR ACIDOSIS AND ALKALOSIS ON THE ELECTRICAL COUPLING

In 1977, Turin and Warner found that when cells of Xenopus embryos were exposed

TABLE II

EFFECT OF 2-4-DINITROPHENOL (DNP) ON MEMBRANE RESISTANCE PER UNIT LENGTH (r_m), INTRACELLULAR LONGITUDINAL RESISTANCE PER UNIT LENGTH (r_a), SPACE CONSTANT (λ) AND INPUT RESISTANCE (R_o) OF PURKINJE FIBRES IMMERSED IN NORMAL TYRODE SOLUTION

| | λ (μm) | | R_o ($\times 10^6 \Omega$) | | r_m ($K\Omega cm$) | | r_a ($M\Omega/cm$) | |
	Normal	DNP	Normal	DNP	Normal	DNP	Normal	DNP
Fibre 1	1500	950	2	3	600	570	26	63
Fibre 2	1575	830	2	3.3	600	547	26.6	79.5
Fibre 3	1685	900	2	2.3	640	414	25	51.1
Fibre 4	1700	1010	2.8	3.4	952	680	32.9	68
Fibre 5	1600	980	1.9	2.4	608	470	23.7	48.9

Values of R_o and λ were experimentally determined. Values of r_m and r_a were calculated as described in Table I. Measurements of λ and R_o were performed between 7 and 10 min after introduction of DNP to the bath. From De Mello, 1979a, with permission of Springer Verlag.

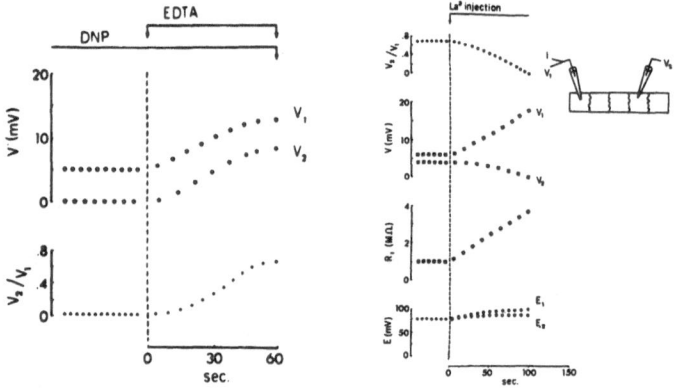

FIGURE 6 *Influence of intracellular injection of EDTA on the electrical coupling of Purkinje cells exposed to DNP for 10-12 min. (average from 5 experiments). Arrow shows start of EDTA injection. $I - 2 \times 10^8$ A, 600 ms, 0.5 Hz. Temperature, 37 °C. From De Mello (1979a), with permission of Springer-Verlag.*

FIGURE 7 *Decoupling of Purkinje cells produced by intracellular injection of La^{3+}. Time-course of V_1, V_2, E_1 and E_2 and coupling coefficient (V_2/V_1). Arrows show start of La^{3+} injection. The points before La^{3+} injection represent control values of each of the electrical parameters. $I = 10^8$ A; 50 ms. duration, 3 Hz. At right diagram showing experiment procedure. From De Mello, 1979c - with permission of Academic Press, London.*

to 100% CO_2, the resting potential was reduced and the electrical coupling abolished. The pH_i dropped from 7.7 to 6.4 on exposure to 100% CO_2. As the intracellular injection of Ca in nerve cells is known to reduce the intracellular pH (Meech and Thomas, 1977), it was suggested that the effect of high $\left[Ca^{2+}\right]_i$ on cell communication might be due to a rise in $\left[H^+\right]_i$.

These observations impelled me to search the influence of intracellular acidosis on the electrical coupling of cardiac cells. For this, H ions were injected electrophoretically into a Purkinje cell and its effect on cell communication investigated. As is shown in Fig. 8, the membrane potential is increased by about 16 mV, V_2/V_1 is gradually reduced and the input resistance increased. Cell decoupling is achieved in about 10 min. (De Mello, 1980b). The intracellular injection of H^+ increases r_a by 650% and reduced r_m by 45% (see Table III).

TABLE III

EFFECT OF INTRACELLULAR INJECTION OF H^+ ON SPACE CONSTANT, INPUT RESISTANCE, r_m AND r_a OF PURKINJE FIBRES

	λ **(mm) control	H^+ inj.	*R_o (KΩ) control	H^+ inj.	r_m (KΩcm) control	H^+ inj.	r_a (MΩ/cm) control	H^+ inj.
Fibre 1	1.65	0.37	470	1110	150	82	5.8	60
Fibre 2	1.75	0.43	510	980	175	85	6	45.5
Fibre 3	1.58	0.38	485	1150	145	79.8	6.4	55
Fibre 4	1.71	0.52	390	860	132	89	4.5	33

Measured with two microelectrodes. Voltage recording was about 50 µm from polarizing electrode.
**Space constant was measured by recording the amplitude of electrotonic potentials generated by constant current pulse at 3 different distances from polarizing electrode (200 to 1.000 µm).*
Both measurements (R_o and λ) were made between 6 and 8 minutes after beginning of H^+ injection. From De Mello, 1980b, with permission of Academic Press, London.

On the other hand, an increase in intracellular pH elicited by the intracellular injection of OH ions, causes a quick and appreciable increment in the electrical coupling of cardiac cells (De Mello, unpublished). Similar enhancement of cell communication is produced by NH_4Cl (see Fig. 9 - De Mello, unpublished), which is known to increase pH_i (Boron and De Weer, 1976). Weingart and

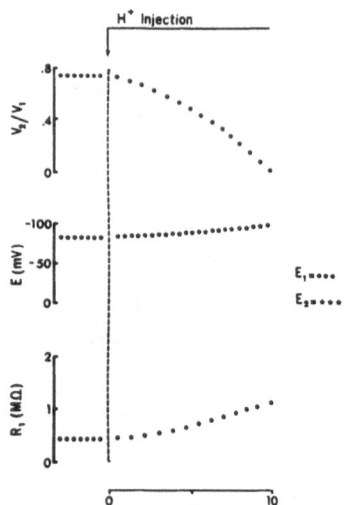

FIGURE 8 *Effect of intracellular injection of H^+ on the electrical coupling of canine Purkinje cells (average from 5 experiments). Time-course of input resistance (R_1), E_1, E_2 and coupling coefficient (V_2/V_1). Arrows shows start of H^+ injection represent control values of each of the electrical parameters. $I - 10^{-8}$ A; 60 ms duration, 5 Hz. R_1 was measured with voltage recording microelectrode impaled about 50 m away from polarizing electrode. Measurements of R_1 made with a balanced bridge circuit showed changes in the same direction. From De Mello (1980b), with permission of Academic Press, London.*

Reber (1979) also reported a decrease in r_a with NH_4Cl in sheep Purkinje fibres.

The question is - can H ion, by itself, change the junctional resistance? Lea and Ashley (1978) found a rise in free $[Ca^{2+}]_i$ in barnacle muscle exposed to 100% CO_2. In Chironomus salivary gland, cell acidification increases $[Ca^{2+}]_i$ (Rose and Rick, 1978).

It is not feasible at this moment to know how dependent is the decoupling action of low pH_i on a rise in free $[Ca^{2+}]_i$. The possibility exists that H ion can alter the junctional resistance by itself, and in part, through the release of Ca intracellularly.

Concerning the effect of Ca on junctional resistance, preliminary studies indicate that NH_4Cl does not alter the effect of intracellular Ca injection on the electrical coupling (De Mello, unpublished), what suggests that Ca is, by itself, enough to change the junctional conductance.

The finding that the intracellular injection of La^{3+} (which is known to inhibit the ejection of H linked to Ca uptake by mitochondria - Mela, 1968; Lehninger, 1966) causes electrical uncoupling, not only indicates that the H/Ca transport in mitochondria is not necessarily involved on the action of this cation but also means that strong positive charges influence the junctional permeability directly.

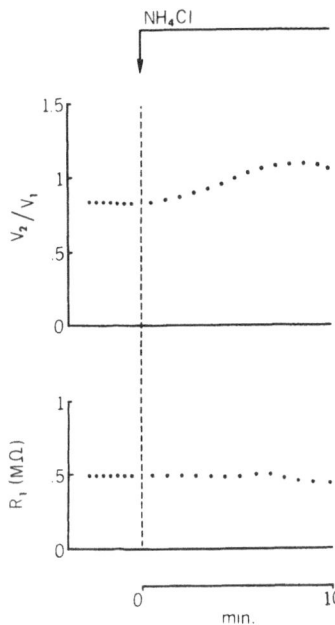

FIGURE 9 *Effect of NH_4Cl (20 mM) on the coupling coefficient (V_2/V_1) and input resistance (R_1) of Purkinje cells (average from 6 experiments). V_1 and V_2 — same as in Fig. 9. Temperature — 37 °C. (De Mello, unpublished).*

CELL-TO-CELL COMMUNICATION IN THE SINOATRIAL AND ATRIOVENTRICULAR NODES

The sinoatrial node is composed of small cells (15-20 μm in length; 5-8 μm in diameter), organized as functional units.

Electrophysiological studies (see Dudel and Trautwein, 1958) provided evidence that these units are electrically coupled.

The spread of electrical current in this tissue, is, however, limited by a small space constant (465 μm - Bonke, 1973).

Although scarce, gap junctions have been identified between pacemaker cells (Masson-Pevet, 1979). The mean area of these junctions, is nevertheless, small-

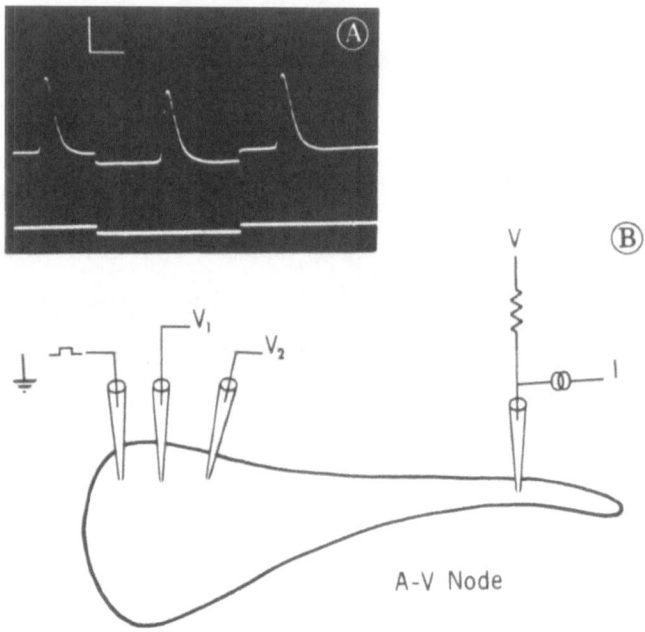

FIGURE 10 (A) Top: Change in membrane potential of a nodal cell from the AN layer elicited by an inward current pulse injected into another cell from the same layer. Bottom: Rectangular inward current pulse (10^{-6} A, 400 ms duration). Vertical line, 35 mV; horizontal line, 93 ms. (B) This drawing that is not to an exact scale, shows, at left, the procedure used to measure the electrical coupling of nodal cells with intracellular microelectrodes. From De Mello, 1977b, with permission of Springer Verlag.

er than those found in myocardial fibres (Masson-Pevet, 1979).

When fluorescein (mol. wt. 320) is injected into sinus node cells and the tissue is observed under a fluorescent microscope, no apparent diffusion of the dye is seen (De Mello, 1980a). Longitudinal movement of the dye can be detected in the sinoatrial ring bundle, or in atrium fibres (De Mello, 1980a). These findings seem to indicate that the diameter of the hydrophyllic channel or its number is much smaller in the sinoatrial node than in myocardial or Purkinje fibres.

Since the resting potential of true pacemaker cells is smaller than those recorded in node cells located near crista terminalis (Paes de Carvalho, De Mello and Hoffman, 1959), it is reasonable to conclude that the permeability of the gap junctions, inside the node, or the number of channels between apposing cells, is not enough to avoid the establishment of ionic gradients inside the sinoatrial node. The existance of a high intracellular resistance in this tissue is probably essential to the preservation of the pacemaker function since the abolishment of ionic barriers would result in an equal value of resting potential in pacemaker and atrial cells.

How then, pacemaker cells can be electrically coupled and at the same time present different resting potentials? A possible explanation is that the intensity of active ionic extrusion (Na, for instance) is distinct in different area of the sinoatrial node, keeping the membrane polarization at dissimilar levels, despite the presence of high conductance gates between the cells.

In the atrioventricular node the cells are electrically coupled (see Fig. 10), but the space constant here is also small (430 μm - De Mello, 1977b). The small value of λ seems to be due, in part, to a high intracellular resistance. As it can be seen in Table IV, r_a is about 4 times larger in the A-V node than in the atrium. This finding might be related to the rare occurrence of gap junctions in this tissue (James and Sherf, 1968).

The delay of impulse conduction in the A-V node seems then greatly due to a high intracellular resistance along the pathway of conduction. The high value of r_a makes the propagation of the impulse extremely vulnerable to variations in resistance on the non-junctional membrane. A small decrease in this resistance, for instance, can be enough to cause cell decoupling. This seems to be the mechanism by which acetylcholine blocks the A-V conduction (De Mello, 1977b). On the other hand, it is reasonable to assume that at least, part of the depressant

action of ouabain on A-V conduction is due to a rise in r_a (see De Mello, 1976;
Weingart, 1977).

REFERENCES

Bonke, F.I.M.: Electrotonic spread in the sinoatrial node of the rabbit heart.
      Pfluegers Arch., 339: 17-23, 1973.
Boron, W.F. and De Weer, P.: Intracellular pH transients in squid giant axons
      caused by CO_2, NH_3 and metabolic inhibitors. J. Gen. Physiol., 67:
      91-112, 1976.
De Haan, R. and Hirakow, R.: Synchronization of pulsation rates in isolated
      cardiac myocytes. Exp. Cell Res., 70: 214-220, 1972.
De Mello, W.C.: Electrical uncoupling in heart fibres produced by intracellular
      injection of Na or Ca. The Physiologist, 17: 3, 1974.
De Mello, W.C.: Effect of intracellular injection of calcium and strontium in
      cell communication in heart. J. Physiol. (London), 250: 231-245, 1975.
De Mello, W.C.: Influence of the sodium pump on intercellular communication in
      heart fibres: effect of intracellular injection of sodium ion on electri-
      cal coupling. J. Physiol. (London), 263: 171-197, 1976.
De Mello, W.C.: Intercellular communication in heart muscle. In:
      Intercellular Communication, De Mello, W.C., ed., Plenum Press, New York,
      pp. 87-125, 1977a.
De Mello, W.C.: Passive electrical properties of the AV node. Pfluegers Arch.,
      371: 135-139, 1977b.
De Mello, W.C.: Effect of 2-4-dinitrophenol on intercellular communication in
      mammalian cardiac fibres. Pfluégers Arch., 380: 267-276, 1979a.
De Mello, W.C.: On the decoupling action of ouabain. The Physiologist, 22: 4,
      1979b.
De Mello, W.C.: Effect of intracellular injection of La^{3+} and Mn^{2+} on electri-
      cal coupling of heart cells. Cell Biol. Intern. Rep., 3: 113-119,
      1979c.
De Mello, W.C.: Intercellular communication and junctional permeability. In:

Membrane Structure and Function, Vol. 3, Bittar, E.E., ed., John Wiley and Sons, New York, pp. 127-170, 1980a.

De Mello, W.C.: Influence of intracellular injection of H^+ on the electrical coupling in cardiac Purkinje fibres. Cell Biol. Intern. Rep., 4: 51-55, 1980b.

Dudel, J. and Trautwein, W.: Der Mechanismus der Automatischen Rhythmischen Impulsbildung der Herzmuskelfaser. Pfluegers Arch., 267: 553-565, 1958.

Glitsch, H.G. and Reuter, H.: The effect of internal sodium concentration on calcium fluxes in isolated guinea-pig auricles. J. Physiol. (London), 209: 25-43, 1970.

Gorman, A.L.F. and Herman, A.: Internal effects of divalent cations on potassium permeability in molluscan neurons. J. Physiol. (London), 296: 393-410, 1979.

Imanaga, I.: Cell-to-cell diffusion of Procion Yellow in sheep and calf Purkinje fibers. J. Memb. Biol., 16: 381-388, 1974.

James, T.N. and Sherf, L.: Ultrastructure of the human atrioventricular node. Circulation, 37: 1049-1070, 1968.

Keeter, J.S., Deschenes, M., Pappas, G.D. and Bennett, M.V.L.: Fine structure and permeability studies of a rectifying electrotonic synapse. Biol. Bull., 147: 485, 1974.

Lea, T.J. and Ashley, C.C.: Increase in free Ca^{2+} in muscle after exposure to CO_2, Nature, 275: 236, 1978.

Lehninger, A.L.: Dynamics and mechanism of active ion transport across the mitochondria membrane. N. Y. Acad. Sci., 137 (2): 700-707, 1966.

Masson-Pevet, M.: The fine structure of cardiac pacemaker cells in the sinus node and in tissue culture. Thesis, Rodopi Press, Amsterdam, 1979.

Meech, R.H. and Thomas, R.C.: The effect of calcium injection on the intracellular sodium and pH of snail neurones. J. Physiol. (London), 265: 867-879, 1977.

Mela, L.: Interactions of La^{3+} and local anesthetic drugs with mitochondria, Ca^{++} and Mn^{++} uptake. Archiv. Biochim. Biophys., 123: 286-293, 1968.

Paes de Carvalho, A., De Mello, W.C. and Hoffman, B.: Electrophysiological evidence for specialized fiber types in rabbit atrium. Am. J. Physiol., 196: 483-488, 1959.

Pollack, G.H.: Intercellular coupling in the atrioventricular node and other tissues of the rabbit heart. J. Physiol. (London), 225: 275-298, 1973.

Reuter, H. and Seitz, H.: The dependence of calcium efflux from cardiac muscle on temperature and external ion composition. J. Physiol. (London), 195: 451-470, 1968.

Rose, B. and Loewenstein, W.R.: Permeability of cell junction depends on local cytoplasmic calcium activity. Nature (London), 254: 250, 1975.

Rose, B. and Rick, R.: Intracellular pH, intracellular free Ca and junctional cell-cell coupling. J. Membr. Biol., 44: 337-415, 1978.

Turin, L. and Warner, A.: Carbon dioxide reversibly abolishes ionic communication between cells of early amphibian embryo. Nature, 270: 56, 1977.

Weidmann, S.: The diffusion of radiopotassium across intercalated disks of mammalian cardiac muscle. J. Physiol. (London), 187: 323-342, 1966.

Weingart, R.: The permeability to tetraethylammonium ions of the surface membrane and intercalated disks of sheep and calf myocardium. J. Physiol. (London), 240: 741-762, 1974.

Weingart, R.: The action of ouabain on intercellular coupling and conduction velocity in mammalian ventricular muscle. J. Physiol. (London), 264: 341-365, 1977.

Weingart, R. and Reber, W.: Influence of internal pH on r_i of Purkinje fibres from mammalian heart. Experientia, 35: 929, 1979.

TABLE IV

PASSIVE ELECTRICAL CONSTANTS OF THE ATRIO-VENTRICULAR NODE AND RIGHT ATRIAL MUS-CLE OF THE RABBIT[a]

	Input resist. ($K\Omega$)	Space constant (μm)	r_m ($K\Omega cm$)	r_a ($M\Omega/cm$)	R_m (Ωcm^2)	C_m ($\mu F/cm^2$)	τ (ms)
A-V node	880[c] (± 75)	430 (± 44)	75.5 (± 7.8)	40.9 (± 9)	3400[d] (± 288) 9000[c] ($+ 765$)	1	3.4[d] (± 0.5)
	(10)	(7)	(7)	(7)	(10)		(10)[c] (± 1.2) (10)
Atrial muscle	320 (± 42)	660[c]	42.2 (± 6.4)	9.6 (± 7)	3800 (± 270)	1.3[b]	5 (± 0.7)
	(10)		(7)	(10)	(10)		(7)

[a]Standard error of the mean is given by $\pm$ figures. In brackets, the number of preparations. [b]From Pags de Carvalho et al. (1969). [c]From cells of the N layer. [d]From AN cells. [e]Bonke (1973). (From De Mello, 1977b, with permission of Springer Verlag).

ELECTRICAL CELL COUPLING IN RABBIT SINO ATRIAL NODE AND ATRIUM

EXPERIMENTAL AND THEORETICAL EVALUATION

Feliksas F. Bukauskas, Aron M. Gutman, Klemensas J. Kisunas
and Romualdas P. Veteikis

INTRODUCTION

Intercellular coupling has hitherto been scrutinized nearly in every myocardial structure and at many phylogenetic levels, the human heart being not excepted (Barr, 1969; Bonke, 1973; Bredikis et al., 1976, 1978; Bukauskas et al., 1977a, 1977b; De Mello, 1977; Johnson and Tille, 1961; Sakson et al., 1974; Seyama, 1976; Tanaka and Sasaki, 1966; Weidmann, 1970). The most popular approach in cell to cell coupling studies has been the measurement of passive electrical properties, viz. input resistance and space constant of electrotonic decay. To evaluate these parameters with regard to cell coupling theoretical models are needed which simulate the passive electrical properties and which take into account the actual build up of myocardial tissue as good as possible.

Myocardial tissue is obviously a three-dimensional anisotropic syncytium. A generalized solution of the problem is hardly possible and usable for evaluation of the electrical parameters of the tissue. The main theoretical point in the approach we are using lies in dealing, whenever possible, with the syncytium as a continuous medium. Inhomogeneity does not enter at this point; for transitional zones therefore the results should be used with caution.

In this paper individual parts of the myocardium are considered as an continuous anisotropic medium. Cell coupling and input resistance was evaluated using the two micro-electrode technique, while electrotonic spread of current was measured using the suction electrode. In this way we were able to estimate the electrical parameters of cells and of tissue and the space constants of electrotonic decay along the three natural axes of the tissue $(\lambda_x, \lambda_y, \lambda_z;$ x, longitudinal;   y, transversal and z, perpendicular to the wall of the atrium).

EXPERIMENTAL

On rabbits, weighing 1.5 to 2.0 kg, and anesthetized with Nembutal (40 mg/kg i.v.), thoracotomy was performed;   the heart was removed and placed into oxygenated Tyrode solution. As quickly as possible the right atrial wall and the sino-atrial area were excised.   The preparation was placed into a perfusion chamber and perfused from the top and from the bottom with a standard Tyrode solution containing: NaCl 136 mM, KCl 2.7 mM, $CaCl_2$ 1.8 mM, $MgSO_4$ 0.5 mM, NaH_2PO_4 4.6 mM, $NaHCO_3$ 14 mM, glucose 2 g/l, pH = 7.35.   Before reaching the chamber the saline was gassed with a mixture of 95 % O_2 and 5 % CO_2 and passed through a heating coil.   A temperature of 37 $^{\circ}$C and a pO_2 of 500 mm Hg were maintained.

The following parameters reflecting the passive electrical properties were measured $-\lambda_x$, λ_y, λ_z, and R_{in}, the input resistance.   Intercellular electrical coupling was measured also with the two micro-electrode technique.

To estimate λ_z and to correct λ_x and λ_y the following experiment was performed.   The most homogeneous locus was identified on the trabeculae of the right atrium.   A suction electrode was placed on the endocardial side (Bonke, 1973;   Sakson et al., 1974), internally perfused with isotonic KCl to which Chicago sky blue was added.   The suction electrode was used for intracellular hyperpolarization of the preparation.   The electrotonic decay along and across the fibers was studied with micro-electrodes.   Thereafter the suction electrode was removed, leaving a stained spot at the locus of stimulation.   Half an hour later after complete recovery of the action potentials, another suction electrode of appropriate shape was placed with utmost precision, at the place of the stained dot, this time from the epicardial side of the preparation.   Again the electrotonic spread along and across the fibers was recorded.

In another series of experiments the preparation was at first polarized from the epicardial side and records were taken from the endocardial side;   then the preparation was turned over and the polarization was applied to the same locus from the endocardial side while the recordings were made at the epicardial side. We have not observed any significant differences between the two techniques of measurement, therefore we will not distinguish between them. Following the experiment, a cut was made in the area of interest and atrial wall thickness was estimated with the aid of a microscope. This protocol was kept in twelve experiments. The average thickness of the preparations was 190 μm (150 to 250 μm).Since the tissue is known to be fully oxygenated down to 200 to 250 μm (Pearson et al., 1949; Cranefield and Greenspan, 1961) our preparations perfused from both sides, should have been oxygenated well enough.

The input resistance of cardiac fibres was measured with double barrel micro-electrodes (Johnson and Tille, 1961) with a tip outer diameter not exceeding 0.5 μm. One barrel served for current injection into a cell, the other was used to pick up the resulting voltage drop across the cell membrane. Square current pulses with an amplitude of 20 to 50 nA and a duration of 50 to 100 ms were used. The input resistance was calculated from the relationship

$$R_{in} = \frac{V_i - V_e}{I_o} \tag{1}$$

where V_i and V_e are the voltage drops with the micro-electrode tip inside and outside the cell respectively; I_o is the intensity of the injected current.

In order to verify some theoretical inferences obtained by us earlier (Bukauskas et al., 1975, 1977b), we have carried out experiments aimed at estimating cell to cell electrical coupling with the aid of glued-together micro-electrodes. The tips of micro-electrodes were positioned 10 to 15 μm apart from each other and glued together with wax. The distance between the micro-electrode tips, r_{el}, was checked in Tyrode's by injecting a square pulse of 0.1 to 0.5 μA into one electrode, and measuring the resulting voltage drop, ΔV, with the other pipette. The value of r_{el} was obtained from

$$r_{el} = \frac{I_o \rho_T}{4 \pi \Delta V} \tag{2}$$

where ρ_T is the resistivity of the Tyrode's solution. The micro-electrode pairs were used only if r_{el} did not exceed 15 μm. While measuring cell-to-cell coupling, the intensity of the current injected was 25 nA for true pacemakers in the SA node and 50 nA for atrial trabeculae. R_{in} and electrical coupling were measured at the same locus. Additionally 37 experiments were done aimed at estimation of passive electrical properties of the SA nodal area.The results are presented as mean $\pm$ SE of the mean.

RESULTS

I. ANALYSIS OF THE ELECTROTONIC SPREAD
Equation for a continuous anisotropic medium.

Consider a three dimensional excitable medium made up of units contacting through junctional membrane. Let the intracellular compartment of the syncytium be characterized by anisotropic resistivities, $\rho_x \neq \rho_y \neq \rho_z$, along the principal directions of the resistivity tensor. The resistivities ρ_x, ρ_y and ρ_z encompass the myoplasmic resistivity, ρ_{pl}, and those of the intercellular junctions, for the intracellular current spread along the x, y and z axes; also it is assumed that the resistivity of the junctional membrane is evenly distributed over the entire length of the cell. A corollary is that

$$\rho_x = \rho_{kx} + \rho_{pl}, \; \rho_y = \rho_{ky} + \rho_{pl}, \; \rho_z = \rho_{kz} + \rho_{pl},$$

where ρ_{kx}, ρ_{ky} and ρ_{kz} are resistivities of the "distributed" junctional membranes along the x, y and z axes. Suppose the intercellular space to have zero potential and the cells to display cable properties.

Now, assume there is a current source in the intracellular compartment. According to Bukauskas et al., (1975), the following equation of continuous medium holds for the lengths manifold those of the fibers

$$\lambda_x^2 \frac{d^2V}{dx^2} + \lambda_y^2 \frac{d^2V}{dy^2} + \lambda_z^2 \frac{d^2V}{dz^2} = V \tag{3}$$

where $V = V(x, y, z)$ stands for electrotonic potential.

Within the normalized coordinate system $\bar{x}$, $\bar{y}$, $\bar{z}$, where $\bar{x} = x/\lambda_x$, $\bar{y} = y/\lambda_y$ and $\bar{z} = z/\lambda_z$, equation (3) would assume the canonical expression

$$\frac{d^2V}{d\bar{x}^2} + \frac{d^2V}{d\bar{y}^2} + \frac{d^2V}{d\bar{z}^2} = V \tag{4}$$

For the case of infinite space $(\bar{x}, \bar{y}, \bar{z})$, with spherical symmetry the solution of equation (4) is (Bukauskas et al., 1975)

$$V(\bar{r}) = C \, e^{-\bar{r}} / \bar{r} \tag{5}$$

Further we will need an expression for the two dimensional case $(\bar{x}, \bar{y})$. In this instance (Bukauskas et al., 1974)

$$V(\bar{r}) = C' \, K_o(\bar{r}) \tag{5a}$$

C and C' are constants, $K_o(\bar{r})$ is a zero Bessel function of the second kind with imaginary argument and

$$\bar{r} = \left(\frac{x^2}{\lambda_x^2} + \frac{y^2}{\lambda_y^2} + \frac{z^2}{\lambda_z^2} \right)^{1/2} \tag{6}$$

For Eq. 5a insert $z = 0$ into eq. 6.

Similar solutions for current spread in isotropic media have been reported by Barr (1969) and Purves (1976).

An indispensable condition for a spherically symmetrical solution is that the electrode be either a sphere in $\bar{x}$, $\bar{y}$, $\bar{z}$ coordinates, i.e. an ellipsoid with axes proportional to λ_x, λ_y and λ_z, or a point source, i.e $\bar{r}$ should be a multiple of the electrode dimensions. If so the value of λ_x can easily be obtained from equations (5) and (6)

$$\lambda_x = \frac{\lambda_{xe}}{1 + \ln \dfrac{x_o}{X_o + \lambda_{xe}}} \qquad (7)$$

where λ_{xe} is the distance at which the electrotonic potential is decayed e-fold, and x_o the shortest distance on the x-axis from the point of recording to the electrode midpoint.

As evident from (7), λ_{xe} would in all cases be less than the true value of λ_x.

Experimental and theoretical data concerning electrotonic spread on the two sides of the atrial preparation.

Figure 1 shows averaged data of electrotonic spread along and across the fibers on the two sides of the preparation. It can be seen that in the vicinity of the source there is a clear cut difference between the potentials on both sides as well as a prominent anisotropy.

For intracellular polarization of myocardial tissue we have used suction-electrodes with an orifice diameter of r_{se} = 150 μm. Because one can not rule out the possibility of current flow from the suction electrode to deep layers of the tissue, the prediction of the shape of an equivalent electrode is quite a speculative matter. Therefore, at the initial stage of modelling, we restricted the analysis by considering the case of a semi-ellipsoid, the half axes of which were in x, y, z -coordinates, $a_x = a_y = r_{se}$ = 150 μm and a_z any value ranging from 0 to 150 μm. In $\bar{x}, \bar{y}, \bar{z}$ coordinates the ellipsoid will have half-axes as follows:

$$A_x = r_{se}/\lambda_x, \ A_y = r_{se}/\lambda_y, \ \text{and} \ 0 \le A_z \le r_{se}/\lambda_z \ \text{(Fig. 2B)}.$$

Now, we will consider an excitable isotropic medium, infinite on the $\bar{x}, \bar{y}$ plane and restricted by two planes perpendicular to the $\bar{z}$ -axis, intersecting with it at the points $\bar{z} = 0$ and $\bar{z} = -d$ (distances given in λ). We will analyse the electrical field V $(\bar{x}, \bar{y}, \bar{z})$ produced by a semi-ellipsoidal current source with its geometrical centre at the point (0, 0, 0) and principal axes parallel to $\bar{x}, \bar{y}$ and $\bar{z}$ (Fig. 2B). Let the boundary conditions on the planes perpendicular to the $\bar{z}$ - axis be

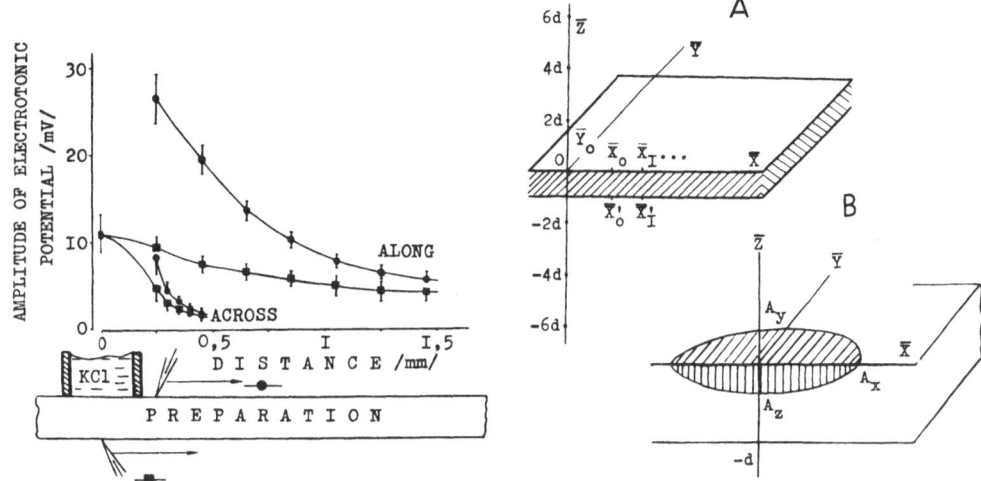

FIGURE 1 *Averaged data for the electrotonic potential distribution on the both sides of a right atrium preparation. Means (n = 12) and S.E. are given.*

FIGURE 2 *The diagram showing the premises used in the theoretical computation of the electrotonic spread on the both side of a preparation for the instance of an infinite excitable medium restricted within two parallel planes, $\bar{z} = 0$ and $\bar{z} = -d$. $\bar{x}_o$, $\bar{x}_1$, $\bar{x}'$, $\bar{x}'_1$, ... stand for locations along the $\bar{x}$-axis of the pick-up electrode tip. $\bar{y}_o$, a similar location on the $\bar{y}$-axis, closest to the current electrode. (part A) B. A blown-up view of the origin of axes with the ellipsoid current source shown; A_x, A_y and A_z being its half-axes.*

$$\frac{dV}{d\bar{z}}\bigg|_{\substack{\bar{z}\,=\,o \\ \bar{z}\,=\,-d}} = 0$$

that is, suppose there is no current flow across the planes. We will use the reflection method to fulfill the boundary conditions.

Suppose the planes $\bar{z} = 0, -d$ to be mirrors. Then the semi-ellipsoidal source would reflect on the plane $\bar{z} = 0$ assuming the shape of an ellipsoid; the latter would reflect on the plane $\bar{z} = -d$ resulting in an identical ellipsoid, with its geometrical centre at the point $\bar{z} = -2d$. This one produces on the plane $\bar{z} = 0$ a third ellipsoid source with its geometrical centre at the point $\bar{z} = 2d$, and so on. Thus obtaining a solution is reduced to solving eq. (4) in non-restricted medium with an infinite sequence of ellipsoid sources, with their centres on the $\bar{z}$-axis at $\bar{z} = \pm 2nd$, $n = 0, 1, 2, \ldots$ (fig.2A)

Since we could but speculate on the actual shape and physical properties of the source, we neglected strict boundary conditions on the electrode plane and tackled the problem by substituting a set of uniform point sources on the ellipsoid's surface for the suction electrode.

To save computations, we started with obtaining, from eq. (5a) estimates for λ_x and λ_y via the two-dimensional approach, $\lambda_x = 1200 \,\mu m$ and $\lambda_y = 120 \,\mu m$. Then, taking these values as correct, we estimated λ_z by computing, as described above, the distribution of the potential over the $\bar{x}$ and $\bar{y}$ axes, with $\bar{z} = 0, -d$.

The experimental data for electrotonic spread were normalized and plotted together with the computed curves. Fig. 3 shows the results obtained for various values of λ_z. When the electrotonus is measured on the same side as the electrode is placed $(\bar{z} = 0)$ the decay is a relatively weak function of λ_z. The relationship becomes much stronger with the electrotonic decay measured on the reverse side of the preparation $(\bar{z} = -d)$. The best fit is obtained with $\lambda_z \simeq \lambda_y$. With the accuracy of the present measurements a further variation of λ_x and λ_y would be not justified.

Thus we can consider $\lambda_x \gg \lambda_y \simeq \lambda_z$; the magnitude of λ_x is in the mm range, while λ_y is an order of 0.1 mm.

II. ELECTRICAL COUPLING BETWEEN ADJACENT CELLS

THEORY OF THE INPUT RESISTANCE

While estimating R_{in} in micro-electrode studies, a model for a three-dimensional infinite medium can be used, because the thickness of the bathing solution layer is some tens of times larger as compared to the dimensions of the individual fibers.

The expression for R_{in} reported by us earlier (Bukauskas et al., 1975)

$$R_{in} \cong \rho /4\pi r_o \tag{8}$$

where r_o is the electrode radius and ρ is the resistivity of the interior of the

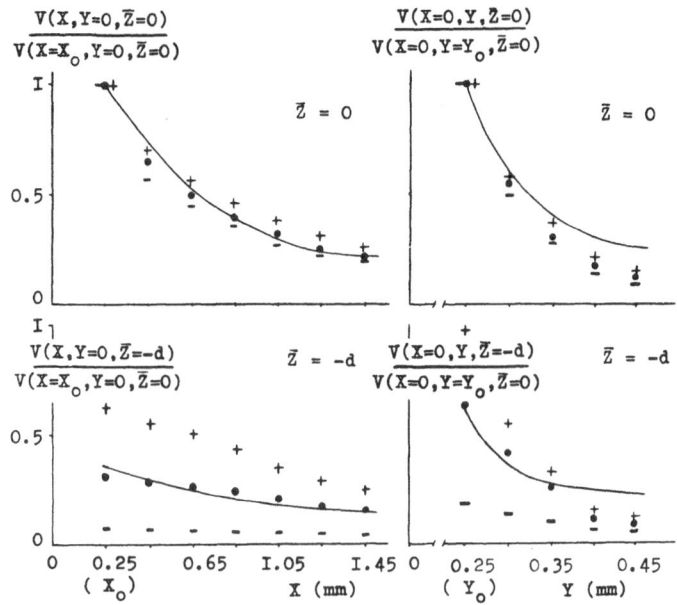

FIGURE 3 *Plots of the experimental (solid curves) and theoretical data for an ellipsoid source with the half-axes $a_x = a_y = 150$ m, $a_z = 70$ m. The theoretical data were obtained with $\lambda_z = 60$ µm (horizontal bars), 120 µm (solid circles), and 220 µm (crosses). The abscissa shows distance to the midpoint of the current electrode, mm; on the ordinate, normalized, with regard to locations x_o and y_o (along the x-axis and the y-axis respectively), values of the electrotonic potential have been plotted.*

syncytium, holds only for r_o much larger than the cell dimensions. To determine the actual R_{in}, in a case when a continuous model should be rejected **a priori,** we shall analyze a hypothetical tissue, consisting of tightly packed spherical cells coupled to each other via low-resistance junctions (Fig. 4). Suppose current to be injected in cell A which flows in all directions by passing through the junctional membranes separated, on the average, by a distance 2 r_c (r_c = cell radius).

We neglected the fact that, with tightly packed cells, the interjunctional distance might be slightly different from 2 r_c. So the tissue could be roughly approximated by surfaces of spherical units with radii r_c $(2n-1)$, $n = 1, 2, \ldots$ and resistivities equaling R_k, the resistivity of the junctions distributed over

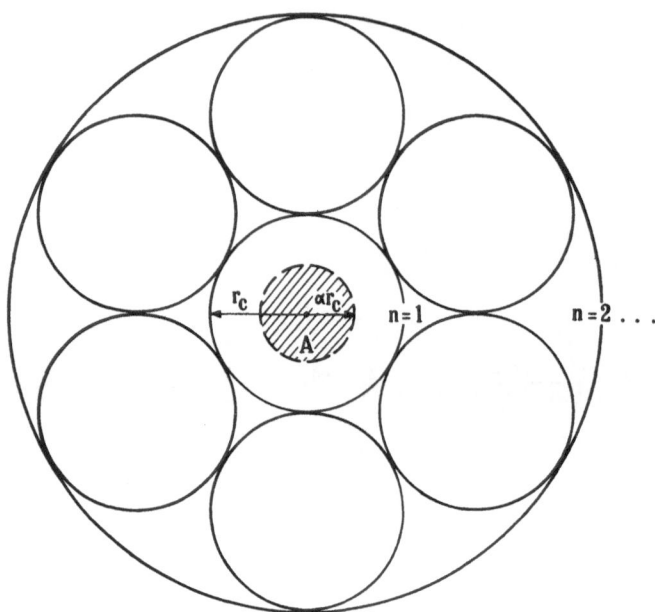

FIGURE 4 *The arrangement of the spherical units in a model representation of the medium. A, the cell, of radium r_c, from which potential is picked up; αr_c, the volume outside which the estimation of the input resistance is accomplished utilizing the 3-dimensional model for a continuous medium. n, radius number of the junctional membrane.*

the whole cell surface. The spheres are filled with continuous material having the resistivity of the myoplasm, ρ_{pl} . From Bukauskas et al. (1977b)

$$R_{in} = \frac{\rho_{pl}}{4\pi r_o} + \sum_{n=1}^{\infty} \frac{R_k}{4\pi r_c^2 (2n-1)^2} \qquad (9)$$

$$R_{in} = \frac{\rho_{pl}}{4\pi r_o} + \frac{\pi^2}{8} \frac{R_k}{4\pi r_c^2} \tag{9b}$$

where r_o is the tip separation of a double barreled micro-electrode.

As stated above, R_{in} was determined as the ratio of the difference between the extracellular and intracellular potentials to the current injected. Hence, the term $\rho_T/4\pi r_o$, which denotes the input resistance of the Tyrode's solution and is referred to as inter-electrode coupling resistance (Tanaka and Sasaki, 1966) should be subtracted from (9a) and (9b). (9b) transforms then into

$$R_{in} = \frac{\rho_{pl} - \rho_T}{4\pi r_o} + \frac{\pi^2}{8} \frac{R_k}{4\pi r_c^2} \tag{10}$$

To make use of the three-dimensional theory for continuous medium in micro-electrode estimation of R_{in}, we will use an equivalent electrode with a radius αr_c. Assuming the resistivity within the equivalent electrode to be equal to ρ_{pl} and that of the continuous material outside the electrode to $\rho = \rho_{pl} + R_k/2r_c$, we get

$$R_{in} = \frac{\rho_{pl} - \rho_T}{4\pi r_o} - \frac{\rho_{pl}}{4\pi r_c \alpha} + \frac{\rho}{4\pi r_c \alpha} \tag{11}$$

From the right hand side of equations (10) and (11) we obtain $\alpha = 4/\pi^2$, i.e. for the electrode with a radius $r_o = 4 r_c/\pi^2$ the expression for a continuous syncytium (8) holds, if one neglects the resistance of the myoplasm inside the equivalent electrode.

According to Bukauskas et al. (1975; 1977a; 1977b), the estimates for parameters reflecting passive electrical properties of the tissue consisting of tightly packed oblong cells coupled by highly permeable junctions can be obtained as follows:

$$\rho_x = F - R''_{in} \left(\left(\frac{\lambda_y}{\lambda_x} \right)^4 x_c y_c^2 \right)^{1/3} \frac{8}{\pi} \tag{12}$$

$$\rho_y = \rho_z = F - R''_{in} \left(\left(\frac{\lambda_x}{\lambda_y} \right)^2 x_c y_c^2 \right)^{1/3} \frac{8}{\pi} \tag{13}$$

$$R_m = F \frac{8 \ R''_{in}}{\pi \ b} \left(\lambda_x^2 \lambda_y^4 x_c y_c^2 \right)^{1/3} \tag{14}$$

in which $1 \leq F \leq 2$ depending on whether current flows out to all surrounding cells $(F = 2)$ or only in one direction $(F = 1)$, and b is volume to surface area ratio and

$$R''_{in} = R_{in} - \frac{\rho_{pl} - \rho_T}{4\pi r_o} + \frac{\pi \rho_{pl}}{16(x_c y_c^2)^{1/3}} \tag{15}$$

From the comparison of the two approaches to the estimation of R_{in} it can be inferred that R_{in} measured via a micro-electrode can be used also in the case of an anisotropic tissue, provided the myoplasmic resistance of the peri-electrode material is subtracted and "the effective radius of the micro-electrode" is assumed to be approximately $4(x_c y_c^2)^{1/3}/\pi^2$.

If one disregards the resistance of the myoplasm surrounding the micro-electrode tip, 80 % of the R_{in} (the second term in (10)) should be accounted for by the junctional membrane of the central unit A (Fig. 4.), the first term upon expansion of the sum of (9a). Consequently the potential drop over the cells adjacent to A should be approximately fivefold. This inference was verified in our experiments with glued-together micro-electrodes in the area

of true pacemakers in the SA node.   The imaginary line drawn through the
micro-electrode tips would have the same direction of the major axes of the
fibers, i.e. one parallel to the crista terminalis (Masson-Pevet, 1979).   The
results of the measurement are presented in the form of histograms (Fig. 5,
upper panel).   It can be seen that the mean value of the electrotonic potential
in adjacent cells (glued-together micro-electrodes, black columns) was 3.0 +
0.5 mV (n = 19).   The corresponding potential in the same sinus node cell was
27.0 + 1.0 mV (n = 54).   The data obtained in the SA node, as a whole, do fit
the isotropic model with concentric spheres.

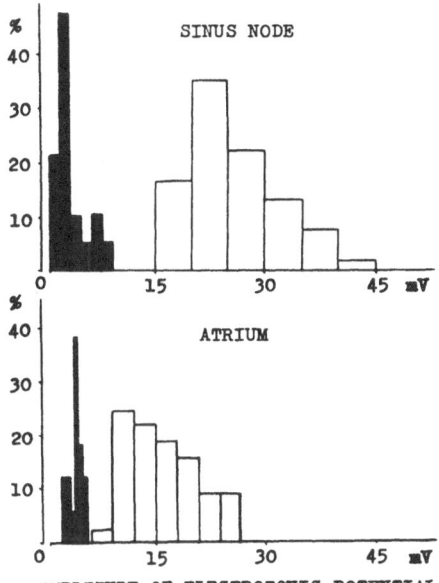

FIGURE 5 *Histograms for the potential*
drops recorded, in the zone of true SA
nodal pacemakers and in the atrial tra-
beculae, with two sealed-together pi-
pettes (black columna) and
double-barreled microelectrodes (empty
columns). The current injected was _2.5
x 10^{-8} A (SA node and 5 x 10^{-8} A
(atria).

In the more anisotropic trabecular tissue with larger cells and better
electrical coupling, it follows from (9b), (10) and (15) that the respective potential drop over the adjacent units should be approximately sevenfold.   The experimental evidence was as follows: the mean value of the electrotonic potential in the adjacent cells was 3.9 + 0.2 mV (n = 16), the potential in the unit
into which the current was injected was equal to 16.1 + 0.8 mV (n = 37).   One
of the reasons for discrepancies between the theoretical and experimental   data

might be the greater extent of anisotropy in the trabeculae as compared with the
SA node (cf. below). In the case of infinite anisotropy, the one-dimensional
cable theory can be used, in which instance the expected potential drop would
not be greater than twofold.

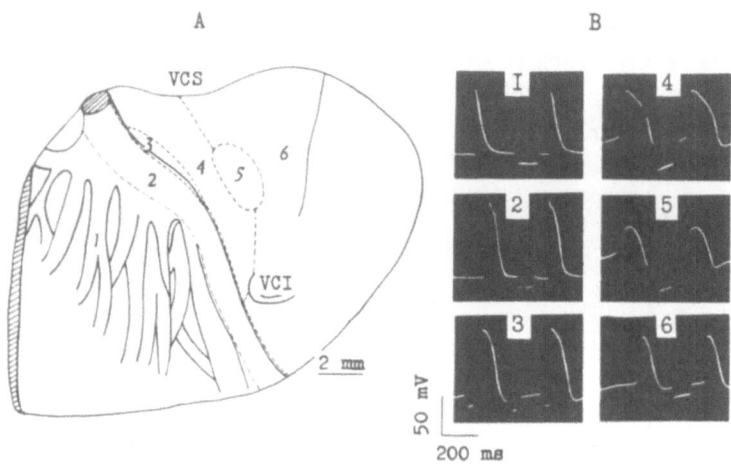

FIGURE 6 A. *The arbitrary division of the SA node area. (Modified from Masuda, Paes de Carvalho (1977)). 1, trabeculae of the right atrium; 2, crista
terminalis; 3, area of the excitation transition from the SA node to crista
terminalis (the sinoatrial junction); 4, a perinodal area lying between the
zone of true pacemakers and crista terminalis; 5, the zone of true pacemakers;
6, a perinodal area lying between the zone of true pacemakers and interatrial
septum; VCS, vene cava superior; VCI, vena cava inferior.*
B. *Sample recordings of the input resistance characteristic of various parts of
the SA node area. The current pulse used was 5 x 10^{-8} A in 1 and 2 and 2.5 x
10^{-8} A in 3, 4, 5 and 6.*

III. PASSIVE ELECTRICAL PROPERTIES OF THE SA NODE AREA

The experimental and theoretical approaches developed above were used to investigate the passive electrical properties of the SA node extensively. The space
constant of electrotonic decay was measured both parallel to (λ_x) and normal to
(λ_y) the crista terminalis; in the crista terminalis itself and in atrial trabeculae the space constant was measured parallel to the longitudinal axis of the
fibres (λ_x) and perpendicular to them (λ_y). The SA node region and adjacent
area was divided into the following parts : (1) the trabeculae of the right

atrium, (2) the crista terminalis, (3) the area of excitation transition from
the SA node to the crista terminalis, (4) a perinodal area between the zone of
true pacemakers and crista terminalis, (5) the zone of true pacemakers and (6) a
perinodal area between the latter zone and the interatrial septum (fig. 6A.).
The action potential shape and the maximal positive value of delay between the
action potentials in the SA node and the crista terminalis (Hoffman 1965) served
as criteria for true pacemakers. Zone 3 was outlined according to Masuda and
Paes de Carvalho (1975); Sano and Iida (1968); Sano and Yamagishi (1965);
Sano et al., 1966; the perinodal area's 4 and 6 were identified after Strauss
and Bigger, (1972).

Fig. 6B shows representative recordings of the R_{in} measurement in various
parts of the SA node area. R_{in} values of 300 to 400 kOhms were characteristic
for atrial tissue; in the zone of latent and true pacemakers R_{in} ranged between
0.5 and 1.0 MOhm. The mean values for R_{in} an the space constants of electrotonic decay are given in Table I. It can be seen that R_{in} had the largest value
(1050 kOhm) in the zone of true pacemakers and decreased in the direction of the
crista terminalis as well as the interatrial septum, i.e. moving towards the
area of latent pacemakers.

In the SA node area the electrotonic decay was always less pronounced along
the x-axis as compared to the y-axis ($\lambda_{xe} > \lambda_{ye}$), i.e. the electrotonic anisotropy was characteristic of all the SA node areas ($a_e = \lambda_x / \lambda_y$).

In the crista terminalis a_e equaled 16.3; in the trabeculae it amounted to
11.6; in the SA node it ranged from 1.4 to 3.9.

The shortest space constants, in the x-direction, were obtained for the
zone of true pacemakers. An increase was observed with transition to the area
of latent pacemakers, both toward the interatrial septum and towards the crista
terminalis. Our λ_y, for the true pacemaker zone, was one fourth of the value
reported by Seyama (1976). Although we do not have a sound explanation for this
discrepancy, we feel that differences in experimental conditions might be the
cause; e.g. the preparation in the work cited was not spontaneously active,
hence an electrophysiological identification of the true pacemaker zone was impossible.

Noteworthy is the finding that, in the SA node area, there were no inhomogeneities found in space constant both in the true and latent pacemaker region.
This area was also devoid of loci characterized by an abrupt drop of electroton-

TABLE I

MEAN VALUE AND VARIATION RANGES FOR THE SPACE CONSTANTS
AND THE INPUT RESISTANCE IN VARIOUS PARTS OF THE
RABBIT SA NODE AREA

The area of recording	λ_{xe} $\mu m \pm SEM$	λ_x μm	λ_{ye} $\mu m \pm SEM$	λ_y μm	R_{in} $kOhms \pm SEM$
1. Trabeculae of the right atrium	670+40 425÷850 n=11	1220	90+9 60÷130 n=8	105	3222+16 180÷500 n=37
2. Crista terminalis	790+60 550÷1100 n=11	1420	76+6 50÷125 n=13	87	370+16 200÷650 n=42
3. Area of excitation transition from the SA node to the crista terminalis	460+30 300÷625 n=11	750	150+15 55÷350 n=25	190	600+40 200÷1350 n=42
4. Peridonal area by the crista termi- nalis	425+25 200÷625 n=21	670	160+17 80÷270 n=12	218	750+38 300÷1650 n=60
5. Zone of true pace- makers	325+22 140÷520 n=22	468	160+16 85÷280 n=14	205	1050+40 700÷2000 n=54
6. Perinodal area by the interatrial septum	450+50 250÷725 n=11	720	340+45 250÷460 n=5	527	450+28 200÷900 n=36

n, the size of sample

ic potential.   Ultrastructural   investigations have suggested the existence of local inhomogeneities at small distances (Trautwein and Uchizono, 1963).   To check this   suggestion, in a few experiments, electrotonic spread was measured every 10 μm along the y-axis. We did not find abrupt drops of electrotonic po- tential at a short range of distances.

For the calculation of the resistivities of the interior of the syncytium (ρ_x, ρ_y) the membrane specific resistance R_m and the specific junctional dis- tributed resistance R_k, (equations (12) to (15)) were used, as well as theoreti- cal inferences from the analysis of the isotropic model, as far as the extent of the electrotonic and geometrical (length to diameter ratio) anisotropies are small in the zone of true SA nodal pacemakers and do not differ significantly from each other.

For the sake of simplicity, let the true pacemaker units from the SA node be ellipsoid shaped, with the major half-axis x_c = 10 μm and the minor one y_c = 3 μm; taking the infoldings of the excitable cell membrane into account, the surface area amounts 1×10^{-5} cm^2; the area of nexus is equal to 2×10^{-8} cm^2 (Masson-Pevet, 1979). While calculating the resistivity of the "distributed" junctional membrane, R_k, and the resistivity of the nexuses, R_n, we will make use of the inferences from the theoretical analysis of the isotropic model in that the input resistance is primarily determined by the junctions of a cell. In estimating R_k and R_n, the assumption was made that a cell might or might not have neighbours and nexuses from above (F = 1 or 2 in eq. (12) to (14)). The corresponding values obtained were R_k = 4 - 8 Ohm.cm^2 and R_n = 0.008 - 0.016 Ohm.cm^2. These data are in quite good accordance with those obtained by Matter (1973), who reported a R_n value of 0.025 Ohm.cm^2. When ρ_{pl} = 120 Ohm.cm (Schanne, 1969), ρ_T = 64 Ohm.cm (Sperelakis and MacDonald, 1964) and r_o - 0.5 μm, we calculate for the zone of true pacemakers in the SA node the following values: ρ_x = 400 to 800 Ohm.cm, ρ_y = 2000 to 4000 Ohm.cm and R_m = 20.000 to 40.000 Ohm.cm^2.

DISCUSSION

A variety of models for continuous and discrete media have been used for the analysis of syncytial properties of myocardium (Smolyaninov, 1980). Whatever the model, one-dimensional (Hodgkin and Rushton, 1946), two-dimensional (Bukauskas et al., 1974; Kukushkin et al., 1974) or three-dimensional (Bukauskas et al., 1975; Purves, 1976), infinite space has regularly been postulated. As our measurements of the electric field distribution on both sides of a preparation show, the most acceptable approximation for the electrotonic spread in real cardiac structures, is a three-dimensional anisotropic medium of finite thickness. With this model, electrotonic decay in the two directions normal to the fibre axis was found to be of the same order of magnitude. Obviously, in

some particular cases, the model can be simplified; thus, for very thin plane
layers, it is reasonable to use a two-dimensional anisotropic model, while for
thick plane layers, the infinite three-dimensional model is more expedient, etc.
With regard to the input resistance, when measured with micro-electrodes, it is
more reasonable to use a three dimensional model, provided the effective radius
of the current electrode is used.

Our results indicate that a relatively good intercellular coupling is inherent to all parts of the SA node. We failed to find loci with an abrupt drop
in electrotonic potential. This points to the fact that the block zone, found
under normal conditions in the SA node (Sano and Yamagishi, 1965; Bleeker
et al., 1980) should be primarily accounted for by the excitable properties of
the cells, and not by weak cell to cell coupling. The same explanation is valid
for the low velocity of excitation propagation in this area.

Looking ahead, it should be of interest to investigate the electrotonic potential spread in the direction of the z-axis in the area of the SA node. This
could probably shed some light on the causes giving rise to the discrepancy
between our estimates of λ_x and λ_y and those of other investigators (Seyama,
1976). It also would give a better insight into processes associated with the
electrical activity in the cells from the SA node.

REFERENCES

Barr, L.: Electrical transmission between the cells of vertebrate cardiac muscle. In: Comparative Physiology of the Heart: Current Trends. McCann,
F.V., ed., Birkenhauser Verlag, Basel and Stuttgart, pp. 102-110, 1969.

Bleeker, W.K., Mackaay, A.J.C., Masson-Pevet, M., Bouman, L.N. and Becker,
A.E.: Functional and morphological organization of the rabbit sinus node.
Circ. Res., 46: 11-22, 1980.

Bonke, F.I.M.: Electrotonic spread in the sinoatrial node of the rabbit heart.
Pfluegers Arch., 339: 17-23, 1973.

Bredikis, J.J., Bukauskas, F.F., Muckus, K.S. and Puodzius, S.S.: Ontogenetic
pecularities of the electrical activity in cardiac fibres of human embryo.

J. Evol. Biochem. Physiol. (Leningrad), 14: 43-48, 1978.

Bukauskas, F.F., Kukushkin, N.I. and Saxon, M.E.: Model of two-dimensional anisotropic syncitium. Biofizika, 19: 712-716, 1974.

Bukauskas, F.F. and Veteikis, R.P.: Passive electrical properties of AV node region of rabbits heart. Biofizika, 22: 449-504, 1977a.

Bukauskas, F.F., Veteikis, R.P. and Gutman, A.M.: A model for passive three-dimensional anisotropic syncitium as continuous medium. Biofizika, 20: 1083-1086, 1975.

Bukauskas, F.F., Veteikis, R.P., Gutman, A.M. and Mutskus, K.S.: Intercellular electrical coupling in the sinoatrial node of rabbit's heart. Biofizika, 22: 108-112, 1977b.

Cranefield, P.F. and Greenspan, K.: The rate of oxygen uptake of quiescent cardiac muscle. J. Gen. Physiol., 44: 235-247, 1961.

De Mello, W.C.: Passive electrical properties of the atrioventricular node. Pfluegers Arch., 371: 135-139, 1977.

Hodgkin, A.L. and Rushton, W.A.H.: The electrical constants of a crustacean nerve fibre. Proc. Roy. Soc. London, B133: 444-479, 1946.

Hoffman, B.F.: Atrioventricular conduction in mammalian hearts. Ann. N.Y. Acad. Sci., 127: 105-112, 1965.

Johnson, E.A. and Tille, J.: Investigations of the electrical properties of cardiac muscle fibres with the aid of intracellular double-barrelled electrodes. J. Gen. Physiol., 44: 443-467, 1961.

Kukushkin, N.I., Bukauskas, F.F. and Saxon, M.E.: II. Model of two-dimensional anisotropic syncitium. Biofizika, 19: 888-893, 1974.

Masson-Pevet, M.A.: The fine structure of cardiac pacemaker cells in the sinus node and in tissue culture. (Doct. Thesis), Rodopi, Amsterdam, 1979.

Masuda, M.O. and Paes de Carvalho, A.: Sinoatrial transmission and atrial invasion during normal rhythm in the rabbit heart. Circ. Res., 37: 414-421, 1975.

Matter, A.: A morphometric study on the nexus of rat cardiac muscle. J. Cell Biol., 56: 690-696, 1973.

Pearson, O.H., Hastings, A.B. and Bunting, H.: Metabolism of cardiac muscle: utilization of C^{14} labelled pyruvate and acetate by heart slices. Amer. J. Physiol., 158: 251-260, 1949.

Purves, R.D.: Current flow and potential in a three-dimensional syncitium. J.

Theor. Biol., 60: 147-163, 1976.

Sakson, M.E., Bukauskas, F.F., Kukushkin, N.I. and Nasonova, V.V.: Study of electrotonic distribution on the surface of cardiac structures. Biofizika, 19: 1045-1049, 1974.

Sano, T. and Iida, Y.: Sinoatrial connection and wandering pacemaker. J. Electrocardiol., 1: 147-153, 1968.

Sano, T. and Yamagishi, S.: Spread of excitation from the sinus node. Circ. Res., 16: 423-430, 1965.

Sano, T., Yamagishi, S. and Iida, Y.: Several aspects on the spontaneous activity of the sinus node and its spread. Jap. Circ. J., 30: 134-138, 1966.

Schanne, O.F.: Measurement of cytoplasmic resistivity by means of the glass microelectrodes. In: Glass microelectrodes, Lavallee, M., Schanne, O.F. and Herbert, N.C., eds., Wiley Sons, New York-London-Sydney-Toronto, pp. 299-321, 1969.

Seyama, I.: Characteristics of the rectifying properties of the sino-atrial node cell of the rabbit. J. Physiol. (London), 255: 379-397, 1976.

Smolyaninov, V.V.: Mathematical models of biological tissues (in Russian), Nauka, Moscow, 1980.

Sperelakis, N. and Macdonald, R.L.: Ratio of transverse to longitudinal resistivities of isolated cardiac muscle fiber bundle. J. Electrocardiol., 7: 301-314, 1974.

Strauss, H.C. and Bigger, J.T.: Electrophysiologic properties of the rabbit sinoatrial perinodal fibers. Circ. Res., 31: 490-506, 1972.

Tanaka, I. and Sasaki, Y.: On the electrotonic spread in cardiac muscle of the mouse. J. Gen. Physiol., 49: 1089-1110, 1966.

Trautwein, W. and Uchizono, K.: Electron microscopic and electrophysiologic study of the pacemaker in the sinoatrial node of the rabbit heart. Z. Zellforsch., 61: 96-109, 1963.

Weidmann, S.: Electrical constants of trabecular muscle from mammalian heart. J. Physiol. (London), 210: 1041-1054, 1970.

DISCUSSION BY SILVIO WEIDMANN

From letter by Silvio Weidmann, Berne, to Feliksas Bukauskas, Kaunas,
10 February 1981.
In your theory as applied to a 3-dimensional network, the resistance of the surface membrane seems to drop out, leaving internal resistivity (myoplasmic lumped
with nexal) as practically the only determinant for the measured input resistance (R_{in}).   I now have the problem in reconciling your model with the models
published by Berkinblit et-al. (1965, 1). In their Fig. 2, they plot input
resistance as a function of membrane resistivity (R_m) for different types of
networks. Whatever their assumptions, there is a slight dependence of R_{in} on
R_m.   Does the apparent discrepancy reflect a difference of assumptions?   My mathematical knowledge is not sufficient to decide on this point, and I should   be
grateful if you could check on this question.

From letter by F. Bukauskas to S. Weidmann
6 March 1981.
Fig 2 of Berkinblit et al. (1965) reflects the dependence of input   resistance
(R_{in}) on membrane resistivity (R_m) for syncytia of various configurations and
for various distances of   the   "branching points".   Our   approximation for   a
3-dimensional syncytium is comparable only to the case of the cubical network of
Berkinblit et al. Their lowest curve of Fig. 2 shows that R_{in} is almost constant   when   branching   points are 200 µm apart and when R_m exceeds 1000 Ohmcm^2.
If they had assumed more realistic cell lengths (10 - 20 µm for SA node) the dependence of R_{in} on R_m would be ven less pronounced.   There is thus no contradic-
tion between our theory and the theory by Berkinblit et al.

From letter by S. Weidmann to F. Bukauskas,
24 May 1981.
I feel revieled that an apparent controversy is settled.   It   seems   important
that   investigators interested in changes of cell-to-cell coupling under various
experimental conditions be aware of this particular prediction.   For   instance,
if constant current pulses are injected into a cell of a 3-dimensional syncytium

and voltage displacement is measured from the same cell, an increase of R_{in} can only   mean   an increase of cell-to-cell or cytoplasmic resistance, regardless of possible changes (within limits) of R_m.

Reference :   Berkinblitt, M.B., Kovalev, S.A., Smolyaninov, S.S., Chailakhyan, L.M.:   The electrical structure of myocardial tissue. Doklady Akademii Nauk SSSR 163: 741-744, 1965.

GAP JUNCTION STRUCTURE IN COUPLED AND UNCOUPLED CONDITIONS

Camillo Peracchia

INTRODUCTION

Activities such as heart contraction, uterus contractures at labor, simultaneous firing of groups of neurons, as well as a variety of cooperative cellular functions would be ineffective in the absence of a system for direct cell-to-cell communication. This system, known as cell coupling, relies on the presence of specialized cell junctions called gap junctions, nexuses, maculae communicantes, coupling junctions, etc. (Peracchia, 1980).

In the heart three types of intercellular junctions have been described (Staehelin, 1974). Two of them, fasciae adherentes and maculae adherentes (spot desmosomes), function as strong, adhesive linkages between cells; the other, gap junctions, provides intercellular pathways for small molecules (Fig. 1).

The communicating property of gap junctions in heart has been clearly demonstrated by studies on the reversible effects of hypertonic solutions on electrical coupling and gap junction integrity (Barr et al., 1965). In these solutions the membranes of gap junctions became separated, being pulled apart by the cell shrinkage, and simultaneously the intercellullar electrical resistance increased dramatically. Moreover the noncommunicating property of fasciae and maculae adherentes was demonstrated by the effects of hypertonic solutions low in Ca^{++} or chloride (Dreifuss et al., 1966; Kawamura and Konishi, 1967). These solutions in fact, while causing membrane separation at fasciae and maculae adherentes, maintained gap junctions and electrical coupling intact.

More recently elegant demonstrations of the involvement of gap junctions in electrical coupling of heart muscle cells have been provided by evidence that the establishment of cell contact, either directly or via heterologous cells, induces beating synchrony in cultured myocardial cells (Goshima, 1969, 1970; Hyde et al., 1969; DeHaan and Hirakow, 1972; Lawrence et al., 1978).

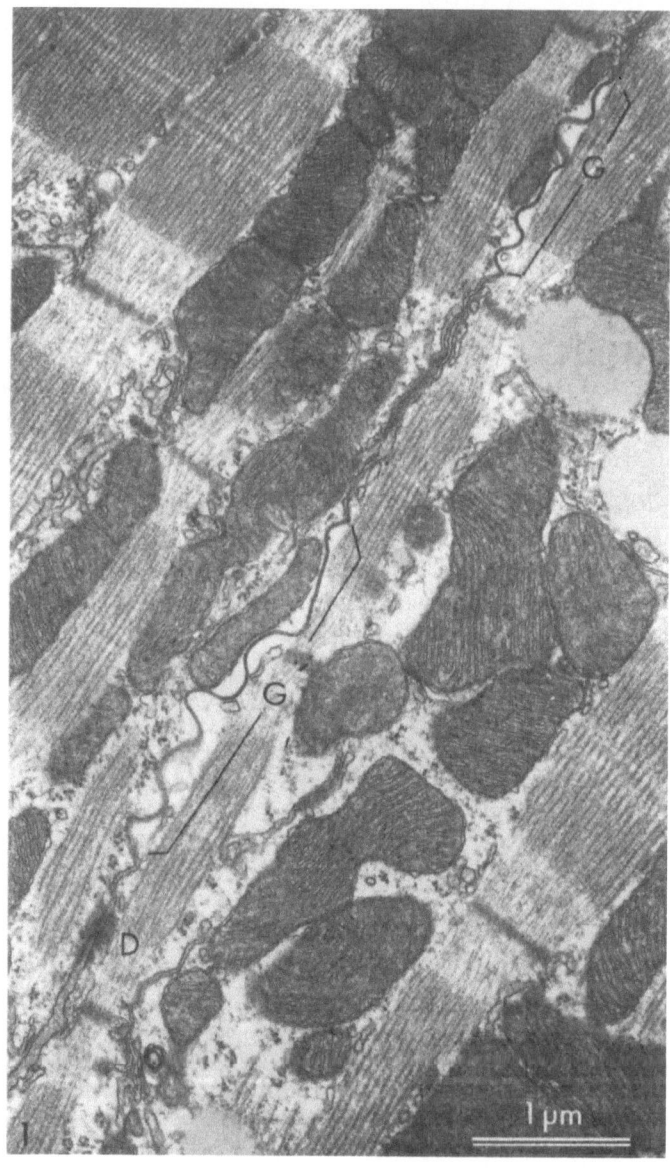

FIGURE 1 *Rat heart. Two longitudinally sectioned myofibers are joined by extensive gap junctions (G) and a spot desmosome (D).*

Synchronous beating is provided by newly formed gap junctions because myocardial cells do not acquire synchrony (Goshima, 1969) when they are connected via mouse L cells, which are incapable of forming gap junctions (Goshima, 1970) and of establishing electrical (Gilula et al., 1972) and metabolic (Pitts, 1971) coupling with normal cells.

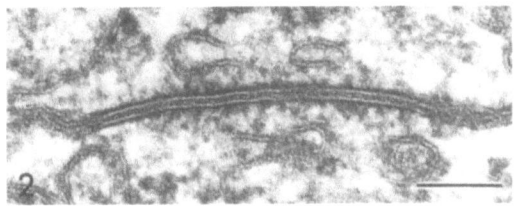

FIGURE 2 *Rat stomach. Cross sectional profile of a gap junction between epithelial cells. At the junction the membranes appear separated by an extracellular space 2–3 nm wide. The overall thickness of the junction is 18 nm. Bar = 100 nm.*

For establishing synchronous electrical activation of neighbouring cells the only requirement is intercellular free diffusion of small ions (Weidmann, 1966; Bennett et al., 1967; Weingart, 1974; Politoff et al., 1974; Ledbetter and Lubin, 1979). There is evidence, however, that also larger molecules of a molecular weight not greater than 1000 (in vertebrates), including aminoacids, nucleotides, oligosaccharides and second messengers, are indeed exchanged from cell to cell (Pitts, 1971, 1977; Tsien and Weingart, 1974; Lawrence et al., 1978; Flagg-Newton et al., 1979), which makes cell coupling a more mysterious, yet more provocative, aspect of tissue function. These molecules travel across the cell boundaries via well insulated intercellular channels approximately 1.5 nm in diameter, located in the intramembrane particles of gap junctions.

Differently from other membrane channels, the intercellular channels are usually stable in an open state, but can be closed in a variety of circumstances through a mechanism believed to be activated by divalent cations (Loewenstein, 1975; DeMello, 1980; Peracchia, 1980) and, possibly, also by hydrogen ions (Turin and Warner, 1977, 1980). The occlusion of intercellular channels and

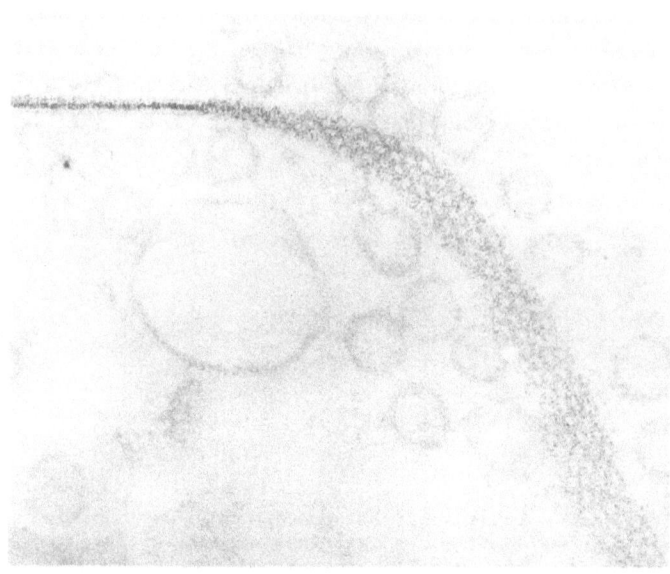

FIGURE 3 *Crayfish ganglion. Gap junction between lateral giant axons negative-ly stained with lanthanum hydroxide. The tracer fills the extracellular space producing an electron opaque layer at the center of cross sectioned regions of the junction (upper left corner) and a polygonal network where the junction is obliquely sectioned (right half of micrograph). The electron opaque network surrounds the protruding ends of the intramembrane particles (the electron transparent spots), staining them negatively. Bar = 100 nm.*

consequently the cell uncoupling, is known mainly as a safety mechanism which allows healthy cells to isolate themselves from damaged neighboring cells, but it might play a role in a number of pathological events including cardiac arrhythmias.

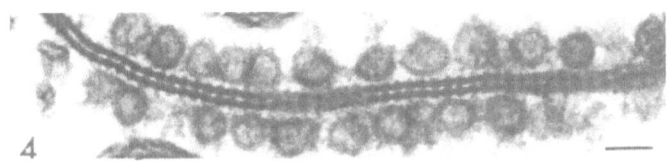

FIGURE 4 *Crayfish ganglion. Cross sectional profile of a gap junction between lateral giant axons. Notice that the intramembrane particles are visible as electron opaque beads repeating every 20 nm along the profile of each membrane and binding to similar beads of the adjacent membrane across the gap. Both surfaces of the junction are coated with a layer of 70-100 nm vesicles whose function is yet to be determined. Bar = 100 nm.*

GAP JUNCTION STRUCTURE

For the most part, the surface of a cell is separated from that of a neighboring cell by an extracellular space 10-15 nm thick. There are regions, however, where the plasmamembranes come in close apposition to each other. Some of these regions are belt-like structures which seal the extracellular space along the entire cell perimeter, where apical and lateral cell surfaces meet. These, known as tight junctions or zonulae occludentes, provide a barrier between luminal and lateral compartments of the epithelial extracellular space. Other regions, gap junctions, are disc-like regions where the membranes appear separated by a narrow extracellular space.

At first, gap junctions were described as areas of tight membrane apposition, with complete obliteration of the extracellular space (Sjostrand et al., 1958; Karrer, 1960a, b; Dewey and Barr, 1962), and, because of the apparent fusion of the two outer membrane layers, were frequently confused with zonulae occludentes. A distinction between the two types of junction was made possible by the introduction of "in block" staining with uranyl salts (Farquhar and Palade, 1965). Due to the increased electron opacity of the membranes stained with uranyl, the presence of an extracellular "gap" 2-3 nm wide (Fig. 2), became obvious (Revel and Karnovsky, 1967).

The reality of the gap was demonstrated unequivocally by its permeability to an extracellular tracer, lanthanum hydroxide (Revel and Karnovsky, 1967) (Fig. 3). However, in spite of an apparently uninterrupted gap the cells are

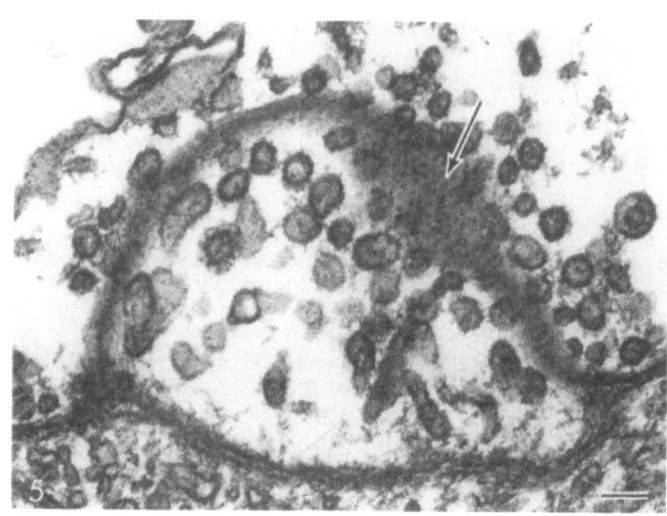

FIGURE 5 *Crayfish ganglion. Gap junction between lateral gians axons. In obliquely or tangentially sectioned junctions the intramembrane particles are visible as electron opaque spots (arrow) arranged in a polygonal array. Bar = 100 nm.*

indeed attached to each other at numerous spots where intramembrane particles, protruding from the external membrane surfaces come in contact with each other bridging the gap. Due to their low electron opacity, the particles usually are not seen in sections. In one case, however, they have been clearly demonstrated by a special fixation and staining procedure (Peracchia, 1973a) (Figs. 4 and 5).

Rare images of particles spanning the electron transparent layer of the membrane (Peracchia, 1980) and evidence from the freeze-fracture behavior of gap junction particles (Peracchia, 1973b; Hanna et al., 1978) have suggested that the particles occupy the entire membrane thickness. Recently, this feature has been demonstrated by X-ray diffraction studies on isolated mouse liver gap junctions (Caspar et al., 1977; Makowski et al., 1977). These studies also provided definite evidence for the presence of a lipid bilayer surrounding the intramembrane particles.

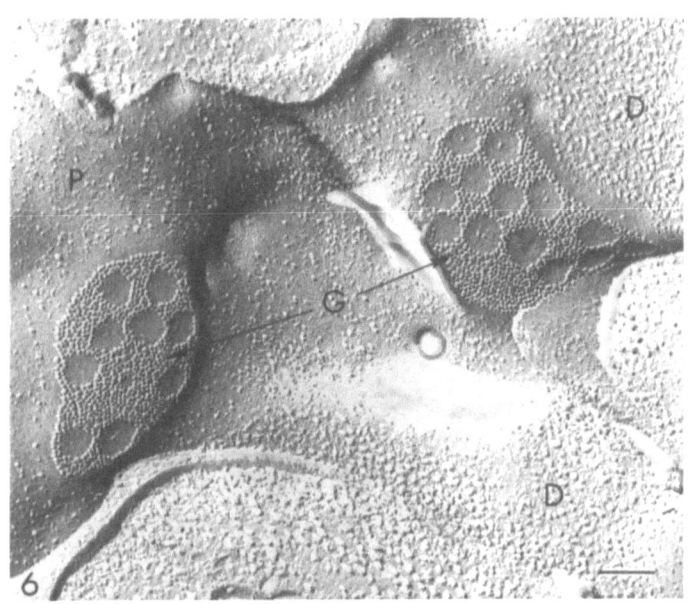

FIGURE 6 *Calf heart. Freeze-fractured gap junctions (G) display 8 nm particles polygonally packed in discrete regions of protoplasmic fractured surface, face P (P). The junctions shown here contain circular, slightly concave areas 70 nm in diameter. They are mostly particle free, although some display one or two central particles. These structures, whose function is unknown, are common in lower vertebrate hearts, but are rare in mammalian hearts. It is possible that they are composed of caveolar membrane (Peracchia, 1980). D = desmosomes.   Bar = 100 nm.*

The particles are organized in the plane of the membrane in polygonal arrays (Figs. 3 and 5). This characteristic, first noticed in gap junctions of goldfish brain fixed with potassium permanganate (Robertson, 1963) was soon confirmed in mammalian heart and liver junctions negatively stained and studied either in thin sections (Revel and Karnovsky, 1967) or in isolated fractions (Benedetti and Emmelot, 1968).

The tridimensional architecture of gap junctions and some characteristics of the structure of intercellular channels have been defined by freeze-fracture. As other membranes (Branton, 1966), gap junction membranes fracture down the middle, splitting the lipid bilayer into two monolayers. In the process, the

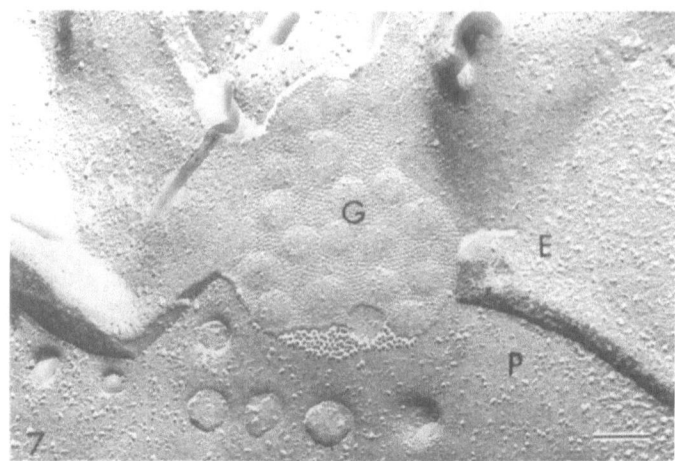

FIGURE 7 *Calf heart. The fractured face of the exoplasmic leaflet, face E (E) displays, at gap junctions (G), polygonal arrays of pits, representing the com- plementary images of particles fractured away with the protoplasmic leaflet. In this micrograph the junction is fractured in steps, such that a few particles of one membrane, face P (P) and most of the pits of the apposed membrane are seen. Bar = 100 nm.*

intramembrane particles are pulled out of one of the leaflets, and remain at- tached to the other one.

In vertebrate and most of the invertebrate gap junctions the particles re- main with the protoplasmic leaflet, appearing as bumps on the P fractured face (Fig. 6), and leave complementary pits on the exoplasmic face (E face) (Fig. 7). In the crayfish, as in other arthropods, while most of the particles frac- ture with the exoplasmic leaflet (Fig. 8), some fracture with the protoplasmic (Peracchia, 1973b) (Fig. 9).

This peculiar fracture property, aside from supporting the concept that the par- ticles span the entire thickness of the membrane and protrude from both membrane surfaces (Peracchia, 1973b; Hanna et al., 1978) has given us the chance to study both the cytoplasmic (Fig. 8) and the extracellular (Fig. 9) end of the particles. On both ends most of the particles displayed a 2.5 nm central de- pression (Figs. 8 and 9) (Peracchia, 1973b; Peracchia, 1980) supporting previ-

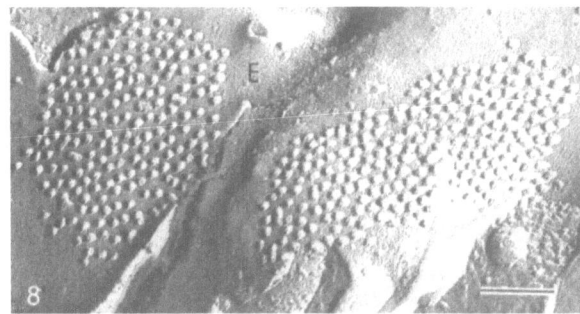

FIGURE 8 Crayfish ganglion. In crayfish, as in most of the Arthropods, gap junction particles remain with the exoplasmic leaflet, face E (E). The two gap junctions shown here display 12-14 nm particles irregularly packed at 18-20 nm (center-to-center distance). Some of the particles show a central indentation believed to represent the cytoplasmic end of the channel. Bar = 100 nm.

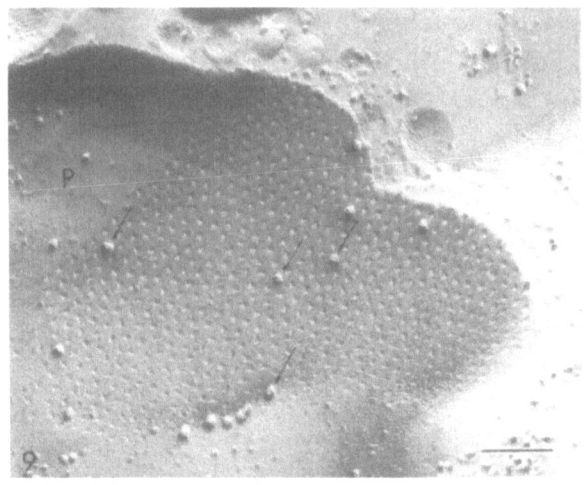

FIGURE 9 Crayfish ganglion. On P faces (P) crayfish gap junctions display a polygonal array of pits; they are the complementary images of particles which have fractured away with the exoplasmic leaflet. A few pits contain particles which have remained attached to the protoplasmic leaflet. Some of the particles (arrows) display central indentations believed to represent the external ends of the channels. Bar = 100 nm.

ous hypotheses (Payton et al., 1969b; McNutt and Weinstein, 1970) for the location of intercellular channels at the center of particles (Fig. 10).

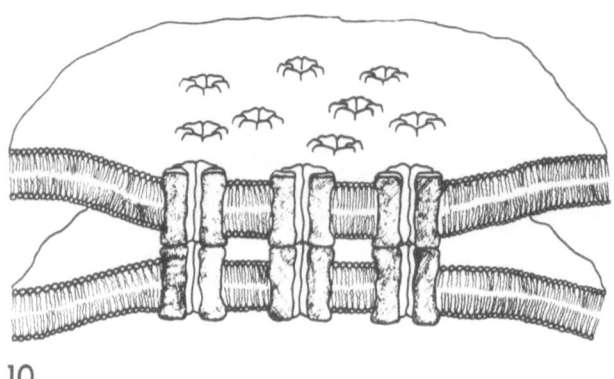

10

FIGURE 10 Tentative model of gap junction structure in coupled conditions.
*Intramembrane particles composed of six subunits span the membrane thickness and
bind to similar particles of the adjoined membrane. 1.5 - 2 nm channels are located at the center of the particles. The particles are grouped in a disordered
array at a center-to-center distance of 10 nm (vertebrates). The particles are
interspaced by a lipid bilayer.*

        Images from freeze-fractured (Peracchia, 1973b, 1974; Hama and Saito,
1977) and from lanthanum (Peracchia, 1973a) or phosphotungstate (Peracchia,
1973b) negatively stained gap junctions have shown that the particles are composed of six main subunits radially arranged around the central channel (Peracchia, 1980) (Fig. 10). The six subunit composition of the intramembrane particles has recently been confirmed by data from low dose electron microscopy of
isolated junctions (Zampighi and Unwin, 1979; Unwin and Zampighi, 1980).   This
study has also indicated that the subunits may be tilted with respect to an axis
perpendicular to the membrane and has provided some evidence for two conformational structures of the particles, possibly related to different functional
states.

        A peculiar resistance of gap junction membranes to certain detergents have
made possible the isolation of fairly pure gap junction fractions from mammalian
liver (Benedetti and Emmelot, 1968; Goodenough and Stoekenius, 1972; Evans and

Gurd, 1972), lens (Dunia et al., 1974; Alcala et al., 1975) and heart (Kensler and Goodenough, 1980). Polycrilamide gel electrophoreses of junctions solubilized with sodium dodecyl sulfate (SDS-PAGE) have indicated the presence of a major polypeptide component of M.W. 26,000-28,000 in liver and lens junctions (see Peracchia, 1980, as a review). The only study on heart junctions on the contrary reports bands at M.W. 38,000, 31,000, 33,500 and possibly a diffuse one at 47,000. Whether this diversity is indeed due to an intrinsic difference in molecular structure rather than to a different preparative procedure is not known at present.

Limited information is available on gap junction lipid composition. Preliminary studies have shown some similarity between gap junction and plasma-membrane lipids, the only difference being a high amount of cholesterol (Evans and Gurd, 1972; Caspar et al., 1977; Herzberg and Gilula, 1979; Henderson et al., 1979) and virtual absence of sphingomyelin (Hertzberg and Gilula, 1979) in gap junction membranes.

GAP JUNCTION AND CELL UNCOUPLING

Already in the last century, heart muscle, differently from skeletal muscle, was known to recover from mechanical injury to some of its cells. This phenomenon, known as "healing over" (Engelmann, 1877; Rothschuh, 1951; Weidmann, 1952; Deleze, 1965, 1970; DeMello et al., 1969 etc.) was believed to depend on the capacity of ruptured cells to reseal. However, in 1965 Deleze noticed that "healing over" takes place only if the extracellular medium contains calcium. This important information came at the time when evidence for the involvement of calcium ions in cell uncoupling was accumulating (Loewenstein, 1966; Nakas et al., 1966; Loewenstein et al., 1967). Thus, it seemed likely that "healing over" could result from uncoupling between injured and uninjured cells rather than from membrane resealing. More recently this concept has been strongly supported by evidence for the penetration of lanthanum or procion yellow in injured cells after complete "healing over" (Baldwin, 1977; Bernardini et al., 1980) and by the observation that procion yellow, a dye (M.W. 550) known to diffuse rapidly across gap junctions (Payton et al., 1969b; Imanaga, 1974; Rae, 1974 etc.), does not diffuse from injured to uninjured cells (Bernardini et al., 1980).

Knowledge of the capacity of gap junction channels to close off upon cell injury, or treatments which raise the intracellular calcium concentration $\left[Ca^{++}\right]_i$, has stimulated great interest among membranologists. Electrophysiologists, electronmicroscopists and crystallographers have concerted their efforts in an attempt to define the uncoupling factors and the mechanism by which the intercellular channels close off.

In early studies cell uncoupling was always believed to follow a complete separation of the junctional membranes (Barr **et al.,** 1965, 1968; Asada and Bennett, 1971; Pappas et al., 1971). However, there were cases in which the electrical resistance between cells increased without obvious evidence for disappearance of gap junctions (Payton et al., 1969a; Pappas et al., 1971; Politoff and Pappas, 1972). These data suggested that, in some cases, finer structural changes in gap junctions may take place (Peracchia, 1973a).

A correlation between changes in intercellular electrical resistance and changes in gap junction structure was first reported in crayfish (Peracchia and Dulhunty, 1974, 1976). Here, the gap junctions between axons uncoupled by Ca^{++}-chelation or inhibition of the metabolism changed their particle packings from disordered arrays, in coupled conditions, to tight crystalline arrays in uncoupled conditions. A decrease in particle diameter and gap thickness were also detected. Similar changes in particle packing and particle diameter were soon reported also in mammalian stomach and liver exposed to uncoupling treatments such as inhibition of metabolism or hypoxia (Peracchia, 1977) (Figs. 11 and 12) and, more recently, gap junction crystallization has been confirmed in ciliary epithelium (Raviola et al., 1978), heart (Baldwin, 1979; Dahl and Isenberg, 1980), pancreas (Meda et al., 1980; Petersen et al., 1980) and lens (Peracchia, 1978; Peracchia et al., 1979) following various uncoupling circumstances. In some of the mammalian studies electrical uncoupling was monitored electrophysiologically (Dahl and Isenberg, 1980; Petersen et al., 1980); however, only in crayfish have the changes in gap junction structure been detected in the very cells in which the electrical uncoupling was monitored (Peracchia and Dulhunty, 1974, 1976).

In mammalian heart the particles of gap junctions between cells uncoupled

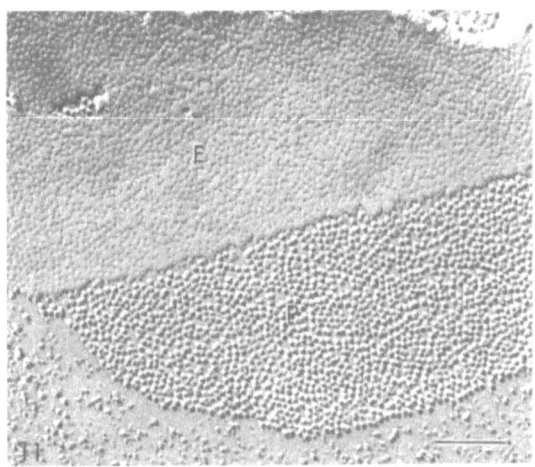

FIGURE 11 Rat liver. In samples fixed rapidly by vascular perfusion most of gap junctions display disordered arrays of particles on the P face (P) and pits on E face (E) at 10 nm center-to-center distance. Bar = 100 nm.

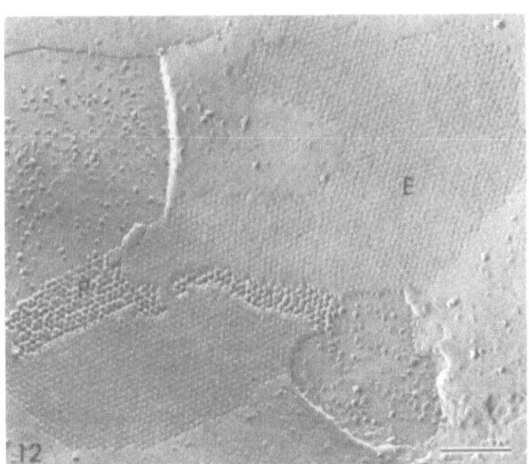

FIGURE 12 Rat liver. In samples fixed by vascular perfusion 15 minutes after animal death, particles and pits form crystalline arrays with a periodicity of approximately 8.5 nm. These arrays are similar to those produced in gap junctions of various vertebrate and invertebrate tissues with uncoupling treatments and are believed to follow an increase in $[Ca^{++}]_i$ and/or $[H^+]_i$ resulting from tissue hypoxia. P = P face; E = E face. Bar = 100 nm.

by mechanical injury were seen to crystallize in small domains separated by particle free isles (Baldwin, 1979); this pattern of crystallization was believed to reflect early uncoupling stages. Typical of early stages were also believed to be crystalline packings containing particles slightly larger than those of coupled junctions (Dahl and Isenberg, 1980), as packings with smaller particles, similar in size to those described in stomach junctions after one hour exposure to a metabolic inhibitor (Peracchia, 1977), were seen only at later times. Dahl and Isenberg (1980) interpreted the particle enlargement to reflect channel occlusion and the particle shrinkage to be a secondary phenomenon. However, all the data on changes in particle diameter should be taken with great caution as small variations in particle size cannot be reliably measured in freeze-fracture replicas, due to artifacts like plastic deformation, surface contamination and inconsistency in platinum depostion and platinum-carbon ratio.

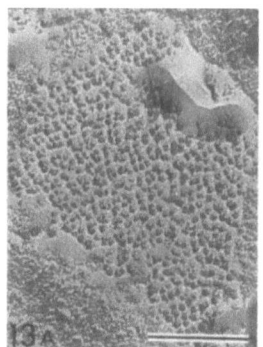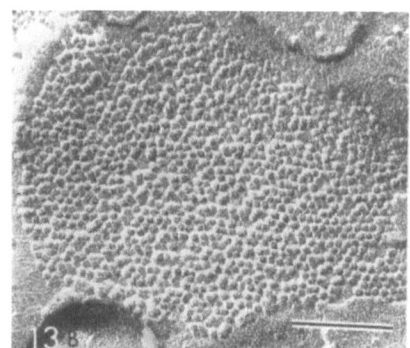

FIGURE 13 Dog heart. Purkinje fibers of ventricular bundles rapidly frozen in liquid nitrogen (Peracchia and Peracchia, 1980b) and freeze-fractured without glutaraldehyde fixation and cryoprotective treatment. The physiological state of dissected Purkinje dibers, determined with field stimulation, varies greatly due to dissection damage. Gap junctions with disordered particle arrays (A) as well as crystalline junctions (B) are often seen in the same sample indicating that, while some cells are still coupled, others have uncoupled. The coexistance of both junction types in unfixed samples indicates that changes in particle packing are not affected by glutaraldehyde fixation. Bar = 100 nm.

In the past, questions have been rasied about the ultrastructural data on changes in gap junctions with functional uncoupling in view of the fact that glutaraldehyde fixation, usually employed in these experiments, causes itself electrical uncoupling (Politoff and Pappas, 1972; Bennett, 1973). Recently, however, similar changes in particle packing with uncoupling have been obtained in samples prepared for freeze-fracture without glutaraldehyde fixation (Raviola et al., 1978; Baldwin, 1979; Peracchia and Peracchia, 1980b; Dahl and Isenberg, 1980) (Figs. 13A and B), thus we feel that glutaraldehyde uncouples cells by a different mechanism, which does not involve particle crystallization. On the other hand, Raviola et al., (1978) feel that glutaraldehyde fixation indeed crystallizes gap junction particles, since, in their samples, gap junctions of ciliary epithelium were consistently crystalline unless prepared for freeze-fracture without glutaraldehyde. However, if this were the case, one should expect virtually all gap junctions yet studied to be crystalline, as they are all glutaraldehyde fixed. Clearly this is not the case, as demonstrated quantitatively in a number of studies (Peracchia and Dulhunty, 1974, 1976; Hama and Saito, 1977; Peracchia, 1977, 1978; Baldwin, 1979; Dahl and Isenberg, 1980).

Undoubtedly, gap junction crystallization is a phenomenon closely associated with cell uncoupling. But, is it an intergral part of the uncoupling mechanism or simply a parallel phenomenon? Still this question cannot be fully answered; however, recent data (Peracchia, 1980) on the crystallizing effects of various uncoupling agents on isolated junctions, strongly supports the intimate relationship between crystallinity and uncoupling.

The junctions between lens fibers offer a unique sample for studying the direct effect of uncoupling agents on gap junction structure because they can be isolated with the configuration of coupled junctions, namely with disordered particle arrays (Fig. 14), if the isolation medium contains EDTA. Isolated lens fiber junctions reversibly crystallize upon exposure to solutions with a $[Ca^{++}]$ of 5.10^{-7} M or higher (Peracchia, 1978; Peracchia and Peracchia, 1980a) (Figs. 15 and 16) or a $[Mg^{++}]$ greater than 1.10^{-3} M at pH 7, as well as to Ca^{++}, Mg^{++}-free solutions with a $[H^+]$ of 3.10^{-7} M or higher (pH 6.5 or lower) (Peracchia and Peracchia, 1980a,b). Interestingly, these values are close to those known to affect cell coupling (Loewenstein, 1975; Weingart, 1977; Turin and Warner, 1977, 1980), which supports the hypothesis that gap junction crystallinity reflects the occlusion of intercellular channels by a direct interaction between uncoupling agents and gap junction components.

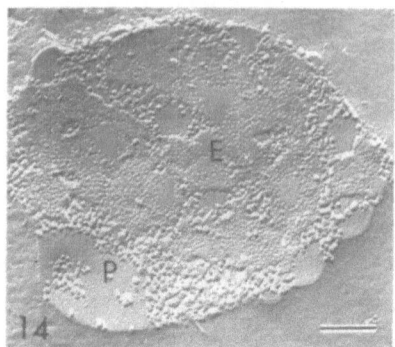
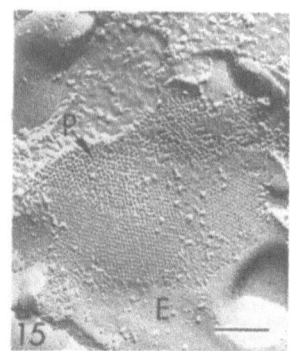

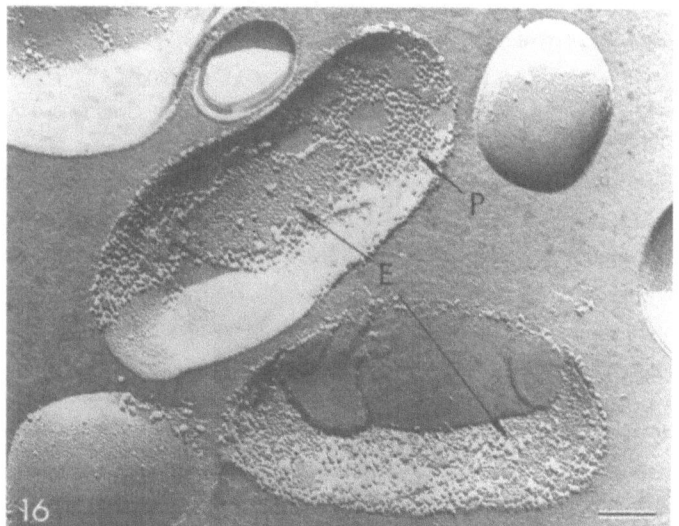

FIGURE 14 Calf lens. *Gap junctions isolated from lens fibers in the presence of EDTA at pH 7 display disordered arrays of particles and pits. P = P face; E = E face. Bar = 100 nm.*

FIGURE 15 Calf lens. *Gap junctions isolated from lens fibers in the presence of EDTA at pH 7 crystallize upon exposure to Ca^{++}-EDTA solutions (pH 7) in which the [Ca^{++}]is 5.10^{-7} M or higher. P = P face; E = E face.*

FIGURE 16 Calf lens. *Most of the gap junctions isolated in EDTA and subsequently exposed to Ca^{++} solution (as in Fig. 14) recover the appearance of control junctions (disordered particle arrays) upon incubation in Ca^{++}, Mg^{++}-free solutions buffered to pH 7.5. P = P face; E = E face. Bar = 100 nm.*

The calcium effects on lens junctions, recently confirmed by others (Alcala et al., 1979; Kistler and Bullivant, 1980b), have been criticized by Goodenough (1979) on the basis of lack of evidence for the capacity of lens fiber junctions to crystallize in intact cells and to uncouple physiologically. Recently, however, widespread crystallization has been obtained in intact lens fiber junctions by a treatment which increases the intracellular calcium content (Peracchia et al., 1979) and evidence for lens fiber uncoupling has been provided by the demonstration of a rapid return of ^{42}K efflux rate to control values, following mechanical injury in Ca^{++} containing media (Bernardini et al., 1980). Fiber uncoupling is also supported by the observation that procion yellow invades injured cells even 20 minutes after injury, but does not diffuse directly from injured to uninjured cells (Bernardini et al., 1980).

The calcium induced crystallinity is not a phenomenon peculiar to lens junctions; indeed, particle crystallinity has been recently obtained also in gap junctions of rat stomach epithelium upon exposure to a Ca^{++} ionophore (Lilly, A23187) (Peracchia and Peracchia, 1980a). Curiously, while Ca^{++} and Mg^{++} caused the particles of isolated lens gap junctions to crystallize into hexagonal arrays, low pH treatments produced rhombic and orthogonal particle packings. According to Kistler and Bullivant (1980a) membranes with orthogonal arrays are not gap junctions but individual membranes of different origin, and orthogonal arrays can be induced by trypsin digestion at pH values ranging from 5.5 - 8. Since in our samples unequivocal evidence for the junctional nature of these arrays was consistently obtained (Peracchia and Peracchia, 1980b) we feel that trypsin digestion and/or the different isolation procedure employed by Kistler and Bullivant (1980a) may have caused the crystalline junctional membranes to separate. The successful induction of orthogonal arrays by trypsin is interesting, as trypsin has been shown to cause electrical uncoupling (Loewenstein, 1966), and it raises the possibility that junctional crystallinity may also result from the loss of some protein components. The coexistance of rhrombic, orthogonal and hexagonal arrays in lens fiber junctions, and other peculiar structural characteristics, have suggested that the particles composing these junctions may be made of four rather than six main subunits (Peracchia and Peracchia, 1980b).

The mechanism by which divalent cations, and possibly hydrogen ions, close the channels is not yet known. As a hypothesis it has been proposed (Peracchia

et al., 1979; DeMello, 1980; Peracchia, 1980) that both gap junction particle crystallization and channel occlusion result from the neutralization of negatively charged sites on the membrane, followed by conformational changes.
Since Ca^{++} is the most effective of all the divalent cations, yet tested, in
causing cell uncoupling and junction crystallization, and the effectiveness of
the other divalent cations is higher, the closer they are to the crystalline radius of Ca^{++} (0.99 Å), we have suggested that the gap junction protein site is
similar, in size, to the crystalline diameter of Ca^{++} and is endowed with two
net negative charges (Peracchia et al., 1979; Peracchia, 1980). This would
explain why none of the monovalent cations, aside from H^+, are effective. On
the contrary, trivalent cations similar in size to Ca^{++} are expected to be more
effective that Ca^{++}, due to greater attraction to the negatively charged sites.
Indeed, La^{+++} (crystalline radius: 1.15 Å), iontophoretically injected in cardiac Purkinje fibers, seems to cause uncoupling faster than Ca^{++} (DeMello,
1979). The particles of disordered arrays are believed to be kept separated by
electrostatic forces and neutralization of negatively charged sites on the protein is expected to cause the particles to clump into tight crystalline arrays
and cause a conformational change in the protein resulting in channel occlusion.

A previous model has suggested that the channels close at the extracellular
end of the particles (Makowsky et al., 1977). This model was based on X-ray
diffraction patterns, recorded from isolated liver junctions after trypsin
digestion, indicating an increase in protein density in the extracellular region
and a decrease in gap thickness. However, these data do not provide evidence
for changes in channel size and there is no reason to believe that trypsin
digestion causes channel occlusion in isolated junctions.

In our model (Peracchia et al., 1979; Peracchia, 1980) we have proposed
that the channels close at their cytoplasmic end (Fig. 17) because an extracellular tracer, lanthanum hydroxide, which penetrates the channels of uncoupled
junctions of crayfish from the gap, does not infiltrate them completely, but
stops abruptly at a depth of 4-6 nm from the external end of the particles,
leaving the cytoplasmic halves of the channels unstained (Peracchia, 1980). A
similar staining behavior has recently been reported in isolated liver junctions
stained with uranyl acetate (Zampighi et al., 1980), which is consistent with
this hypothesis because isolated liver junctions are believed to be in an uncoupled state as a result of cell disruption during tissue homogenization (Perac-

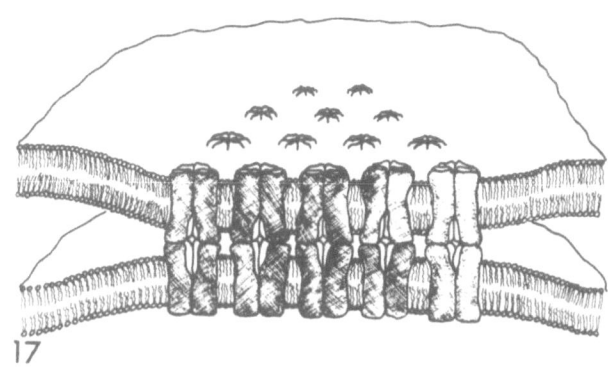

FIGURE 17 *Tentative model of gap junction structure in uncoupled conditions. The channels are believed to close at their cytoplasmic end as a result of conformational changes in particle proteins. These changes are believed to follow neutralization of negatively charged sites by divalent cations or H^+. This is also believed to induce the particles to aggregate into tight crystalline arrays as the particles are likely to be kept separated by electrostatic repulsion.*

chia, 1980).

A detailed model for channel occlusion has recently been proposed by Unwin and Zampighi (1980). Here, the channels are believed to close at their cytoplasmic end as a result of a rotation and tilting of the six subunits composing the channels framework. This model is based on the observation of two conformational architectures in isolated liver gap junctions, negatively stained with uranyl acetate and examined by low dose electronmicroscopy. Indeed, this would be an exciting piece of information were it not for the unphysiological way by which the two conformational states were obtained, namely short versus prolonged washing of the junctions following detergent treatment. Unfortunately the authors did not attempt to test the effects of known uncoupling agents such as divalent cations or H^+, thus, until further evidence is provided, the physiological meaning of these data remains dubious.

Supported by NIH grant (GM 20113).

REFERENCES

Alcalá, J., Kuszak, J., Katar, M., Bradley, R.H. and Maisel, H.: Relationship of intrinsic and peripheral proteins to chicken lens gap junction morphology. J. Cell Biol., 83 (2, pt. 2): 269a, 1979.

Alcalá, J., Lieska, N. and Maisel, H.: Protein composition of bovine lens cortical fiber cell membranes. Exp. Eye Res., 21: 581-595, 1975.

Asada, Y. and Bennett, M.V.L.: Experimental alteration of coupling resistance at an electrotonic synapse. J. Cell Biol., 49: 159-172, 1971.

Baldwin, K.M.: The fine structure of healing over in mammalian cardiac muscle. J. Mol. Cell Cardiol., 9: 959-966, 1977.

Baldwin, K.M.: Cardiac gap junction configuration after an uncoupling treatment as a function of time. J. Cell Biol., 82: 66-75, 1979.

Barr, L., Dewey, M.M. and Berger, W.: Propagation of action potentials and the structure of the nexus in cardiac muscle. J. Gen. Physiol., 48: 797-823, 1965.

Barr, L., Berger, W. and Dewey, M.M.: Electrical transmission at the nexus between smooth muscle cells. J. Gen. Physiol., 51: 347-368, 1968.

Benedetti, E.L. and Emmelot, P.: Hexagonal array of subunits in tight junctions separated from isolated rat liver plasma membranes. J. Cell Biol., 38: 15-24, 1968.

Bennett, M.V.L.: Function of electrotonic junctions in embryonic and adult tissue. Fed. Proc., 32: 65-75, 1973.

Bennett, M.V.L., Dunham, B. and Pappas, G.D.: Ion fluxes through a "tight junction". J. Gen. Physiol., 50: 1094a, 1976.

Bernardini, G., Peracchia, C. and Venosa, A.: Uncoupling of lens fibers. J. Cell Biol., 87 (2, pt. 2): 207a, 1980..

Branton, D.: Fracture faces of frozen membranes. Proc. Natl. Acad. Sci. U.S.A., 55: 1048-1056, 1966.

Caspar, D.L.D., Goodenough, D.A., Makowski, L. and Phillips, W.C.: Gap junction structures. I. Correlated electron microscopy and X-ray diffraction. J. Cell Biol., 74: 605-628, 1977.

Dahl, G. and Isenberg, G.: Decoupling of heart muscle cells: correlation with increased cytoplasmic calcium and with changes of nexus ultrastructure. J. Memb. Biol., 53: 63-75, 1980.

DeHaan, R.L. and Hirakow, R.: Synchronization of pulsation rates in isolated cardiac myocytes. Exp. Cell Res., 70: 214-220, 1972.

Délèze, J.: Calcium ions and the healing over of heart fibers. In: Electrophysiology of the Heart, Taccardi B. and Marchetti, G., eds., Pergamon Press, Oxford, England, pp. 147-148, 1965.

Délèze, J.: The recovery of resting potential and input resistance in sheep heart injured by knife or Laser. J. Physiol. (London), 208: 547-562, 1970.

DeMello, W.C.: Effect of intracellular injection of La^{+++} and Mn^{++} on electrical coupling of heart cells. Cell Biol. Int. Rep., 3: 113-119, 1979.

DeMello, W.C.: Intercellular communication and junctional permeability. In: Membrane Structure and Function, Vol.3, Bittar, E.E., ed., John Wiley and Sons, Inc., New York, pp. 127-170, 1980.

DeMello, W.C., Motta, G. and Chapeau, M.: A study on the healing over of myocardial cells of toads. Circ. Res., 24: 475-487, 1969.

Dewey, M.M. and Barr, L.: Intercellular connection between smooth muscle cells: the Nexus. Science (Wash., D.C.), 137: 670-672, 1962.

Dreifuss, J.J., Girardier, L. and Forssman, W.G.: Etude de la propagation de l'excitation dans le ventricule de rat au moyeu de solutions hypertoniques. Pfluegers Arch., 292: 13-33, 1966.

Dunia, I., Sen Gosh, C., Benedetti, E.L., Zweers, A. and Bloemendal, H.: Isolation and protein pattern of eye lens fiber junction. FEBS Lett., 45: 139-144, 1974.

Engelman, T.W.: Vergleichende Untersuchungen zur Lehre von der Muskel- und Nervenelectrizitaet. Pfluegers Arch., 15: 116-148, 1877.

Evans, W.H. and Gurd, J.W.: Preparation and properties of nexuses and lipid enriched vesicles from mouse liver plasmamembranes. Biochem. J., 128: 691-700, 1972.

Farquhar, M.G. and Palade, G.E.: Cell junctions in amphibian skin. J. Cell Biol., 25: 263-291, 1965.

Flagg-Newton, J.L., Simpson, I. and Loewenstein, W.R.: Permeability of the cell-to-cell membrane channels in mammalian cell junction. Science, 205: 404-407, 1979.

Gilula, N.B., Reeves, O.R. and Steinbach, A.: Metabolic coupling, ionic coupling and cell contacts. Nature (Lond.), 235: 262-265, 1972.

Goodenough, D.A.: Lens gap junctions: A structural hypothesis for non-regulated low resistance intercellular pathways. Invest. Ophtalmol., 18: 1104-1122, 1979.

Goodenough, D.A. and Stoeckenius, W.: The isolation of mouse hepatocyte gap junctions. Preliminary chemical characterization and X-ray diffraction. J. Cell Biol., 54: 646-656, 1972.

Goshima, K.: Synchronized beating of and electrotonic transmission between myocardial cell, mediated by heterotypic strain cells in monolayer culture. Exp. Cell Res., 63: 124-130, 1969.

Goshima, K.: Formation of nexuses and electrotonic transmission between myocardial and FL cells in monolayer cultures. Exp. Cell Res., 63: 124-130, 1970.

Hama, K. and Saito, K.: Gap junctions between the supporting cells in some acoustico-vestibular receptors. J. Neurocytol., 6: 1-12, 1977.

Hanna, R.B., Keeter, J.S. and Pappas, G.D.: The fine structure of a rectifying electrotonic synapse. J. Cell Biol., 79: 764-773, 1978.

Henderson, D., Eibl, H. and Weber, K.: Structure and biochemistry of mouse hepatic gap junctions. J. Mol. Biol., 132: 193-218, 1979.

Hertzberg, E.L. and Gilula, N.B.: Isolation and characterization of gap junctions from rat liver. J. Biol. Chem., 254: 2138-2147, 1979.

Hyde, A., Blondell, B., Matter, A., Cheneval, J.P., Filloux, B. and Girardier, L.: Homo and heterocellular junctions in cell cultures: an electrophysiological and morphological study. Prog. Brain Res., 31: 283-311, 1969.

Imanaga, I.: Cell-to-cell diffusion of procion yellow in sheep and calf Purkinje fibers. J. Memb. Biol., 16: 381-388, 1974.

Karrer, H.E.: Cell interconnections in normal human cervical epithelium. J. Biophys. Biochem. Cytol., 7: 181-183, 1960a.

Karrer, H.E.: The striated musculature of blood vessels. II. Cell interconnections and cell surface. J. Biophys. Biochem. Cytol., 8: 135-150, 1960b.

Kawamura, K. and Konishi, T.: Ultrastructure of the cell junction of heart muscle with special reference to its functional significance in excitation conduction and in the concept of "disease of intercalated discs". Japan. Circ. J., 31: 1533-1543, 1967.

Kensler, R.W. and Goodenough, D.A.: Isolation of mouse myocardial gap junctions. J. Cell Biol., 86: 755-764, 1980.

Kistler, J. and Bullivant, S.: Lens gap junctions and orthogonal arrays are unrelated. FEBS Lett., 111: 73-78, 1980a.

Kistler, J. and Bullivant, S.: The connexon order in isolated lens gap junctions. J. Ultrastruct. Res., 72: 27-38, 1980b.

Lawrence, T.S., Beers, W.H. and Gilula, N.B.: Transmission of hormonal stimulation by cell-to-cell communication. Nature (Lond.) 272: 501-506, 1978.

Ledbetter, M.L. and Lubin, M.: Transfer of potassium. A new measure of cell-cell coupling. J. Cell Biol., 80: 150-165, 1979.

Loewenstein, W.R.: Permeability of membrane junctions. Ann. N.Y. Acad. Sci., 137: 441-472, 1966.

Loewenstein, W.R.: Permeable junctions. Cold Spring Harbor Symp. Quant. Biol., 40: 49-63, 1975.

Loewenstein, W.R., Nakas, M. and Socolar, S.J.: Junctional membrane uncoupling: permeability transformations at a cell membrane junction. J. Gen. Physiol., 50: 1865-1891, 1967.

Makowski, L., Caspar, D.L.D., Phillips, W.C. and Goodenough, D.A.: Gap junction structures. II. Analysis of the X-ray diffraction data. J. Cell Biol., 74: 629-645, 1977.

McNutt, N.S. and Weinstein, R.S.: The ultrastructure of the nexus. A correlated thin-section and freeze-cleave study. J. Cell Biol., 47: 666-688, 1970.

Meda, P., Perrelet, A. and Orci, L.: Gap junctions and beta-cell function. Horm. Metab. Res. Suppl. (in press), 1980.

Nakas, M., Higashino, S. and Loewenstein, W.R.: Uncoupling of an epithelial cell membrane junction by calcium-ion removal. Science (Wash., D.C.), 151: 89-91, 1966.

Pappas, G.D., Asada, Y. and Bennett, M.V.L.: Morphological correlates of increased coupling resistance at an electrotonic synapse. J. Cell Biol., 49: 173-188, 1971.

Payton, B.W., Bennett, M.V.L. and Pappas, G.D.: Temperature-dependence of resistance at an electrotonic synapse. Science (Wash., D.C.), 165: 594-597, 1969a.

Payton, B.W., Bennett, M.V.L. and Pappas, G.D.: Permeability and structure of junctional membranes at an electrotonic synapse. Science (Wash., D.C.),

166: 1641-1643, 1969b.

Peracchia, C.: Low resistance junctions in crayfish. I. Two arrays of globules in junctional membranes. J. Cell Biol., 57: 54-65, 1973a.

Peracchia, C.: Low resistance junctions in crayfish. II. Structural details
and further evidence for intercellular channels by freeze-fracture and negative staining. J. Cell Biol., 57: 66-76, 1973b.

Peracchia, C.: A structure-function correlation in gap junctions of crayfish.
Proc. Int. Cong. Electron Microsc., 8th Canberra, II, 226-227, 1974.

Peracchia, C.: Gap junctions: structural changes after uncoupling procedures.
J. Cell Biol., 72: 628-641, 1977.

Peracchia, C.: Calcium effects on gap junction structure and cell coupling.
Nature (London), 271: 669-671, 1978.

Peracchia, C.: Structural correlates of gap junction permeation. Int. Rev.
Cytol., 66: 81-146, 1980.

Peracchia, C., Bernardini, G. and Peracchia, L.L.: Uncoupling mechanism: a
hypothesis. J. Cell Biol., 83: (2, pt. 2): 86a, 1979.

Peracchia, C. and Dulhunty, A.F.: Gap junctions: structural changes associated with changes in permeability. J. Cell Biol., 63: (2, pt. 2): 263a,
1974.

Peracchia, C. and Dulhunty, A.F.: Low resistance junctions in crayfish:
structural changes with functional uncoupling. J. Cell Biol., 70:
419-439, 1976.

Peracchia, C. and Peracchia, L.L.: Gap junction dynamics: reversible effects
of divalent cations. J. Cell Biol., 87: 708-718, 1980a.

Peracchia, C. and Peracchia, L.L.: Gap junction dynamics: reversible effects
of hydrogen ions. J. Cell Biol., 87: 719-727, 1980b.

Petersen, O.H., Findlay, I., Meda, P., Laugier, R. and Iwatsuki, N.: Control
of cell-to-cell communication in exocrine glands by the intracellular hydrogen ion concentration. In: Hydrogen Ion Transport In Epithelia,
Schulz, I., ed., Elsevier (North Holland Press), pp. 227-234, 1980.

Pitts, J.D.: Molecular exchange and growth control in tissue culture. In:
Growth Control in Cultures, Wolstenholme, G.E.W. and Knight, J., eds.
Churchill Livingstone, London, pp. 89-105, 1971.

Pitts, J.D.: Direct communication between animal cells. In: International
Cell Biology, Brinkley, B.R. and Porter, K.R., eds., The Rockefeller Un-

iversity Press, New York, pp. 43-49, 1977.

Politoff, A. and Pappas, G.D.: Mechanism of increase in coupling resistance at electrotonic synapses of the crayfish septate axon. Anat. Record., 172: 384-385, 1972.

Politoff, A., Pappas, G.D. and Bennett, M.V.L.: Cobalt ions cross an electrotonic synapse if cytoplasmic concentration is low. Brain Res., 76: 343-346, 1974.

Rae, J.L.: The movement of procion dye in the crystalline lens. Invest. Ophtalmol. Vis. Sci., 13: 147-150, 1974.

Raviola, E., Goodenough, D.A. and Raviola, G.: The native structure of gap junctions rapidly frozen at 4 ^{o}K. J. Cell Biol., 79 (2, pt. 2): 229a, 1978.

Revel, J.P. and Karnovsky, M.J.: Hexagonal array of subunits in intercellular junctions of the mouse heart and liver. J. Cell Biol., 33: C7-C12, 1967.

Robertson, J.D.: The occurrence of a subunit pattern in the unit membranes of club endings in Mauthner cell synapses in Goldfish brains. J. Cell Biol., 19: 201-222, 1963.

Rothschuh, K.E.: Ueber den funktionellen Aufbau des Herzens aus elektrophysiologischen Elementen und ueber den Mechanismus der Erregungsleitung im Herzen. Pfluegers Arch., 253: 238-251, 1951.

Sjostrand, F.S., Andersson-Cedergren, E. and Dewey, M.M.: The ultrastructure of the intercalated discs of frog, mouse and guinea pig cardiac muscle. J. Ultrastruct. Res., 1: 271-287, 1958.

Staehelin, L.A.: Structure and function of intercellular junctions. Int. Rev. Cytol., 39: 191-283, 1974.

Tsien, R.W. and Weingart, R.: Cyclic-AMP: cell-to-cell movement and inotropic effect in ventricular muscle, studied by a cut-end method. J. Physiol. (London), 242: 95P-96P, 1974.

Turin, L. and Warner, A.E.: Carbon dioxide reversibly abolishes ionic communication between cells of early amphibian embryo. Nature (London), 270: 56-57, 1977.

Turin, L. and Warner, A.E.: Intracellular pH in early Xenopus embryos: its effect on current flow between blastomeres. J. Physiol. (London), 300: 489-504, 1980.

Unwin, P.N.T. and Zampighi, G.: Structure of the junction between communicating cells.   Nature (London), 283:   545-549, 1980.

Weidmann, S.: The electrical constants of Purkinje fibres.   J.   Physiol.
     (London), 118:   348-360, 1952.

Weidmann, S.: The diffusion of radiopotassium across intercalated discs of mam-
     malian cardiac muscle. J. Physiol. (London), 187:   323-343, 1966.

Weingart, R.: The permeability to tetraethylammonium ions of the surface mem-
     brane and the intercalated disks of sheep and calf myocardium. J.
     Physiol. (London), 240:   741-762, 1974.

Weingart, R.: The actions of ouabain on intercellular coupling and conduction
     velocity in mammalian ventricular muscle. J. Physiol. (London), 264:
     341-365, 1977.

Zampighi, G. and Unwin, P.N.T.: Two forms of isolated gap junctions. J. Mol.
     Biol., 135:   451-464, 1979.

Zampighi, G., Corless, J.M. and Robertson, J.D.: On gap junction structure.
     J. Cell Biol., 86:   190-198, 1980.

FORMATION AND GROWTH OF MYOCARDIAL GAP JUNCTIONS:

IN VIVO AND IN VITRO STUDIES

Daniel Gros, Ian Lee and Cyril E. Challice

INTRODUCTION

As early as 1966, Loewenstein proposed a model for direct cell-to-cell coupling that could permit ions and small hydrophilic molecules to move between cells (see Loewenstein et al., 1978a). The morphological structure which would fulfill such a role remained a matter for speculation until Revel and Karnovsky (1967) used the lanthanum impregnation technique to distinguish, without ambiguity, between tight (occluding junctions) and gap junctions. Later, gap junctions were identified as plaques of closely aggregated transmembrane particles in freeze-fracture studies (McNutt and Weinstein, 1970). Their molecular structure was studied by high resolution transmission electron microscopy and low angle X-ray diffraction (Staehelin, 1974; Caspar et al., 1977; Makowsky et al., 1977; Bennett and Goodenough, 1978; Zamphighi and Unwin, 1979). Recently, Unwin and Zampighi (1980) have confirmed that the communicating unit (i.e., "connexon") is a hexameric polymer which spans the membrane and would possess a central channel. It has been speculated that rotational displacement of the subunits to glide against each other, represents the mechanism whereby the channel is opened and closed. Biochemical analyses of gap junctions isolated from different organs have provided some data about their lipid and protein components (Dunia et al., 1974; Goodenough, 1975 and 1979; Duguid and Revel, 1976; Broekhuyse et al., 1976; Ehrhardt and Chaveau, 1977; Caspar et al., 1977; Hertzberg and Gilula, 1979; Henderson et al., 1979), but investigators are not unanimous concerning the molecular weight of the main polypeptide components of these junctions.

The existence of nexuses is now established throughout phylogeny, proving their functional importance. Their presence and abundance have been correlated with the capacity for the intercellular transfer of molecules (fluorescent dyes, labelled cations, nucleotides, amino-acids and other metabolites), and the transmission and regulation of hormonal stimulation and growth control (see Sheridan, 1976; Griepp and Revel, 1977; Larsen, 1977a; Bennett and Goodenough, 1978; Lawrence et al., 1978; Loewenstein, 1978). There has been a steady growth of evidence over the past few years that gap junctions represent the morphological specialization responsible for cell-to-cell metabolic and electronic coupling. Thus gap junctions between myocardial cells (which are excitable cells) are structures of primary importance in enabling them to transmit an action potential (thus stimulating contraction) between each other.

Gap junctions have been observed and described in the adult cardiac muscle of animals in all classes of vertebrates (McNutt, 1970; Cobb, 1974; Mazet and Cartaud, 1976; Mazet, 1977a and b; Kensler et al., 1977; Sibata, 1977; Shibata and Yamamoto, 1977 and 1979) and they are present in all the tissues of the organ: ventricular, atrial, conductive tissues, and also the sinoatrial node (Masson-Pevet et al., 1978). Although the ultrastructure and the distribution of the gap junctions in the adult heart has provided the subject of numerous studies, relatively little is known about gap junctions in the embryonic and developing heart. The present work was undertaken to investigate the formation of gap junctions between developing myocardial cells, both in vivo (in embryonic mouse myocardium) and in vitro (between chick myocardial cells in culture). Reports of parts of these studies have been published previously (Gros et al., 1978, 1979 and 1980a; Lee and Challice, 1980).

MATERIALS AND METHODS

IN VIVO STUDIES
Embryonic hearts at 10, 12, 14 and 18 days post coitum (dpc) were obtained from pregnant mice. Adult hearts were taken from 3-month old female mice. The specimens were treated as described previously by Gros et al. (1978) before to be fractured using a Balzers freeze-etch apparatus.

IN VITRO STUDIES

Dissociated myocardial cells from 7-day embryonic chicks were plated on 9 mm diameter polystyrene discs in airtight vials as described by Lee and Challice (1980). Cultures were incubated at 37 $^{\circ}$C for three different durations: 6, 24 and 48 hours. The cells covering the polystyrene discs were freeze-cleaved in situ according to the method described by Fujisawa and Morioka (1977) and adapted to a Balzers apparatus.

ELECTRON MICROSCOPY AND MORPHOMETRY

Cleaned replicas were examined with a Hitachi HU11Cs, Siemens Elmiskop 1a, or AEI 6 B electron microscope. The microscopes were calibrated using a germanium-shadowed carbon replica (54,864 lines/inch). For in vivo investigations the measurements of the surfaces of the gap junctions were all performed from micrographs of both P and E fracture faces, at 90,000 magnification. Single linear gap junctions were not included in the calculations. The smallest macular junctions measured consisted of from 8 to 10 closely packed particles. For in vitro investigations, because of the smaller size of gap junctions than in vivo, the measurements of the size distributions of gap junctions were made by counting the number of gap particles packed in junctional complexes. These measurement were performed from micrographs of magnification ranging from 25,000x to 45,000x. Minimum junctional size was arbitrarily set at 3 gap particles.

RESULTS

GAP JUNCTIONS IN DEVELOPING MOUSE CARDIAC MUSCLE

P and E fracture faces of embryonic and adult myocardial cells are studded with intramembranous particles distributed at random. Their density (number of particle/μm^2) does not change during development (Gros et al., 1980b). For fixed specimens, their density ranges, on average, from 1400 to 1500 particles/μm^2 for PF faces and from 225 to 285 for EF faces. Besides these intramembranous particles, various arrays of gap particles may be observed, both in fixed and unfixed specimens, and it is believed that they represent successive steps in the assembly of the gap junctions.

At 10 dpc, four types of gap junctions may be categorized.   These   various types of junctions are also found in the hearts of 12 and 14 dpc mice.

1.   Single chains of 9 nm particles on the PF faces or linear arrays of pits   on the   EF   faces (see Gros et al., 1978).   These single chains seem to be formed by the alignment of larger particles of 10-11 nm diameter (Fig.   1).

The regions where the linear arrays are generated are sometimes   identical   with the   "formation plaques" defined by Johnson et al. (1974).   The chains of particles may be branched, or associated with other in such a way that they form   a circle (see   Fig.   3 from a 12 dpc embryonic heart).   Aggregates of 2 or 3 rows may also be observed (Fig.   2).   The linear arrays are sometimes   associated   at

FIGURE 1   *10 dpc mouse embryonic   heart   unfixed   specimen.   P   fracture   face. Besides   small   aggregates of gap particles (arrowheads) note the lining of free gap particles (arrows) larger than the one incorporated in   clusters   and   which will probably form linear arrays. Bar scale, 0.2 μm.*

FIGURE 2   *10 dpc mouse embryonic heart.   Unfixed specimen.   P   and   E   fracture face (PF_1 and EF_2).   Small gap junction (arrowhead) and linear array formed by 2 rows of particles (arrow).   The reduction of the   extracellular   space   (es)   is clearly seen at the level of the linear array. Cyt_2, cytoplasm.   Bar scale, 0.2 μm.*

FIGURE 3   *12 dpc mouse embryonic   heart.   Fixed   specimen.   P   fracture   face. Association of single chains of gap particle. Bar scale, 0.2 μm.*

FIGURE 4   *14 dpc mouse embryonic   heart.   Unfixed   specimen.   P   fracture   face. Arrowhead   indicates a linear array of gap particles.   Notice in the right upper corner   a short chain of particles (black arrow)   associated   at   its   ends   with small   clusters.   Close to this junction, notice a stream of particles (parallel to the white arrow) which seems   to   converge   towards   another   junction.   Bar scale, 0.2 μm.*

FIGURE 5   *14 dpc mouse embryonic heart.   Unfixed   specimen.   P   fracture   face. Gap junctions with central particle-free zones (arrows).   Bar scale, 0.2 μm.*

FIGURE 6   *14 dpc mouse embryonic heart.   Unfixed   specimen.   E   fracture   face. Gap   junctions with a pit-free zone (bend arrows) and two "arms" (black arrows). Arrowheads indicate the regular arrangement of pits which permits to recognize a gap junction on the EF faces.   Bar scale, 0.2 μm.*

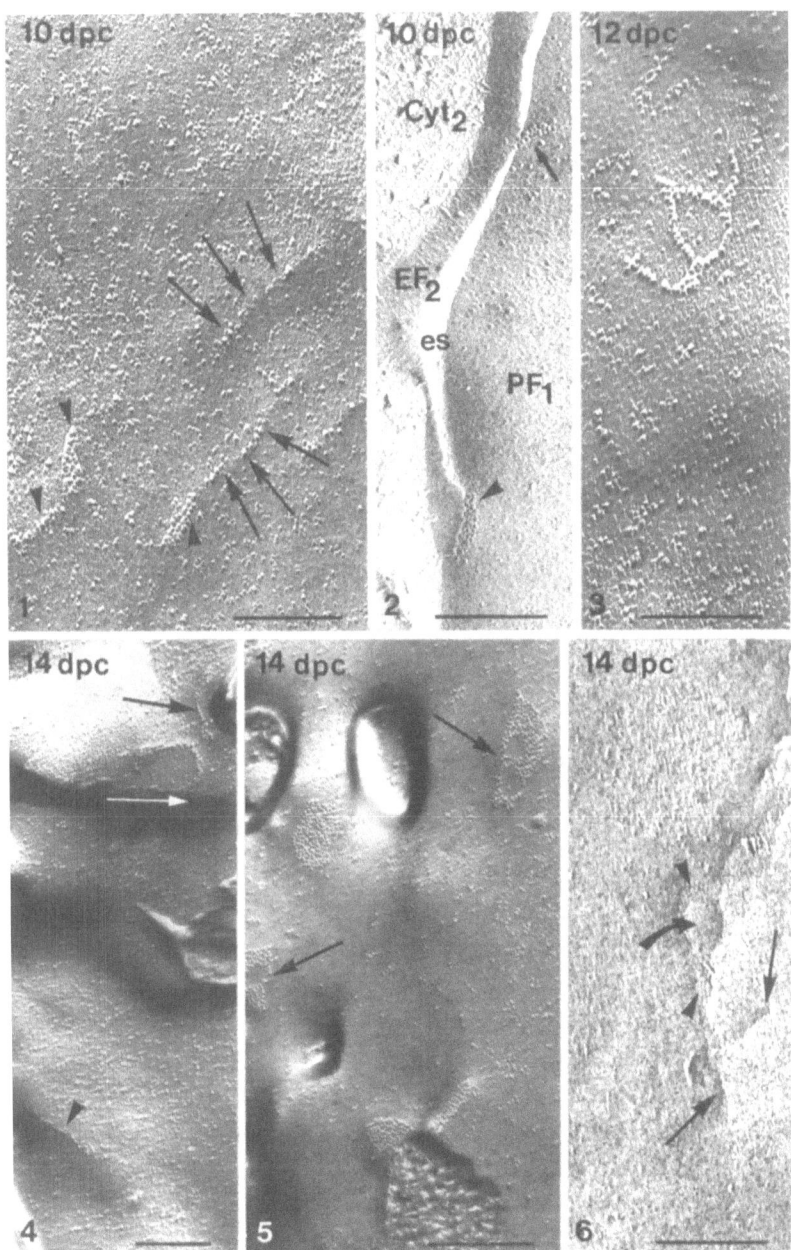

their ends with loosely organized clusters of particles (Fig. 4 from a 14 dpc embryonic heart).

2. Aggregates of gap particles on the PF faces with one, two, or three "arms" which seem to be formed by the successive addition of single gap particles. These latter are observed beside the junction in a kind of stream (see Fig. 4 from a 14 dpc embryonic heart; also Gros et al., 1980a). Corresponding images on the EF faces are found (Gros et al., 1978).

3. Aggregates of gap particles with one, two, or three central particle-free zones (see Fig. 5 from a 14 dpc embryonic heart; also Gros et al., 1978 and 1980a). On the EF faces, gap junctions with central pit-free areas are observed (see Fig. 6 from a 14 dpc embryonic heart).

4. Small hexagonal arrays of particles with a 9 nm center-to-center spacing with the corresponding EF faces showing similar arrays of depressions. These structures are referred to as "adult-type junctions".

TABLE I

DIVERSITY OF THE GAP JUNCTIONS IN THE DEVELOPING MOUSE HEART

Stage of development	10 dpc	12 dpc	14 dpc	18 dpc	Adult
Linear arrays	+	+	+	–	–
	(11%)	(34%)	(8.5%)		
Macular gap junctions					
+ with "arms"	+	+	+	–	–
+ with particle-free zones	+	+	+	–	–
+ small (without particle-free zones or "arms"	+	+	+	+	+
+ large (without particle-free zones or "arms")	–	–	+	+	+

Usually two or three of these categories of junctions, and sometimes all of them, may be found in the same area. At this stage of development (10 dpc) 11 % of the junctions are in the form of linear arrays.

The above description applied to both 12 and 14 dpc hearts with only slight modification. At 12 dpc (Fig. 3), gap junctions are more numerous than at 10 dpc, and the linear arrays of gap particles are abundant (34 % of the overall total of junctions observed). By 14 dpc (Fig. 4, 5 and 6), the chains of particles have become rare (8.5 %) whereas the other types of gap junctions are relatively numerous. At 18 dpc (Fig. 7) and also at the adult stage (Figs. 8

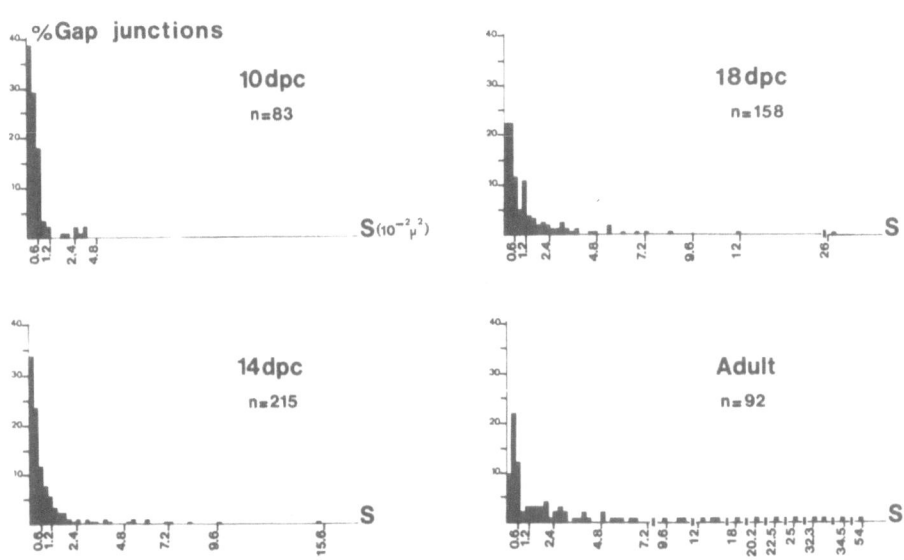

HISTOGRAMS I *Histograms showing the size distribution of gap junctions in the embryonic mouse heart at 10, 14 and 18 day post-coitum (dpc) and in the adult heart. Abscissa, area, S, of gap junctions; class interval: 0.3×10^{-2} μm^2. Ordinate, percentage of the ratios, number of gap junctions in class intervals/total number of gap junctions observed at each stage (n). Preparations from these hearts were used at each stage. Unfixed specimens. (From Gros et al., J. Cell Sci., 30: 45-61, 1978, reproduced by permission).*

and 9) linear gap junctions and junctions with "arms" or central particle (or pit)-free regions are no longer observed, all the junctions being of the "adult-type". However, variations in the arrangement of the gap particles are found. Some junctions show the classical hexagonal array, whereas in others this pattern is not obvious. At 18 dpc in particular, some junctions are formed by strands of particles leaving between them narrow spaces devoid of particles (Fig. 7). At the adult stage, in the largest gap junctions, sometimes a part of a junction may exhibit the hexagonal pattern whereas the remainder does not. In close proximity to these nexuses of the "adult-type", 10-11 nm particles are sometimes present (see Gros et al., 1978). The above observations are summarized in Table I.

Set of histograms I shows the distribution of the area (S) of the gap junctions through 4 stages examined. At 10 dpc the area of the gap junctions ranges from 0.1 to 3×10^{-2} μm^2; at 14 dpc, from 0.1 to 15×10^{-2} μm^2; at 18 dpc from 0.1 to 26.3×10^{-2} μm^2 and at the adult stage from 0.1 to 54×10^{-2} μm^2. These results, which demonstrate the growth of the gap junctions, can be expressed in a more significant manner. They can be separated into two classes: class I with $S \leq 0.5 \times 10^{-2}$ μm^2 and class II with $S > 0.5 \times 10^{-2}$ μm^2; the number 0.5×10^{-2} representing the median area of all the gap junctions measured (N = 548). These results, presented in Table II, show that the percentage of small gap junctions decreases as cells become more and more differentiated.

GAP JUNCTIONS BETWEEN CHICK MYOCARDIAL CELLS IN CULTURE

The density of the intramembranous particles does not seem to change between 6 and 48 hours of culture. This density is about 1480 particles/μm^2 on the P fracture faces.

The diverse types of gap junctions observed in the developing heart are also found in the cultures of chick myocardial cells. In the 6 and 24 hour cul-

FIGURE 7 *18 dpc mouse embryonic heart. Unfixed specimen. P and E fracture face (PF_1 and EF_2). The E faces of the junctions (arrows) have been in part cleaved away. Note that the junctions are formed by strands of particles leaving in between them narrow spaces free of particles. Bar scale, 0.5 μm.*

FIGURE 8 *Adult mouse heart. Unfixed specimen. P fracture face. Plasma membrane region with small gap junctions (arrows). Bar scale, 0.5 μm.*

FIGURE 9 *Adult mouse heart. Fixed specimen. The cleaving process has revealed both the PF and EF faces (PF_1 and EF_2) of a gap junction. A part of the cytoplasm is also seen (Cyt. 1). On the top of gap particles small pits are sometimes observed (circles). They indicate the presence of a central channel in the gap particles. Bar scale, 0.25 μm.*

FIGURE 10 *6 hour culture of chick myocardial cells. Fixed specimen. Region of gap junction formation. The two kinds of gap junctions observed in the 6 and 24 hours cultures are present in this micrograph: linear arrays (arrows) and small clusters. Note the 10-11 nm particles in close proximity to the clusters (arrowheads). Bar scale, 0.5 μm.*

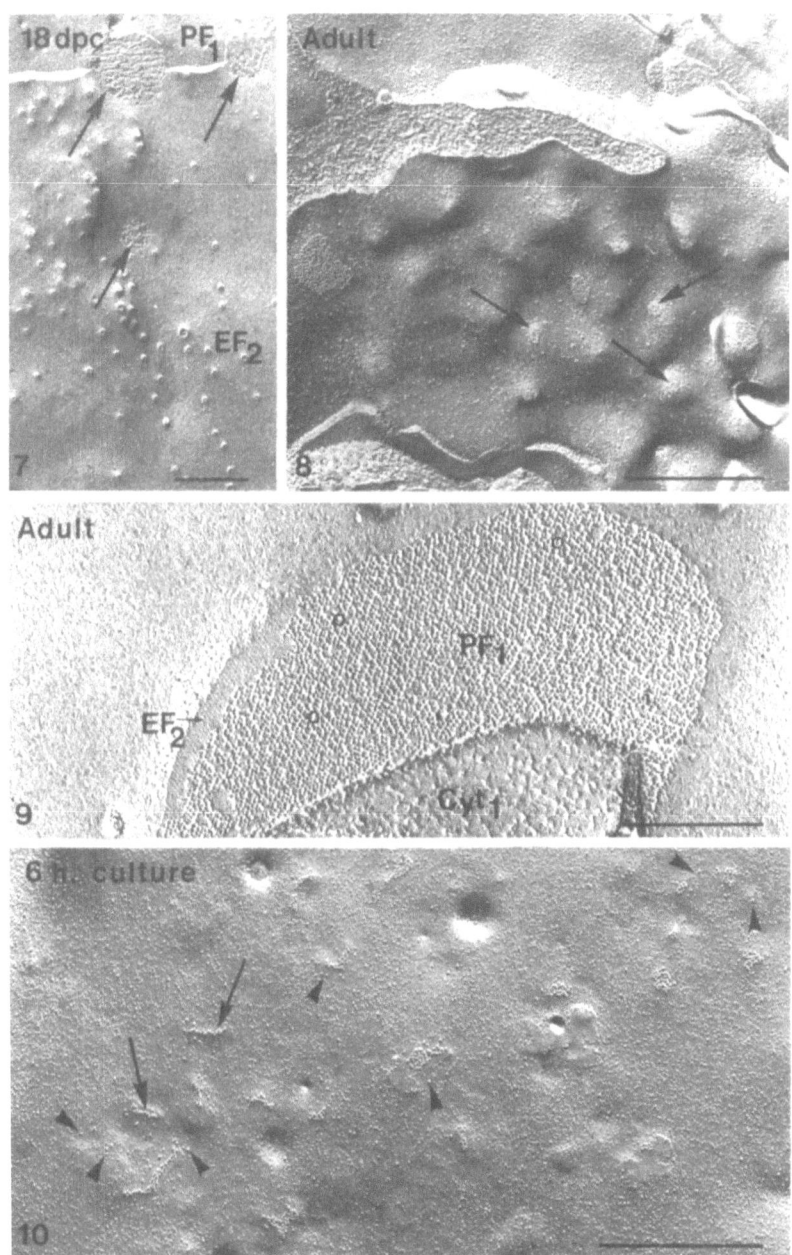

tures, gap junctions are in the form of single linear arrays and small clusters
of particles (Fig. 10). The frequency of occurrence of single linear gap junctions is 9.6 % and 9.8 % for the 6 and 24 hour cultures respectively. In the 48
hour cultures (Fig. 11 to 14) another form of gap junction appears: one with a
central particle (or pit)-free zone. These are usually composed of one, two or
three rows of particle forming a ring (Fig. 14). Such junctions sometimes have
"arms", formed by chains of particles. In the 48 hour cultures the frequency of
occurrence of linear arrays is 32.6 %.

TABLE II

*DISTRIBUTION OF GAP JUNCTIONS BETWEEN CLASS I (S $\leq$ 0.5 x 10^{-2} μm^2)
AND CLASS II (S > 0.5 X 10^{-2} μm^2), IN DEVELOPING MOUSE HEART*

	Area of the gap junctions (μm^2)	
	S $\leq$ 0.5 x 10^{-2}	*S > 0.5 x 10^{-2}*
10 dpc	*67%*	*33%*
14 dpc	*57%*	*43%*
18 dpc	*44%*	*56%*
Adult	*31%*	*69%*

In the "formation plaques" where the gap junctions are generated, the line-

*FIGURE 11 to 14 48 hour cultures of chick myocardial cells. Fixed specimens. P
and E fracture faces (PF$_1$ and EF$_2$).*

*FIGURE 11 Very beginning of the formation of gap junctions from 10-11 nm parti-
cles (arrowheads). These particles are present in the plasma membrane, close to
each other, but without any particular arrangement (zone 1), then they start to
line up (zone 2). Zone 1 represents a "formation plaque" as defined by Johnson
et al. (1974). Bar scale, 0.5 μm.*

*FIGURE 12 Single chains of gap particles. Notice they are all orientated in the
same direction as it is generally the case. Large particles (circle) are close
to the linear arrays in which they will be probably incorporated. Bar scale, 1
μm.*

*FIGURE 13 Linear arrays (arrows), branched chains (arrowhead) and small cluster
of gap particles (asterisks). Bar scale, 0.5 μm.*

*FIGURE 14 Linear array (arrowhead) and small clusters of gap particles (aster-
isks). Note also the gap junction with a central particle-free region (white
arrow). Bar scale, 0.5 μm.*

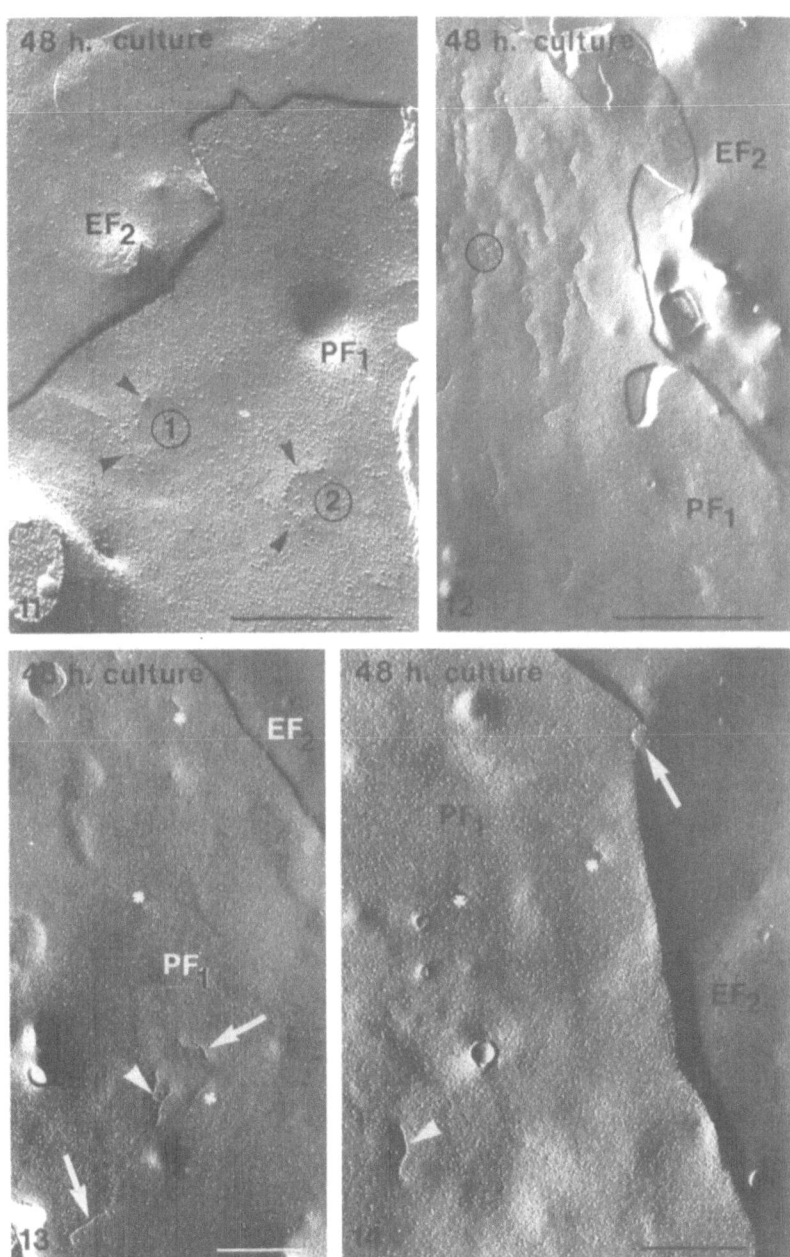

D. Gros **et al.**

ar arrays seem to form from the aligment of large particles (10-11 nm) as has been previously described for the mouse developing heart (Fig. 11). These 10-11 nm particles are also found in close proximity with clustered gap particles (Fig. 10). In the aggregates the hexagonal pattern of gap particles is seen, but sometimes a part of the junction exhibits the hexagonal ordering whereas the other part does not. The above observations are summarized in Table III.

TABLE III

DIVERSITY OF THE GAP JUNCTIONS IN CULTURES OF CHICK MYOCARDIAL CELLS

Duration of culture	6 hours	24 hours	48 hours
Linear arrays	+ (9.6%)	+ (9.8%)	+ (32.6%)
Macular gap junctions + with "arms" and/or central particle-free zones	-	-	+
+ small (without "arms" or central particle-free zones)	+	+	+

Set II of the histograms shows the distribution of the size S of the gap junctions for the three durations of culture examined; the size of the junctions being evaluated as the number of particles comprising the junction. The percentage of small junctions decreases slightly as the duration of culture increases. These results are also shown in Table IV. The junctions have been catalogued into two classes: class I with a size $S \leq 10$ particles, and class II with $S > 10$ particles, the number of 10 particles representing the median size of the overall number of gap junctions observed (N = 842). The size of the junctions is comparable in the 6 and 24 hour cultures, but in the 48 hour cultures the percentage of large gap junctions ($S > 10$ particles) is significantly increased.

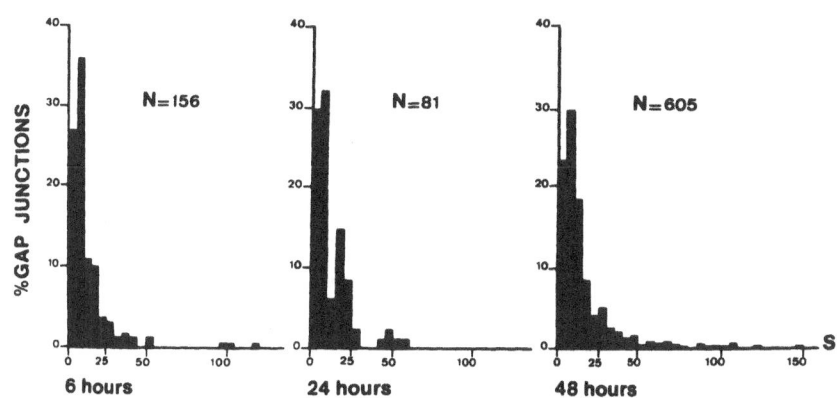

HISTOGRAMS II *Histogram showing the size distribution of gap junctions in 6, 24 and 48 hour cultures of chick myocardial cells. Abscissa, size, S, of gap junction; class interval: 5 gap particles. Ordinate, percentage of the ratios, number of gap junctions in class intervals/total number of gap junctions observed at each stage(n). 8, 13, and 9 preparations were used for 6, 24, and 48 hour cultures, respectively. Fixed specimens.*

TABLE IV

DISTRIBUTION OF GAP JUNCTIONS BETWEEN CLASS I (S ≤ 10 GAP PARTICLES) AND CLASS II (S < 10 PARTICLES) IN CULTURES OF CHICK MYOCARDIAL CELLS

	Size of the gap junctions (number of particles)	
	S ≤ 10 particles	*S < 10 particles*
6 hour cultures	*62.8%*	*37.2%*
24 hour cultures	*62.9%*	*37.1%*
48 hour cultures	*52.6%*	*47.4%*

DISCUSSION

The present study has confirmed the existence of gap junctions in mouse embryonic heart as early as 10 dpc, and also in cultures of myocardial cells, where they had been previously identified in a number of studies (Masson-Pevet et al., 1976; Mazet, 1977a; Larsen, 1977b; Lee and Challice, 1980). Two particular points of interest arise from this investigation; in both the devel-

oping myocardium and in cultures of differentiating cardiac muscle cells, the
gap junctions, (i) increase in size with time and (ii) show a wide structural
diversity.

The results clearly demonstrate that the gap junctions increase progressively in size as cells differentiate (see histograms and Tables II and IV).
For the developing mouse myocardium the histograms relate to unfixed specimens
but it has been demonstrated that fixation does not change the size distribution
of gap junctions (Gros et al., 1978). The size distribution of gap junctions
in the adult mouse myocardium is parallel with that reported by Shibata and Yamamoto (1979) in adult rat, sparrow, and lizard; they all show the existence of
a continuous spread of size from small junctions to large ones. However, species differences in size must be noticed. In the mouse adult heart the largest
gap junctions observed have an area of 0.5 μm^2. In the rat they are much
larger: 7.7 μm^2; but in contrast, they are much smaller in the sparrow and the
lizard: 0.11 μm^2 and 0.12 μm^2 respectively. In cultures of chick myocardial
cells (48 hours), the largest junctions are only 0.012 μm^2 ($\sim$ 150 gap particles).

The structural diversity of gap junctions has been reviewed by Larsen
(1977b) who concluded that the variations may reflect differences in the developmental and/or functional activities of this structure. As will be discussed
later, phylogenic origins may also be involved. In the present case, this variability is interpreted as representing ontogenic steps in gap junction formation. Such a hypothesis is supported by three observations: (i) the progressive increase in size of the junctions with time, (ii) the presence of 10-11 nm
isolated particles (considered as gap particle precursors); (iii) the disappearance (Table I) or the appearance (Table III) of certain kinds of junctions
as cells differentiate and junctions grow. For example, the linear junctions or
the junctions with central particle-free zones observed in the early embryo, are
no longer seen at 18 dpc and adult. In contrast, the junctions with a central
particle-free zone appear only in the 48-hour cultures and are not seen before
in the 6 and 24 hour cultures. The first available study suggesting the structural variation of gap junctions to reflect their development was that of Pinto
da Silva and Gilula (1972). Later this hypothesis was taken up again by most
other authors studying gap junctions in regeneration or differentiation.

The process of development of gap junctions suggested by the present study begins with aligment of 10-11 nm particles present in the "formation plaques" defined by Johnson et al. (1974). In both types of biological material investigated the observation of these "formation plaques" was, however, rare. They were first observed by Johnson et al. (1974) in cultures of Novikoff hepatoma cells and then reported to be present in regenerating liver (Yancey et al., 1979; although their presence is contraversial, see Yee and Revel, 1978), developing embryos (Revel, 1974; Decker and Friend, 1974; Decker, 1976a), granulosa cells (Albertini et al., 1975; Gilula, 1977), and cultured differentiating tumor cells (Decker, 1976b).

The large 10-11 nm particles have been postulated to represent the precursors of the 9 nm gap particles (Johnson et al., 1974). Assuming that the particles have dimensions which reflect accurately the size of the structure that they represent, there is a reduction of these structures as gap junctions form. According to Revel et al. (1978) this reduction could be the result of a proteolytic cleavage prerequisite for induction of formation of junctions. The earliest forms of gap junctions as such are formed of lines of particles or clusters of a few particles. The linear arrangements have been described by most authors who have investigated the formation of gap junctions (Pinto da Silva and Gilula, 1972; Benedetti et al., 1974; Decker and Friend, 1974; Decker, 1976a; Anderson and Albertini, 1976; Fujisawa et al., 1976; Mazet, 1977a and b; Griepp et al., 1978) and therefore they appear to be characteristic of immature differentiating junctions. In the next step, at the ends of the linear arrays, small aggregates would develop either by a coiling of the chain or by accretion of other gap particles. Such aggregates would act as nucleation sites or as "seeds", which would then grow by incorporation of individual particles, or linear arrays, or both. Nexuses with "arms" (or a central particle-free zone) would represent an intermediate stage in the formation of junctions before assuming their adult shapes. It might be speculated that the free end of a junction arm, carried away by the moving surrounding molecules, could contact the "body" of that junction, and become bound to the packed particles, thus enclosing an internal particle-free zone. Incorporation of new gap particles and/or structural modification would then lead to adult-type nexuses. These junctions could possibly proceed to grow, either by incorporation of new gap particles, or by fusion with others, or both. (Elias and Friend, 1976; Yee and Revel, 1978; Yancey et al., 1979).

The successive stages which describe the formation of gap junctions are consistent with the observations reported in the results, but another possibility has to be considered. During the process of liver regeneration, hepatocyte gap junctions undergo a cycle of disappearance and reappearance, then subsequently increase in size until about 48 hours after partial hepatectomy (Yee and Revel, 1978; Yancey et al., 1979). These junctions reappear as small clusters of particles and never in the form of linear arrays. Thus, at least in the renegerating liver, the development of gap junctions by-passes the linear array stage. Such a direct developmental process can also be considered in the present investigation, since, at the beginning of the formation of junctions, besides the linear arrays, small clusters of a few particles are observed. That process could be parallel with the former, although situations intermediate between the two may occur, such as fusion of linear arrays with small clusters, or with aggregates of gap particles.

In the present study, the variations in gap junction shape have been related to their formation and development. However, atypical junctions, like the one described in the embryonic mouse heart and in the cultures of chick cardiac muscle cells, have also been observbed in the adult heart of fish, amphibians, reptiles, and birds (Mazet and Cartaud, 1976; Mazet, 1977 a and b; Kensler et al., 1977; Shibata, 1977; Shibata and Yamamoto, 1979). In Xenopus (for example) adult-type gap junctions are represented only by single circles of particles; in the frog, the most advanced junctions are anastomosed circles of particles (Mazet, 1977 a and b). Junctions with "arms" and/or a central particle-free zone have been described in the lizard and the sparrow (Shibata and Yamamoto, 1979). Thus, there are remarkable differences between mammalian and non-mammalian adult-type myocardial gap junctions, and these differences are related to phylogeny.

The sequence of events of gap junction formation has been described from freeze-fractured specimens. Because of treatments imposed by the technique (fixation, cryoprotection) the junctions were frozen under conditions where they were likely physiologically uncoupled. Raviola et al. (1980) have shown that connexons of adult gap junctions rapidly frozen at $4\,^{\circ}K$ under conditions consonant with a low-resistance, exhibit a great variability in clustering and are even sometimes "randomly arrayed making precise identification of the junctional domain difficult" (Goodenough, 1980). These recent results indicate the necessity for caution in the interpretation of the sequence of events described. Nevertheless, it holds true that gap junctions increase progressively in size as myocardial cells differentiate, and this supports the demonstration by Loewenstein et al. (1978b) of steps in junction permeability during junction formation. On the other hand the model proposed by Unwin and Zampighi (1980) makes intercellular conductivity dependent only on the number of connexons present, and their arrangement into arrays in gap junctions is not a factor.

ACKNOWLEDGEMENTS

This work was supported by DGRST grants, The Natural Science and Engineering Research Council of Canada, The Alberta Heart Foundation, and the CNRS/NRCC scientific exchange programme.

REFERENCES

Albertini, D.F., Fawcett, D.W. and Olds, P.J.: Morphological variations in gap junctions of ovarian granulosa cells. Tissue and Cell, 7: 389-405, 1975.

Anderson, E. and Albertini, D.F.: Gap junctions between the oocyte and companion follicle cells in the mammalian ovary. J. Cell Biol., 71: 680-686, 1976.

Benedetti, E.L., Dunia, I. and Bloemendal, H.: Development of junctions during differentiation of lens fibres. Proc. Natl. Acad. Sci. USA, 71: 5073-5077, 1974.

Bennett, M.V.L. and Goodenough, D.A.: Gap junctions, electrotonic coupling, and intercellular communication. Neurosci. Res. Prog. Bull., 16: 373-486, 1978.

Broekhuyse, R.M., Kuhlmann, E.D. and Stols, A.H.: Lens membrane. IV. Isolation and characterization of the main intrinsic polypeptide (MIP) of bovine lens fiber membranes. Exp. Eye Res., 23: 365, 1976.

Caspar, D.L.D., Goodenough, D.A., Makowski, L. and Phillips, W.C.: Gap junction structures. I. Correlated electron microscopy and x-ray diffraction. J. Cell Biol., 74: 605-628, 1977.

Cobb, J.L.S.: Gap junctions in the heart of the teleost fish. Cell Tissue Res., 154: 131-134, 1974.

Decker, R.S.: Hormonal regulation of gap junction differentiation. J. Cell Biol., 69: 669-686, 1976a.

Decker, R.S.: Adrenocorticotropic hormone (ACTH) - induced formation of gap junctions between differentiating Y-1 tumor cells in vitro. J. Cell Biol., 70: 412a (Abstr.), 1976b.

Decker, R.S. and Friend, D.S.: Assembly of gap junctions during amphibian neurulation. J. Cell Biol., 62: 32-47, 1974.

Duguid, J. and Revel, J.P.: The protein components of the gap junction. Cold Spring Harbor Symp. Quant. Biol., 40: 45-47, 1976.

Dunia, I., Sem, K.C., Benedetti, E.L., Zweers, A. and Bloemendal, H.: Isolation and protein of eye lens fiber junctions. FEBS letters, 45: 139-144, 1974.

Ehrhart, J.C. and Chauveau, J.: The protein component of mouse hepatocyte gap junctions. FEBS Letters, 78: 295-299, 1977.

Elias, P.M. and Friend, D.S.: Vitamin-A-induced mucous metaplasia. An in vitro system for modulating tight and gap junction differentiation. J. Cell Biol., 68: 173-188, 1976.

Fujisawa, H., Morioka, H., Nakamura, H. and Watanabe, K.: Gap junctions in the differentiated neural retinae of newly hatched chickens. J. Cell Sci., 22: 597-606, 1976.

Fujisawa, H. and Morioka, H.: A simple method for freeze-cleaving of cells grown on plastic culture dish. Cell Struct. Funct., 2: 361-365, 1977.

Gilula, N.B.: Gap junctions and cell communication. In: Int. Cell Biol., Brinkley, E. and Porter, K., eds., Rockefeller Univ. Press, New York, pp. 61-69, 1977.

Goodenough, D.A.: Methods for the isolation and structural characterization of hepatocyte gap junctions. In: Methods in Membrane Biology, Vol. 3, Korn, E.D., ed., Plenum Publishing Corp., New York, pp. 51-80, 1975.

Goodenough, D.A.: Lens gap junction: A structural hypothesis for nonregulated low-resistance intercellular pathways. Invest. Ophtalmol. Vis. Sci., 18: 1104-1122, 1979.

Griepp, E.B., Peacock, J.H., Bernfield, M.R. and Revel, J.P.: Morphological and functional correlates of synchronous beatng between embryonic heart cell aggregates and layers. Exp. Cell Res., 113: 273-282, 1978.

Griepp, E.B. and Revel, J.P.: Gap junctions in development. In: Intercellular Communication, De Mello, W.C., ed., Plenum Publishing Corp., New York, pp. 1-14, 1977.

Gros, D., Mocquard, J.P., Challice, C.E. and Schrével, J.: Formation and growth of gap junctions in mouse myocardium during ontogenesis. A freeze-cleave study. J. Cell Sci., 30: 45-61, 1978.

Gros, D., Mocquard, J.P., Challice, C.E., and Schrével, J.: Formation and growth of gap junctions in mouse myocardium during ontogenesis. Quantitative data and their implications on the development of intercellular communication. J. Mol. Cell. Cardiol., 11: 543-554, 1979.

Gros, D., Mocquard, J.P., Schrével, J. and Challice, C.E.: Assembly of gap junctions in developing mouse cardiac muscle. In: Perspectives in Cardiovascular Research, vol. 5, Pexieder, T., ed., Raven Press, New York, pp. 285-298, 1980a.

Gros, D., Potreau, D. and Mocquard, J.P.: Myocardial plasma membrane during ontogenesis: Density and size of intramembranous particles. J. Cell Sci., 43: 301-317, 1980b.

Henderson, D., Eibl, H. and Weber, K.: Structure and biochemistry of mouse hepatic gap junctions. J. Mol. Biol., 132: 193-218, 1979.

Hertzberg, E.L. and Gilula, N.B.: Isolation and characterization of gap junctions from rat liver. J. Biol. Chem., 254: 2138-2147, 1979.

Johnson, R.G., Hammer, M., Sheridan, J. and Revel, J.P.: Gap junctions between reaggregated Novikoff hepatoma cells. Proc. Natl. Acad. Sci. USA, 71: 4536-4540, 1974.

Kensler, R.W., Brink, P. and Dewey, M.M.: Nexus of frog ventricle. J. Cell Biol., 73: 768-781, 1977.

Larsen, W.J.: Gap junctions and hormone action. In: Transport of Ions and Water in Epithelia, Walls, B.J., Oschman, J.L., Moreton, D. and Gupta, B., eds., Academic Press, London, pp. 333-363, 1977a.

Larsen, W.J.: Structural diversity of gap junctions. Tissue and Cell, 9:

373-394, 1977b.

Lawrence, T.S., Beers, W.H. and Gilula, N.B.: Transmission of hormonal stimulation by cell-to-cell communication. Nature (London), 272: 501-506, 1978.

Lee, I. and Challice, C.E.: A freeze-cleave study of the influence of cyclohexamide on the development of gap junctions in vitro. IRCS Medical Sci., 8: 49-50, 1980.

Loewenstein, W.R.: Permeability of membrane junctions. Ann. N.Y. Acad. Sci., 137: 441-472, 1966.

Loewenstein, W.R.: The cell-to-cell membrane channel in development and growth. In: Differentiation and Development, Ahmad, F., Russell, T.R., Schultz, J. and Werner, R., eds., Academic Press, New York, pp. 399-409, 1978.

Loewenstein, W.R., Kanno, Y. and Socolar, S.J.: The cell-to-cell channel. Fed. Proc., 37: 2645-2650, 1978a.

Loewenstein, W.R., Kanno, Y. and Socolar, S.J.: Quantum jumps of conductance during formation of membrane channels at cell-to-cell junction. Nature (London), 274: 133-136, 1978b.

Makowski, L., Caspar, D.L.D., Phillips, W.C. and Goodenough, D.A.: Gap junction structures. II. Analysis of the x-ray diffraction data. J. Cell Biol., 74: 629-645, 1977.

Masson-Pevet, M., Bleeker, W.K., Mackaay, A.J.C., Gros, D. and Bouman, L.N.: Ultrastructural and functional aspects of the rabbit sinoatrial node. In: The Sinus Node. Structure, Function and Clinical Relevance, Bonke, F.I.M., ed., Martinus Nijhoff, The Hague, pp. 195-211, 1978.

Masson-Pevet, M., Jongsma, H.J. and De Bruijne, J.: Collagenase- and trypsin-dissociated heart cells: A comparative ultrastructural study. J. Mol. Cell. Cardiol., 8: 747-757, 1976.

Mazet, F.: Mise en évidence et étude des variations morphologiques des gap-junctions dans les tissues électriquement couplés. Applications aux tissus cardiaques. Thèse de Doctorat d'Etat, University of Paris XI (Orsay), France, 1977a.

Mazet, F.: Freeze-fracure studies of gap junctions in the developing and adult amphibian cardiac muscle. Devel. Biol., 60: 139-152, 1977b.

Mazet, F. and Cartaud, J.: Freeze-fracture studies of frog atrial fibres. J. Cell Sci., 22: 427-434, 1976.

McNutt, N.S.: Ultrastructure of intercellular junctions in adult and developing
    cardiac muscle. Am. J. Cardiol., 25: 169-182, 1970.

McNutt, N.S. and Weinstein, R.S.: The ultrastructure of the nexus. A corre-
    lated thin-section and freeze-cleave study. J. Cell Biol., 47: 666-688,
    1970.

Pinto da Silva, P. and Gilula, N.B.: Gap junctions in normal and transformed
    fibroblasts in culture. Exp. Cell Res., 71: 393-401, 1972.

Raviola, E., Goodenough, D.A. and Raviola, G.: Structure of rapidly frozen gap
    junctions. J. Cell Biol., 87: 273-279, 1980.

Revel, J.P.: Contacts and junctions between cells. SEM Symp., 28: 447-461,
    1974.

Revel, J.P., Griepp, E.B., Finbow, M. and Johnson, R.: Possible steps in gap
    junction formation. Zoon, 6: 139-144 (Proc. Symp. "Formshaping Move-
    ments in Neurogenesis", Uppsala, Sept. 1977), 1978.

Revel, J.P. and Karnovsky, M.J.: Hexagonal array of subunits in intercellular
    junctions of the mouse heart and liver. J. Cell Biol., 33: C7-C12, 1967.

Sheridan, J.D.: Cell coupling and cell communication during embryogenesis. In:
    The Cell Surface in Animal Embryogenesis and Development. Poste, G. and
    Nicolson, G.L., eds., Elsevier/North-Holland Biomedical Press, Amsterdam,
    pp. 409-447, 1976.

Shibata, Y.: Comparative ultrastructure of cell membrane specializations in
    vertebrate cardiac muscles. Arch. Histol. Jap., 40: 391-406, 1977.

Shibata, Y. and Yamamoto, T.: Gap junctions in the cardiac muscle cells of the
    lamprey. Cell Tissue Res., 178: 477-482, 1977.

Shibata, Y. and Yamamoto, T.: Freeze-fracture studies of gap junctions in ver-
    tebrate cardiac muscle cells. J. Ultrastructure Res., 67: 79-88, 1979.

Staehelin, L.A.: Structure and function of intercellular junctions. Int. Rev.
    Cytol., 39: 131-283, 1974.

Unwin, P.N.T. and Zampighi, G.: Structure of the junction between communicat-
    ing cells. Nature (London), 283: 545-549, 1980.

Yancey, B.S., Easter, D. and Revel, J.P.: Cytological changes in gap junctions
    during liver regeneration. J. Ultrastructure Res., 67: 229-242, 1979.

Yee, A.G. and Revel, J.P.: Loss and reappearance of gap junctions in regener-
    ating liver. J. Cell Biol., 78: 554-564, 1978.

Zampighi, G. and Unwin, P.N.T.: Two forms of isolated gap junctions. J. Mol.

Biol., 135: 451-464, 1979.

INTERCELLULAR COUPLING BETWEEN EMBRYONIC HEART CELL AGGREGATES

David E. Clapham and Robert L. DeHaan

INTRODUCTION

Heart tissue is a functional syncytium composed of individual cells (Sjöstrand and Andersson, 1954) connected by nexuses (Barr et al., 1965; Fawcett and McNutt, 1969). Since electrical current flows across cell membranes and from cell to cell, rate and rhythm in normal whole heart must be regulated at the cellular level by intercellular resistance as well as by excitable membrane characteristics. Consequently changes in intercellular resistance may cause arrhythmias or changes in rate.

Numerous ulstructural studies have demonstrated the presence of nexuses, or gap junctions, in heart tissue. Work with invertebrate cells and simple tissue has characterized the gap junction as a proteinaceous, $\simeq 10^{10}$ Ohm channel spanning the intercellular space to provide electrical and molecular communication between cells. (For review see Gilula, 1977; Loewenstein, 1975). The gap junction may lower membrane resistance from many KOhm.cm^2 to less than 1 Ohm.cm^2. Junctional patency may depend on transcellular voltage (Spray et al., 1979), intracellular Ca^{++} (Rose and Loewenstein, 1976), or intracellular pH (Turin and Warner, 1977; Rose and Rick, 1978).

Embryonic heart cells have the striking attribute of developing synchrony when placed in contact as single isolated cells (Cavanaugh, 1955; DeHaan and Hirakow, 1972), as monolayers (Jongsma, 1972), or as spherical aggregates (DeHaan and Fozzard, 1975). Synchrony between aggregates of embryonic ventricular heart cells develops within minutes with a delay between the leading and entrained action potentials averaging $\simeq 125$ ms (Ypey et al., 1979). The synchronization and consequent reduction in delay between entrained action potentials is a result of a decrease in junctional resistance between aggregates (Clapham et al., 1980). We postulate that junctional resistance is a function of developing gap junctional channels between apposed heart cells. By analogy, delays in normal adult heart tissue may be a function of number of gap junctions between cells as well as excitable membrane characteristics. Alterations in the cellular environment, such as increase in intracellular Ca^{++} (DeMello, 1975; Weingart, 1977), may decrease the number of open junctional channels resulting in decreased electrical coupling and arrhythmias.

RESULTS

LATENCY MEASUREMENTS

Chick ventricle is dissociated by a multicycle trypsinization process to yield individual ($\simeq 10\mu$) cells. The cells are gyrated for 48 hours to form 100 μ - 300 μ spherical aggregates of several thousand cells. Aggregates behave, for our purposes, as single, large heart cells. For low-frequency, low-voltage signals, the aggregates are virtually isopotential (Clapham, 1979; Clay et al., 1979). Aggregates beat spontaneously in 1.3 mM K^+, but can be made quiescent by addition of 10^{-6} M TTX (V_r = -50 mV). Aggregates are quiescent in 4.8 mM K^+ (V_r = -80 mV), but a train of action potentials can be elicited by a short depolarizing pulse. In some experiments in 1.3 mM K^+, physical contraction is inhibited by preincubation in cytochalasin B with little alteration of electrical activity. In general, for a 150 μ aggregate, the input resistance is three to four times lower in 4.8 mM K^+ (1 - 2 MOhm) than in 1.3 mM K^+ (4 - 5 MOhm).

Aggregates are easily manipulated into apposition with $\simeq$ 10 μ (ID) suction electrodes. Both intracellular and extracellular electrodes monitor electrical activity and both may be used to inject current pulses. Action potentials measured intracellularly (MDP - 90mV, overshoot +30 mV) are measured extracellularly as 1 - 2 mV "extracellular spikes" proportional to the first derivative of the action potential (Clapham, 1979). Latency (L) is defined as the delay in milliseconds between the fastest parts of the upstroke of two synchronized action potentials of apposed aggregates. We will define synchrony as the condition in which action potentials from two apposed aggregates are entrained with a fixed or slowly changing time delay between leading and following action potentials.

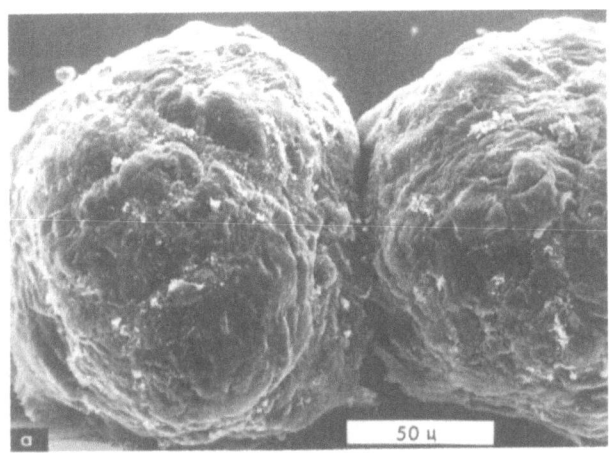

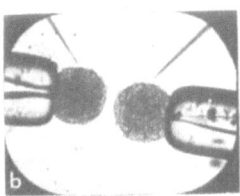

FIGURE 1a *Scanning electron micrograph of a pair of apposed aggregates. Bar scale = 50 μ. Courtesy of Dr. C. Adkison.*
FIGURE 1b *Aggregates are held by suction pipettes attached to micromanipulators. Current may be injected via suction electrodes or microelectrodes. Scale = 100 μ.*

When two aggregates of heart cells, each beating at inherently different rates, are apposed gently (Figure 1), they begin to alter each other's normally regular rate within a few minutes and synchronize to a common rate a few minutes later. When observed under the microscope at first synchrony, there may be no discernible delay between aggregates. However, when electrical activity is measured via suction electrodes applied to independent aggregates (Figure 2), and the process repeated, the moment of first synchrony is found to correspond to a delay ranging between 20 and 200 ms. Thereafter the delay (Latency, L) is found to decrease exponentially to less than 1 ms in 5 to 30 minutes (Figure 3)

(Ypey et al., 1979).

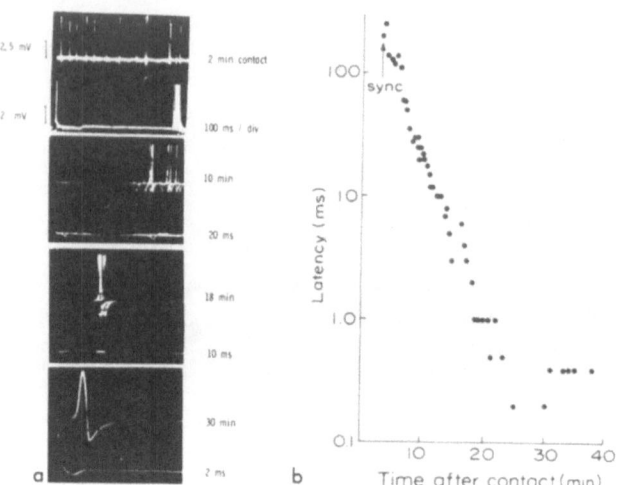

FIGURE 2a *Extracellular spikes recorded from coupling aggregates. In each panel the oscilloscope is triggered by the spikes recorded from the aggregate of the bottom trace. About 15 successive sweeps are superimposed in each frame. The numbers on the right are the time after contact and the time scale for each panel. Two minutes after contact aggregates are beating independently. By 10 minutes after contact the aggregates have synchronized with a mean latency of ≈ 130 ms. By 30 minutes after synchrony the latency has decreased to ≈ 3 ms with little variability about the mean.*
FIGURE 2b *Examples of the decline in latency for a pair of aggregates in 1.3 mM K⁺. Note log scale. Different experiment from 2a.*

The process of entrainment of two aggregates may be divided for descriptive purposes into phases of (1) no synchrony; (2) partial synchrony; and (3) synchrony. Separated aggregates, beating independently, have remarkably constant beat rates. Interbeat interval variability is dependent on size of cluster (Clay and DeHaan, 1979), but is extremely regular for the 100 μ - 200 μ aggregates used in these experiments (± 10 ms). When aggregates are attached to suction electrodes and pushed together, they quickly return to stable, independent beat rates with little rate variation. Within minutes, however, both aggregates begin to display rate disturbances with each aggregate's action potential, producing depolarization in its neighbor (Ypey et al., 1979). One

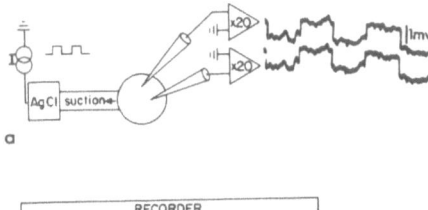

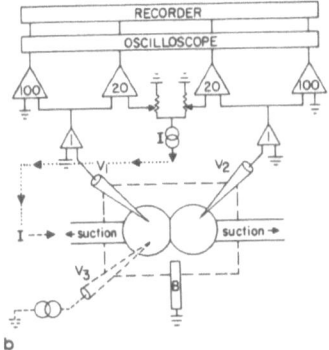

a

b

FIGURE 3 (a) *Uniformity of voltage response in a single aggregate to a series of 5-s current pulses injected via a suction electrode. Two voltage electrodes in the aggregate measure the same potential, regardless of orientation or separation distance. One microelectrode was then used to inject current to obtain the input resistance of the isolated aggregate. Aggregate input resistance varied with size and K and ranged from 0.5 to 4 MOhm for the preparations studied here. (b) Diagrammatic representation of measurement system. Suction electrodes were used for current injection and micromanipulation of aggregates. Two microelectrodes (V₁, V₂)* (V_1, V_2) *were used to measure response to current pulses applied via one suction electrode in most cases. In some experiments, a third microelectrode was used (V₃)* (V_3) *for current injection in lieu of the suction electrode. Slight offset from current drop across the agar bridge (B) to ground was balanced as shown. High gain (X100) amplifiers are AC-coupled. From Clapham, Shrier and DeHaan (1980), courtesy J. Gen. Physiol.*

aggregate may entrain the other for a few beats before reverting to complex beat interaction. "Partial synchrony" refers to this stage of variable interaction. After two to five minutes of partial synchrony, the smaller aggregates (higher input resistance) usually is entrained to the rate of the larger aggregate, with a latency of 20 - 200 ms (1.3 mM K^+). From the time of first synchrony, the latency declines approximately exponentially ($\tau = 18 \pm 11$ min) to a plateau at about 1 ms latency (Ypey et al., 1979). In contracting aggregates, occasional regression to longer latencies occurs (i.e., 20 → 70 ms). These disruptions are thought to be breaks in attachment of cells. In these cases, L recovers to

its previous level within 10 to 30 beats. As L decreases, beat-to-beat variation in L declines markedly. Whereas fluctuations in latency of 40 ms commonly
occur at L = 200 ms, at L = 1 ms, fluctuations are on the order of 0.5 ms (Ypey
et al., 1979). After reaching an L of approximately 0.5 - 1 ms, further decline in L is extremely slow. In one experiment, L declined to 0.5 ms only
after 10 hours at an L less than 1 ms. Apposition for many hours leads to a
gradual migration of cells filling the appositional area.

　　　Table I shows accumulated data for the decline in L in aggregates pressed
into apposition and monitored via suction electrodes. There is a large degree
of variability in the rates of synchrony and decline. One pair of
≃ 100 μ aggregates reached synchrony 1 minute after apposition. Several factors play a role in the onset of synchrony and rate of decline of L. First,
time to synchrony is directly related to appositional area and inversely proportional to the input resistance of the aggregates (Clapham et al., 1980).
Second, the amount of pressure used to apposed aggregates seems to speed synchrony, although this has not been quantified. Third, physical contraction
seems to delay the synchronization process. When contraction is prevented with
pretreatment of aggregates by cytochalasin B, synchronization proceeds at a
slightly faster rate. It is probable that junctions in contracting preparations
are occasionally disrupted by mechanical forces. Fourth, increasing K^+ from 1.3
mM to 4.8 mM slows synchrony.

TABLE I

	number of pairs	aggregate diameter (microns)	diameter of contact area (microns)	time to 1st synchrony (minutes) t_s	latency at 1st synchrony L_s (ms)	time constant (minutes) τ_s
1.3 mM K_o^+	18	*1 168±34 *2 102±29	120±33	12.9±9	90.22±58	18.7±16.7
1.3 mM K_o^+ cyto B	9	*1 158±24 *2 178±24	127±53	8.1±3.7	127±53	3.6±1.4
4.8 mM K_o^+	11	*1 158±26 *2 155±18	109±26	31.1±12	38±29	49±21

In 4.8 mM K^+ L can be measured by applying a short pulse, initiating a train of
beats. Latencies are then measured between action potentials after termination

of the current. In 4.8 mM K$^+$, time to synchrony and subsequent decrease in L proceed more slowly, in part reflecting a decrease in input resistance of the apposed aggregates (Clapham et al., 1980). In a few pairs measured in 1.3 mM K$^+$ with 10^{-6} TTX, latency progressed at a rate intermediate between 1.3 mM K$^+$ and 4.8 mM K$^+$.

Measurements of synchrony may provide a useful tool in studying the effect of membrane and cell surface changes on junction formation. Aggregates preincubated in cholesterol (Clapham and Lantz, unpublished) showed no appreciable alteration in t_s or decline in L. However, surface-active proteases decrease the time to synchrony of aggregates apposed between glass plates, as observed by eye (Williams and DeHaan, 1978; DeHaan et al., 1980).

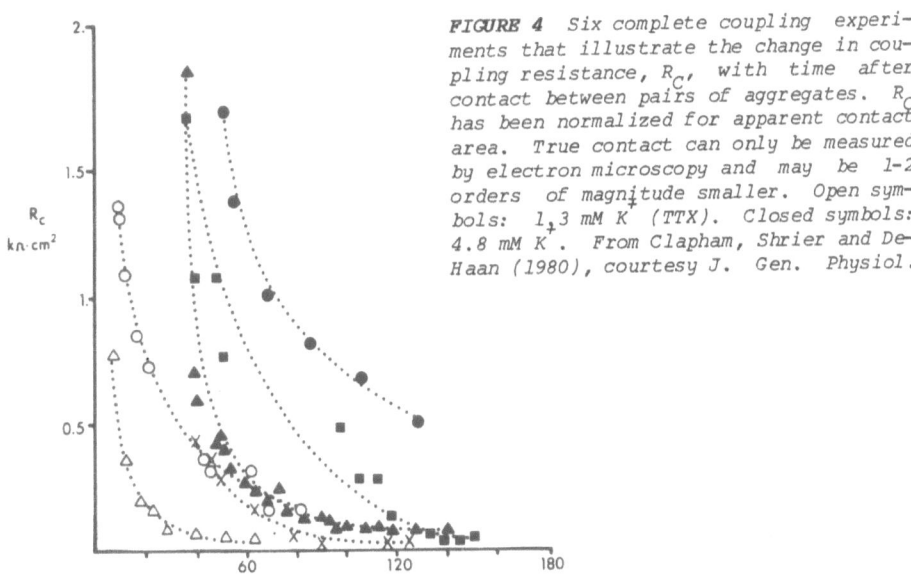

FIGURE 4 *Six complete coupling experiments that illustrate the change in coupling resistance, R_c, with time after contact between pairs of aggregates. R_c has been normalized for apparent contact area. True contact can only be measured by electron microscopy and may be 1-2 orders of magnitude smaller. Open symbols: 1.3 mM K$^+$ (TTX). Closed symbols: 4.8 mM K$^+$. From Clapham, Shrier and DeHaan (1980), courtesy J. Gen. Physiol.*

COUPLING RESISTANCE MEASUREMENTS

Despite the descriptive utility of L measurements, action potential synchrony is regulated by the coupling resistance (R_c) between aggregates. Synchrony of aggregates requires the exchange of current across junctional areas driven by the voltage differences created by action potentials. R_c may be measured between quiescent aggregates as a function of time after apposition (Figure 3). Current pulses (I) are injected into one of two apposed aggregates to produce a small transmembrane voltage change (ΔV_1). Several minutes after apposition, a voltage drop also appears across the cell membrane of the second aggregates (ΔV_2). By measuring the input resistance of each aggregate before and after apposition, the junctional or coupling resistance (R_C) may be derived (see Clapham et al., 1980). Current may be injected into aggregates via intracellular electrodes. When extracellular electrodes are used, most of the current shunts across the intercellular space to ground. However, enough current is driven intracellular-ly to produce a uniform voltage deflection of 1-5 mV (Figure 3a) across the cell membranes of the aggregate. When quiescent aggregates (1.3 mM K^+ with TTX or 4.8 mM K^+) are placed in apposition and pulses continuously injected, R_C is seen to decline in a manner similar to the decline in L (Fig. 4).

In several experiments, pulses were injected continuously to measure R_C while at intervals of several minutes, short, larger current pulses were used to elicit a train of action potentials. Latencies were then measured between ac-tion potentials. Figure 5 shows the decline in L compared with the decline in R_C in one experiment. L declines from 100 ms to 0.8 ms over 160 minutes. Coupling resistance could not be measured until R_C was $\simeq$ 12 MOhm. R_C then de-clined at the same rate as L to 0.4 MOhm. Figure 6 shows action potentials delay (L) as a function of R_C from two experiments. There is a linear relation-ship between L and R_C at two different K^+ concentrations (Clapham et al., 1980).

In one pair of nonbeating aggregates, one of the aggregates was briefly stimulated to produce a train of action potentials. At an early phase of cou-pling, the aggregate acting as the pacemaker initiated beating in the entrained aggregate in a rate-dependent manner. During rapid beating, a five to one block occurred. As beating slowed, the entrained aggregate followed each action po-tential with an L of 50 ms. Nineteen minutes later, two aggregates were per-fectly entrained even at fast rates, when measured L was 20 ms (Clapham et al., 1980).

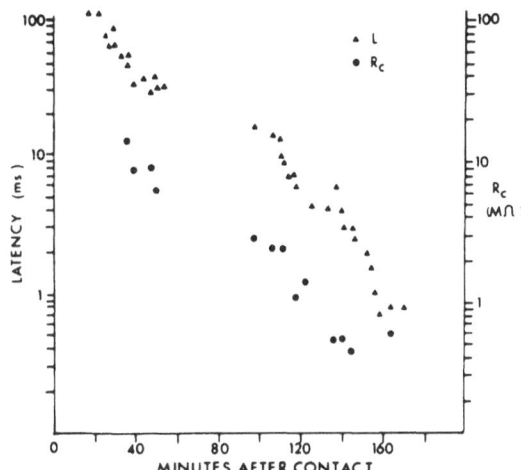

FIGURE 5 *L and R_C plotted against time after contact for one aggregate pair (K^+ = 4.8 mM). Note semilogarithmic scale. The gap in data between t_s = 50-90 min represents multiple penetrations with a microelectrode to regain a puncture. Coupling has been "set back" but is regained as the same slope. r_1 = 80 μ. R_1 = R_2 = 1.5 MOhm. r_a = 60 μ. From Clapham, Shrier and DeHaan (1980), courtesy J. Gen. Physiol.*

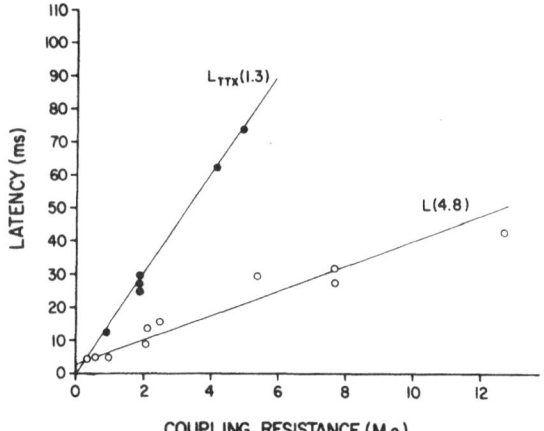

FIGURE 6 *Correlation of R_C and L for one pair of aggregates in 4.8 mM K (o) and a different pair in 1.3 mM K (TTX) (●). Slopes are 3.7 ms/MOhm and 16 ms/MOhm respectively. Modified from Clapham, Shrier and DeHaan (1980), courtesy J. Gen. Physiol.*

DISCUSSION

The results of our studies show that apposition of embryonic heart cell aggregates leads to synchronization of beating through a decrease in junctional resistance. The delay between action potentials in synchronous aggregates decreases linearly with junctional resistance.

The nexus is believed responsible for electrotonic coupling between individual myocardial cells. Typical ultrastructural characteristics of the nexus have also been demonstrated between cells within embryonic ventricular cell aggregates by transmission electron micrography and by freeze-fracture electron micrographs (DeHaan et al., 1980). We interpret our findings of pulse and action potential synchrony between newly apposed aggregates as a result of formation of resistive intercellular gap junctions between aggregates. It is doubtful that 1-5 mV pulse transmission, as well as action potential synchrony, could be achieved by extracellular potassium accumulation with depolarization. Experiments using cytochalasin B to halt mechanical beating while maintaining electrical activity (Ypey et al., 1979) exclude mechanical theories of entrainment.

We have treated aggregates of embryonic ventricular cells as if each aggregate behaved as a single large cell. For low frequency, low voltage changes an aggregate is virtually isopotential (Clay et al., 1979; Clapham, 1979). During the fastest part of the action potential, delays of 48 ± 20 µsec across a distance of $\simeq 165$ µ in an aggregate can be measured (Clapham, 1979). Since latencies between well-coupled aggregates are on the order of 1 ms, inhomogeneities within each aggregate by comparison are insignificant. Input resistance measurements are made before apposition and after separation of the aggregates to assure membrane resistance stays constant. The cell membranes of both aggregates are assumed to be unchanged except for the formation of low-resistance junctions in the relatively small area of new apposition. Thus, a simple three-resistor model (R_C, R_1, R_2) suffices for DC measurements in coupling aggregates.

The relation between R_C and L is analogous to the well-known strength duration curve in that R_C determines the size of the stimulation current (strength) and L is the time to initiation of the action potential (duration). When R_C is large, L is long and depends on the nonlinear kinetics of the heart membrane.

At short latencies, L depends simply on the membrane time constants.

When pulses in the linear range of voltage are injected into one of a pair of quiescent aggregates, the current passing into the second aggregate is limited by the coupling resistance alone. Of course, no delay occurs in the initiation of the pulse in the second aggregate, since the two aggregates are connected only by linear elements. The pulse charges according to the time constant of the membrane. However, in spontaneously beating aggregates the relationship is more complicated. Time to threshold in an aggregate is again a function of the nonlinear kinetics of excitable membranes. Furthermore, the stimulating current is not constant but depends on the voltage difference between respective action potentials at any point in time. Each aggregate passes current to the apposed aggregate at different times in its cycle. Biophysical characterization of synchronization may best be accomplished by constant current injection in spontaneously beating heart preparations.

Excitable cells of muscle and heart have been modelled as coupled oscillators linked by pure resistance (Torre, 1976; Linkens and Datardina, 1977; Berkenblit et al., 1975). The mathematically modelled cells reach entrainment as resistance is progressively decreased and exhibit constant phase shifts (corresponding to latency) at first synchrony. However, in the model systems the phase shift can be progressively reduced without further reduction in coupling resistance. Our experiments show that in embryonic heart tissue R_C decreases dramatically with time, paralleling the decrease in L. This implies that continued addition of gap junctions dominates the progression of synchrony rather than entrainment at constant resistance.

Gap junction channels are modelled as 10^{10} Ohm pores spanning the intercellular space (e.g., Loewenstein, 1975). Since we have measured R_C as a function of time we may speculate about the rate of channel formation with synchrony. Clapham et al., (1980) plotted G_C ($1/R_C$) as a function of time after contact. The rate of channel formation varied from linear to exponential in experiments. In all cases, G_C rose to a plateau of $\simeq 10^{-2}$ S/cm^2 (total apparent contact area). Assuming macular gap junctions occupy 0.3 % of the total face (DeHaan et al., 1980), specific junctional conductances are on the order of 3 S/cm^2. At the time of first synchrony, when R_C is $\simeq 20$ MOhm between aggregates, 500 channels ($1/(20.10^6 \times 10^{-10})$) would have formed in an 8.10^{-5} cm^2 ($\simeq 100$ apposed cells) for a density of five channels/cell. To an R_C of 1 MOhm, 10,000 channels must now span the interaggregate space (100 channels/cell). Note that perfect apposition of two cardiac cell membranes without channels over an equal area of contact would yield a resistance of $\simeq$ 125 MOhm (assuming a specific membrane resistance of 20 KOhm.cm^2). Thus, very few channels are needed, theoretically, for synchrony of aggregates. Single cells would easily be entrained to a common rhythm by one channel (Clapham et al., 1980). Morphometric analysis of nexal areas in rat ventricle (Mitter, 1973), sheep Purkinje fiber (Mobley and Page, 1972), and mouse ventricle (Gros et al., 1979) reveal thousands of junctional subunits per cell on average. Such a large number of channels certainly represents a surplus with respect to the function of electrical synchrony.

Tissue properties of cardiac preparations add to the difficulty of studying ell membranes. Changes may occur simultaneously in cell-to-cell coupling as ll as across the cell membrane upon addition of various drugs or changes in extracellular milieu. In effect, one is studying current flow via two par-pathways - the cell membrane and the nexus - with only one vantage point. assumption is generally made that either intercellular impedance alone or mbrane impedance alone is changed by the experimental manipulation. re several lines of evidence that indicate the gap junction channel is a tructure. Injection of Ca^{++} into Chironomus salivary gland cells at er than 10^{-5} M causes a rapid decrease in junctional membrane perme-and Loewenstein, 1976). In dog Purkinje fibers, intracellular in-$^{++}$ produced a rapid reduction in electrical coupling which reversed DeMello, 1975). Wier (1980) measured aequorin light response to try and intracellular release and found intracellular Ca^{++} levels . Localized peak concentrations were probably much greater. oted that 2.10^{-6} M ouabain caused a four-fold increase in esistance in bovine ventricular trabeculae. He postulat-increase in internal Ca^{++} uncoupled cells. Both decreases lular pH can lead to elevation of intracellular Ca^{++} between Chironomus salivary gland cells (Rose and Rick, gradients may also result in cell uncoupling. permeability to dye are markedly decreased by trans-mV in either direction in isolated pairs of eres (Spray et al., 1979).

Myocardial injury secondary to anoxia or ischemia produce many of the circumstances that are implicated in uncoupling. Intracellular pH decreases (Case et al., 1969) and intracellular Ca^+ probably rises (Nayler et al., 1979) after ischemia. Extracellular K^+ rises to levels as high as 8 to 9 mEq/liter, even when measured in cardiac venous drainage (Downar et al., 1977). Local increases in concentrations of K^+ in clefts surrounding myocardium are propably much higher. Potassium accumulation creates local depolarization and changes in action potential duration (Kline and Morad, 1978). Within 15 minutes after coronary occlusion in isolated porcine and canine hearts, Janse et al. (1980) found that maximal current flows occurred across the ischemic border when normal cells had repolarized and ischemic cells had not. Ventricular premature beats followed in such regions when injury currents were largest.

Interestingly, TenEick et al. (1976) observed that arrhythmias were more likely to occur in the first 20 minutes after ischemia, despite a lack of change in the shape of the action potential. We have observed that changes in cell-to-cell coupling may occur without changes in the shape of the action potential. In experiments with bovine ventricular trabeculae, Wojtczak (1979) reported that longitudinal resistance rose three-fold under anoxia and 20-fold when tissue was exposed to both low O_2 and epinephrine. Further evidence that ischemia results in cellular uncoupling comes from electron microscopic studies. Changes in the ultrastructure of nexuses seen in freeze fracture have been observed after myocardial ischemia in dogs (Ashraf and Halverson, 1978). Frank et al. (1980) measured a decrease in the number of intramembranous particles in the myocardial membrane after anoxia in rabbit myocardia. In addition to direct effects on gap junctions, ischemia alters the other branch of the parallel circuit: the membrane resistance. Increasing extracellular K^+ decreases membrane resistance. This may result in failure of propagation in nerve as an effect of the "loading" of low resistance in the area (Joyner et al., 1980).

We have shown simply that delays of over 100 ms may result between cultured embryonic ventricular cells due to high coupling resistance alone. No depression of action potential upstroke velocity, input resistance, or changes in other nonjunctional membrane characteristics occurred in our experiments. We postulate that weak electrotonic interactions may occur in areas of damaged myocardium where closing junctional channels have resulted in high coupling resistance. Since delays of 100 ms can occur at a single cell interface, microreentry is possible. Small, isolated areas of myocardium may also give rise to ec-topic foci coupled at a wide range of delays.

At early stages of coupling, functional similarities exist between the junctional area of apposed aggregates and the A-V node (nodal delay $\simeq$ 40 ms). Rate-dependent block can be demonstrated between poorly coupled aggregates (Clapham et al., 1980) and delays (L) as long as 200 ms occur at large values of R_C. Measuring only at the opposite poles of two apposed aggregates, one might assume the delay resulted from distributed slow tissue conduction (10^{-4} m/s) rather than from one high-resistance interface. Conduction velocities in A-V node have been measured as low as 0.02 m/s (Hoffman et al., 1959). Morphologic studies by James and Sherf (1968), DeFelice and Challice (1969), and Kim and Baba (1971), as well as dye studies by Pollack (1976), show a relative paucity of gap junctions in the A-V node. A high intracellular resistance of 40.9 MOhm/cm in rabbit A-V node (compared to 9.6 MOhm/cm in atria) may reflect the low number of junctions (DeMello, 1977). However, in the A-V node, slow conduction is not associated with as large a fluctuation in delay as those between newly apposed aggregates (Ypey et al., 1979). A hypothesis to explain nodal slow conduction would combine nodal cells with only moderately high cou-pling resistance and slow nodal upstroke velocities. Cell-to-cell delays of only a few milliseconds would yield slow conduction with only small fluctuations in conduction velocity.

REFERENCES

Ashraf, M. and Halverson, C.: Ultrastructural modifications of nexuses (gap junctions) during early myocardial ischemia. J. Mol. Cell. Cardiol., 10: 263-269, 1978.

Barr, L., Dewey, M.M. and Berger, W.: Propagation of action potentials and the structure of the nexus in cardiac muscle. J. Gen. Physiol., 48: 797-823, 1965.

Berkinblit, M.B., Kalinin, O., Kovalev, S.A. and Chilakhyan, L.M.: Study with the Noble model of synchronization of the spontaneously active myocardial cells bound by a highly permeable contact. Biofizika, 20: 121-125, 1975.

Case, R.B., Nasser, M.G. and Crampton, R.S.: Biochemical aspects of early myocardial ischemia. Am. J. Cardiol., 24: 766-775, 1969.

Cavanaugh, M.W.: Pulsation, migration and division in dissociated chick embryo heart cells in vitro. J. Exp. Zool., 128: 573, 1955.

Clapham, D.E.: A whole tissue model of the heart cell aggregate: electrical coupling between cells, membrane impedance and the extracellular space. Doctoral dissertation, Emory University, Atlanta, Georgia USA, 1979.

Clapham, D.E., Shrier, A. and DeHaan, R.L.: Junctional resistance and action potential delay between embryonic heart cell aggregates. J. Gen. Physiol., 75: 633-654, 1980.

Clay, J.R. and DeHaan, R.L.: Fluctuations in interbeat interval in rhythmic heart cell clusters. Biophys. J., 28: 377-390, 1979.

Clay, J.R., DeFelice, L.J. and DeHaan, R.L.: Current noise parameters derived from voltage noise and impedance in embryonic heart cell preparations. Biophys. J., 28: 169-184, 1979.

DeFelice, L.J. and Challice, C.E.: Anatomical and ultrastructural study of the electrophysiological atrioventricular node of the rabbit. Circ. Res., 24: 457-474, 1969.

DeHaan, R.L., Williams, E.H., Ypey, D.L. and Clapham, D.E.: Intercellular coupling of embryonic heart cells. In: Mechanisms of Cardiac Morphogenesis and Teratogenesis: Perspectives in Cardiovascular Research, Pexieder, T., ed., Raven Press, New York, pp. 299-316, 1980.

DeHaan, R.L. and Fozzard, H.A.: Membrane responses to current pulses in spheroidal aggregates of embryonic heart cells. J. Gen. Physiol., 65: 207-222, 1975.

DeHaan, R.L. and Hirakow, R.: Synchronization of pulsation rates in isolated cardiac myocytes. Exp. Cell Res., 70: 214-220, 1972.

DeMello, W.C.: Effect of intracellular injection of calcium and strontium on cell communication in heart. J. Physiol. (London), 250: 231-245, 1975.

DeMello, W.C.: Passive electrical properties of the atrioventricular node. Pfluegers Arch., 371: 135-139, 1977.

Fawcett, D. and McNutt, N.S.: The ultrastructure of the cat myocardium I. Ventricular papillary muscle. J. Cell Biol., 42: 1-45, 1969.

Frank, J.S., Beydler, S., Kreman, M. and Rau, E.E.: Structure of the

freeze-fractured sarcolemma in the normal and anoxic rabbit myocardium.
Circ. Res., 47: 131-143, 1980.

Gilula, N.B.: Gap junctions and cell communication. In: International Cell
Biology 1966-1977, Brinkley, B.R. and Porter, K.R., eds., The Rockefeller
University Press, New York, pp. 61-69, 1977.

Gros, D., Mocquard, J.P., Challice, C.E. and Schrevel, J.: Formation and
growth of gap junctions in mouse myocardium during ontogenesis:
quantitative data and their implications on the development of intercellular common reaction. J. Mol. Cell. Cardiol., 11: 543-554, 1979.

Hoffman, B.F., Paes de Carvalho, A., DeMello, W.C. and Cranefield, P.:
Electrical activity of single fibers of the atrioventricular node. Circ.
Res., 2: 11-18, 1959.

James, T.N. and Sherf, L.: Ultrastructure of the human atrioventricular node.
Circulation, 37: 1049-1070, 1968.

Janse, M.J., Van Capelle, F.J., Morsink, H., Kleber, A.G., Wilms-Schopman, F.,
Cardinal, R., D'Almoncourt, C. and Durrer, D.: Flow of "injury" current
and patterns of excitation during early ventricular arrhythmias in acute
regional myocardial ischemia in isolated porcine and canine hearts. Circ.
Res., 47: 151-165, 1980.

Joyner, R.W., Westerfield, M. and Moore, J.W.: Effects of cellular geometry on
current flow during a propagated action potential. Biophys. J., 31:
183-194, 1980.

Jongsma, H.J. and Van Rijn, H.E.: Electrotonic spread of current in monolayer
cultures of neonatal rat heart cells. J. Memb. Biol., 9: 341-360, 1972.

Kim, S. and Baba, N.: Atrioventricular node and Purkinje fibers of the guinea
pig heart, Am. J. Anat., 132: 339-353, 1971.

Kline, R. and Morad, M.: Potassium efflux and accumulation in heart muscle.
Biophys. J., 16: 367-380, 1976.

Linkens, D.A. and Datardina, S.: Frequency entrainment of coupled
Hodgkin-Huxley type oscillators for modeling gastrointestinal electrical
activity. IEEE Trans. Biomed. Eng., 24: 362-365, 1977.

Loewenstein, W.R.: Permeable junctions. Cold Spring Harbor Symposium on Quantitative Biology, 40: 49-63, 1975.

Matter, A.: A morphometric study on the nexus of rat cardiac muscle. J. Cell
Biol., 56: 690-696, 1973.

McNutt, N.S. and Weinstein, R.S.: Membrane ultrastructure at mammalian intercellular junctions. Prog. Bioph. Mol. Biol., 26: 45-101, 1973.

Mobley, B.A. and Page, E.: The surface area of sheep cardiac Purkinje fibers.
J. Physiol. (London), 220: 547-563, 1972.

Nayler, W.G., Poole-Wilson, P.A. and Williams, A.: Hypoxia and calcium. J.
Mol. Cell. Cardiol., 11: 683-706, 1979.

Rose, B. and Loewenstein, W.R.: Permeability of a cell junction and the local
cytoplasmic free ionized calcium concentration: a study with aequorin. J.
Memb. Biol., 28: 87-119, 1976.

Sachs, H.G. and DeHaan, R.L.: Embryonic myocardial cell aggregates: volume
and pulsation rate. Devel. Biol., 30: 233-240, 1973.

Sjöstrand, F.S. and Andersson, E.: Electron microscopy of the intercalated
discs of cardiac muscle tissue. Experimentia, 10: 369-370, 1954.

Spray, D.C., Harris, A.L. and Bennett, M.V.L.: Voltage dependence of junctional conductance in early amphibian embryos. Science, 204: 432-434, 1979.

TenEick, R.E., Singer, D.H. and Solberg, L.E.: Coronary occlusion effect on
cellular electrical activity of the heart. Med. Clin. North Am., 60:
49-67, 1976.

Torre, V.: A theory of synchronization of heart pacemaker cells. J. Theor.
Biol., 61: 55-71, 1976.

Turin, L. and Warner, A.: Carbon dioxide reversibility abolishes ionic communication between cells of early amphibian embryo. Nature, 270: 56-57,
1977.

Weingart, R.: The actions of ouabain on intercellular coupling and conduction
velocity in mammalian ventricular muscle. J. Physiol. (London), 264:
341-365, 1977.

Wier, W.G.: Calcium transients during excitation-contraction coupling in mammalian heart: aequorin signals of canine Purkinje fibers. Science, 207:
1085-1087, 1980.

Ypey, D.L., Clapham, D.E. and DeHaan, R.L.: The development of electrical coupling and action potential synchrony between aggregates of embryonic heart
cells. J. Memb. Biol., 51: 75-96, 1979.

INTERCELLULAR COUPLING BETWEEN CARDIAC CELLS AND ITS DISTURBANCES

Jacek Wojtczak

A decrease in the degree of cell-to-cell coupling in heart muscle may induce disturbances of the synchronous discharge in the pacemaker region, produce slow conduction or even conduction block. It is thus desirable to study the processes which could modulate this cell-to-cell coupling under normal and pathological conditions.

In any quantitative study of cell-to-cell coupling it is usual to use either papillary muscles or trabeculae since these approximate to a one-dimensional cable and avoid the complex three-dimensional cable problems inherent in studies in intact hearts. The method used in this study depends on measuring longitudinal current distribution in muscle trabeculae immersed in silicon oil (see Weidmann, 1970; Wojtczak, 1979). The modification used by Wojtczak enabled tension to be measured simultaneously with the changes in internal resistance.

In this method,

$$\frac{V_i}{V_o} = \frac{r_i}{r_o}$$

where V_i, V_o, r_i and r_o are the numerical values of the internal and external potential, and the internal and external longitudinal resistance respectively. On the assumption that r_o is constant and that the extracellular space is 30% of the bundle, the specific internal longitudinal resistance (R_i) can be calculated (for further details see Wojtczak, 1979).

Using this method the influence of various factors on cell-to-cell coupling has been investigated and will now be described.

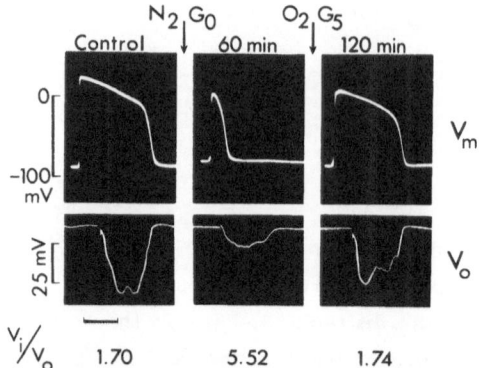

FIGURE 1 *Effects of hypoxia (N_2) in glucose-free Tyrode's solution (G_O) and of subsequent reoxygenation of Tyrode's solution containing 5 mM of glucose (O_2G_5). Upper panel: transmembrane action potential (V_m) recorded at relatively slow sweep speed. Time mark corresponds to 200 ms. Lower panel: initial deflection of biphasic external action potential (V_O). The same time mark in this case corresponds to 20 ms. At the bottom of the figure the ratio of the numerical values for intracellular potential (V_i) to extracellular potential (V_O) is shown. The values of other electrical parameters during control, after 60 minutes of hypoxia, and on reoxygenation, respectively, were as follows: action potential duration 443 ms, 131 ms, 402 ms; action potential amplitude 113 mV, 85 mV, 95 mV. From Wojtczak (1979) with permission of the American Heart Association.*

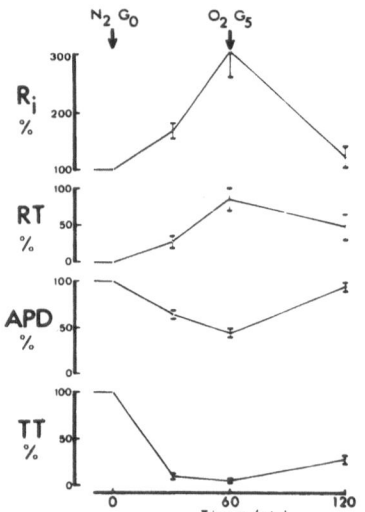

FIGURE 2 *Changes of internal longitudinal resistance (R_i), resting tension (RT), action potential duration (APD) and twitch tension (TT) after 30 to 60 minutes of hypoxia in glucose-free Tyrode's solution (N_2G_O) and after 60 minutes of subsequent reoxygenation in Tyrode's solution containing 5 mM glucose (O_2G_5). The points on the curves represent percent change from values during control (100%) expressed as means ± SE from 11 experiments. The increase in RT was expressed as the percent of the control twitch tension. From Wojtczak (1979) with permission of the American Heart Association.*

HYPOXIA/ISCHAEMIA

Because of the increasing frequency of ischaemic heart disease this has become an important clinical problem. To study hypoxia in muscular trabeculae the partial pressure of oxygen was reduced to very low values by perfusing both Tyrode's solution and the silicon oil in the bath with 95% N_2, 5% CO_2 except when measurements were taken to avoid mechanical artefacts. This experimental set-up does not closely mimic ischaemia since the possibility exists for end products of metabolism as well as for K ions to diffuse from extracellular space to the perfusion fluid. Glycolysis is known to be stimulated transiently in early ischemia and to be blocked as intracellular pH decreases (Rovetto et al., 1973). Glycolytic energy production was reduced as far as possible by omitting glucose from the perfusate when muscles were subject to hypoxia. Fig. 1 shows that exposure of bovine ventricular muscle to hypoxic, glucose-free solution for 60 minutes resulted in a moderate drop of resting potential, a pronounced shortening of the action potential duration, a decrease in its amplitude and a significant increase of internal longitudinal resistance (R_i), as judged from the increase of the ratio V_i/V_o. These changes were reversible on reoxygenation.

The collected results showing changes in R_i, resting tension (RT), action potential duration and twitch tension during hypoxia and subsequent recovery are shown in Fig. 2. It is characteristic of these results that an increase in R_i is associated with the development of a contracture. On reoxygenation, while the changes in R_i were reversible, the relaxation was incomplete.

R_i is the sum of both nexal and cytoplasmic resistance, so a change in R_i can mean either a change in cytoplasmic or nexal resistance or both. Cytoplasmic resistance in hypoxia probably decreases, for it has been shown in cardiac muscle that hypoxia lowers the internal pH (Lavalee and Webb), 1963), and under these conditions in skeletal muscle there is a decrease in cytoplasmic resistance (Meves and Voelkner, 1958). An influence of total ionic concentration on cytoplasmic resistance seems unlikely for Nayler and Seabra-Gomes (1976) have found that in hypoxia the loss of potassium is balanced by a gain of sodium. Thus it seems reasonable to conclude that the measured changes in R_i reflect changes in the nexal resistance during hypoxia.

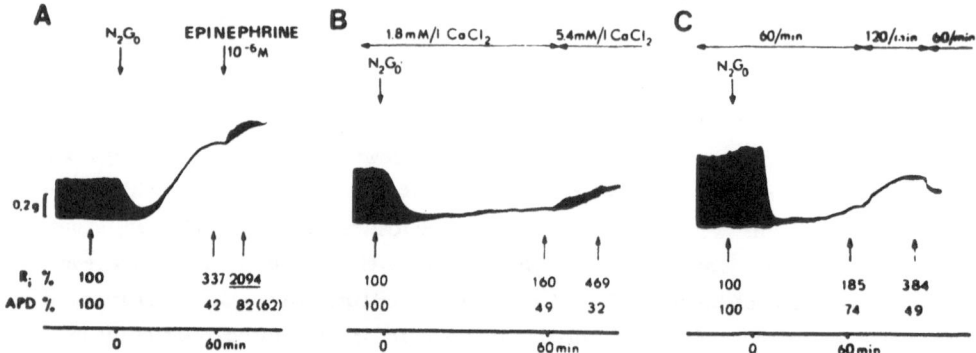

FIGURE 3 *A: Influence of epinephrine administered after 1 hour of hypoxia in glucose-free Tyrode's solution. Further explanations in the text. B: Influence of an increase in CaCl$_2$ concentration in the perfusion fluid after 1 hour of hypoxia in glucose-free Tyrode's solution. C: Effects of an increase in the frequency of stimulation after 1 hour of hypoxia in glucose-free solution. During control and the 1-hour hypoxic period, the muscle was stimulated at a rate of 60/min. The rate was subsequently increased to 120/min. The measurements of R$_i$ and APD were done immediately after restoration of the frequency of stimulation to 60/min. From Wojtczak (1979) with permission of the American Heart Association.*

EPINEPHRINE, EXTRACELLULAR CALCIUM AND STIMULATION RATE

During hypoxia it was found that epinephrine, elevated extracellular calcium or increased stimulation rate could further increase R$_i$ and the resting tension, the effects of epinephrine being especially pronounced (Fig. 3). The drug increased R$_i$ by a factor of 20; the action potential duration shortened by hypoxia was initially prolonged before decreasing to pre-epinephrine values.

The increase in R$_i$ was accompanied by a sudden decrease in conduction velocity. In some experiments a splitting of the action potential into a spike and a slow wave occurred prior to an irreversible block of conduction. As is shown in Fig. 4, the cell in which the recordings were made could still respond with a normal action potential when the mode of stimulation was changed from point stimulation at one end to longitudinal field stimulation. The reason for this behavior could lie in the fact that with point stimulation at one end the conducted action potential might not induce sufficient current to adequately depolarize a

LOCAL STIMULATION

5x10⁻⁶M **ADRENALINE**

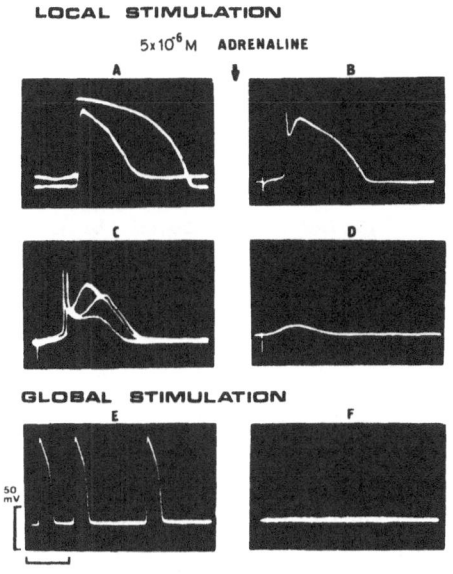

GLOBAL STIMULATION

FIGURE 4 Influence of high concentration of epinephrine (B-F) on the hypoxic transmembrane potentials. A: Two superimposed action potentials - control (C) and after 60 min of hypoxic, glucose-free perfusion (H). B: Addition of epinephrine induces prolongation of the action potential and a small hyperpolarization after 10 min of perfusion. C: Changes in the configuration of the action potential plateau after 15 min of perfusion. D: After 20 min the cell is inexcitable. The recordings in A-D were made in a trabecular muscle which was stimulated at one end by means of small, shielded bipolar electrodes. When the mode of stimulation was changed (large, extracellular electrodes at each end of the preparation), the cell could still respond with an action potential (E) and then after 5 min (F) it became irresponsive. Time mark corresponds to 200 ms for A-D and 1 s for E-F (Wojtczak, 1976, unpublished results).

decoupled cell. This would not be the case with field stimulation. However, it must be pointed out that failure of the action potential to propagate cannot be excluded.

CYCLIC AMP AND ARRHYTHMIAS

The epinephrine-induced electrical uncoupling reflected by the large increase in R_i could be important to explain the rhythm disturbance arising during myocardial infarction accompanied by high catecholamine release and by increased adrenergic drive. It is well documented that epinephrine by its action on beta-receptors can increase the intracellular level of cyclic adenosine monophosphate (cAMP). Recently Opie and coworkers (see Opie et al., 1979) have shown that the level of cAMP is increased in the myocardial tissue during ischaemia and this increase correlates with the onset of ventricular fibrillation. A direct link between these two events is still missing, but I would suggest that the deleterious effects of catecholamines on cell-to-cell coupling induced in energy-depleted cells might be of prime importance.

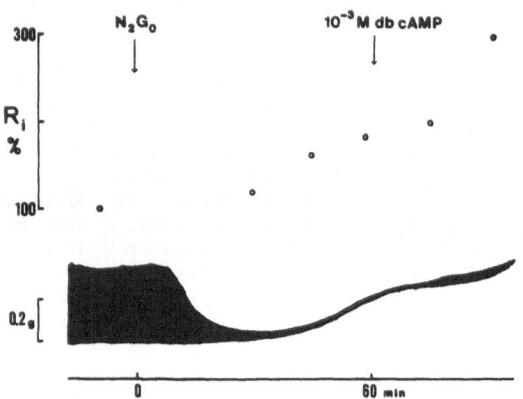

FIGURE 5 *Effects of the dibu-tyryl-cyclic adenosine mono-phosphate (DBcAMP) on the internal longitudinal resistance (R_i) and the force of contraction of cat trabecular muscle exposed to hypoxic, glucose-free (N_2G_0) perfusion (Wojtczak, 1979, unpublished results).*

As an additional argument, the effect of cAMP on electrical coupling in hypoxic muscle is shown in Fig. 5. DBcAMP applied after one hour of hypoxia increased the rate of rise of R_i, transiently increased the force of the twitches and increased the rate of rise of the contracture. These effects are in agreement with a deleterious arrhythmogenic action of intracellular cAMP accumulation.

The data shown above were obtained in hypoxic heart muscle. Since hypoxia is one of the components of ischaemia, cardiac ischaemia may be accompanied by intercellular uncoupling. As in hypoxic muscle, hearts rendered ischaemic develop contractures (McGregor et al., 1975). It would follow from the present experiments that under conditions of energy depletion regions in contracture should be looked upon as being partially uncoupled. Recently, Ashraf and Halverson (1978), in a freeze fracture study of ischaemic heart tissue, have found changes in gap junction morphology which could underlie the changes in electrical coupling.

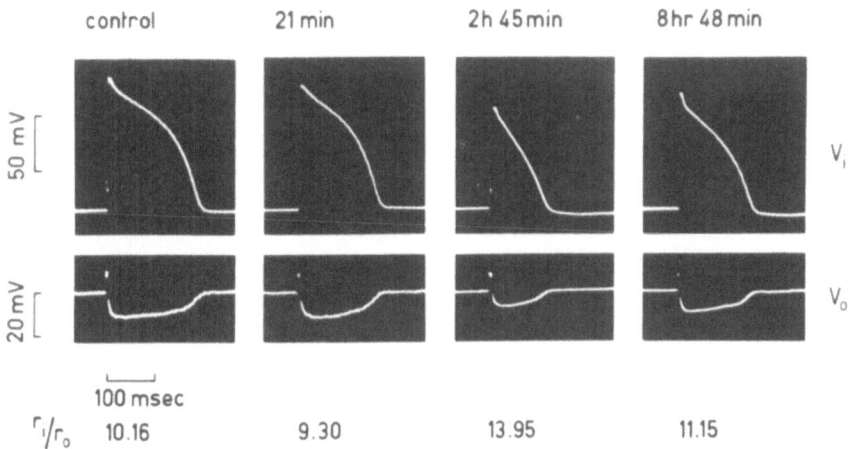

| control | 21 min | 2h 45min | 8hr 48min |

50 mV V_i

20 mV V_o

100 msec

r_i/r_o 10.16   9.30   13.95   11.15

FIGURE 6 *Reversible effects of ouabain on the action potential and the ratio of internal and external longitudinal resistance (r_i/r_o). Exposure to 10^{-6} M ouabain for a period of 2 hr 45 min resulted in a reversible shortening of the action potential duration by 43% and a reversible increase of r_i by 38% (Weingart, 1975, unpublished results, with permission).*

OUABAIN

The effects of ouabain on cell-to-cell coupling have been investigated by Weingart (1977), and Fig. 6 (Weingart, unpublished) shows the effects of exposure to ventricular muscle to 10^{-6} M ouabain for nearly three hours. This exposure resulted in a shortening of the action potential duration and a decrease in its amplitude. From the changes in V_i/V_o it could be calculated that R_i had increased by 38%. These changes were reversible, but exposure of the preparation to higher concentrations produced more marked changes which were irreversible. These changes are shown in Fig. 7 together with the time course of changes in slack length which mirrors the development of a contracture.

Fig. 8 shows that there is a correlation between the shortening of the slack length and a decrease of the conduction velocity. This decrease in the conduction velocity could be explained by the alterations in the maximal rate of rise of the action potential, the amplitude of the action potential, the membrane capacity and the sum, respectively, of the internal and external longitudinal resistance per unit distance ($r_i + r_o$). Weingart (1977) showed that about

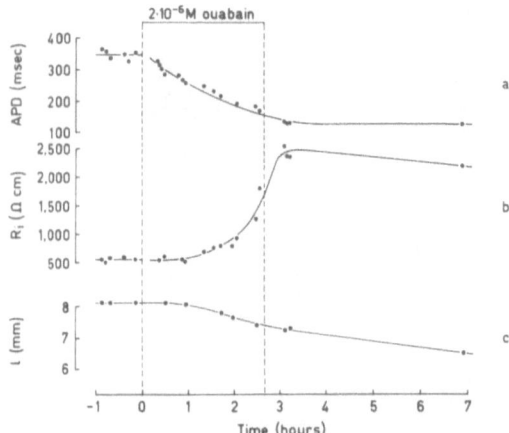

FIGURE 7 *Irreversible effects induced by a toxic ouabain concentration. A: exposure to 2 x 10⁻⁶ M ouabain for 2 hr 40 min led to a dramatic shortening of the action potential duration by 62%. B: large increase of R_i by 325%. C: shortening of the slack length. All three parameters were irreversibly affected. From Weingart (1977) with permission.*

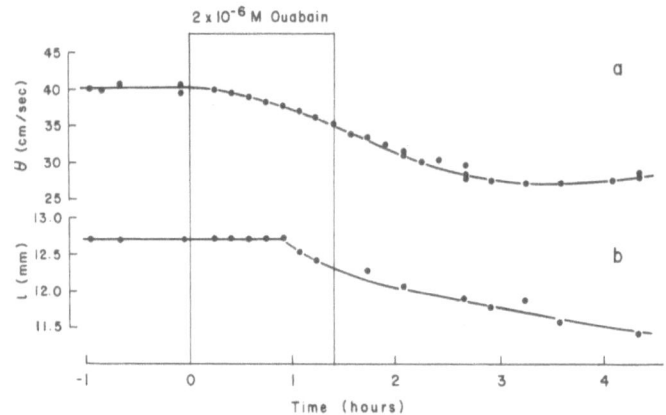

FIGURE 8 *A: time course of the action of ouabain on the conduction velocity, Θ. B: the preparation's slack length, l. The muscle bundle was exposed to 2 x 10⁻⁶ M ouabain for 85 min, as indicated by the horizontal line over A. This treatment resulted in a gradual decrease of Θ which started right after the application of the drug and a delayed shortening of the length of the preparation. From Weingart (1977) with permission.*

60% of the decrease of conduction velocity could be accounted for by the experimentally determined increase of R_i. He also showed that the increase of R_i induced by the toxic doses of ouabain is very much dependant on the extracellular
concentration of calcium (Fig. 9). The higher the extracellular calcium, the
shorter the ouabain exposure period necessary for the preparation to reach a
certain degree of uncoupling.

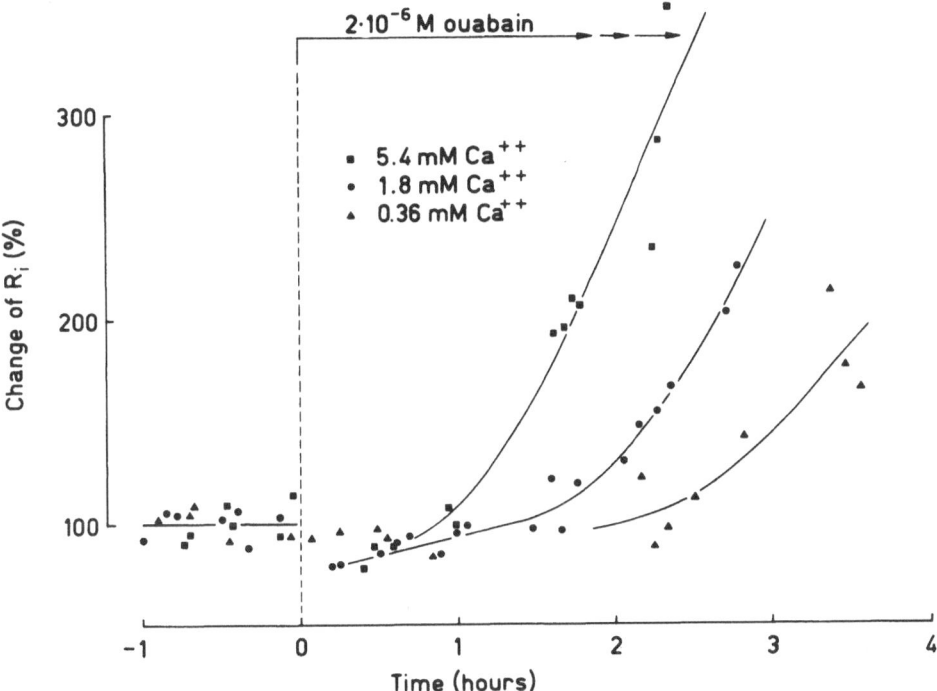

FIGURE 9 *Modification of the ouabain-induced decoupling by* $[Ca]_o$. *The normalized changes in R_i are plotted against time. The symbols represent single determinations from three different experiments which were carried out at control
$[Ca]_o$ of 1.8 mM (●), at 0.36 mM $[Ca]_o$ (▲), and at 5.4 mM $[Ca]_o$ (■). As a standard ouabain concentration, 2 x 10⁻⁶ M was administered. Time t = 0 hr marks
the beginning of the exposure to the drug, the horizontal arrows on top indicate
its end (the lower the $[Ca]_o$, the longer the ouabain exposure). After an initial decrease, which was absent in the experiment at 0.36 mM $[Ca]_o$, R_i progressively increased in a dose-dependent fashion. From Weingart (1977) with permission.*

UNCOUPLING Ca OR H (OR OTHERS)?

The data of Weingart (1977) strongly suggest that an increase in intracellular calcium is responsible for ouabain-induced uncoupling as the effects are potentiated by increased extracellular calcium. Furthermore, there is a rather close relationship between the time course of uncoupling and the development of a contracture. If we assume that a contracture is an adequate measure for calcium accumulation inside the cell, then the hypoxia-induced uncoupling may also be caused by an increased intracellular calcium concentration since alterations in the level of resting tension and R_i follow each other reasonably closely. This correlation was most marked during the potentiation of uncoupling and contractures induced by either epinephrine, DBcAMP, elevated extracellular calcium or increased rate of stimulation. The experiments of De Mello (1975), who injected Ca into Purkinje fibres, also support the idea of a Ca-mediated uncoupling.

Since a twitch can reach the same amplitude as a contracture associated with decoupling (see Fig. 3), the question arises if decoupling could occur during an action potential. This seems unlikely for as shown in Fig. 10 (an experiment by Weidmann, 1970), there is no change in the amplitude of the square wave applied during the action potential indicating a consistency of R_i.

This conclusion is supported by the results of Weingart (1977) and Wojtczak (1979), who found that increasing twitch tension (in contrast to contracture tension) did not alter R_i. The most likely explanation for this is that the increase in calcium during a twitch does not reach the region of the nexus.

Recently, it has been reported that intracellular hydrogen ions may play a role in the control of nexus conductance. Turing and Warner (1977) found that amphibian embryo cells would uncouple if the bathing fluid was gassed with 100 % CO_2. Moreover, Weingart and Reber (1979), by measuring intracellular pH with the microelectrode in cardiac Purkinje fibres, demonstrated that the changes in R_i closely follow the changes of intracellular pH. R_i is lowered during intracellular alkalinization and is increased during acidification. In a seperate study Hess and Weingart (1980), using Ca-sensitive microelectrodes, have found that the cellular alkalinization was accompanied by an increase of intracellular calcium. These recent findings would rather speak against calcium as being the only factor responsible for uncoupling. Furthermore, a direct effect of the lack of ATP on the nexal junctions cannot be excluded. However, if this were

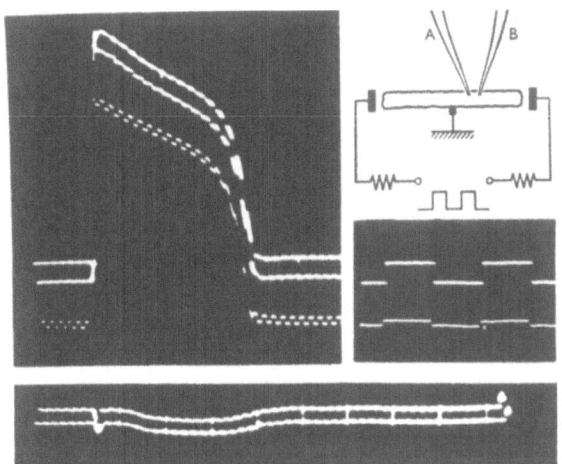

FIGURE 10 *Measurement of longitudinal resistance during the action potential. Diagram illustrates position of micro-electrodes. Lowest trace is a differential record between intracellular electrode A and intracellular electrode B, showing no appreciable change of square-wave amplitude (6 mV) throughout a cardiac cycle. The two upper records were taken simultaneously, and immediately after the differential trace. The action potential with the smaller superimposed square-wave was derived between A and earth, that with the larger square-wave between B and earth. The two traces (bundle at rest) are displayed again on the right, using a faster time base. Pulse frequency was 50/s throughout the experiment. Duration of action potentials: 340 ms. Amplitude of action potentials: 112 mV. From Weidmann (1970) with permission.*

so, then it has to be assumed that the nexus permeability is energy-dependent.

Other factors which would influence the junctional electrical resistance also have to be considered, e.g. cyclic nucleotides. I have found (Wojtczak, 1979; unpublished) that derivates of cAMP and cGMP have no effect on the internal longitudinal resistance of normal muscles, unlike the effects previously described for hypoxic muscle. Contrary results have been found by Hax and co-workers (1973), who showed that DBcAMP could lower intercellular resistance in insect glandular tissue. The effects appear then to be species-dependent or organ-dependent.

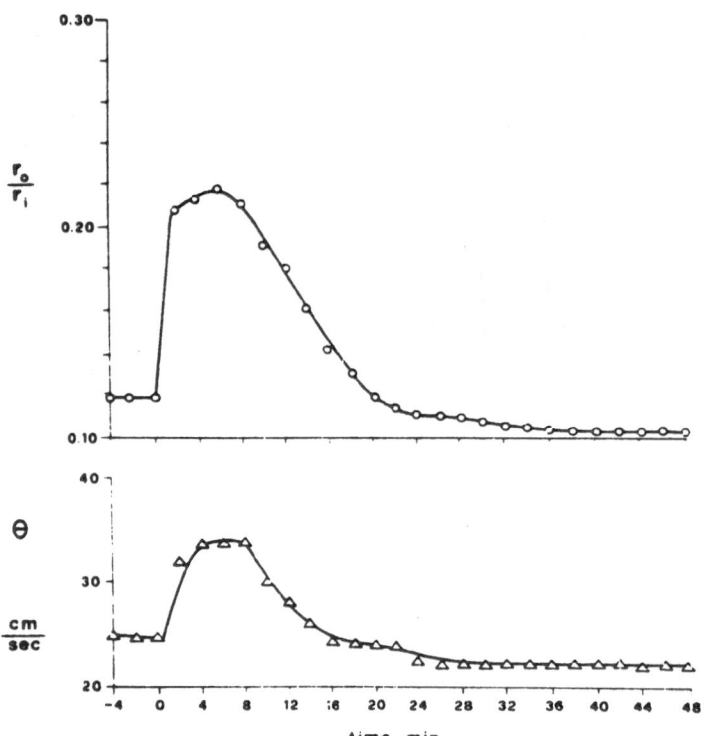

FIGURE 11 *Effect of an exposure to angiotensin II (30 nM). Conduction velocity (lower trace) increases in parallel to an increase of r_o/r_i (upper trace), the latter ratio representing a decrease of r_i. The peak effect occurs within 6-8 min followed by a decrease to below control values during the next 30 min. From Hermsmeyer (1980), with permission of the American Heart Association.*

ANGIOTENSIN II

Up to now I have described several factors which can lead to an increase in R_i but have not discussed any mediator capable of reducing R_i. While the increase in R_i induced by catecholamines during hypoxia can be prevented by propranolol or verapamil (Wojtczak, 1979; unpublished), they do not reverse the increase in R_i induced by hypoxia alone. However, angiotensin II has recently been shown by Hermsmeyer (1980) to be capable of reducing R_i in normal cardiac muscle. This decrease in R_i was accompanied by an increased conduction velocity as shown in Fig. 11.

In conclusion, it appears that the nexal permeability is controlled by numerous factors including calcium, hydrogen ions and polypeptides.

REFERENCES

Ashraf, M. and Halverson, C.: Ultrastructural modifications of nexuses (gap junctions) during early myocardial ischemia. J. Mol. Cell. Cardiol., 10: 263-269, 1978.

De Mello, W.C.: Effect of intracellular injection of calcium and strontium on cell communication in heart. J. Physiol. (London), 250: 231-245, 1975.

Hax, W., van Venrooij, G. and Vossenberg, J.: Cell communication: a cyclic-AMP mediated phenomenon. J. Memb. Biol., 19: 253-266, 1974.

Hermsmeyer, K.: Angiotensin II increases electrical coupling in mammalian ventricular myocardium. Circ. Res., 47: 524-529, 1980.

Hess, P. and Weingart, R.: Intracellular free calcium modified by pH_i in sheep cardiac Purkinje fibres. J. Physiol. (London), 307, 60P, 1980.

Lavallee, M. and Webb, J.L.: Mesure directe de l'acidose cellulaire sur le muscle cardiaque au cours de l'anoxie (abstr.). Memorias del IV Congreso Mundial de Cardiologia, Mexico, 5: 249, 1963.

MacGregor, D.C., Wilson, D.J., Tanaka, S., Holness, D.E., Lixfeld, W., Silver, M.D., Rubis, L.J., Goldstein, W. and Gunstensen, J.: Ischemic contracture of the left ventricle. J. Thor. Cardiovasc. Surg., 70: 945-954, 1975.

Meves, H. and Voelkner, K.G.: Die Wirkung von CO_2 auf das Ruhemembranpotential und die elektrischen Konstanten der quergestreiften Muskelfaser. Pfluegers Arch., 265: 457-476, 1959.

Nayler, W. and Seabra-Gomes, R.: Effect of methylprednisolone sodium succinate on hypoxic heart muscle. Cardiovasc. Res., 10: 349-358, 1976.

Opie, L.H., Nathan, D. and Lubbe, W.: Biochemical aspects of arrhythmogenesis and ventricular fibrillation. Amer. J. Cardiol., 143: 131-147, 1979.

Rovetto, M.J., Whitmer, J.T. and Neely, J.R.: Comparison of the effects of anoxia and whole heart ischemia on carbohydrate utilization in isolated working rat heart. Circ. Res., 32: 669-711, 1973.

Turin, L. and Warner, A.: Carbon dioxide abolishes ionic communication between cells of early amphibian embryo. Nature, 270: 56-57, 1977.

Weidmann, S.: The diffusion of radiopotassium across intercalated disks of mammalian cardiac muscle. J. Physiol. (London), 187: 323-342, 1970.

Weingart, R.: The actions of ouabain on intercellular coupling and conduction velocity in mammalian ventricular muscle. J. Physiol. (London), 264: 361-365, 1977.

Weingart, R. and Reber, W.: Influence of internal pH on r_i of Purkinje fibres from mammalian heart. Experientia, 35: 929, 1979.

Wojtczak, J.: Contractures and increase in internal longitudinal resistance of cow ventricular muscle induced by hypoxia. Circ. Res., 44: 88-95, 1979.

ECTOPIC ACTIVITY IN THE EARLY PHASE OF REGIONAL

MYOCARDIAL ISCHEMIA

Michiel J. Janse and Frans J.L. van Capelle

INTRODUCTION

The studies of Harris and coworkers some 40 years ago established the existence
of different phases of arrhythmias following occlusion of a coronary artery in
animal experiments (Harris and Rojas, 1943; Harris, 1950). Within minutes following coronary artery ligation, ventricular premature beats, ventricular tachycardia and ventricular fibrillation occur, the last arrhythmia being responsible
for the sudden death of the animals in Harris' experiments, and also accounting
for the great majority of sudden death in people with coronary artery disease
outside the hospital (Myerburg et al., 1980). This early phase of arrhythmias
lasts only for 10 to 30 minutes and is followed by a period that is relatively
free of arrhythmias. A late phase of ectopic activity ensues after 5 to 12
hours, during which ventricular premature beats and tachycardia dominate and
ventricular fibrillation occurs infrequently. This phase may last for several
days.

Thus, the malignant arrhythmias caused by ischemia occur very early after
cessation of blood flow to a part of the ventricles, and, as Harris observed:
"each fibrillation was initiated by a paroxysm of ventricular ectopic systoles
accelerating in frequency" (Harris, 1950). Harris indicated that the ectopic
discharges originated "at the boundary between the fully ischemic and normally
circulated area of muscle" (Harris, 1950). He also suggested that the injury
current flowing at that boundary could be a factor contributing to the occurrence of ectopic activity.

The present paper is limited to the ectopic activity occurring in the first
10 minutes after coronary artery occlusion. The changes in electrical activity,

as recorded with microelectrodes and DC extracellular electrodes, will be described. Secondly, mapping experiments, in which the sequence of activation was studied by recording DC extracellular potentials from 60 sites simultaneously in intact hearts, are discussed. By using DC recording methods, not only could the activation pattern during different arrythmias be analyzed, but also the strength of the injury currents in different phases of the cardiac cycle be estimated. From these experiments it emerged that both a "focal" mechanism and re-entry are responsible for the early ischemic arrythmias. The last part of this paper will be devoted to a discussion of the "focal" mechanism. Computer simulations will be described to illustrate various posibilities with which the findings in intact hearts can be explained.

METHODS

The methods are described in detail elsewhere (Janse et al., 1980). In essence, hearts of pigs and dogs were isolated and perfused according to the Langendorff technique with a mixture of modified Tyrode solution and blood. Regional ischemia was produced by placing a clamp on the left anterior descending coronary artery. DC extracellular electrograms were recorded simultaneously from 60 epicardial or intramural sites. The electrodes consisted in principle of cotton silk wicks soaked in isotonic saline. The saline was in contract with a chlorided silver wire, which was connected to a buffer amplifier with a high input impedance. A differential input DC amplifier measured the potential at each wick with respect to the DC potential of the aortic root. Different electrode arrangements were used: terminals were either spaced regularly on the epicardial surface within a rectangle at interterminal distances varying from 1.5 to 4 mm, or irregularly so that a large part of the heart was covered. After an initial 20-fold amplification, the signals were led into a high speed A/D converter (maximal sampling frequency 130 kc/s) and written into a circular buffer in the memory of a PDP 11-34 computer. In most instances samples were taken every 8 ms (sometimes every ms). During the experiment signals were monitored. When an event (spontaneous premature beats, ventricular fibrillation) occurred, a button could be pushed so that the signals of the preceding 2 seconds were transferred to a high speed digital tape recorder. Analysis of the data was performed using the same computer by means of an interactive program, where the signals were displayed on a megatek graphic display and moments of activation could be indicated using a joy stick. Zero potentials were obtained from control signals and DC-potential values could be obtained at any desired moment of the cardiac cycle.

Transmembrane potentials were recorded from the subepicardium using "floating" microelectrodes; as a reference a second floating microelectrode was used, located in the extracellular space as close as possible to the intracellular electrode. The recording of DC extracellular potentials, using an electrode with regularly spaced terminals, enabled us to construct isopotential maps. From such maps, the distribution of current sources (transmembrane current flowing out of the cells) and current sinks (transmembrane current flowing into cells) could be calculated. To determine the source or sink current at a particular site C, we used the potential values of the 8 surrounding sites.

$$
\begin{array}{ccc}
B1 & A1 & B2 \\
A2 & C & A3 \\
B3 & A4 & B4
\end{array}
$$

The source current:

$$
i = - \frac{4 \sum_{k=1}^{4} V(AK) + \sum_{k=1}^{4} V(BK) - 20\, V(c)}{6\rho L^{2}} \; A/m^{3}
$$

in which V is the DC potential at each site, ρ is the specific resistance of the tissue (we used a value of 400 Ohm cm), L is the distance between sampling points and 6 is a geometrical factor.

THE COMPUTER MODEL

We have developed a computer model (van Capelle and Durrer, 1980) which consists of an arbitrary number of excitable elements. The behaviour of the individual elements is determined by a set of functions and parameters which can be adjusted in order to bring about electrophysiological characteristics such as automaticity and duration of the refractory period. In this way a library of elements

with different electrophysiological properties was created, from which elements
could be extracted for use in subsequent multielement simulation studies.

For a simulation run, up to 650 elements can be connected in various ways.
Since different types of element may be present in the same simulation the interaction of different cell types may be studied. The geometrical arrangement
of the elements, together with the values of the coupling resistances between
the elements and the sizes of the individual elements (that is, their membrane
area), is specified interactively using a graphic screen and a joystick. A simulation may be interrupted at all times to change the configuration and it may
be restarted from an earlier point in time.

Since the differential equations controlling the behaviour of the elements
have to be solved for many elements simultaneously, we had to use a very primitive model for the underlying mechanism. Two voltage-current relations $i(V)$
describe the behaviour of the membrane. $i_0(V)$ has a region of negative chord
conductance and is therefore able to generate an action potential upstroke. The
other current, $i_1(V)$, is used to carry the membrane back to its resting potential. An excitability parameter Y, which assumes values between 0 (maximal excitability) and 1 (complete inexcitability) determines how much of each current
is switched on at a particular time. Y acts simply as a weighing factor and the
instantaneous voltage-current relation of the complete membrane is thus given by
$i(V) = Y\, i_1(V) + (1-Y)i_0(V)$. Y itself moves toward a steady state value
$Y_{inf}(V)$, an S shaped curve which corresponds with maximal excitability for values of V which are more negative than the resting potential and with inexcitability for positive values of V. The membrane is now characterized by the two
equations:

$$C\ dY/dt = -\ Yi_1(V) - (1-Y)i_0(V) + i_{ex}$$

$$T\ dY/dt = Y_{inf}(V) - Y$$

where C is the membrane capacitance, T the time constant of the
activation/inativation process and i_{ex} the current entering the element through
its connections with other elements.

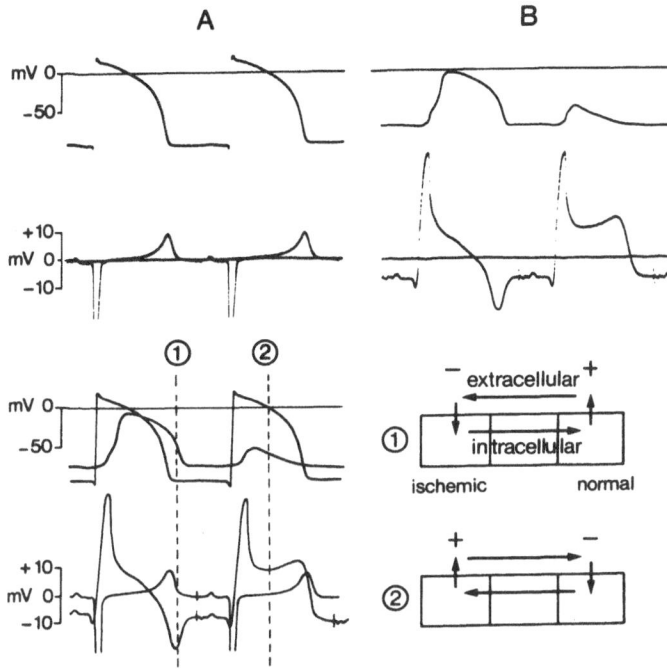

FIGURE 1 *A(left): transmembrane potentials (upper tracing) and local DC extra-cellular electrograms (lower tracings) before coronary occlusion. B(right) alternation in action potential amplitude and duration 5 minutes after coronary artery occlusion. Note that the smaller action potentials give rise to a large ST-elevation; negative T wave reflects long action potential duration, positive T wave a short duration. In diagram, normal and ischemic potentials are super-imposed and current flow between ischemic and normal cells is schematically dep-icted at moments one and two (dotted lines). (Reproduced with permission from J. Cinca, M.J. Janse, H. Morena, J. Candell, V. Valle and D. Durrer, Chest 77: 499-505, 1980).*

RESULTS

Fig. 1 shows transmembrane potentials and local DC extracellular electrograms from the subepicardium of the left ventricle of an isolated porcine heart before (A) and 5 minutes after occlusion of the left anterior descending coronary ar-tery (B). Zero lines in the transmembrane potential recording were obtained when both microelectrodes were in the extracellular space; zero potential in the extracellular recording is the DC potential of the aortic root. The characteristic changes caused by ischemia are: 1) a reduction in resting membrane potential, which in the extracellular signal is evident as a depression of the TQ-segment, 2) a reduction in amplitude and rate of rise of the action potential upstroke, resulting in delayed activation (late intrinsic deflection in the electrogram) and elevation of the ST-segment, 3) alternation in action potential amplitude and duration, leading to alternation in the ST-segment and the T wave. Such alternation progresses into 2:1 responses, until between 6 and 15 minutes after occlusion, the ischemic cells show absence of action potentials at resting membrane potentials of -60 to -65 mV (Kleber et al., 1978). The corresponding extracellular complex during this phase of unresponsiveness is completely monophasic.

Action potentials duration of ischemic cells shortens. However, when alternation or 2:1 responses develop, every second action potential lengthens, and, also because of the delayed activation of the ischemic cells, repolarization occurs later than it does in normally perfused cells. In the lower part of Fig. 1, the potentials before and after occlusion are superimposed, using P wave as time reference. Assuming that potentials recorded before occlusion are representative of those of non inschemic myocardium after occlusion, the flow of current between ischemic and normal myocardium in different phases of the cardiac cycle is schematically depicted in the diagram. At moment 1), when repolarization of the ischemic cells is delayed, the intracellular compartments on the ischemic side of the border are positive with respect to the intracellular compartments of the non ischemic side of the border. Consequently, a local current circuit is set up which gives rise to current sources on the non-ischemic side, and to current sinks at the ischemic side. The injury current flowing across the ischemic border during the negative T wave tends to depolarize the normal cells adjacent to the border, and we believe this current to exert an arrhythmogenic effect.

In our experiments, following abrupt occlusion of the left anterior descending coronary artery, ventricular premature beats occurred in 75%, ventricular tachycardia defined as a run of ectopic beats of 8 or more in 45%, and ventricular fibrillation in 32% of the occlusions, all within 2 to 8 minutes.

Fig. 2 shows three selected DC extracellular electrograms recorded 5 minutes after coronary occlusion from an isolated porcine heart. A is from normal

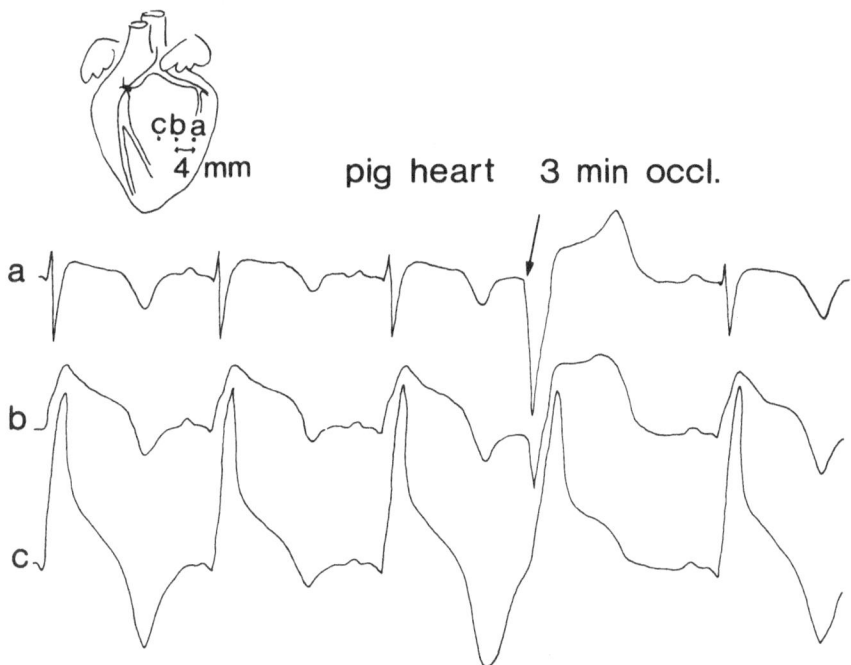

pig heart   3 min occl.

FIGURE 2 *Three DC extracellular electrograms recorded from subepicardial sites 4 mm apart in an isolated perfused porcine heart 3 minutes after occlusion of the left anterior descending coronary artery (see inset). Note alternation in T wave in c, monophasic complexes indicating local inexcitability in b, and early premature activity (arrow) in a which is close to the border between ischemic and normal tissue. (See text for discussion).*

myocardium close to the border (note the iso-electric-TQ- and ST-segments), b and c are from ischemic myocardium. The three signals were recorded from electrodes 4 mm apart. The complexes at b are nearly completely monophasic, indicating that the tissue at b is practically inexcitable. The signals at c show the characteristic alternation in T wave. Note that the premature intrinsic deflection at a is not preceded by an R wave, as it is during the beats propagated from the atrium (arrow). This figure contains several of the most characteristic features of ventricular premature beats in the acute phase of ischemia: 1) earliest activity occurs in the non-ischemic tissue close to the border with ischemic tissue, 2) just before the ectopic impulse, the central ischemic area

displays delayed repolarization as is evident from the pronounced negative T
wave, 3) a zone of inexcitability is interposed between the central ischemic
area still showing activity (usually alternating, or 2:1 responses) and the
non-ischemic myocardium.

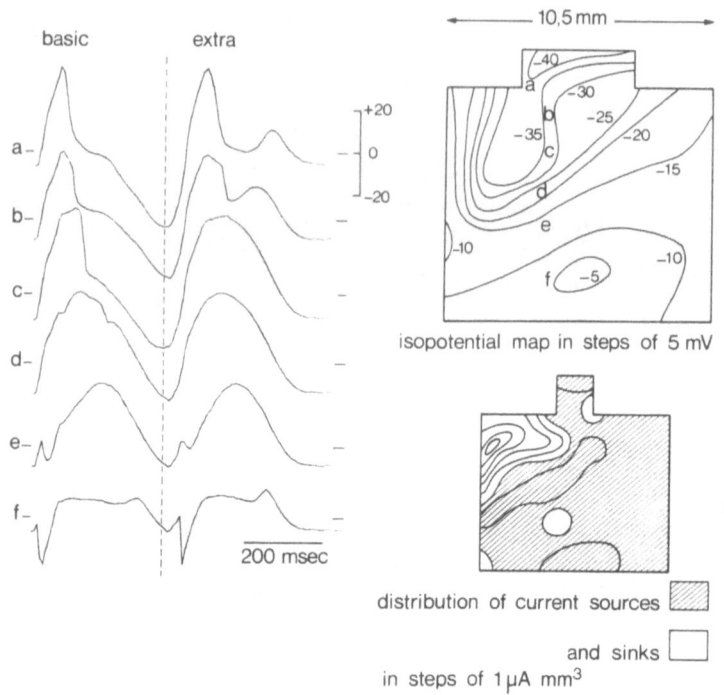

FIGURE 3 *Six selected DC electrograms recorded during a propagated beat from
the atrium (basic) and spontaneous ventricular premature beat (extra) 4 min
after coronary artery occlusion. Note negative T wave in a, b and c, inexcitability in d, and earliest premature activity in f. In right upper panel the
area of about 1 cm^2 is indicated from which 60 DC electrograms were simultaneously recorded at 1.5 mm intervals. The potential distribution in that area
during the moment indicated by the dotted line in the recordings is depicted by
isopotential lines. In the lower right panel, the distribution of current
sources and sinks at that moment is depicted (the area is now smaller since current source and sink values cannot be calculated for points at the edges of the
electrode grid).*

Fig. 3 shows 6 selected DC electrograms recorded from sites located 1.5 mm
apart. The multiple electrode covered an area of about 1 cm^2 and the terminals

were arranged regularly at 1.5 mm intervals within the space indicated in the right part of the figure. As in Fig. 2, the basic beat propagated from the atrium preceding the spontaneous premature beat (marked "extra") has a deep negative T wave (sites a, b, c and d). Site f, although still in the ischemic area, is closer to the border than the other sites, as is evident from the small degree of TQ segment depression and ST-segment elevation, and the early intrinsic deflection, in comparison with the complexes recorded from a to e. Site d is inexcitable since it shows a monophasic extracellular complex. The DC potential distribution in the extracellular space is shown at the moment indicated by the dotted line: over a distance of 7.5 mm, a gradients of circa 35 mV exists. In the lower panel, the distribution of current sources and sinks at that moment is indicated (the area is smaller since source and sink currents cannot be calculated for points at the edge of the grid). Current sources close to the border are in the order of 2 $\mu A/mm^3$. In other experiments we have determined the current sources in front of a wavefront propagating as a broad wave through normal myocardium, and found values in the order of 5 $\mu A/mm^3$ (Janse et al., 1980). In other words, the injury current flowing across the ischemic border just before the emergence of a spontaneous premature beat is about half as strong as the electrotonic currents associated with propagation of a broad wavefront through normal myocardium.

In Fig. 4, AC extracellular electrograms, recorded from intramural electrodes in a dog heart are shown at two different time scales. From top to bottom we see signals recorded from the normal subendocardium close to the ischemic border in which Purkinje activity can be seen (arrows), then signals from non-ischemic endocardium and epicardium showing only deflections caused by myocardial activity, and finally electrograms recorded from ischemic subepicardium. A spontaneous ventricular premature beat (1^e extra) initiates a bout of ventricular tachycardia (B) which finally degenerates into ventricular fibrillation (C). As can be seen from the signals in which the time scale is expanded, Purkinje activity precedes myocardial activity both during basic beats propagated from the atrium, and during the initial beats of the tachycardia. Only when at beats 71 and 72 of the arrhythmia ventricular fibrillation has developed, does the activity of the Purkinje cells occur clearly later than depolarization of adjacent myocardium. Note also that during the tachycardia the sequence of activation is from endocardium to epicardium and that activity of the ischemic su-

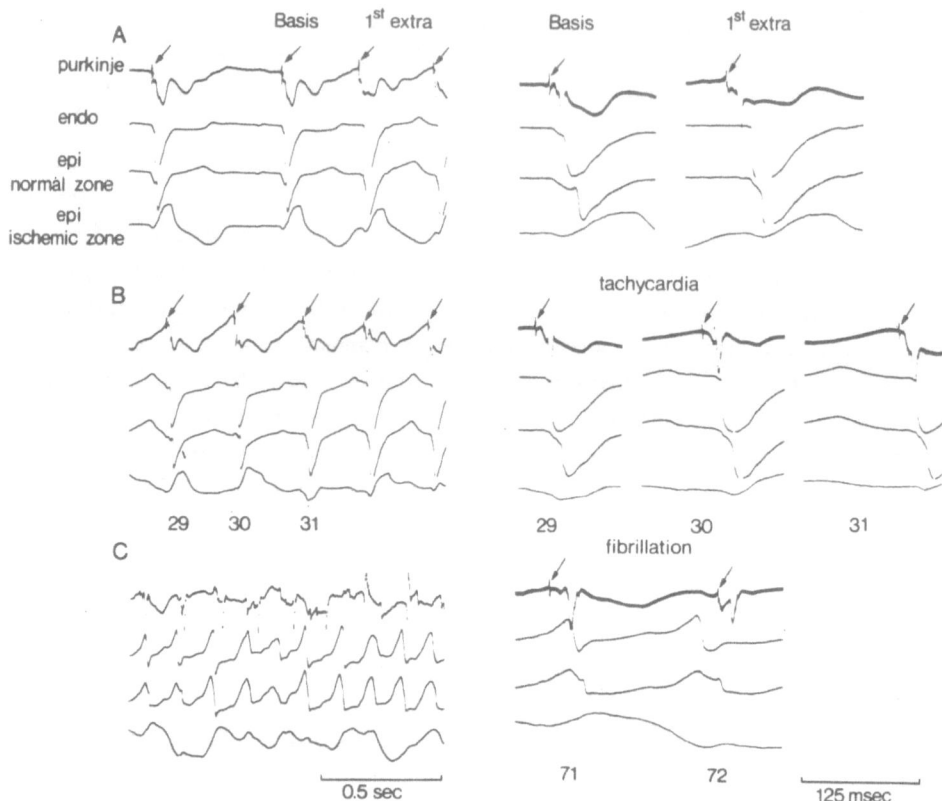

FIGURE 4 *Four AC recordings of extracellular potentials in an isolated canine heart at two different time scales. In A 2 basic beats propagated from the atrium are followed by 2 spontaneous premature beats ("extra") 5 min after coronary artery occlusion. These premature beats initiate a bout of ventricular tachycardia (B) which finally degenerates into ventricular fibrillation after the 71th ectopic impulse. In the top trace, recorded from the non-ischemic subendocardium close to the ischemic border, activity caused by depolarization of Purkinje fibers can be seen (arrows). In the 2nd and 3rd trace, myocardial activity from the non-ischemic subendocardium and subepicardium is recorded, and the lowest tracing was recorded from the ischemic subepicardium. Note that both during normally propagated, and ectopic beats during the tachycardia phase, Purkinje activity precedes myocardial activity.*

bepicardium occurs later than that in non ischemic subepicardium.

In Fig. 5, the sequence of activation during 2 ectopic beats, occurring after 4 minutes of regional ischemia, is depicted. An epicardial electrode was used in which the 60 terminals were spaced as indicated, and activity was recorded from both ischemic and non ischemic myocardium. Isochrones separate areas activated within the same 20 ms interval; time zero was arbitrarily chosen. Beat A was the third of ventricular tachycardia which eventually degenerated into ventricular fibrillation. Early activity, as during the first two ectopic impulses, occurred in the non ischemic part. The electrophysiological border, defined as the site where the TQ-segments of basic beats propagated from the atrium become negative (in other words, the zone where resting membrane potentials become depolarized) is indicated in B by the heavy dotted line. The ectopic activity invades the ischemic tissue but is blocked in the central area. Two wavefronts bypass this area of block and join on the left side of the area covered by the electrode. The wavefront ending at 120 ms in A retrogradely invades the area of unidirectional block and continues at 140 ms in beat B. Again two wavefronts circle around a central area of block. The lower is blocked at 240 ms, the upper wave continues till 300 ms. At that point the recording ended and we do not know how the arrhythmia continued. When somewhat later a new 2 seconds period of recording started, the heart was fibrillating.

In Fig. 6, the characteristic pattern of activation during ventricular fibrillation is shown. In contrast to the large circus movements present in the early phase of the arrhythmia, now multiple activation fronts are simultaneously present. Time zero was arbitrarily chosen. The wavefront in the upper part of the area under the electrode describes an S shaped pattern in the three successive "activations" shown. In the first panel a small circus movement is counter clockwise completed around a small area of block, the diameter being in the order of 5 mm. In the second panel, the wavefront curves to the left, and in the third panel a clockwise circusmovement is set up. However, complete circus movements during fibrillation are the exception rather than the rule. Usually, multiple wavelets follow tortuous paths along different islets of conduction block. Somêtimes wavefronts collide, somtimes they join and summate. Areas which at one moment show conduction block, can conduct the impulse the next moment. By and large the activation pattern bears a striking resemblance to that in the computer study of Moe about atrial fibrillation (Moe, 1962).

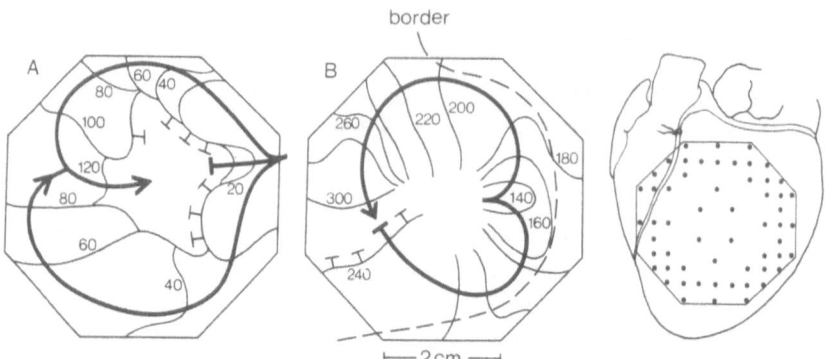

ventricular tachycardia

FIGURE 5 *Pattern of excitation during 2 beats of a spontaneous ventricular ta-chycardia, after 4 min of ischemia in an isolated porcine heart. In the right panel, the multiple electrode is shown, sutured onto the anterior surface of the ventricles. Each dot represents an electrode terminal. 60 DC electrograms were recorded simultaneously, and the pathways of excitation are shown by the two maps of the area covered by the electrode in which isochrones separate areas ac-tivated within the same 20 ms interval. Time zero was arbitrarily chosen. Thick lines with arrows indicate general direction of wavefront, transverse bars indicate conduction block. Dotted line in B indicates border between ischemic and normally perfused myocardium. Note that in A, earliest activity is found on the normal side of the border, and that 2 wavefronts bypass an area of unidirec-tional block, which in B is retrogradely invaded, resulting in re-entry.*

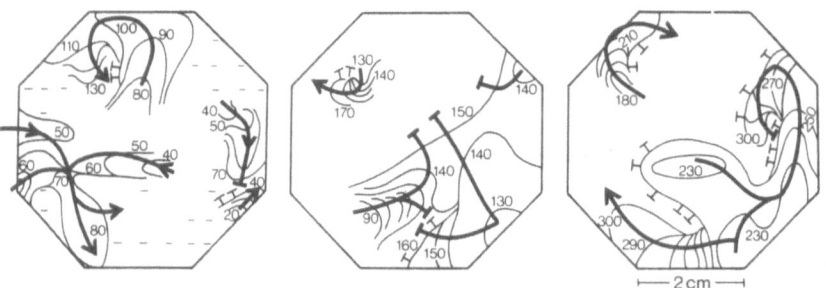

FIGURE 6 *Patterns of activation in three successive "beats" of the same ar-rhythmia shown in Fig. 5 at a later stage. Multiple wavefronts are present, and multiple re-entry can be observed. The wavefront in the upper part of the area covered by the electrode describes a S-shaped pathway in three successive "activations". This fragmentation into multiple re-entrant wavelets is charac-teristic for ventricular fibrillation.*

RE-ENTRY AND FOCUS

There is no doubt that re-entry occurs in the later phases of ventricular tachy-cardia and that single circus movements of fairly large dimensions, diameters being in the order of 1 to 2 cm, are responsible for the continuation of the ar-rhythmia. When the circulating wavefront finds in its front tissue with such a low level of excitability that the circle cannot be completed, the tachycardia ends and sinus rhythm is restored. When on the other hand, the single circus movement is fragmented into multiple wavelets, which can describe full circles of small diameter, but more frequently worm their way through many zones of tem-porarily inexcitable cells, the arrhythmia will not end spontaneously. For fi-brillation to occur, the ischemic tissue must of course have a reduced level of excitability, and must conduct the impulse slowly, but it must not be totally inexcitable. It is no coincidence that after some 10 to 15 minutes the majority of ischemic cells is completely inexcitable and fibrillation does not occur any more. Certain drugs, such as lidocaine, exaggerate and accelerate the reduction in action potential amplitude and upstroke characteristics of ischemic cells. Lidocaine is not able to prevent premature beats and ventricular tachycardia during ischemia, but it is able to prevent ventricular fibrillation, by shorten-ing the period during which multiple re-entry in the ischemic myocardium can occur.

The ectopic impulses which initiate re-entrant arrhythmias seem to have a "focal" origin. The experimental findings from intact hearts concerning the genesis of single or multiple premature beats in the setting of acute ischemia can be summarized as follows: 1) earliest activity was found in the normal tis-sue adjacent to the electrophysiological border zone, 2) no evidence was found for propagating activity bridging the gap between latest activity during the last beat conducted from the atrium and earliest ectopic activity, 3) whenever Purkinje activity was recorded, it preceded myocardial activity in ectopic beats, 4) very often the ectopic beats occurred just after a deep negative de-flection was recorded from the ischemic area. Current sources during this phase on the non-ischemic side of the border were half as strong as current sources in front of a wavefront propagating with a large margin of safety through normal myocardium.

Schematically, the anatomical situation can be described as follows: the normal subendocardium, containing strands of Purkinje fibres, is separated by a

zone of inexcitable ischemic tissue from the more centrally located ischemic myocardium showing, for example, 2:1 responses. Every second action potential in
the central ischemic area is long, and its moment of activation is delayed, so
that repolarization occurs later than in the normal Purkinje fibers on the other
side of the inexcitable border. Electrotonic current flowing through the inexcitable border zone tends to depolarize the normal Purkinje fibers, where,
indeed earliest ectopic activity is observed. Several mechanisms could be considered.

REFLECTION

The term reflection has been used to describe a form of reexcitation in a linear
bundle where two excitable ends are separated by an area of depressed conduction. In such a segment showing no gross branching or loops, reflection would
require the impulse to find a circuitous re-entrant pathway within the depressed
segment (Wit et al., 1972). In essence, it would be very much like the
re-entrant model first proposed by Schmitt and Erlanger in 1929. A second type
of reflection has been proposed by Cranefield et al. (1971) based on the notion that the cardiac action potential is composed of two components. The slow
component may propagate in the depressed segment in the absence of the fast component and initiate a fast response in the distal end, which could retrogradely
travel back over the same fibers which in the forward direction only conducted
the slow component. If either type of reflection would occur within the ischemic border, one would expect to find signs of local activity in the extracellular
signals, bridging the gap between proximal (normal tissue), delayed activity in
the distal end (central ischemic area) and premature activity in the proximal
part, and this we did never find.

A third type of reflection has been described in which the central segment
was depressed to such an extent as to become inexcitable, and was only capable
of transmitting purely passively electrotonic potentials (Antzelevitch et al.,
1980). In that study, the central segment was made inexcitable by a sucrose
gap, and transmission of electrotonic potentials was manipulated by varying the
shunt resistance between proximal and distal end. Such electrotonic potentials
influenced spontaneous phase 4 depolarization in the distal end: when subthreshold electrotonic depolarizations fell early in the spontaneous cycle, the emergence of the spontaneous action potentials was delayed, when it fell late in the

cycle, phase 4 depolarization was speeded up and the action potential occurred earlier then expected. By then, repolarization in the proximal end had occurred, and the action potential "captured" by electrotonic transmission through the gap gave rise to an electrotonic depolarization in the proximal end, which, if properly timed in the repolarization phase, could initiate an extrasystole. Although in all experiments, electrotonic deflections modulated spontaneous diastolic depolarization, it was stated that extrasystoles due to the reflection could occur in the absence of spontaneous impulse formation.

COMPUTER SIMULATION

In order to gain some insight in the mechanisms that may be involved in reflection, several computer simulations were performed. Since no differentiation between fast and slow currents can be made in our model, possibility 2 mentioned above was not considered. Re-entry over spatially distinct pathways can easily be evoked in the model and has been reported elsewhere (van Capelle and Durrer, 1980). Therefore we concentrate here on the third possibility; the occurrence of retrogradely conducted activity following antegradely transmitted electrotonic impulses when a high resistance gap is present.

It turned out that we could not simulate the phenomenon using non-automatic elements, but it could be done easily if some degree of overt of latent automaticity was present. In figure 7 the simplest case using non-automatic elements is depicted. Two elements are coupled through a high resistance connection. In panel A conduction through this high resistance gap fails, whereas it is just succesful in panel B. The action potential configuration in the latter case is not unfamiliar; we observed a "foot" in the distal action potential and a delay of the repolarization of the proximal one. The question now may be posed whether it would be possible to delay the distal action potential long enough to bring about a reexcitation of the proximal one instead of merely a delay of its repolarization. The answer is no, and the reason for it, on reflection, is clear. Using the electrical circuit shown in the inset we note that the time derivate of V_2 disappears during the top of the local response when conduction just fails. At that moment no current passes through the membrane capacitance C_2 and consequently V_1 and V_2 are related by $V_1/V_2 = R_c/(R_2 + R_c)$ at that time. Since R_c must be chosen high in order to delay the local reponse as much as possible, V_1 must be considerably larger than V_2, which is close to the threshold.

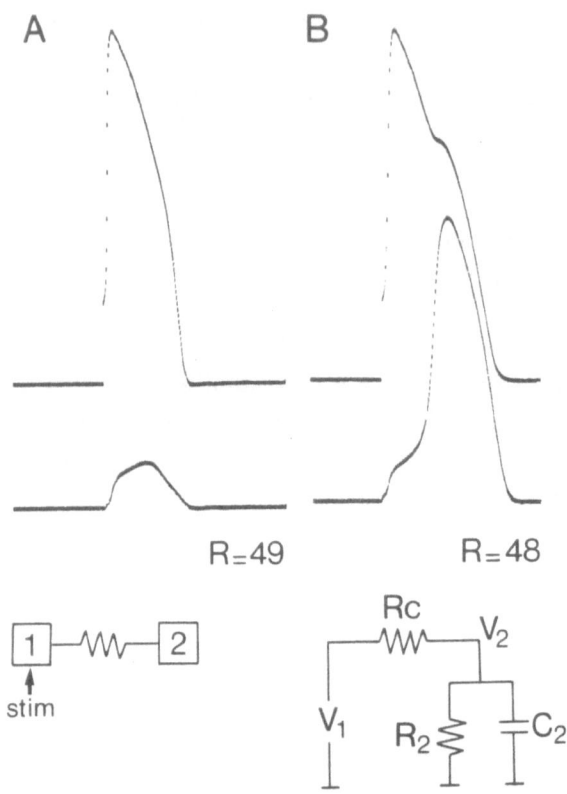

FIGURE 7 *Influence of marginally successful conduction on
the shape of the action potentials. Two non-automatic elements are coupled by a resistance. Element 1 (upper
trace) is stimulated. Panel
A: conduction block. Only a
local response is visible in
element 2. Panel B:
marginally successful conduction. The action potential of
element 2 shows a "foot" and
the action potential of element 1 is lengthened because
of the delayed activation of
element 2. Inset: equivalent
electrical circuit when the
potential of element 2 is
subthreshold.*

Therefore, if element 2 fires at all, it can only do so at an instant when V_1 is
still far above the threshold voltage, resulting merely in a delay of the repolarization of V_1. An additional mechanism to delay the activation of the distal
element thus seems to be necessary to evoke reflection. This we could realize
by the inclusion of a certain amount of automaticity at the distal end.
It has to be pointed out at this point that the automaticity of pacemaker elements in the model can be modified by variations in the amount of coupling
between these elements and non-automatic elements. An example is given in Fig.
8 where the action potentials of a non-pacemaker element (element 1) and a pacemaker element (element 2) are displayed for various values of the coupling resistance. If there is no coupling (panel A) element 1 is silent and the pacemaker fires at its intrinsic rate. When the coupling is sufficiently tight

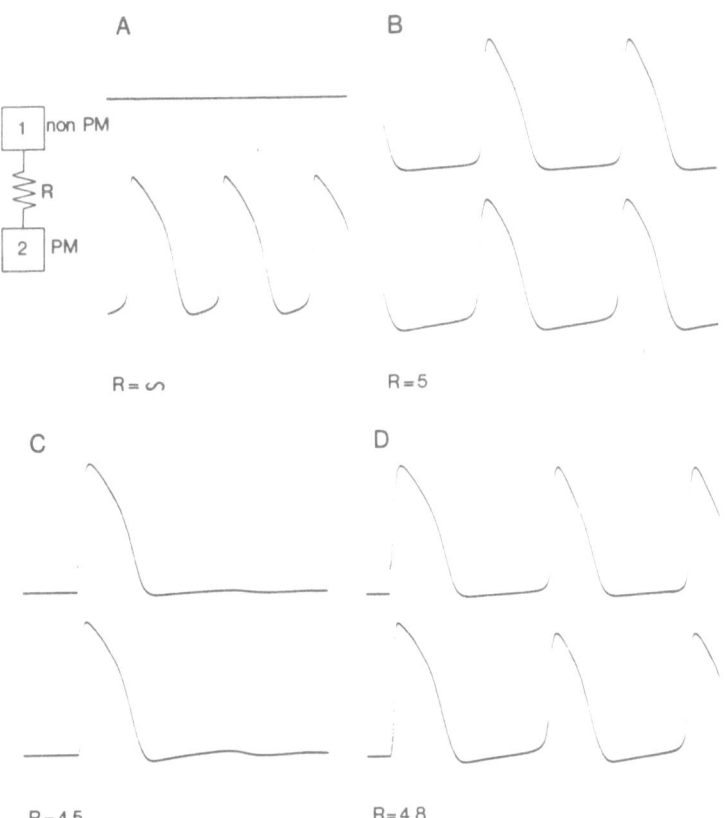

FIGURE 8 *Latent pacemaker activity. A non-pacemaker element (1) and a pacemaker (2) are coupled through a resistance R. Panel A: R is infinite, element 1 is silent and element 2 fires at its intrinsic rate. Panel 2: Tight coupling is present and the elements fire in unison. The frequency is much lower than in A. Panel C: At even tighter coupling the ensemble becomes silent. On stimulation both elements fire and subthreshold oscillatory activity follows the action potentials. Panel D. At critical values of the coupling resistance automaticity is turned on after stimulation of the previously silent ensemble.*

(panel B) the two elements fire practically in unison. In this case differences in shape between the action potentials disappear and it is hard to tell from the registrations which element is the pacemaker and which is the non automatic cell. The rate of diastolic depolarization is slower than that of the pacemaker cell firing on its own, resulting in a lower frequency of the ensemble. The reason for this is that the non-pacemaker element has a resting potential which is more negative than the pacemaker during all or the larger part of phase 4, and that it supplies a hyperpolarizing current to the pacemaker cell. If the coupling is made even tighter (and supposing the non pacemaker cell is large enough to supply the required current) this hyperpolarizing current can be large enough to prevent the pacemaker cell to reach its threshold, and the ensemble loses its overt-automaticity. It can however be stimulated, and in that case we observe a single activation which is followed by subthreshold after depolarizations (panel C). If the amount of coupling between both elements assumes a critical value, a conditionally stable system may result, in the sense that automatic impulse generation may be turned on by stimulus (panel D). Incidentally, it may also be turned off again when the stimulus is properly timed (not shown).

Returning now to the reflection problem, Fig. 9 depicts an example where the distal side of the gate was made automatic by the addition of a pacemaker element. The size of element 1, the proximal side of the gap, was somewhat reduced in order to obtain a unidirectional block across the gap, only retrograde activity being conducted succesfully. Activity originating in the ensemble consisting of elements 2 and 3, the distal end of the gap, is thus propagated to element 1. Upon stimulation of this element, it is seen that a local response occurs in 2, which brings the ensemble close to threshold and these elements fire after a short additional delay. This activity is in turn conducted back toward element 1, thus mimicking the experimental observations reported by Antzelevitch et al. (1980). A similar situation is illustrated in Fig. 10. In this case the pacemaker was coupled to a short cable consisting of three non pacemaker cells. The coupling of the pacemaker was so tight that it could not fire spontaneously. Again only a subthreshold response could be conducted antegradely over the gap on stimulation of element 1. This local response was of sufficient magnitude to trigger the pacemaker and retrograde propagation of the resulting action potential across the gap ensued. The present mechanism of reflection therefore also can work if no overt pacemaker activity is present: although latent pacemaker activity seems to be required in that case.

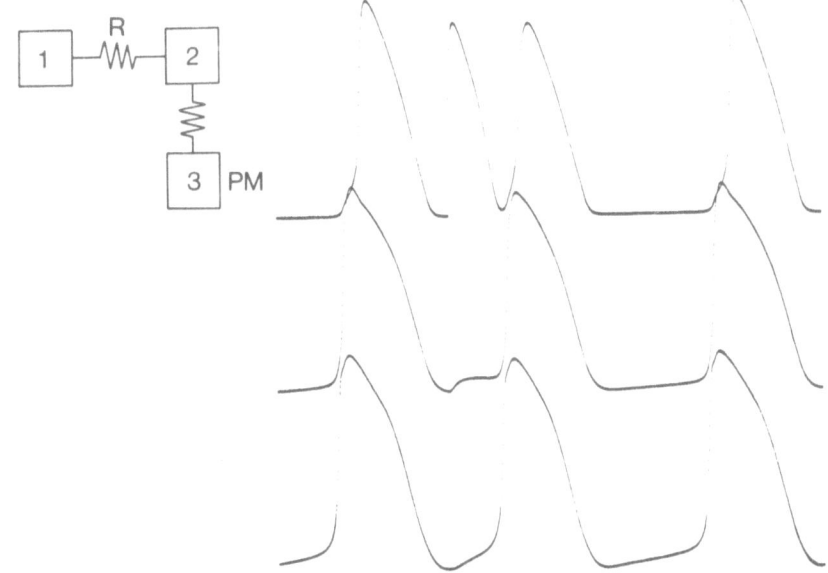

FIGURE 9 *Reflection in the presence of overt automaticity.   A high-resistance gap R separated a non-automatic element (1) and an automatic ensemble (2 and 3). Only unidirectional conduction (2 → 1) is possible through the gap.   Element 3 is a pacemaker. Activations originating in this element are conducted back to element 1. Stimulation of element 1 (upper trace, second action potential) results in a local response in 2 which precipitates the next pacemaker action potential.   This activation is conducted backward resulting in a closely coupled activation in element 1.   After that normal pacemaker activity resumes.*

AUTOMATICITY TRIGGERED BY INJURY CURRENTS

Since in our experiments the border zone seems to be completely inexcitable when extrasystoles originate from the normal side of the border, we were interested whether latent automaticity might play a similar role in case the conduction block through the gap was bidirectional. In the simulations pertaining to this case, the high-resistance gap used in the previous simulations was replaced by a gap consisting of an inexcitable element which was coupled through low resistance connections with both compartments. The inexcitable element is of a special kind, lacking the regenerative current $1_0(V)$ and having a resting potential zero. This completely depolarized element constitutes essentially a leakage pathway to the extracellular space through an RC filter. When coupled to excitable elements it tends to depolarize them, thereby inactivating their regenerative inward current.

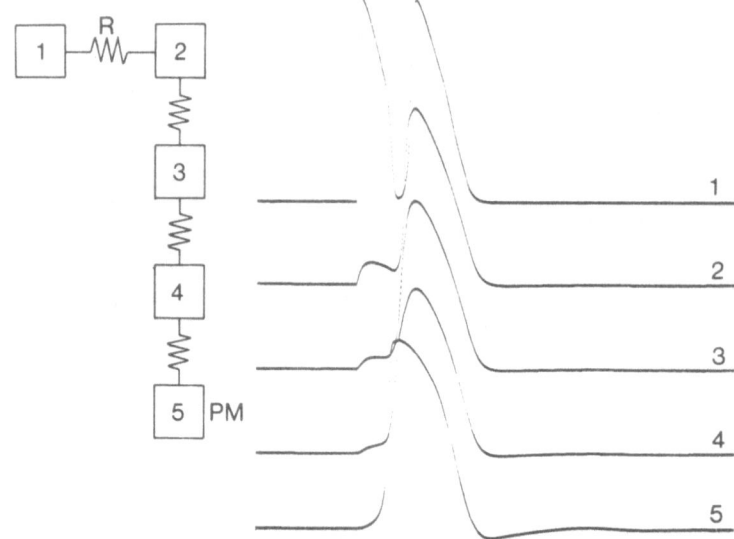

FIGURE 10 *Reflection in the presence of latent automaticity. The high-resistance gap R separates the non automatic element 1 from elements 2-5. 5 is a pacemaker element but its automaticity is suppressed by the non-pacemaker elements 2,3 and 4. Conduction through the gap is unidirectional. Upon stimulation of element 1 only a local response ensues at the other side of the gap. This local response triggers the pacemaker and the resulting activity is conducted back across the gap.*

Elements 2, 3 and 4 in Fig. 11 form a similar inexcitable gap, elements 1 and 3 being largely inactivated by the depolarized element 2. In addition, a long string of normal excitable non pacemaker elements connects both sides of the gap, ensuring that activity on either side of the gap can be conducted through this loop to the other side.

The conduction delay through the loop can be modified changing the coupling resistances in the loop. At one side of the gap a pacemaker element is added. This element does not fire spontaneously because of its tight coupling with two relatively large non-pacemakers, but it does show subthreshold oscillatory activity following activation. In panel A a stimulus is applied to element 1.

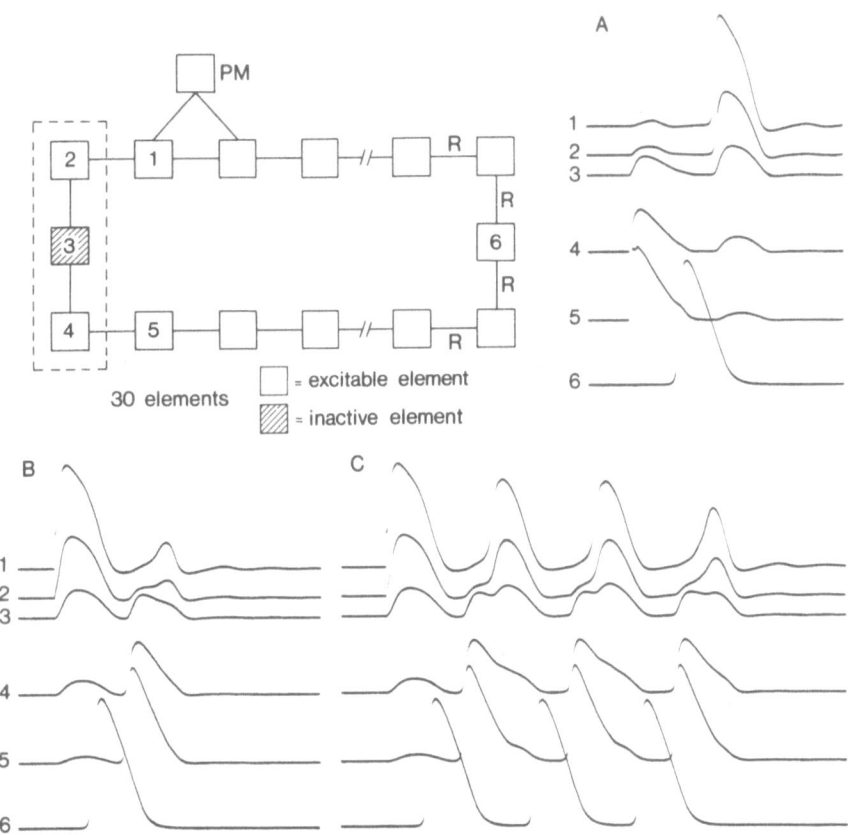

FIGURE 11 Enhancement of latent automaticity through a gap with bidirectional conduction block. Elements 2-4 form an inexcitable gap as described in the text. Both sides of the gap are also connected by a long string of excitable non-automatic elements. The conduction delay through this loop can be modulated by variations of the coupling resistance R of the elements in the loop. Latent automaticity is present at one side of the gap as a result of the addition of a pacemaker element (PM). Panel A: element 5 is stimulated. No propagation of activity occurs through the gap, only local responses being visible in elements 1 and 2. The activity is conducted through the loop however (element 6) and reaches element 1. It is blocked in the gap, and subthreshold afterpotentials appear in element 1. Panel B: Stimulation of element 1. Conduction through the gap fails, but element 5 is reached through the loop. The local response at the other side of the gap enhances the afterdepolarization in element 1. Panel C: Same as panel B, with a slightly larger conduction delay in the loop. The afterdepolarization in element 1 now reaches threshold, and a short run of extrasystoles results.

There is no conduction over the gap, only a local response being visible in element 5, but somewhat later the opposite side of the gap is activated through the loop. Note the subthreshold oscillations in element 5. In panel B the stimulus is applied to element 5. Again conduction fails to cross the gap and again the opposite side is activated later by the wavefront which travels through the loop. This wavefront is blocked in the gap, but this time the local response ensuing in element 4-5 can be in a position to magnify subthreshold depolarizations which are present in those elements at the same time. In panel B this did not result in activation of the elements, but when the conduction velocity of the loop was depressed a bit single or multiple (panel C) extrasystoles could be evoked.

We realize quite well that computer simulations offer no proof regarding mechanisms occurring in intact hearts. Yet, they do point to possibilities which would be very difficult to find in intact hearts. A major point raised by the computer simulations is that automaticity may be latent, and therefore not apparent by phase 4 depolarization in normally conducted beats of even after a short period of asystole. Automaticity may only become manifest by a properly timed subthreshold depolarization. The "current of injury" may well provide such a trigger. Whether there are other factors associated with acute ischemia which promote automaticity in Purkinje fibers close to ischemic myocardium is difficult to say. One may speculate that stretch, caused by systolic bulging of the ischemic myocardium, can induce automaticity (Kaufmann and Theophile, 1967); catecholamine release might also contribute. On the other hand, the extracellular K^+ concentration on the normal side of the border, which in our experiments was 4,5 mM, might counteract the induction of automaticity. Since the ischemic border is large, and the area where latent automaticity may be present and could be triggered into repetitive focal activity could be very small, it seems a hopeless undertaking to prove the reality of the mechanism depicted in Fig. 11.

That other effects, such as shown in Fig. 7, could occur at the ischemic border seems more than plausible, and these could also contribute to the occurrence of arrhythmias. In certain areas where the impulse is conducted with difficulty into the ischemic zone, proximal action potentials (i.e. in non ischemic tissue) will be long, in other areas where conduction fails they will be short. Such dispersion in refractory periods will obviously facilitate the occurrence of re-entry in and around the border zone.

REFERENCES

Antzelevitch, C., Jalife, J. and Moe, G.K.: Reflection as a mechanism of re-entrant arrhythmias and its relationship to parasystole. Circulation, 61: 182-191, 1980.

Capelle, F.J.L. van, and Durrer, D.: Computer simulation of arrhythmias in a network of coupled excitable cells. Circ. Res., 47: 454-466, 1980.

Cranefield, P.F., Klein, H.O. and Hoffman, B.F.: Conduction of the cardiac impulse. I. Delay, block and one-way block in depressed Purkinje fibers. Circ. Res., 28: 199-219, 1971.

Harris, A.S.: Delayed development of ventricular ectopic rhythms following experimental coronary occlusion. Circulation, 1: 1318-1328, 1950.

Harris, A.S. and Rojas, A.G.: The initiation of ventricular fibrillation due to coronary occlusion. Exp. Med. and Surg., 1: 105, 1943.

Janse, M.J., van Capelle, F.J.L., Morsink, H., Kleber, A.G., Wilms-Schopman, F., Cardinal R., Naumann d'Alnoncourt, C. and Durrer, D.: Flow of "injury" current and patterns of excitation during early ventricular arrhythmias in acute regional myocardial ischemia in isolated porcine and canine hearts. Evidence for 2 different arrhythmogenic mechanisms. Circ. Res., 47: 151-165, 1980.

Kaufman, R. and Theophile, U.: Automatie-foerdernde Dehnungseffekte an Purkinje Faeden, Papillarmuskeln und Vorhoftrabekeln von Rhesus-Affen. Pluegers Arch., 297: 174-189, 1967.

Kleber, A.G., Janse, M.J., van Capelle, F.J.L. and Durrer, D.: Mechanisms and time course of S-T and T-Q segment changes during acute regional myocardial ischemia in the pig heart determined by extracellular and intracellular recordings. Circ. Res., 42: 603-613, 1978.

Moe, G.K.: On multiple wavelet hypothesis of atrial fibrillation. Arch. Int. Pharmacodyn Ther., 140: 183-188, 1962.

Myerburg, R.J., Conde, C.A., Sung, R.J., Mayorga-Cortes, A., Mallon, S.M., Sheps, D.A., Appel, R.A. and Castellanos, A.: Clinical, electrophysiologic and hemodynamic profile of patients resuscitated from prehospital cardiac arrest. Am. J. Med., 68: 568-576, 1980.

Schmitt, F.O. and Erlanger, J.: Directional differences in the conduction of the impulse through heart muscle and their possible relation to extrasystolic and fibrillary contractions. Am. J. Physiol., 87: 326-347, 1928/29.

Wit, A.L., Hoffman, B.F. and Cranefield, P.F.: Slow conduction and re-entry in the ventricular conducting system. I. Return extrasystole in canine Purkinje fibers. Circ. Res., 30: 1-10, 1972.

SECTION THREE

ESTABLISHMENT OF CARDIAC RHYTHM

IN VITRO MODELS OF ENTRAINMENT OF CARDIAC CELLS

Robert L. DeHaan [*]

INTRODUCTION: THE PACEMAKER CONCEPT

In science, our concepts of reality are dependent largely on the material upon which we perform experiments. The ways in which we "explain" the physical and biological universe around us, our conceptual models, are derived from our experimental models. However, the converse is also true. We are often led to discover new or better experimental models by the need to test a novel hypothesis. Thus, science progresses apace with our ability to develop models, both experimental and conceptual. The history of the biological sciences is replete with examples.

As we try to show in the following sections, the evolution of our ideas of how the heart generates its steady rhythm is no exception to the generalization that hypothesis and experiment interact. Before the turn of the present century, when neuromuscular interactions were first recognized the heart was supposed to be driven by neural elements leading to, or embedded within the cardiac muscle. Later, when the property of automaticity was described in the sino-auricular tissues at the venous end of the heart, the ventricle was thought to be driven by the sinus region. At a third conceptual stage, with better methods for maintaining heart tissue in vitro and more information about the conditions required, it was demonstrated that all parts of the organ were capable of exhibiting spontaneous rhythmic contractions under different specified conditions and with different intrinsic beat rates. The idea of the driving function of the sinus was then altered from a triggering mechanism to a

[*] This article was largely written in the Laboratoire de Physiologie comparee, Universite de Paris-Sud, Orsay, France through the hospitality of Prof. Edouard Coraboeuf.

pace-setter. The sinus was supposed to coordinate the disparate intrinsic rhythms of the various parts of the heart to its own (highest) rate. This is the pacemaker concept as it is generally found (implicitly or explicitly) in modern textbooks of physiology and cardiology. To this point, the pacemaker concept was unidirectional. A pacemaker region was supposed to drive or pace other parts of the heart at its intrinsic rate, but was not itself affected in the process. Within the past few decades, however, further improvements have been made in experimental techniques for isolating and maintaining heart cells and tissue in more nearly optimal conditions in vitro, for reassembling cells into tissue-like configurations, and for recording the various parameters of their electrical activity both in vivo and in vitro. Furthermore conceptual models derived from electric circuit theory and the equations for coupled oscillators have been applied with increasing succes to cardiac function. The result that has begun to emerge gives a new twist to the pacemaker concept. As has been noted by some of the contributors to this volume (Scott, 1979; Winfree, 1980; Ypey et al., 1980), pacemaker function may not be unidirectional, but is more probably interactive. A pacemaker region does not alone determine the pulsation rate of the tissue with which it is in contact; it is itself modified by interaction with that issue. It is mainly this evolution of the pacemaker concept from unidirectional to interactive, as new and hopefully more informative experimental models of cardiac tissue have become available, that I would like to explore in this article.

HISTORY OF THE PACEMAKER IDEA: THE ADULT HEART AS THE MODEL

Although Aristotle and many of the ancients had observed the spontaneous beating of animal hearts, perhaps the first in vitro model of cardiac tissue was prepared some 350 years ago by William Harvey (1628) when he cut the heart out of a pigeon. Keeping the organ moist in a drop of saliva in the palm of his hand, he noted that it continued beating without external stimulus. Moreover, when he cut the heart into several pieces with a sharp blade, he reported that after a brief pause, each piece resumed beating independently. Harvey was obviously struck by the spontaneous rhythmicity of these fragments of cardiac muscle. He noted that pieces of atrium had higher inherent rates than did fragments of ventricular muscle. But he made no mention of the question of how the independent rhythms of these pieces had been coordinated in the intact organ. Nor does he wonder in his writings whether the fastest beating piece might have been driving the slower regions. That idea, the pacemaker concept, had to wait for its formulation nearly 300 years, till shortly before the turn of the present century.

The idea that the region of heart tissue with the most rapid intrinsic rhythm sets the pace for, or drives, other portions of the heart arose primarily from three kinds of experiments, employing physical isolation techniques, electrical recording and methods for modifying the beat rate. For an informative discussion of this early literature, and the instrumentation employed, see Lewis (1920). Eyster and Meek also traced the evidence in support of the pacemaker concept in an extensive review (1921).

In the frog heart at low temperature, the progression of the wave of contraction from the sinus to atria to ventricle is readily seen. When Stannius (1852) applied a tight ligature between the sinus and atria, the sinus continued to beat rapidly whereas the atria and ventricle slowed their rate of beating or stopped altogether in diastole. Stannius misinterpreted these results in terms of the prevailing neurogenic model of the origin of the heart beat. However, similar experiments were reported some years later by Bowditch (1871, 1879), by Bernstein (1876) and Gaskell (1880) in their analyses of the role of pressure and nutritional factors in controlling spontaneous activity of the heart. By this time these authors already understood that the beat of the ventricular apex depended upon its connection with "the motor apparatus at the base of the heart" (Bowditch, 1879, p. 107). However, according to Gaskell (1882) all parts of the heart have automaticity, but in different degrees, "this property being most developed at the venous end and least within the ventricles". Erlanger and Blackmann (1907) refined the Stannius approach by cutting the conduction pathways between SA node, the AV node and the His bundle branches, and showed that three independent rhythms were established in rabbit and other mammalian hearts. In most cases, the atria continues to exhibit the most rapid rhythm, the tissue surrounding the AV node took on an intermediate rate, and the ventricles slowed dramatically. These results lent substantial support to the pacemaker hypothesis by suggesting that the sinus region normally drives the slower tissues of the heart at its own frequency, overdriving the local intrinsic rates. This interpretation was further strengthened by electrophysiological data that were beginning to appear at that time.

Koelliker and Mueller (1855) first demonstrated the existence of an electrical change in a beating heart. By observing the twitch of a frog nerve-muscle preparation laid in contact with the heart they demonstrated two distinct electrical discharges with each beat of the ventricle. Following the lead of Du Bois-Reymond (1848) who demonstrated "injury currents" in muscle using a primitive induction device, Engelman (1877) applied a Kelvin type of galvanometer and "rheotome" to investigate the time relations of the electrical wave in the heart. Engelmann (1877) and Sanderson and Page (1880) who worked with capillary electrometers, concluded that excitation in the frog heart arose with each beat near the base of the ventricle and progressed as a wave to the apex. Similar results were obtained by Bayliss and Starling (1892) in the mammalian heart. After Einthoven invented the sensitive string galvanometer (1903) he was able to show on even the earliest electrocardiograms (Einthoven, 1908) that the P wave, associated with the auricular contraction, preceded by some time the ventricular component. In 1906 Keith and Flack discovered the sinoatrial node and described its special histological characteristics. Shortly thereafter Wybauw (1910) and Lewis et al. (1910) were able to record directly from the cardiac surface the earliest point of electrical activity arising in the SA node. They followed the "wave of negativity" as it swept out across the atria to the AV node and ventricles, thus confirming the nodal pacemaker function.

These observations of the normal sequence of events in the cardiac cycle were supplemented with experimental manipulations that demonstrated convincingly that the SA node was the site of origin of the cardiac activation. Engelmann had already shown that when the frog sinus was warmed the entire heart increased in beat rate, whereas a similar effect was not obtained by locally heating the ventricle alone. This approach was later employed with great delicacy by Ganter and Zahn (1912) on the mammalian heart. In cats, goats, dogs and apes they showed that cooling the node itself produced slowing, while warming resulted in acceleration of the whole heart. However, the further their thermal probe was placed from the head of the node, the smaller were the effects. Finally, when Lewis (1910) compared the shape of his galvanometric curves produced by spontaneous heart beats with those from beats generated by artificially stimulating different points on the atria, he showed convincingly that the auricular complex of stimulated contraction resembled that of a spontaneous beat only if the stimulating surface electrode was placed over the SA node. On the basis of these investigations, Lewis and his colleagues (Lewis et al., 1910; Lewis, 1910) were apparently the first to apply the phrase "the pacemaker of the heart" to the SA node.

DIFFERENTIATION OF PACEMAKER FUNCTION:
THE EMBRYONIC HEART AS THE MODEL

The vertebrate heart begins beating at a very primitive stage in embryonic development when only the conoventricular portion of the cardiac tube has differentiated (Johnstone, 1925; Davis, 1927; Patten and Kramer, 1933; DeHaan and O'Rahilly, 1978 for review). The more posterior portions of the heart are each added in turn as development progresses. As each new region forms it brings to the organ tissues with different physiological properties. The action potential recorded from cells in the early ventricle, atria and sinoatrial tissues differ in ways that anticipate the definitive differences of the adult organ (Meda and Ferroni, 1959; for review see DeHaan, 1980). Each new region is also different in its intrinsic rate of contraction. In the chick heart for example, the beat starts at about 36 hrs of incubation in the right caudal margin of the newly fused primitive ventricular tube. The first beats are weak and irregular but the heart soon develops a rhythmic slow rate of 30-40 beats/minute. Over the next few hours, as more caudal portions of the heart tube differentiate the heart rate increases. By the time dextral looping of the ventricle is accomplished (at stage 11-12) the spontaneous rhythm is 80-90 beats/minute. By about 60 hrs of incubation, when the sinoatrial tissue has differentiated the heart normally beats 110-120 times/minute.

This sequence of events was only vaguely understood by workers in the 19th century, but Gaskell (1882) associated the differences in "rhythmic power" in different region of the adult heart with the degree to which they retained embryonic characteristics, an idea which underlies much comtemporary thinking about excitable-cell physiology (for discussion, see DeHaan, 1980). Moreover, at about the same time that the dominance of the sinus was being demonstrated in the frog heart by ligature isolation experiments, the embryologist Pickering (1893) showed that the conoventricular region of tubular chick embryo heart would slow its spontaneous beat rate when severed from the sinoatrial tissue. This result has since been confirmed by numerous workers (Johnstone, 1924; Lewis, 1924; Patten and Kramer, 1933; Barry, 1942). That is, if the heart tube is cut transversely into three fragments at a stage when its rate is 120 beats/minute, the sinoatrial piece maintains a fast rhythm, but each of the more rostral pieces slows down: the ventricle to about 70 beats/minute and the cono-ventricular segment to 30-40 beats/minute (Barry, 1942; DeHaan, 1963). Further support for the pacemaker role of the sino-atrial tissue was provided by Paff (1936) who transplanted fragments of sino-atrium into the atrial walls of other embryos and found that an ectopic focus always developed, with the transplant controlling the surrounding region of myocardium.

The observed differences in spontaneous beat rate appeared to reside ulti-mately in the cells that comprise each segment of the heart. Single cells iso-lated in tissue culture from embryonic ventricle beat more slowly on average that those from the atria (Cavanaugh, 1955; Norwood et al., 1980). Moreover, ventricle cells re-aggregated into spheroidal clusters beat more slowly than did similar aggregates prepared from atrial tissue (Sachs and DeHaan, 1973).

Further evidence that the local rate is an intrinsic property (though modi-fied by regional differences in tissue chemistry, geometry, and - at later stages - by innervation) came from observations showing that different rhythms are coded into the cells of the embryo well before the heart itself forms. At stage 5-6, before the heart differentiates, the embryo can be cut into fragments containing either the anterior, middle, or posterior portion of the cardiogenic crescent, the regions destined to form, respectively, the conoventricular, atri-oventricular, and sinoatrial parts of the heart. Such fragments maintained in vitro continued their normal development to form vesicles of rhythmically contractile heart tissue, with beat rates that averaged 35 beats/minute for the rostral fragments to 115 beats/minute for vesicles of prospective sinoatrial tissue (DeHaan, 1963). When these vesicles were impaled with microelectrodes, the slowly-beating tissue showed action potentials typical of conus, the vesi-cles with intermediate rates had ventricle-like action potentials, and the fastest fragments exhibited pacemaker potentials characteristic of sinoatrial tissue (Le Douarin et al., 1966).

The gradual increase in its spontaneous beat rate as the heart develops, when viewed in the light of the pacemaker concept as it was emerging in the physiological literature, suggested to early workers that as each new portion of the heart differentiated, with a higher intrinsic rate, it would act as pacemaker for the rest of the organ. Thus one would expect to see, during cardiac embryogenesis, a sequence of pacemaker regions progressing more and more caudally as the posterior portions of the heart were added (Patten, 1949).

Johnstone (1925) initially reported that when the right edge of the conoventricular portion of the newly formed heart tube first starts its weak beat in the 9-somite chick embryo, it serves as its own pacemaker. However, using microsurgical techniques, DeHaan (1959) demonstrated that when the left and right primordia were prevented from fusing, the beat started earlier and with a faster rate on the left side than on the right. He postulated that therefore at early stages the left side should dominate. When Van Mierop (1967) succeeded in impaling the small fragile cells of the very early heart with microelectrodes he found that the source of the action potential was not in the beating ventricle. In the 11 somite heart, for example, he recorded a small pacemaker-like action potential in the unfused left atrioventricular wall - that was not itself contractile - which preceded the ventricular action potential by as much as 100 ms. Even in the 8 somite embryo, before any portion of the heart started to beat, he recorded action potentials that originated in the left atrio-ventricular primordium. Van Mierop's observation of electrical activity in the 8 somite heart has recently been elegantly confirmed with the aid of potential sensitive dyes applied to embryos of the same stage (Fujii et al., 1980).

Two questions then remain unresolved for the normal heart: 1) During early cardiac development, when the heart first starts to beat, is the conoventricular region driven by an external pacemaker and if not, when does that condition develop? 2) Does a pacemaker region drive the remainder of the heart at its intrinsic rate, or does the driven tissue act back on the pacemaker area?

These questions can be answered by microsurgical manipulation of the chick embryo in culture. In a series of studies previously unpublished, embryos were incubated in ovo for 24 hrs, to stage 6-8 (Hamburger and Hamilton, 1951). They were then explanted ventral side up on their vitelline membranes by the

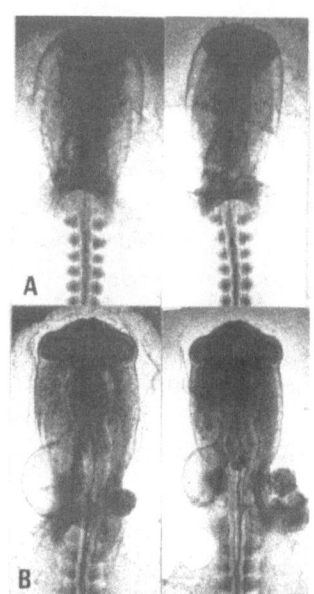

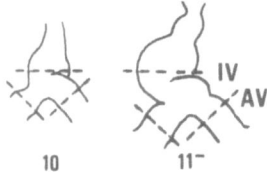

FIGURE 1 *Tracings of hearts from a 10-somite and a 12-somite embryo. The broken lines show the pattern of cuts that were made. The single horizontal cut
(IV) at the point of the future interventricular sulcus separated conoventricular tissue from prospective left ventricle and sinoatrial rudiments. The more
caudal V-shaped cuts (AV) separated the entire formed conoventricular tube from
the caudal undifferentiated regions.*

FIGURE 2 *Embryos photographed from the ventral side just before and after mi-
crosurgery. A. 10-somite embryo with an IV cut. B. 12-somite embryo with an
AV cut. The stub of the left atrial rudiment attached to the curved ventricle
has drawn in under it and is not distinguishable.*

technique of New (1955) modified as described earlier (DeHaan, 1967). The embryos were covered with a layer of Klearol mineral oil to prevent evaporation,
and maintained at $37 \pm 0.3\ ^{\circ}C$ on the heated stage of a dissecting microscope.
In this conditions they could be cleaned, accurately staged, and allowed to develop in vitro under constant observation to stage 10^-, when 9 somite pairs
had formed but before contractile activity had begun, or to later stages. At
the desired stage the body wall over the cardiac region was carefully torn away

without disturbing the heart and the spontaneous beat rate of the intact organ was counted with a stopwatch. With a sharpened tungsten needle cuts were then made according to the patterns shown in Fig. 1, which diagrams hearts from a 10 somite (stage 10) and a 12 somite (stage 11⁻) embryo. Either a V-shaped pair of cuts was made (AV) to separate the entire formed heart tube from more caudal undifferentiated regions, or a single horizontal cut (IV) was used to separate conus and prospective right ventricle from prospective left ventricle and sino-atrium. With practise the cuts could be made cleanly and without excessive tearing or stretching of the remaining tissue (Fig. 2).

The results of such operations on 62 embryos are summarized in Table I. At the earliest stage (10⁻) when the heart had not yet begun to beat or was exhibiting only its first weak irregularly-timed twitches, rhythmic beating began in the isolated conoventricular portion of the heart at the same time and at about the same rate as stage-matched unoperated pairs. In these cases, during the time observed (about 60 minutes) no additional cardiac tissue differentiated caudal to the cuts. In embryos operated just after the heart had begun beating (stage 10-11⁻) the rate of the isolated conoventricle was not significantly different from the pre-operation rate. In one of these cases which was observed after two hours, a small mass of tissue had differentiated posterior to the cut which was beating with a regular rhythm of 50 beats/minute, while the conoventricular portion rostral to the cut was beating at 34 beats/minute. When cuts were made at later stages (10⁺ - 11⁺) according to the IV pattern, tissue both rostral and caudal to the cut resumed beating within a few minutes and achieved a stable rate within 30 minutes. In every case, the rostral conoventricle beat more slowly than the pre-cut intact heart rate whereas the caudal tissue had a faster rhythm. In only two cases at stage 11-11⁺ when an AV cut was made was there enough tissue left caudal to the operation site to resume beating. But in both of these, the same pattern emerged.

Thus, it would appear from these results that Johnstone (1925) was correct. When the beat first appears in the 9-somite embryo, the stimulus arises in the caudalmost region of the conoventricular portion of the heart tube, which is not itself yet contractile. But the firing rate of the caudal part is no faster than the intrinsic rate of the rostral contractile region, as demonstrated by its autonomy after isolation. Over the next few hours however, as more caudal ventricular and atrial tissues begin to differentiate these regions drive the

TABLE I

DEMONSTRATION OF PACEMAKER CONTROL BY SURGICAL
SEGMENTATION OF THE EARLY BEATING HEART

Stage	N	R of intact heart	Location of cut	Rate after cut conoventr.	sinoatr
10^-	8	$0^{(2)}$	$^{-(3)}$	$31.2 \pm 4.1^{(1)}$	-
10^-	8	0	AV	28.0 ± 7.2	0
$10_+ - 11^-$	15	34.1 ± 7.8	$AV^{(4)}$	37.2 ± 8.1	$50.0^{(5)}$
$10^+ - 11_+$	14	50.5 ± 2.5	IV	45.3 ± 6.1	$66.3 \pm 3^{(6)}$
$11 - 11_+$	13	70.7 ± 4.0	AV	56.7 ± 3.5	$79.0^{(6)}$
$11 - 11_+^{(7)}$	12	70.1 ± 4.2	IV	35.0 ± 15.6	73.5 ± 7.8
$18 - 19^{(7)}$	33	143.3 ± 4.3	AV	86.4 ± 5.2	161.3 ± 6.2

(1) Sham operated control embryo in which the body wall was torn and the heart was mechanically disturbed but not cut. Rate counted within 60 minutes after first beat. Mean ± S.E.

(2) The hearts of 3 of these intact embryos were exhibiting occasional weak twitches before cutting.

(3) A V-shaped cut was made just caudal to the atrioventricular sulcus, to separate the formed conoventricular tube from the caudal prospective sinoatrial tissue.

(4) A horizontal cut in the location of the interventricular sulcus was made to separate conus and prospective right ventricle from prospective left ventricle and caudal differentiating SA tissue.

(5) Single case

(6) Mean of two cases

(7) The intact heart was dissected from 3-day embryos and maintained in medium 8/8 (4.5 mM K^+) for 30-60 min before the spontaneous beat rate was determined. Atria and ventricles were seperated by a cut at the AV constriction and their rates were counted 1 hr later.

more rostral heart tube, as the original pacemaker idea suggested. But contrary to that concept, at any given stage the region serving as pacemaker does not set a heart rate equal to its own intrinsic rhythm. The intact rate is intermediate between the free-running rate of the pacemaker and the slower intrinsic rhythm of the driven tissue. Even in the 3-day embryo (stage 18-19) the intact heart has a slower spontaneous beat rate than the isolated atria (Table I). Thus, the answers to the two questions posed above appear to be that (1) pacemaker function arises in the embryonic chick heart within 2-3 hrs after the first beats (about stage 10^+), and (2) when it does, it is not unidirectional but interactive.

MECHANISMS OF INTERACTION: CELLULAR MODELS

The main prediction of a simple unidirectional pacemaker model is that the coordinated rhythm of the intact heart - or any system of cardiac cells or tissues - should equal the intrinsic rate of the fastest zone, or even of the fastest cell. As soon as techniques for the isolation and maintenance of heart cells in vitro became available, evidence began to accumulate indicating that that prediction was not valid.

In 1912 Burrows explanted the whole hearts of chick embryos into plasma clots and was able to maintain them in apparently healthy condition, beating rhythmically for 3-8 days. Later studies (Lewis, 1920) on explants of cardiac fragments and myocytes separated by teasing the tissue demonstrated that pieces of tissue or even single cells could beat in isolation. Fischer (1924) was the first to report that when two independently beating fragments of heart tissue were placed in contact in culture they took on a synchronous pulsation rate after a day or two of incubation. Extending these observations to the single-cell level, Garofolini (1927) noted that one beating cell influences the rate of a neighbor with which it makes contact , but he did not observe that the pair synchronized at the initial rate of the faster cell. We have documented elsewhere the gradual improvements during the past 50 years in methods for embryo and organ culture (DeHaan, 1967a) and techniques of isolating and maintaining single heart cells in culture (DeHaan, 1967b). When Cavanaugh (1955) dissociated embryonic chick hearts into their component cells using a rapid trypsinization procedure, and maintained the cells in an adequate nutrient medium for a few days, she too noted that each of the beating cells initially pulsated with an individual frequency. But her limited data suggested that as the cells established contact and formed small sheet and clusters, their rhythms synchronized at a rate approximately equal to the average of the individual cells in the culture. When we recorded the spontaneous beat rates of 37 pairs of isolated chick heart cells before and immediately after they achieved synchrony, only 10 pairs entrained at a rate equal to that of the initially faster cell ($\pm$ 5 %), whereas the rest took on a rate near that of the originally slow cell, or were faster than the fast or intermediate in their entrained rates (DeHaan and Hirakow, 1972; DeHaan and Sachs, 1972). Thus, fewer than one-third of the cell pairs behaved according to the expectations of the unidirectional pacemaker hypothesis.

Whether a rapidly beating pacemaker cell or region drives neighboring tissues in a unidirectional fashion, or is connected in an interactive way with those tissues depends on the mechanism of cell-cell interaction that exists. DeHaan and Hirakow (1972) examined newly synchronized cell pairs in the electron microscope, and found the cells joined by narrow, punctate regions of close membrane apposition. These zones, which were generally less than 0.1 μm diameter, resembled the primitive gap junctions seen in the newly-beating (stage 10) intact chick (DeHaan and Sachs, 1972; Mazet, 1979) and mouse (Gros et al., 1979) heart. It is now widely held that cardiac tissue behaves like an electrical syncytium in which currents flow from cell to cell through the low-resistance gap junctions (Weidmann, 1952; Pollack, 1976; Weingart, 1977; Bleeker et al., 1980; for review see DeHaan et al., 1980). However it was not apparent that a few points of close membrane apposition between cell pairs provided enough contact surface to mediate cell coupling, or that membrane resistance at these contact points could have fallen sufficiently in the time between initial cell apposition and synchrony to allow current flow between cells, since entrainment was achieved in times that ranged from 4 to 38 minutes with a mean of 16.5 minutes (DeHaan and Hirakow, 1972).

Evidence that only a very small amount of contact surface is required to mediate cell synchronization was provided by the chance observation of pairs of synchronized cells such as that illustrated in Fig. 3A. These cells were separated by a space of 7 μm at their nearest point. Viewed with phase optics at a magnification of 200x they appeared not to be in contact at all. Nonetheless, they were clearly beating in unison, a fact made more obvious by their irregular rhythm. After the cells were fixed and embedded in the culture dish, examination of approximately every third section in a series of 150 thin sections, cut parallel to the bottom of the dish, revealed a single filopodial finger-like

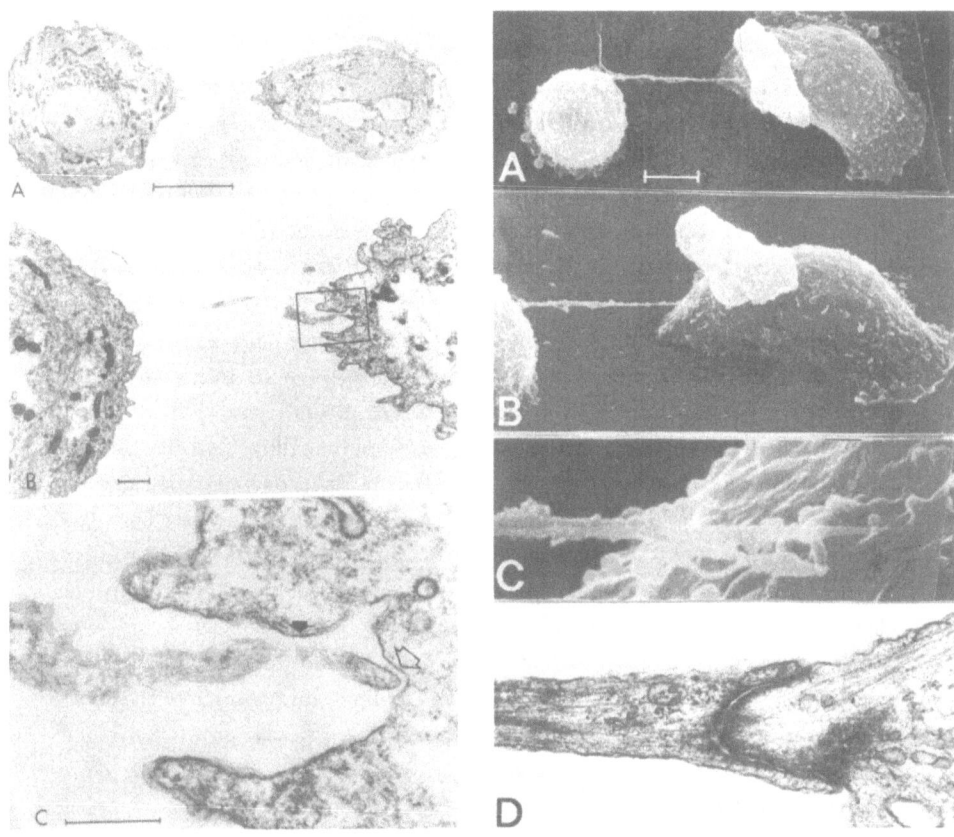

FIGURE 3 *A synchronized pair of chick ventricle myocytes after 24 hrs in culture. The only point of contact was via a cell process that extended across the 7 μm space between the cells. A. Low power micrograph showing both cells. B. An enlarged view of a section that grazes the connecting fiber about midway between the two cells, and provides a more detailed view of the point of contact. C. Further enlargement of the tip of the finger-like process where it contacts the cell on the right. Scales: A = 10 μm, B = 1 μm, C = 0.5 μm (Electron micrographs courtesy of Dr John Rash).*

FIGURE 4 *A different pair of chick ventricular myocytes after 24 hrs in culture, synchronized across a bridging cell process that extends from the left-hand cell to that on the right. A-C. Scanning electron micrographs. D. Transmission electron micrograph of one attachment point, prepared by embedding the same cells after they were observed in the scanning electron microscope. Scale: A, 7 μm; B, 5 μm; C, 0.5 μm; D, 50 nm. (Electron micrscopy courtesy of Dr Max Springer).*

process extending between the two cells. This process was about 0.1 μm in diameter and traversed the space between the upper portions of the cells about 5 μm above the surface of the culture dish (Fig. 3B,C). The area of cell contact was in a region about 50 nm in diameter at the tip of the process. It could be seen in only one section (Fig. 3C), but two adjacent sections on either side were obscured by grid bars. Thus, the vertical dimension of the contact area could be estimated as being no larger than the thickness of five sections (about 100 nm). The cell membranes in the contact zones in the section examined (Fig. 3C) were separated by a space of 20 nm or more. Thus any points of membrane apposition close enough to permit a histologically defined gap junction must have been located in the obscured sections, and could have been no larger than about 50 nm in either vertical or horizontal dimension. A second similar cell pair was synchronized across a bridging fiber about 15 μm long (Fig. 4A,B). In this case the extended process was about 0.6 μm thick at its proximal end and narrowed to about 0.2 μm near its distal end, before it splayed into four finger-like points of contact (Fig. 4C). One of these revealed several points of close membrane apposition in a single section prepared by embedding the cell after observing them in the scanning electron microscope (Fig. 4D).

Earlier workers have reported that heart cells in culture may be synchronized across fine bridging fibers, on the basis of light microscopic (Lehmkuhl and Sperelakis, 1965) or cinemicrographic (Gross, 1971) observations. Lehmkuhl and Sperelakis (1965) observed synchronously beating cells, separated by distances up to several hundred microns, which were connected by long bridging processes 0.5 - 2.0 μm wide. These authors argued that such cells could not be electrotonically coupled because of the problem of "impedance mismatching". However, on the basis of more recent measurements of the electrical properties of heart cells in culture, we can show that pairs of cells such as those illustrated can exhibit strong interactions (DeHaan, Rash and Springer, unpublished).

Ventricle cells dissociated from 7-day embryonic chick heart by standard techniques (DeHaan, 1967, 1970) and maintained in suspension culture, have a mean diameter of 10.8 μm (range 7 - 12.5 μm). Thus mean cell surface, assuming no folding or microvilli is 366 μm^2 (Nathan and DeHaan, 1979). These cells can be reassociated to form spheroidal aggregates (Sachs and DeHaan, 1973) which exhibit virtual voltage homogeneity (DeHaan and Fozzard, 1975; Clay et al., 1979). The input resistance (R_{in}) of these preparations, measured with small hyperpolarizing current pulses, varies with the number of cells in the aggregate (N) as if the membranes of all N cells were connected in parallel with negligible junctional resistance. From such measurements, specific membrane resistance (R_m) of aggregates made quiescent with tetrodotoxin, in medium containing 1.3 mM K^+ was estimated at 18 KOhm.cm^2 (Clay et al., 1979).

Consider a pair of cells of average size and membrane resistance joined by a connecting strand formed of a right cylinder of passive membrane, 0.1 μm in diameter (cross-sectional area, A = 8 x 10^{-11} cm^2) by 10 μm in length (ℓ), filled with a fluid of resistivity ρ = 150 Ohm.cm. Then the bridge resistance (R_b) is the sum of the longitudinal core resistance down the length of the fiber (R_ℓ) plus the junctional resistance (R_j) at the contact point. This simplified model assumes that little current leaks out across the fiber membrane, and that its tip forms a high-resistance seal at the point of contact to prevent current from leaking into the intercellular space. Let the cell from which the fiber extends be the source of rhythmic action potentials, which we model as 80 mV depolarizing rectangular pulses. Under these circumstances:

$$R_\ell = \frac{\rho \ell}{A} = 2 \times 10^9 \text{ Ohm} \tag{1}$$

and the resistance across the membrane that forms the tubular fiber (R_{fm}) is:

$$R_{fm} = \frac{R_m}{A_f} = \frac{1.8 \times 10^4 \text{ Ohm.cm}^2}{3 \times 10^{-8} \text{ cm}^2} = 6 \times 10^{11} \text{ Ohm} \tag{2}$$

(where A_f = the area of the fiber membrane). Thus less than 1 % of the current injected into the proximal end of the fiber from the source cell would leak out along the way to its distal end. R_j can be calculated according to two alternative assumptions: (a) the tip of the fiber that abuts on the driven cell, may be considered as simply a disc of passive membrane 0.1 μm in diameter in which case it would have a resistance of 2.5 x 10^{14} Ohm; or (b) the same disc may be considered to contain a single unit junctional channel (Loewenstein, 1975) of resistance 1 x 10^{10} Ohm, in which case R_j would be 1 x 10^{10} Ohm. In the case (a), R_ℓ is negligible, and effectively R_b = R_j = 2.5 x 10^{14} Ohm. In case (b) the effective resistance is distributed along the fiber as well as at the contact point and $R_b = R_\ell + R_j = 1.2 \times 10^{10}$ Ohm. If the source cell fires an action potential when the driven cell is at rest, the current that would flow along the fiber from one to the other would be:

case (a) $I = (V_1 - V_2)/R_b = 80 \times 10^{-3} / 2 \times 10^{14} = 4 \times 10^{-16}$ A
case (b) $I = (V_1 - V_2)/R_b = 80 \times 10^{-3} / 1.2 \times 10^{10} = 7 \times 10^{-12}$ A

The input resistance (R_{in}) of the driven cell is:

$$R_{in} = \frac{18 \times 10^3 \text{ Ohm.cm}^2}{3.6 \times 10^{-6} \text{ cm}^2} = 5 \times 10^9 \text{ Ohm} \tag{3}$$

In the case (a) with no nexal channels, the voltage response of the driven cell to 4×10^{-16} A of current would be only 2 µV. In case (b), the driven cell would be depolarized by about 33 mV. The model that these calculations are based upon is simplified, in that it does not take into consideration the contact cleft sealing resistance, the voltage dependence of R_{in}, or the fact that both cells of the pairs studied were spontaneously active. Despite these deficiencies, however, two conclusions seem reasonable. Two cells can be synchronized electrotonically across a bridging fiber of the dimensions seen, if the membranes are joined by a point of low-resistance. But the low-resistance junction need be composed of only one or a small number of unit junctional channels. We have shown elsewhere (Williams and DeHaan, 1981) that the cells of a spheroidal aggregate remain well coupled even in the absence of ultrastructurally defined gap junctions. In that case, we drew the same conclusion, that only one or a small number of patent junctional channels were required between each cell to maintain effective electrical coupling. We have also measured directly the fall in junctional resistance between pairs of newly apposed spheroidal aggregates of heart cells, and have shown that these preparations pass enough current to achieve beat synchrony after only about 8 minutes of contact (Ypey et al., 1979), at a time when junctional resistance has a value equivalent to 5 unit junctional channels per apposed cell (Clapham et al., 1980; DeHaan et al., 1980; see below).

If a pair of isolated cells can synchronize their beats by assembling low-resistance junctional channels at points of contact within a few minutes after apposition, it provides a mechanism for the observed coupling of larger clusters, containing tens (Clay and DeHaan, 1979) or thousands (DeHaan and Fozzard, 1975; Clay et al., 1979) of cells. Moreover, in confirmation of a large body of literature (reviewed in McNutt and Weinstein, 1973; DeMello, 1975; Weingart, 1977; DeHaan et al., 1980) it suggests that the cells in all parts of the heart, from the sinus node (Bleeker et al., 1980) to the working ventricle (Fozzard, 1979), may be connected as parallel patches of high-resistance membrane across low-resistance junctions. An equivalent circuit of cardiac tissue based on such a model of heart cell connectivity cannot support a unidirectional pacemaker concept, for in this case the spontaneous rate of the fastest cell in any connected group must inevitably be influenced by the degree of loading (and other electrical properties) of the entire system with which it interacts. Results of studies of the rate relations of intact cardiac systems that exhibit interactions such as "reflection reentry"" (Antzelevitch et al., 1980), "overdrive suppression" (Vassalle, 1971) and a variety of other rhythm influences (Boyett and Jewell, 1980) are consistent with this view, and can be modelled to advantage with in vitro cellular systems.

PACEMAKER FUNCTION IN CULTURED MULTICELLULAR HEART CELL SYSTEMS: REASSEMBLED "TISSUE" AS MODELS

PROPERTIES OF CELL SHEETS AND MASSES

With the development of tissue dissociation and reaggregation procedures (Moscona, 1961) it was demonstrated that isolated heart cells are readily reassociated into tissue-like masses in a variety of geometric configurations. Many of these have proved suitable for studies that focus on one or another specific aspects of heart cell function. Mono- or multi-layer cell sheets are easy to prepare, and to observe at high magnification, for investigation of the effects of cell density, preparative procedures, ionic and nutritional components, and pharmacological agents (Sperelakis et al., 1960; 1972; DeHaan, 1967; 1970; Harary

et al.,   1967;   Speicher   and   McCarl,   1978;   Goshima,   1976;   Sperelakis
et al.,   1976;   Mc Call, 1976;   Mann and Sperelakis, 1979;   Lompre et al.,
1979;   Langer   et al.,   1979;   Jongsma et al.,   1975;   Matter,   1973).
Synthetic   fiber-like   strands   of reassociated heart cells (Lieberman et al.,
1972;   Sachs, 1976) have proven especially useful for ionic flux   studies   (Carmeliet   et al.,   1976);   while cells reassociated into small clusters (Clay and
DeHaan,   1979;   Schanne et al., 1979) or   rounded   masses   (DeHaan   and   Sachs,
1972;   Mc Lean et al., 1976;   DeHaan and Fozzard, 1975;   Clay et al., 1979)
have provided useful information regarding ionic   currents,   and   mechanisms   of
cell interaction.   Indeed, spheriodal aggregates may be especially useful as models of cardiac function because of the ease with which they can be   manipulated
into   interacting pairs or multiaggregate systems (Ypey et al., 1979;   Clapham
et al., 1980;   DeHaan et al., 1980), and because their current-voltage relations   can   be   investigated with good success and remarkable reproducibility by
voltage clamp technique (Nathan and DeHaan,   1978;   1979;   Ebihara   et al.,
1980).

   In all of these configurations, once the preparations recover from the initial effects of the dissociation and reassembly procedures (Le Douarin et al.,
1974; Lompre et al., 1979), they respond to a variety of pharmacological   and
other   environmental   perturbations   in   ways similar to the intact heart muscle
from which they were derived (Goshima, 1976;   Mc Call,   1976;   Lane   et al.,
1977;   DeHaan et al., 1975) although under certain circumstances they may revert   back   to   earlier   embryonic physiological characteristics   (Sperelakis
et al.,   1976;   Sachs et al.,   1973).   When such artificial tissue systems
have been examined in the electron microscope, they have in all   cases   revealed
gap   junctions joining the cells (Purdy et al., 1972;   DeHaan and Sachs, 1972;
Goshima, 1970;   Shimada et al., 1974;   Matter, 1973;   for   review   see   DeHaan
et al., 1980).

   Investigations of a variety of such reassembled systems have emphasized the
interactive nature of heart cell connectivity.   For example, the distribution of
spontaneous pulsation rates of isolated single   chick   heart   cells   in   culture
ranged   from   50 to 290 beats/minute (Sachs and DeHaan, 1973) with only about 5 %
of the cells at the upper end of the skewed Gaussian curve (>200   beats/minute).
Thus,   in   any   assembly   of 100 such cells or more, one would expect to find at
least a few cells in that intrinsically rapid category.   If these   cells   impose

their endogenous rhythm on the rest of the cells in a cluster, the expectation would be that all large aggregates should beat at 200 beats/minute or more, while small clusters would do so on a statistical basis related to the number of cells (N) included in the cluster. However, the observed behavior of cell clusters did not correspond to this prediction (Fig. 5). For clusters of 2-125 cells, mean rate was 133 beats/minute, and did not vary with N (Clay and DeHaan, 1979). Larger aggregates (N= 100-3000) behaved just opposite to the pacemaker prediction. That is, spontaneous rate declined as a function of N (Sachs and DeHaan, 1973).

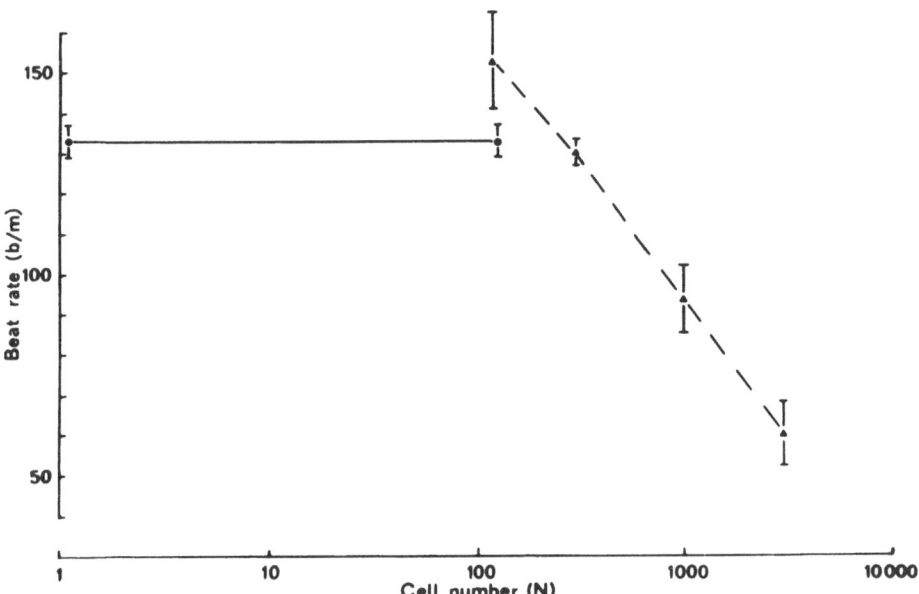

FIGURE 5 *Spontaneous pulsation rate of clusters of 7-day heart cells as a function of the number of cells (N) in each cluster. The horizontal solid line (N = 2-125) is a least squares fit to the data of Clay and DeHaan (1979; fig. 3). The broken line (N = 120-300) is taken from Sachs and DeHaan (1973; fig. 3). Means and standard errors are shown.*

There may be species differences in the degree of interaction between a pacemaker cell and the surrounding cells it influences. Under certain conditions, monolayer cultures of mouse (Goshima and Tonomura, 1969) or rat (Jongsma et al., 1975) heart cells achieved synchronous rates at confluency that approximated those of the fastest beating isolated cells. Moreover, when a confluent sheet of rat heart cells was cut with a needle into two half sheets, one half slowed its rate but the other maintained a rhythm near that of the originally intact culture (Harary and Farley, 1963). These results have since been extended and interpreted in terms of pacemaker function (see Jongsma and Tsjernina, this volume).

Although mammalian cells in monolayer culture behave more like unidirectional pacemakers than do avian cells in their ability to drive surrounding cells at a fast rate, analysis of variance of the interbeat intervals (IBI) in these preparations indicates that the pacemaker is profoundly influenced by its neighbors at the same time it affects their rates. The variability in the synchronized beat rate of multicellular cardiac systems appears to depend upon the number of cells in the system. As reported by Jongsma and his colleagues (Jongsma et al., 1975; Jongsma and Tsjernina, this volume), single rat heart cells beat slowly and irregularly whereas synchronized interconnected multicellular networks increased in their entrained mean rate, but showed a decrease in the variability of consecutive beat intervals. The hypothesis that fluctuation in IBI (σ_{IBI}) is inversely related to N was tested by Clay and DeHaan (1979) with clusters of chick ventricle cells of varying sizes. Whereas the mean IBI of cell clusters in the range N = 1-125 was independent of N (Fig. 5), beat-to-beat fluctuation in IBI decreased approximately as $N^{-1/2}$ (Clay and DeHaan, 1979). This result provided a further argument strongly in favor of the idea that heart cells are joined by low-resistance junctions, and their membranes are connected as parallel resistance-capacitance (RC) circuits.

The evidence presented thus far argues in favor of the idea that heart cells are joined by low-resistance conducting junctions, and that therefore, an electrical signal arising in any cell influences the electrical properties of connected cells and is altered reciprocally by those cells. Thus neither the spontaneous firing rate, the action potential shape, or other electrical properties of a pacemaker cell remain unaltered when that cell is connected to other cells. Such interactive behavior is evident in the pacemaker relations in the early embryonic heart, in the synchronization of isolated pairs of cells, and in the pattern of beat rates of small and large clusters of cells. We will show in a companion paper (Ypey et al., this volume) that the complex electrical interactions involved in the entrainment between pairs of spheroidal aggregates of heart cells, are amenable to phase-response analysis (Ypey et al., 1980).

THE RELATION BETWEEN ACTION POTENTIAL SPREAD AND JUNCTIONAL RESISTANCE

In the intact heart the beat is normally initiated when an action potential arises in the central dominant pacemaker cells of the SA node, and sweeps out through the perinodal cells and surrounding atrial tissue. The spread of current from the active membrane to adjacent segments has been analyzed by many workers, using the cable equations (Hodgkin and Huxley, 1952; Weidmann, 1952) and more complex modes of analysis (for an excellent recent review, see Fozzard, 1979). In simplest terms conduction occurs as the result of a local action potential that raises the adjacent regions of membrane above their threshold for excitation. This concept emphasizes the importance of the passive parameters of the electrotonically connected cells: membrane resistance (R_m) and capacitance (C_m), internal resistance (R_i) which is the sum of longitudinal myoplasmic (R_{my}) and cell-cell junctional or coupling resistance (R_c) and threshold potential (V_{thr}). The question of how stimulus propagation and regional entrainment may be related to cell-cell junctional resistance is an important one in which insights may be gained from the aggregate pair system.

As noted above, when two spontaneously beating aggregates are brought into contact they adhere, but initially each member of the pair beats at its own rhythm, unaffected by its new neighbor. Within a few minutes, however, the aggregates begin to interact and soon their beats synchronize. Each action potential in one aggregate is then faithfully accompanied by an action potential in the other member of the pair. During the early stages of this entrainment the delay or latency (L), between the upstroke of the action potentials in the two aggregates can be as great as 200 ms (Ypey et al., 1979). However, as coupling improves over the next hour or so, L progressively decreases to < 1 ms. By measuring directly the coupling resistance between the aggregates (R_c) we have shown (Clapham et al., 1980; Clapham and DeHaan, this volume) that the decline in L is paralleled precisely by a decrease in R_c (Fig. 6, curve 1). Moreover, additional aggregates can be added in tandem to such a system to form a long chain. Within an hour or two all of these aggregates come to beat synchronously, an entire chain of 20 aggregates or more behaving essentially as a single cardiac fiber (DeHaan et al., 1980).

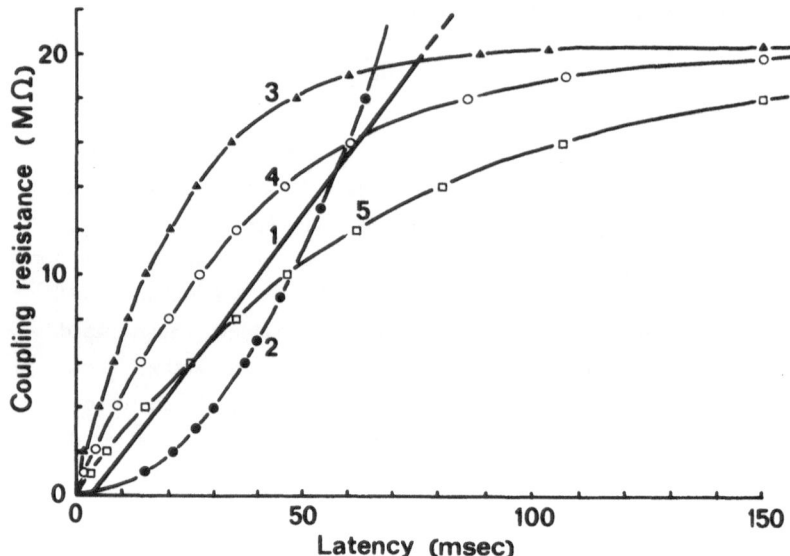

FIGURE 6 *Relation between coupling resistance and action potential latency in aggregate pairs. Curve 1, least-squares fit to the experimental data of Clapham et al. (1980; fig. 9) obtained with aggregates in medium containing 4.8 mM K^+; Curve 2, $L = KR^{1/2}$; Curves 3-5 calculated as described in the text with the following parameters: $R_2 = 2.55$ MOhm; $(V_1 - V_2) = 80$ mV; $V_{rest} = -70$ mV; $V_{th} = -60$ mV; $\tau_m = 22, 40, 70$ ms respectively for curves 3, 4 and 5.*

The passive factors related to conduction of the action potential at constant velocity in a model fiber are generally described by relationships derived with certain simplifying assumptions, from the cable equations:

$$\Theta^2 = \frac{ka}{2R_i C_m} \tag{4}$$

where Θ is conduction velocity (m/s), a is fiber radius (μm), R_i is internal resistance (Ohm.cm), C_m is specific membrane capacitance (μF/cm^2), and k is a constant related to the non-passive properties of the membrane.

Excitability of the membrane must of course be included because conduction is achieved only when an active region brings an adjacent region of resting membrane to threshold for activation of its own inward current system. It had been demonstrated by many workers that Θ is related to action potential size (V_p) and maximal upstroke velocity ($\dot{V}_{max}$) and therefore to inward current density. This relationship can be made explicit by including terms for the action potential characteristics in the equations as for example an equation derived from Hunter et al. (1975):

$$\Theta^2 = \frac{k\,a\,\dot{V}_{max}}{C_m R_i V_p} \tag{5}$$

Since the delay (L) between activation of two points unit distance apart = $1/\Theta$, eq. 5 predicts that $L \propto R_i^{1/2}$. When values for each parameter (measured or estimated) appropriate for 7-day chick ventricle cell aggregates are entered in eq. 5, it is apparent that this equation does not apply directly to a pair or linear chain of aggregates (Fig. 6, curve 2). Because of its geometry such a system is not a simple cable. Nonetheless, it may be instructive to note certain relevant aspects.

When two or more aggregates are brought together to form a pair or chain, the action potential size and shape ($\dot{V}_{max}$ and V_p) do not change, nor does the diameter of the aggregates or specific capacitance of their component membranes, during the subsequent hours while synchrony is achieved. Specific myoplasmic resistance would not change either, but that component of R_i which is attributable to junctional resistance (R_c) at the newly apposed surfaces falls dramatically (Clapham et al., 1980), though not as a square-root function.

An alternative approach to relating L and R_c is with the concept of the strength-duration curve, which is the relation between the duration of a rectangular depolarizing current pulse and the amplitude of such a pulse that is just sufficient to stimulate an action potential. In response to such a pulse, membrane potential in a simple RC-model membrane with uniform potential distribution would rise according to:

$$V_m(t) = I_m R_m (1 - e^{-t/\tau_m}) \tag{6}$$

where $V_m(t)$ is membrane potential (mV) achieved at time t, I_m is the amplitude of the current pulse (nA) injected into the preparation, R_m is the input resistance (MOhm), t is the time after onset of the pulse (ms), and τ_m is the membrane time constant, $r_m c_m$ (ms), where r_m is the specific membrane resistance (Ohm.cm^2), and c_m the specific membrane capacitance (μF/cm^2). The classical description of the strength duration curve for nerve was first derived by Lapicque (1907), who noted that the stimulating current required to excite an action potential varied with the duration of the stimulus. He defined the "rheobasic" current (I_{rh}) as the minimum current that produced an action potential no matter how long the pulse.

It is easy to apply this concept to an aggregate pair by considering the voltage changes in each member of the pair, when one of the aggregates (agg. 1) is beating spontaneously while agg. 2 is quiescent. We can model the action potential recorded in agg. 1 as a rectangular voltage pulse 80 mV in height and 100 ms long, which serves as a constant low-impedance stimulus source. Then the current (I_j) passing across the junction between agg. 1 and agg. 2 would be determined by the instantaneous potential difference between V_1 and V_2 divided by the junctional resistance (R_c). As R_c declines after the aggregates are brought into initial contact, progressively more current crosses the junction. When enough current flows to bring V_2 to threshold within the 100 ms duration of the action potential in A_1 (i.e. $I_j = I_{rh}$) agg. 2 fires its action potential, but with a delay related to the rc-rise time of V_2. As R_c continues to decline, V_2 crosses threshold with every action potential in agg. 1 and the aggregates synchronize, but with a latency described by the strength-duration relationship.

To calculate L as a function of R_c we can modify eq. 6 to conform to the notation of the aggregate system:

$$V_2(t) = I_j R_2 (1 - e^{-t/\tau_m}) \qquad (7)$$

where $V_2(t)$ is the potential in agg. 2 as a function of time after start of the model action potential in agg. 1 and R_2 is R_m of agg. 2. Curves 2-5 (Fig. 6) were calculated from eq. 5 and 7 using membrane parameters for heart cell aggregates (listed in Fig. 6 legend) derived from Clay et al. (1979). Since t represents the delay between the onset of the stimulating pulse (the action potential in agg. 1) and the time at which $V_2 = V_{th}$, then t = L in this model.

As is usual in a strength duration analysis (Fozzard and Schoenberg, 1972; Noble and Stein, 1966) we assumed that membrane potential was stable in the region under consideration (agg. 2; $V_2 = V_{rest}$ = -70 mV) until current began to flow through R_j from the adjacent active segment (agg. 1), and further that threshold potential was constant (V_{th} = -60 mV). A 150 μm diameter aggregate of 7-day embryo ventricle cells in 1.3 mM K^+ has an input resistance of 2.55×10^6 Ohm and a membrane time constant of 22 ms (Clay et al., 1979). These values were used to produce curve 3 (Fig. 6). We reported earlier (Clapham et al., 1980) that when an aggregate pair first achieves synchrony R_c = 20 MOhm and L = 100-200 ms. Curves 1 and 3 cross at R_c = 20 MOhm at L = 75 ms, a bit too short. But as R_c falls the observed L declines at a pace slower than that predicted by curve 3, and at R_c = 16 MOhm, L is declining with a slope that resembles curve 5, based on τ = 70 ms.

There are numerous reasons why the experimentally observed relationship of R_c to L (Fig. 6, curve 1) does not follow that predicted by the classical strength-duration curve. (1) Although aggregates exhibit a surprisingly high level of voltage homogeneity, transmembrane potential does not behave as a simple RC model (Clay et al., 1979; DeHaan and DeFelice, 1978). Moreover the assumption of constant threshold is probably not applicable to real cardiac systems. With short Purkinje fibers, in which voltage distribution was also relatively uniform, the data of Fozzard and Schoenberg (1972) showed that V_{th} for short pulses was less negative than for long ones. (2) The assumption that V_{rest} is stable also would not apply to aggregate pairs. In all experiments reported to date (Ypey et al., 1979; Clapham et al., 1980) both members of the pair were beating spontaneously but at different rates prior to synchrony. (3) Even subthreshold changes of V_m in two aggregates would interact when R_c is relatively low. For example, if R_2 = 2 MOhm and R_c has fallen to 4 MOhm, the subthreshold diastolic depolarization in agg. 1 would be reflected by a depolarization roughly half as large in agg. 2. Thus, if agg. 1 reached threshold at - 60 mV, agg. 2 would no longer be resting at -70 mV, but would already be depolarized to -65 mV. (4) As cardiac membrane approaches threshold during diastolic depolarization R_{in} increases dramatically. This is true for both adult heart cells (Weidmann, 1952; McAllister et al., 1975), and for embryonic heart cell aggregates (Clay et al., 1979). Thus, with high values of R_c and with agg. 2 quiescent, R_2 would be constant. But with low values of R_c, V_2 and

therefore R_2 would change with each diastolic depolarization in agg. 1. (5)
Finally, another difference between a pair or chain of aggregates and an RC
cable is in their physical shape. An aggregate pair is not a right cylinder,
but for many hours retains a dumbell shape. Thus it is necessary to consider
how much of the delay measured as L results from the constriction in the middle
of the "cylinder" rather than from the specific value of R_c at the apposed junctional surfaces (see for example, Khodorov and Timin, 1975).

For all of the above reasons, it should not be surprizing that aggregate
pairs or chains do not behave according to the predictions of the cable equations or the strength interval relationship in their patterns of synchronization. With the aggregate pair system and other reassembled cell models, many of
the relevant membrane parameters can be experimentally controlled or measured
individually, and it is possible to separate R_c from R_i. Since the method of
phase-response analysis predicts accurately the entrainment behavior of heart
cell aggregates (Scott, 1979; Ypey et al., 1980; 1981) and a variety of
other preparations (see below), we are presented with an exciting challenge to
delve further into the mechanisms of action potential propagation and pacemaker
function.

APPLICATION OF MODELS TO INTACT CARDIAC TISSUE:
BACK TO THE ADULT HEART

We have seen that the pacemaker cells, in a variety of in vitro arrangements,
do not drive other heart cells at their own rate. They entrain other cells at a
rate which is determined by the electrical properties of the entire system. In
the course of such entrainment the spontaneous pulsation rate of pairs of
heart-cell aggregates change according to a biphasic phase-response relationship.

Perhaps the most important idea to emerge from the present conference is
that similar complex electrotonic interactions govern the relations between a
pacemaker zone and neighboring elements in adult cardiac tissue. The cells of
the sinoatrial (Sano et al., 1978) and atrioventricular nodes (Mendez and Moe,

1966) exhibit independent intrinsic rates, whose entrainment behavior produces a biphasic phase response relationship. Complex electrotonic interactions have been observed in different regions within Purkinje fibers (Downar and Waxman, 1976; Jalife and Moe, 1976) and at the Purkinje-fiber muscle junction (Mendez et al., 1969). Such interactive behavior and phase-resetting curves also emerge from several recent theoretical models of cardiac rhythm entrainment (Scott, 1979; Ypey et al., 1980; 1981; Capelle and Durrer, 1980; Holden, 1980). Recently the electrotonic interactions between an ectopic pacemaker and the sinoatrial pacemaker across a region of depressed excitability have been analyzed in canine Purkinje fibers (Jalife and Moe, 1979; Antzelevitch et al., 1980). These authors have shown that the entrainment patterns depend on the magnitude of the electrotonic influences among the various segments. By varying the degree of coupling, they produced biphasic phase-response curves and entrainment patterns virtually identical with those predicted and observed during entrainment of embryonic aggregate pairs (Ypey et al., 1980; 1981), and were able to describe the characteristics of reflection in relation to reentrant arrhythmias and parasystole. It seems evident that analyses of cardiac function in both normal and pathological conditions may benefit from continued application of the ideas that (1) heart cells are coupled by electrotonic junctions; (2) the spontaneous activity of a pacemaker region is altered by the surrounding tissues with which it is coupled; and (3) many of the arrhythmic forms of behavior commonly observed in cardiac pathology can be understood in terms of electrotonic interactions between two or more spontaneously active regions that exhibit different phase relations.

ACKNOWLEDGEMENTS

I wish to extend my thanks to Drs Max Springer and John Rash for their help in preparing and photographing the cell pairs illustrated in figures 3 and 4; to Prof. Edouard Coraboeuf for providing me with the generous hospitality of his department during the time most of this manuscript was written; and to Ms Edith Deroubaix, whose many kindnesses included preparation of the illustrations and typing the manuscript.

REFERENCES

Antzelevitch, C., Jalife, J. and Moe, G.K.: Characteristics of reflection as a mechanism of reentrant arrhythmias and its relationship to parasystole. Circulation, 61: 182-191, 1980.

Barry, A.: The intrinsic pulsation rates of fragments of the embryonic chick heart. J. Exp. Zool., 91: 119-130, 1942.

Bayliss, W.M. and Starling, E.H.: On the electromotive phenomena of the mammalian heart. Monthly Internat. J. Anat. and Physiol., 9: 256-281, 1892.

Bernstein, J.: Ueber den Sitz der automatischen Erregung im froschherzen. Zentr. Med. Wiss. (Berlin), 14: 385-387, 1876.

Bleeker, W.K., Mackaay, A.J.C., Masson-Pevet, M., Bouman, L.N. and Becker, A.E.: Functional and morphological organization of the rabbit sinus node. Circ. Res., 46: 11-22, 1980.

Bowditch, H.P.: Ueber die Eigenthuemlichkeiten der Reizbarkeit welche die Muskelfasern des Herzens zeigen. Arb. Physiol. Anstalt (Leipzig), pp. 139-176, 1871.

Bowditch, H.P.: Does the apex of the heart contract automatically. J. Physiol. (London), 1: 104-107, 1879.

Boyett, M.R. and Jewell, B.R.: Analysis of the effects of changes in rate and rhythm upon electrical activity in the heart. Prog. Biophys. Mol. Biol., 36: 1-52, 1980.

Burrows, M.T.: Rhythmical activity of isolated heart muscle cells in vitro. Science, 36: 90-92, 1912.

Carmeliet, E.E., Horres, C.R., Lieberman, M. and Vereecke, J.S.: Developmental aspects of potassium flux and permeability of the embryonic chick heart. J. Physiol. (London), 254: 673-692, 1976.

Cavanaugh, M.W.: Pulsation, migration and division in dissociated chick embryo heart cells in vitro. J. Exp. Zool., 128: 573-590, 1955.

Clapham, D.E., Shrier, A. and DeHaan, R.L.: Junctional resistance and action potential delay between embryonic heart cell aggregates. J. Gen. Physiol., 75: 633-654, 1980.

Clay, J. and DeHaan, R.L.: Fluctuations in interbeat interval in rhythmic heart cell clusters: role of membrane voltage noise. Biophys. J., 28: 377-390, 1979.

Clay, J., DeFelice, L.J. and DeHaan, R.L.: Current noise parameters derived from voltage noise and impedance in embryonic heart cell aggregates. Biophys. J., 28: 169-184, 1979.

Davis, C.L.: Development of the human heart from its first appearance to the stage found in embryos of 20 paired somites. Carnegie Inst. of Washington, Contr. to Embryology, 19: 245-284, 1927.

DeHaan, R.L.: Cardia bifida and the development of pacemaker function in the early chick heart. Devel. Biol., 1: 586-602, 1959.

DeHaan, R.L.: Regional organization of prepacemaker cells in the cardiac primordia of the early chick embryo. J. Embryol. Exp. Morphol., 11: 65-76, 1963.

DeHaan, R.L.: Avian embryo culture. In: Techniques for the Study of Development. Wilt, F.H. and Wessels, N.R., eds., Thomas Y. Crowell, New York, pp. 401-412, 1967a.

DeHaan, R.L.: Regulation of spontaneous activity and growth of embryonic chick heart cells in tissue culture. Devel. Biol., 16: 216-249, 1967b.

DeHaan, R.L.: The potassium sensitivity of isolated embryonic heart cells increases with development. Devel. Biol., 23: 226-240, 1970.

DeHaan, R.L.: Differentiation of excitable membranes. Cur. Topics Devel. Biol., 16: 117-164, 1980.

DeHaan, R.L. and DeFelice, L.J.: Oscillatory properties and excitability of the heart cell membrane. In: Theoretical Chemistry: Advances and Perspectives, Eyring, H., ed., Academic Press, New York, 4: 181-233, 1978.

DeHaan, R.L. and Fozzard, H.: Membrane response to current pulses in spheroidal aggregates of embryonic heart cells. J. Gen. Physiol., 65: 207-222, 1975.

DeHaan, R.L. and Hirakow, R.: The synchronization of pulsation rates in isolated cardiac myocytes. Exp. Cell Res., 70: 214-220, 1972.

DeHaan, R.L. and Sachs, H.G.: Cell coupling in developing systems: the heart-cell paradigm. Current Topics Devel. Biol., 7: 193-228, 1972.

DeHaan, R.L. and O'Rahilly, R.: Embryology of the heart. In: The Heart, Hurst, J.W., Logue, R.B., Schlant, R.C. and Wenger, N.K., eds., McGraw-Hill, New York, pp. 6-18, 1978.

DeHaan, R.L., McDonald, T.F. and Sachs, H.G.: Development of tetrotodoxin sensitivity of embryonic chick heart cells in vitro. In: Developmental and Physiological Correlates of Cardiac Muscle, Lieberman, M. and Sano, T., eds., Raven Press, New York, pp. 155-168, 1975.

DeHaan, R.L., Williams, E.H., Ypey, D.L. and Clapham, D.E.: Intercellular coupling of embryonic heart cells. Perspectives in Cardiovascular Research, vol. 5, Mechanisms of Cardiac Morphogenesis and Teratogenesis, Pexieder, T., ed., Raven Press, New York, pp. 299-316, 1980.

DeMello, W.C.: Effect of intracellular injection of calcium and strontium on cell communication in heart. J. Physiol. (London), 250: 231-245, 1975.

Downar, E. and Waxman, M.B.: Depressed conduction and unidirectional block in Purkinje fibers. In: Conduction System of the Heart, Wellens, H.J.J., Lie, K.I. and Janse, M.J., eds., Stenfert Kroese, Leiden, pp. 393-409, 1976.

Dubois-Reymond, E.: Untersuchungen ueber thierische Electricitaet, Vol. 1, Verlag von G.Reimer, Berlin, 1848.

Ebihara, L., Shigeto, N., Lieberman, M. and Johnson, E.A.: The initial inward current in spherical clusters of chick embryonic heart cells. J. Gen. Physiol., 75: 437-456, 1980.

Einthoven, W.: Ein neues Galvanometer. Annal. Physik. F. IV, 12: 1059, 1903.

Einthoven, W.: Weiteres ueber das Elektrocardiagramm. Arch. Ges. Physiol., 122: 517-584, 1908.

Engelmann, T.: Vergleichende Untersuchungen zur Lehre von der Muskel- und Nervenelektricitaet. Pfluegers Arch., 15: 116-148, 1877.

Erlanger, J. and Blackman, J.R.: A study of relative rhythmicity and conductivity in various regions of the auricles of the mammalian heart. Amer. J. Physiol., 19: 125-174, 1907.

Eyster, J.A.E. and Meek, W.J.: The origin and conduction of the heart beat. Physiol. Rev., 1: 1-43, 1921.

Fischer, A.: The interaction of two fragments of pulsating heart tissue. J.

Exp. Med., 39: 577-583, 1924.

Fozzard, H.A.: Conduction of the action potential. In: Handbook of Physiology: the Cardiovascular System. Sect. 2, Vol. 1. The Heart, Berne, R.M., ed., Amer. Physiol. Soc. Bethesda, Md, pp. 335-356, 1979.

Fozzard, H.A. and Schoenberg, M.: Strength-duration curves in cardiac Purkinje fibers: effects of liminal length and charge distribution. J. Physiol. (London), 226: 593-618, 1972.

Fujii, S., Hirota, A. and Kamino, K.: Optical signals from early embryonic chick heart stained with potential sensitive dyes: evidence for electrical activity. J. Physiol. (London), 304: 508-518, 1980.

Ganter, G. and Zahn, A.: Experimentelle Untersuchungen am Saugetierherzen ueber Reizbildung und Reizleitung in ihrer Beziehung zum spezifischen Muskelgewebe. Arch. Ges. Physiol., 144: 335-392, 1912.

Garofolini, L.: Rhythmical contractions of single heart muscle cells in tissue culture in vitro. J. Physiol. (London), 63: V, 1927.

Gaskell, W.H.: On the tonicity of the heart and blood vessels. J. Physiol. (London), 3: 48-75, 1880.

Gaskell, W.H.: On the rhythm of the heart of the frog and on the nature of the action of the vagus nerve. Phil. Trans. Royal Soc., 3: 993-1033, 1882.

Goshima, K.: Formation of nexuses and electrotonic transmission between myocardial and FL cells in monolayer culture. Exp. Cell Res., 63: 124-130, 1970.

Goshima, K.: Beating of myocardial cells in culture. In: Developmental and Physiological Correlates of Cardiac Muscle, Lieberman, M. and Sano, T., eds., Raven Press, New York, pp. 197-208, 1976.

Goshima, K. and Tonomura, Y.: Synchronized beating of mouse myocardial cells mediated by FL cells in monolayer culture. Exp. Cell Res., 56: 387-392, 1969.

Gros, D., Mocquard, J.P., Challice, C.E. and Schrevel, J.: Formation and growth of gap junctions in mouse myocardium during ontogenesis. J. Mol. Cell. Cardiol., 11: 543-554, 1979.

Gross, W.O.: Reizleitungsphaenomene zwischen Herzmuskelzellen in der Kultur (Film). Anat. Anz., 128: 303-310, 1971.

Hamburger, V. and Hamilton, H.L.: A series of normal stages in the development of the chick embryo. J. Morphol., 88: 49-92, 1951.

Harary, I. and Farley, B.: In vitro studies on single beating heart cells. II: Intercellular communication. Exp. Cell Res., 29: 466-474, 1963.

Harary, I., Seraydarian, M. and Gerschenson, L.E.: Effects of lipids on contractility of cultured heart cells. In: Factors Influencing Myocardial Contractility, Tanz, R.D., Kavaler, F. and Roberst, J., eds., Academic Press, New York, pp. 231-243, 1967.

Harvey, W.: De Motu Cordis. In: Classics of Cardiology (1941), Willius, F.A. and Keys, T.E., eds., Dover, New York, pp. 18-79, 1628.

Hodgkin, A.L. and Huxley, A.F.: A quantitative description of membrane current and its application to conduction and excitation in nerve. J. Physiol. (London), 117: 400-544, 1952.

Holden, A.V.: On the variability of pacemaker activity. Proceedings of the 5th European Meeting on Cybernetic and Systems Research, 1980.

Hunter, P.J., Mc Naughton, P.A. and Noble, D.: Analytical models of propagation in excitable cells. Progr. Biophys. Mol. Biol., 30: 99-144, 1975.

Jalife, J. and Moe, G.K.: Effect of electrotonic potentials on pacemaker activity of canine Purkinje fibers in relation to parasystole. Circ. Res., 39: 801-808, 1976.

Jalife, J. and Moe, G.K.: A biological model of parasystole. Amer. J. Cardiol., 43: 761-772, 1979.

Johnstone, P.N.: Studies on the physiological anatomy of the embryonic heart. I. Bull. Johns Hopkins Hosp., 35: 87-90, 1924.

Johnstone, P.N.: Studies on the physiological anatomy of the embryonic heart. II: An inquiry into the development of the heart beat in chick embryos. Bull. Johns Hopkins Hosp., 36: 299-311, 1925.

Jongsma, H.J., Masson-Pevet, M., Hollander, C.C. and De Bruijne, J.: Synchronization of the beating frequency of cultured rat heart cells. In: Developmental and Physiological Correlates of Cardiac Muscle. Lieberman, M. and Sano, T., eds., Raven Press, New York, pp. 185-196, 1976.

Keith, A. and Flack, M.W.: The auriculo-ventricular bundle of the human heart. Lancet, 2: 359-364, 1906.

Khodorov, B.I. and Timin, E.N.: Nerve impulse propagation along nonuniform fibers. Progr. Biophys. Mol. Biol., 30: 145-184, 1975.

Kölliker, A. and Mueller, H.: Nachweis der negativen Schwankung des Muskelstroms am naturlich sich contrahierende Muskel. Verhandl. J. Physiol.

Med. Gesellsch. in Wurzberg, 6: 528-533, 1855.

Lane, M.A., Sastre, A., Law, M. and Salpeter, M.M.: Cholinergic and adrenergic receptors on mouse cardiocytes in vitro. Devel. Biol., 57: 254-269, 1977.

Langendorff, O.: Studien ueber Rhythmik und Automatie des Froschherzens. Arch. Physiol. (Leipzig), 1: 133, 1884.

Langer, G.A., Frank, J.S. and Nudd, L.M.: Correlation of calcium exchange, structure and function in myocardial tissue culture. Amer. J. Physiol., 237: H239-H246, 1979.

Lapicque, L.: Recherches quantitatives sur l'excitation électrique des nerfs traitée comme une polarisation. J. Physiol. (Paris), 9: 620-635, 1907.

Le Douarin, G., Obrecht, G. and Coraboeuf, E.: Détermination régionales dans l'aire cardiaque présomptive mises en évidence chez l'embryon de poulet par la méthode microélectrophysiologique. J. Embryol. Exp. Morphol., 15: 153-167, 1966.

Le Douarin, G., Renaud, J.D., Renaud, D. and Coraboeuf, E.: Influence of insulin on sensitivity to tetrotodoxin of isolated chick embryo heart cells in culture. J. Mol. Cell. Cardiol., 6: 523-529, 1974.

Lehmkuhl, D. and Sperelakis, N.: Electrotonic spread of current in cultured chick heart cells. J. Cell. Comp. Physiol., 66: 119-133, 1965.

Lewis, M.R.: Muscular contractions in tissue culture. Contr. to Embryol., Carnegie Inst. of Washington, 9: 191-209, 1920.

Lewis, T.: Galvanometric curves yielded by cardiac beats generated in various areas of the auricular musculature. The pacemaker heart. Heart, 2: 23-46, 1910.

Lewis, T.: The Mechanism and Graphic Registration of the Heart Beat. Shaw and Sons, London, 452 pp., 1920.

Lewis, W.H.: The influence of temperature on the rhythm of the isolated heart of the young chick embryo. Bull. Johns Hopkins Hosp., 35: 253, 1924.

Lewis, T., Oppenheimer, A. and Oppenheimer, B.S.: The site of origin of the mammalian heart beat: the pacemaker in the dog. Heart, 2: 147-169, 1910.

Lieberman, M., Kootsey, J.M., Johnson, E.A. and Sawanabori, T.: Slow conduction in cardiac muscle: a biophysical model. Biophys. J., 13: 37-55, 1973.

Loewenstein, W.R.: Permeable junctions. Cold Spring Harbor Sympos. Quant.

Biol., 40: 49-63, 1975.

Lompre, A.M., Poggioli, J. and Vassort, G.: Maintenance of fast sodium channels during primary culture of embryonic chick heart cells. J. Mol.
Cell. Cardiol., 11: 813-825, 1979.

Mann, J.E. and Sperelakis, N.: Further development of a model for electrical
transmission between myocardial cells not connected by low-resistance pathways. J. Electrocardiol., 12: 23-33, 1979.

Matter, A.: A morphometric study on the nexus of rat cardiac muscle. J.   Cell
Biol., 56: 690-696, 1973.

Mazet, F.: Etude ultrastructurale des jonctions présentes dans le myocarde de
poulet. Biol. Cell. (Paris), 29: 27a, 1977.

McAllister, R.E., Noble, D. and Tsien, R.W.: Reconstruction of the electrical
activity of cardiac Purkinje fibers. J. Physiol. (London), 251: 1-59,
1975.

Mc Call, D.: Effect of quinidine and temperature on sodium uptake and contraction frequency of cultured rat myocardial cells. Circ. Res., 39:
730-739, 1976.

Mc Lean, M.J., Renaud, J.F., Sperelakis, N. and Niu, M.C.:   Messenger-RNA induction of fast sodium ion channels in cultured cardiac myoblasts.
Science, 191: 297-299, 1976.

Mc Nutt, N.S. and Weinstein, R.S.: Membrane ultrastructure at mammalian intercellular junctions. Progr. Biophys. Mol. Biol., 26: 45-101, 1973.

Meda, M. and Ferroni, A.: Early functional differentiation of heart muscle
cells. Experientia, 15: 427-428, 1959.

Mendez, C. and Moe, G.K.: Some characteristics of transmembrane potentials of
AV nodal cells during propagation of premature beats. Circ. Res., 19:
993-1010, 1966.

Mendez, C., Mueller, W.J., Meredith, J. and Moe, G.K.: Interaction of
transmembrane potentials in canine Purkinje fiber-muscle junctions. Circ.
Res., 24: 361-372, 1969.

Moscona, A.A.: Rotation-mediated histogenetic aggregation of dissociated cells.
Exp. Cell Res., 22: 455-475, 1961.

Nathan, R.D., and DeHaan, R.L.: **In vitro** differentiation of a fast sodium
conductance in embryonic heart cell aggregates. Proc. Natl. Acad. Sci.
USA, 75: 2776-2780, 1978.

Nathan, R.D. and DeHaan, R.L.: Voltage clamp analysis of embryonic heart cell aggregates. J. Gen. Physiol., 73: 175-198, 1979.

New, D.A.T.: A new technique for the cultivation of the chick embryo in vitro. J. Embryol. Exp. Morphol., 3: 320-331, 1955.

Noble, D. and Stein, R.B.: The threshold conditions for initiation of action potentials by excitable cells. J. Physiol. (London), 187: 129-162, 1966.

Norwood, C.R., Castaneda, A.R. and Norwood, W.I.: Heterogeneity of rat cardiac cells of defined origin in single cell culture. J. Mol. Cell. Cardiol., 12: 201-210, 1980.

Paff, G.H.: Transplantation of sinoatrium to conus in the embryonic heart in vitro. Am. J. Physiol., 117: 313-317, 1936.

Patten, B.M.: Initiation and early changes in the character of the heart beat in vertebrate embryos. Physiol. Rev., 29: 31-47, 1949.

Patten, B.M. and Kramer, T.C.: The initiation of contraction in the embryonic heart. Am. J. Anat., 53: 349-375, 1933.

Pickering, J.W.: Observations on the physiology of the embryonic heart. J. Physiol. (London), 14: 383-466, 1893.

Pollack, G.H.: Intercellular coupling in the atrioventricular node and other tissues of the rabbit heart. J. Physiol. (London), 255: 275-298, 1976.

Purdy, J.E., Lieberman, M., Roggeveen, A.E. and Kirk, R.G.: Synthetic strands of cardiac muscle; formation and ultrastructure. J. Cell Biol., 55: 563-578, 1972.

Sachs, F.: Electrophysiological properties of tissue cultured heart cells grown in linear array. J. Memb. Biol., 28: 373-399, 1976.

Sachs, H.G. and DeHaan, R.L.: Embryonic myocardial cell aggregates; volume and pulsation rate. Devel. Biol., 30: 233-240, 1973.

Sachs, H.G., Mc Donald, T.F. and DeHaan, R.L.: Tetrodotoxin sensitivity of cultured embryonic heart cells depends on cell interactions. J. Cell Biol., 56: 255-258, 1973.

Sanderson, J.B. and Page, F.J.M.: On the time-relations of the excitatory process in the ventricle of the heart of the frog. J. Physiol. (London), 2: 384-435, 1880.

Sano, T., Sawanabori, T. and Adaniya, H.: Mechanism of rhythm determination among pacemaker cells of the mammalian sinus node. Amer. J. Physiol.,

235: H379-H384, 1978.

Schanne, O.F., Ruiz-Ceretti, E., Payet, M.D. and Deslauriers, Y.: Influence of varied Ca^{2+}_o and Na^+_o on electrical activity of clusters of cultured cardiac cells from neonatal rats. J. Mol. Cell. Cardiol., 11: 477-484, 1979.

Scott, S.W.: Stimulation simulations of young yet cultured beating hearts. Ph. D. Thesis, State University of New York at Buffalo, 1979.

Shimada, Y., Moscona, A.A. and Fischman, D.A.: Scanning electron microscopy of cell aggregation: cardiac and mixed retina-cardiac cell suspensions. Devel. Biol., 36: 428-446, 1974.

Speicher, D.W. and Mc Carl, R.L.: Evaluation of a proteolytic enzyme mixture isolated from crude trypsin in tissue disaggregation. In Vitro, 14: 849-853, 1978.

Sperelakis, N.: Electrical properties of embryonic heart cells. In: Electrical Phenomena in the Heart, De Mello, W.C., ed., Academic Press, New York, pp. 1-61, 1972.

Sperelakis, N., Hoshiko, T. and Berne, R.M.: Non-syncytial nature of cardiac muscle: membrane resistance of single cells. Amer. J. Physiol., 198: 531-536, 1960.

Sperelakis, N., Shigenobu, K. and Mc Lean, M.J.: Membrane cation channels: changes in developing hearts, in cell culture and in organ culture. In: Developmental and Physiological Correlates of Cardiac Muscle, Lieberman, M. and Sano, T., eds., Raven Press, New York, pp. 209-233, 1976.

Stannius, H.F.: Zwei Reihen Physiologischer Versuche. I. Versuche am Froschherzen. Arch. f. Anat. und Physiol., pp. 85, 1852.

Van Capelle, F.J.L. and Durrer, D.: Computer simulation of arrhythmias in a network of coupled excitable elements. Circ. Res., 47: 454-466, 1980.

Van Mierop, L.H.S.: Location of pacemaker in chick embryo heart at the time of initiation of heart beat. Amer. J. Physiol., 212: 407-415, 1967.

Vassalle, M.: Automaticity and automatic rhythms. Amer. J. Cardiol., 28: 245-252, 1971.

Weidmann, S.: The electrical constants of Purkinje fibres. J. Physiol. (London), 118: 348-360, 1952.

Weingart, R.: The action of ouabain on intercellular coupling and conduction velocity in mammalian ventricular muscle. J. Physiol. (London), 264:

341-365, 1977.

Williams, E.H. and DeHaan, R.L.: Electrical coupling among heart cells in the
    absence of ultrastructurally defined gap junctions. J. Memb. Biol., 60:
    237-248, 1981.

Winfree, A.T.: The Geometry of Biological Time, Springer-Verlag, New York, 530
    pp., 1980.

Wybauw, M.R.: Sur le point d'origine de la systole cardiaque dans l'oreillette
    droite. Arch. Int. Physiol., 10: 78-89, 1910.

Ypey, D.L., Clapham, D.E. and DeHaan, R.L.: Development of electrical coupling
    and action potential synchrony between aggregates of embryonic heart cells.
    J. Memb. Biol., 51: 75-96, 1979.

Ypey, D.L., Van Meerwijk, W.P.M., Ince, C. and Groos, G.: Mutual entrainment
    of two pacemaker cells. A study with an electronic parallel conductance
    model. J. Theor. Biol., 86: 731-755, 1980.

DISCUSSION BY DENIS NOBLE

I would like to see if I can integrate rather an important result from the first
day's discussion with another important result from the second day's discussion
to explain an important result from the third day's discussion. The important
result from today's discussion is the one that Bob DeHaan described, that is the
fact that you can apparently synchronize a group of cells with only very few or
even a single nexal channel communicating between them. The basis of the calculation is first of all to take one of the results used in the first day's discussion of pacemaker mechanisms. You may be familiar with the fact that those
of us who work on the voltage clamp of cardiac cells often use the equation relating the

$$i_c = -c \, \frac{dV}{dt}$$

rate of change of voltage on the capacitance of the cell to the net-ionic currents that must be flowing to produce that rate of change of voltage. If for example you do that calculation for 0.1 V/s, which is about the rate of the pacemaker depolarization during diastole, you multiply that by the capacitance of the preparation and that will give you the total ionic current flowing during diastole. One of the results that Hilary Brown described in her paper was that if you do that sort of calculation for the sinus node you do indeed get a very similar estimate of ionic current compared to the current you actually record at diastolic potentials under voltage clamp conditions. So this gives one some confidence I think in using this kind of equation. Now, if you do the calculation for about a ten - and I'm not sure what size the cell I should take - but I took a ten micron cell (in diameter) and calculated that would give me about 500 microns squared of cell surface, which is about 5.10^{-6} cm squared. If we make the usual assumption that the capacitance of the membrane is $1 \mu.F/cm^2$ then clearly the capacitance that we should be using in this equation is going to be $5 \times 10^{-6} \mu F$ and we want to multiply that by 0.1 V/s in order to get our estimate of the ionic current flowing during diastole in a single cell. And if you work it out that comes to be of the order of 0.5 pA.

That is the first part of the calculation. I then took the figures that Bob DeHaan gave for the variation in intrinsic rates of single cells. I supposed that we have a couple of cells in which the intrinsic rates are different by say about 100%, which is a pretty large variation. We then suppose that those cells come together; then we are saying that one of the cells might be generating let's say 0.25 pA and the other might be generating 0.5 pA so there is a difference of 0.25 pA between them. To make the currents actually become equal therefore, about half of that difference would have to flow from cell 1 to cell 2, again dealing in orders of magnitude, we want 0.1 pA to flow and you can then ask the question how much voltage will that need across the nexus in order for that current to flow. Actually I had forgotten at the time I did this calculation what the resistance of a single nexal pore was, but that has the virtue that this calculation has got no hidden bias because I had forgotten the figure! So I put the question the other way: I said suppose we wanted to keep the voltages equal to within one millivolt, which seems to me to be about the maximum noise that Bob DeHaan is recording when the cells were very close to being disconnected, then you could say what you would need to have as a conductance for the nexal pores supposing there is only one of them connecting the cells. So we have 10^{-13} amps over 10^{-3} volts siemens of conductance and that comes out to be 10^{-10} siemens. That is the point at which I passed to Bob the question, which was what do people estimate as the resistance of a single nexus pore. He gave me the resistance 10^{10} ohms which fits rather nicely. It seems to me therefore that the result is quite extraordinary because it does mean you can synchronize on the basis even of a single nexal conductance channel.

Now I wonder whether this partly answers the question about the finger of tiny tissue going between the two cells, that DeHaan described. This connection can hardly have had a conductance less than the conductance of a single nexal pore. Doesn't that suggest also that this finger probably could synchronize the cells without difficulty?

SYNCHRONIZATION OF CARDIAC PACEMAKER CELLS BY ELECTRICAL COUPLING

A STUDY WITH EMBRYONIC HEART CELL AGGREGATES AND PACEMAKER CELL MODELS[*]

Dirk L. Ypey, Wilbert P.M. VanMeerwijk and Robert L. DeHaan

INTRODUCTION

When two cardiac pacemaker cells of different intrinsic beat frequencies are coupled electrically by nexal junctions, they exchange current through the nexal conductance. This electrical interaction interferes with the original beat rate of both cells, and if the nexal resistance is low enough, it may result in synchrony, i.e. in a simultaneous or almost simultaneous occurrence (with constant phase difference) of action potentials at the same frequency. This frequency may be different from the intrinsic frequency of either cell (DeHaan and Hirakow, 1972; Ypey et al., 1979). Whether synchrony results, depends both on the properties of the nexal and the non-nexal (excitable) membranes of the cells. For example, two coupled pacemaker cells may require a different nexal conductance to obtain synchrony if one of the two cells changes its intrinsic rate (Ypey et al., 1980).

It has been shown that pacemaker cells from different parts of the rabbit SA-node have different intrinsic rates (Lu et al., 1965; Sano et al., 1978; Mackaay et al., 1980) and probably also other different membrane properties (Mackaay et al., 1980). In addition, the tightness of electrical coupling between SA-nodal cells may vary within the SA-node (Bleeker et al., 1980).

[*] This work was partially supported by the Netherlands Organization for the Advancement of Pure Research, ZWO (D.L.Y.) and NIH Grants HL 17827 and HL 16567 (R.L.D.).

Little is known about how both pacemaker cell membrane properties and electric cell coupling contribute to generate stable SA-nodal rhythms at different
rates (Jongsma et al., 1975). The clinical relevance of this problem is obvious, since a better insight in mutual synchronization of SA-nodal pacemaker
cells will help to understand arrhythmia's arising in a sick SA-node from altered cellular pacemakers and/or electrical communication between the cells.

In order to contribute to a better understanding of mutual synchronization
of a population of electrically coupled pacemaker cells (the SA-node), we have
investigated the mutual synchronization of only two pacemakers, comparing the
behaviour of an electronic and experimental model. The experimental preparation
was a tissue culture model consisting of spontaneously beating spheroidal aggregates (diameter 100 - 200 μm) of ventricle cells dissociated from embryonic
chick hearts (Sachs and DeHaan, 1973). One such an aggregate may be considered
as one large pacemaker cell, since all cells discharge virtually simultaneously
(DeHaan and Fozzard, 1975). In addition, during diastolic depolarization membrane resistance is so much higher than both the nexal and interstitial resistance between the cells, that the membranes of the cells are virtually in parallel during that phase (Clay et al., 1979). Two suction micro-pipets connected
to micromanipulators were used to hold two aggregates and bring them into contact. Extracellular electrodes inside the suction pipets or intracellular electrodes recorded the electric activity of the aggregates. After contact, the two
aggregates developed synchrony within 3 - 30 minutes (Ypey et al., 1979),
while the electrical (nexal) resistance between the intracellular compartments
of the two aggregates declined monotonically (Clapham et al., 1980). These
experiments enabled us to choose pacemakers with different intrinsic rates and
to recognize stages of interaction and entrainment occurring during a synchronization process, in which the nexal resistance was decreasing, while no alterations (presumably) occurred in the pacemaker properties of either aggregate.

The second model used was an electronic, Hodgkin-Huxley type membrane model
of a pacemaker cell. It consisted of a leakage conductance branch, a simplified
Na- and K-conductance branch and a membrane capacitance (for details, see Ypey
et al., 1980). The leakage conductance (conducting the "background" current)
was used to control the intrinsic beat rates of two cell models. We coupled
them by an ohmic resistor representing the nexal resistance. By decreasing the
nexal resistance in small steps from high to low values, the coupling experi-

ments with the heart cell aggregates could be simulated. These experiments enabled us to identify coupling dependent synchronization phenomena for a Hodgkin-Huxley type oscillator (as the cardiac pacemaker cell is), not complicated by time dependent effects. Such effects occur during the aggregate coupling experiments, due, for example, to the continuous decline in nexal resistance, impalement artifacts, spontaneous beat interval fluctuations (Ypey et al., 1979) or overdrive suppression (Lange, 1965).

When developing electric coupling, heart cells have an increasing influence on each other and develop "mutual synchronization". A conceptually simpler experiment is to repetitively stimulate just one cell with increasing current pulse intensities at a frequency higher than the intrinsic frequency. The resulting synchronization is called "unidirectional synchronization". This experiment enabled us to identify synchronization phenomena characteristic for either type of synchronization (Ypey et al., 1980) and to recognize the role of overdrive suppression in cardiac pacemaker cell synchronization.

We found the phase response curve technique very useful as an aid to understand the entrainment phenomena occurring during unidirectional and mutual synchronization. A Phase Response Curve (PRC) is a plot of the phase shift (advance or delay) of an oscillation produced by a single pulse as a function of the phase at which the pulse is applied. (See Fig. 2 and 4). Under certain conditions, unidirectional synchronization of one oscillator and mutual synchronization between two oscillators may be quantitatively described by recurrence relations, derived from the PRC (see Appendix). Since the chronotropic effects of current pulses, as plotted in the PRC, can be interpreted in terms of the ionic pacemaker mechanism (see Noble and DiFrancesco, this volume), the PRC may be used to relate synchronization properties of pacemaker cells to the ionic mechanism of these cells.

Several investigators have used some type of PRC to characterize the phase resetting properties of cardiac pacemakers (Winfree, 1977; Jalife and Antzelevitch, 1979) or to understand irregular pacemaker activity in terms of interaction of pacemaker tissue with discharging neighbouring tissue (Jalife and Moe, 1976; Sano et al., 1978). Scott (1979) was the first to do an extensive study on the applicability of the PRC-technique to cardiac pacemaker cell entrainment and synchronization, in which he elegantly simulated nexal conductance by electronically coupling two spontaneously beating embryonic chick heart cell

agregates. Our observations on unidirectional synchronization of single aggregates and on mutual synchronization of paired aggregates as junctional resistance between them falls, confirm Scott's results.

The present paper focuses on changes in the firing pattern of a pacemaker
cell or cell group reflecting changes in electric coupling to another pacemaker
cell or cell group. Moreover, we will examine to what extent pacemaker cell interactions consist of effects of the action potentials of the cells on each others pacemaker potentials, and to what extent they consist of interactions
between the pacemaker potentials themselves. This kind of analysis yields clues
for the understanding of the effect of nexal resistance on the synchronization
frequency of two pacemaker cells of given pacemaker mechanisms. Finally, we
show how overdrive suppression interferes with heart pacemaker cell synchronization.

ELECTRONIC MODEL EXPERIMENTS ON PACEMAKER CELL SYNCHRONIZATION

UNIDIRECTIONAL SYNCHRONIZATION
Under conditions of weak coupling (i.e. low coupling conductance) mutual pacemaker cell synchronization seems to result mainly from the effects of the action
potentials of each cell on the diastolic depolarizations of the other cell.
(Sano et al., 1978; Ypey et al., 1979; Ypey et al., 1980).

Therefore, we found it useful to analyse synchronization of a pacemaker
cell by current pulses of increasing intensity applied at a frequency higher
than the intrinsic frequency of the cell (Fig. 1). The resulting unidirectional synchronization process may then be compared to mutual synchronization of two
pacemaker cells, which exchange stronger action currents from the firing to the
non-firing cell due to the development of an increasing nexal conductance. This
behavior will form an instructive background for the more complex circumstance
of mutual synchronization between two pacemaker cells.

The period T_d (see Fig. 1) between the driving stimuli (of 50 ms duration)
is 150 ms, less than one half of the period T_s of the free running slower oscillator S (T_{s0} = 340 ms). The intrinsic period of S, T_{s0}, does not fluctuate.

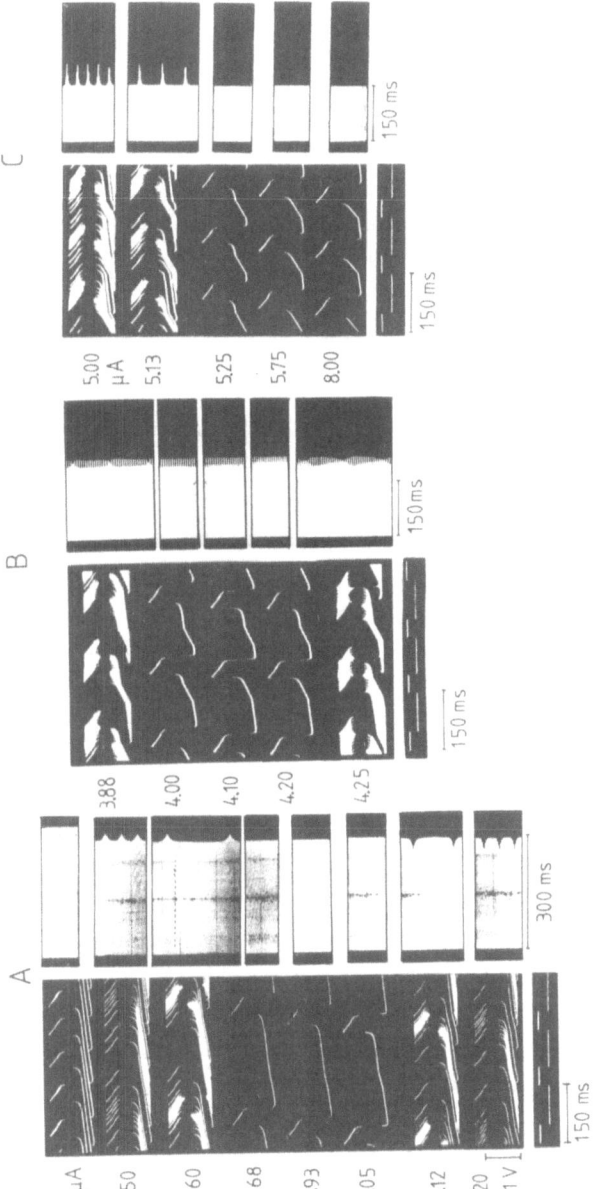

FIGURE 1 Unidirectional synchronization of a model pacemaker cell by current pulses of increasing intensity applied at a rate, faster than the intrinsic rate of the model cell. The left frames of Fig. 1A, B and C show superimposed action potential records (at least ten in most cases) triggered by the current pulses, shown at the bottom. The recordings illustrate the latency behaviour of the cell during synchronization. The intensity of the current pulses was increased in steps from 0 μA to 8.00 μA. Intensity values at which the records were taken are indicated left of the frames. The right hand frames of Fig. 1A, B and C are records of the action potential intervals as a function of time, corresponding to the left hand action potential recordings. Note that the time axis is vertical (calibration in Fig. 1C) and the interval axis is horizontal. The interval recordings illustrate the nature of the interval fluctuations during synchronization. Fig. 1A illustrates the development and disappearance of 2:1 entrainment, Fig. 1B of 4:3 entrainment and Fig. 1C the development of synchrony.

Since the scope is triggered each time after 4 stimulus cycles (600 ms), the delay between that "pulse" and the next action potential at zero current pulses (upper left sweeps of Fig. 1A) increases in constant steps of $2T_{s0} - 4T_d = 80$ ms.

When the current pulse intensity is increased to 0.5 µA, it seems as if S tends to lock to D at a given phase difference, (or latency), since the speed with which the latency increases is no longer constant (as at 0 µA), but fluctuates periodically with a minimal value around 100 ms. At the same time the interval recordings show that $\bar{T}_s$ (the mean T_s) is decreased and that T fluctuates periodically. This phenomenon is also called "beating" and is known as "oscillatory free run" in the field of circadian rhythms (cf. Pavlidis, 1973, pp. 84).

At a current pulse intensity of 0.60 µA, S is almost locked to D in a 1 per 2 fashion with an approximate phase difference of 90 ms. However, this phase difference is not constant. It increases very slowly between 70 and 120 ms, but much faster outside this range. The corresponding interval recording shows that $\bar{T}_s$ is shorter than at 0.5 µA and that this "almost entrainment", also called "fringe entrainment" (Pavlidis, 1973, pp. 84), is characterized by a periodic escape from locking towards the free run period. Other names for this phenomenon are "temporary lock-in", "temporary" or "passing synchronization" (see Pavlidis, 1978), "relative coordination" (Von Holst, 1939), "periodic pulling" (cf. Wever, 1972) or "periodic entrainment" (Ypey et al., 1980). The closer $\bar{T}_s$ is to $2T_d$, the lower the frequency of periodic escape (Fig. 1A, compare pulse intensity of 0.5 µA with 0.6 µA).

From pulse intensities 0.68 µA to 1.05 µA, T_s has exactly the value $2T_d$, so that S is entrained to the first subharmonic of D with a constant phase difference at each intensity. Within this pulse intensity range of subharmonic entrainment, the phase difference declines with increasing pulse intensity. At pulse intensities of 1.12 µA and higher, $\bar{T}_s < 2T_D$ and subharmonic entrainment is lost. Now, the phase difference between S and D decreases continuously, while S periodically escapes subharmonic entrainment to D towards shorter intervals. The escape period is longer, the closer $\bar{T}_s$ is to $2T_D$ (cf. 1.12 µA to 1.20 µA). Thus, fringe entrainment occurs at the two boundaries of subharmonic entrainment.

At the much higher pulse intensity of 5.25 µA (Fig. 1C), S is entrained to

D in a 1 to 1 fashion (synchrony) with a phase difference of $\simeq$ 90 ms. This phase difference again declines with increasing pulse intensities. At pulse intensities slightly below 5.25 μA fringe entrainment can be seen again. The closer $\bar{T}_s$ to T_d, the lower the frequency of periodic escape from synchronization (cf. 5.13 μA to 5.00 μA). The frequency of periodic escape close to the limit of entrainment is equal to the difference between the two mean frequencies of the two oscillators at a given coupling strength (Pavlidis, 1973, pp. 84). An analysis of this beating phenomenon is given by Linkens (1980) for coupled VanderPol oscillators.

At pulse intensities between 1.2 μA and 5.00 μA, the accelerating effect of the pulses on S becomes stronger and $\bar{T}_s$ takes decreasing values between $2T_d$ and T_d. Around many (we found 10) discrete pulse intensity values within this range, locking of S to D was observed in which $\bar{T}_s$ and T_d related as simple integral values m and n. The rational number m:n, which is 1 < m:n < 2 for pulse intensities between 1.2 and 5.00 μA, decreased towards unity for increasing pulse intensities. The range of pulse intensities for which S was stable entrained by D at a given m:n ratio tended to be wider for lower m+n values. Just outside both range limits of m:n entrainment, again fringe entrainment occurred. Fig. 1B illustrates stable entrainment for $\bar{T}_s$: T_d = 4:3 (at 4.00 to 4.20 μA) and the corresponding fringe entrainments (at 3.88 and 4.25 μA) just outside the entrainment limits.

As long as there is stable entrainment, there are as many different action potential latencies (latency = time period between action potential upstroke and the onset of the preceding pulse) and different action potential intervals as there are action potentials in each entrainment cycle P = mT_d = $n\bar{T}_s$). Within the entrainment limits these latencies decrease with increasing pulse intensities. At the same time the pattern of interval fluctuation gradually changes, however, with maintenance of $\bar{T}_s$ (compare 4.00 μA to 4.10 and 4.20 μA in Fig. 1B). A cycle like depicted in Fig. 1B would be called a Wenckebach cycle by cardiologists.

These results can be summarized as follows: When unidirectional coupling of the pacemaker cell to the more frequently "firing" pulse generator became stronger (larger depolarizing pulses), the pacemaker cell monotonically increased its mean rate and passed through successive stable m:n entrainment phases of which the m:n ratios approached closer and closer unity, until synchrony was

established.   Within   each m:n entrainment phase the action potential latencies
decreased.   Each m:n phase was preceded by and followed by a phase of periodic
m:n entrainment (fringe entrainment).

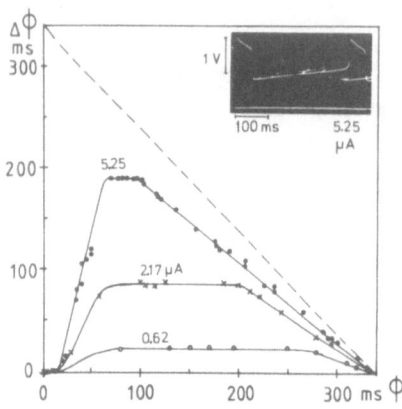

FIGURE 2 *Phase Response Curves (PRC) of the model pacemaker cell of Fig. 1 for three current pulse intensities indicated. The inset illustrates four data points of the 5.25 μA curve from superimposed action potential and pulse recordings, triggered by the action potentials. Both the phase (φ) and the change in phase (Δφ) are in ms. Note that the PRC consists of four parts. Trains of current pulses at 150 ms interval were just able to entrain the model cell in a 2:1 fashion at the pulse intensity of 0.62 μA. Pulses of 2.17 μA (at the same intervals) just caused 5:3 entrainment, while 5.25 μA pulses just caused synchrony.*

UNIDIRECTIONAL SYNCHRONIZATION AND THE PHASE RESPONSE CURVE (PRC)
The Phase Response Curve (PRC) of an oscillation is a plot of the chronotropic
effect of a single current pulse - in terms of the change in phase of the oscillation, $\Delta\phi$, as a function of the phase, ϕ, at which the pulse is applied during
the   cycle.   Fig. 2 illustrates three PRC's of the oscillator S of Fig. 1 for
three stimulus current intensities selected from   the   experiment of Fig. 1.
Both ϕ and $\Delta\phi$ (advance is positive) are in ms, with $0 \leq \phi \leq T_{s0}$ (T_{s0} = 340 ms,
the intrinsic period of S).

The PRC of the model cell consists of four successive   parts   and   exhibits
only phase advances of the oscillation (Fig. 2, inset). During the action potential, when both the sodium and the potassium conductance are high, membrane
conductance   is   high   (Ypey et al., 1980), so that a current pulse having the
duration of the action potential (50 ms) will be   relatively ineffective in
changing the time course of the voltage of the oscillation.   Considerable potassium conductance deactivation occurs within about 10 ms after sodium deactiva-

tion associated with action potential repolarization (Sodium inactivation is not included in the model). Therefore, current pulses at $0 < \phi < 10$ ms (part 1 of the PRC) are still relatively ineffective. When ϕ increases within the range $10 < \phi < 60$ ms, (part 2), the pulse more and more overlaps with the low conductance part of the pacemaker potential, so that the effect of the pulse steeply rises. Since membrane resistance is very high for $\phi > 10$ ms, the membrane simply integrates the current of the pulse. The pacemaker potential itself is the first almost linear part of a slow exponential discharge of the membrane capacitance ($\tau_m \simeq 1$ s) toward the firing threshold. Therefore, the charge applied by the pulse only shifts the pacemaker potential a given amount upwards and the advancing effect of the pulse is independent of ϕ as long as the pulse does not directly trigger the action potential (part 3). In part 4 of the PRC, the pulse discharges the membrane towards threshold, so that the avancing effect must decline with increasing ϕ. Obviously, stronger pulses at a given ϕ cause larger advances and trigger action potentials earlier in the pacemaker potential, so that the plateau in the PRC (part 3) becomes shorter for increasing pulse intensities.

Part 4 would have a slope of -1 (see dashed line in Fig. 2), if the pulse would trigger the action potential instantaneously. The time difference between dashed line and the PRC (part 4) is equal to the latency (L) with which the action potential is triggered by the pulse. Obviously, L depends both on the pulse intensity and on τ_m.

Oscillator S having an intrinsic period of 340 ms can only be driven by repetitive pulses with 150 ms intervals, if each pulse can advance S at least 190 ms. Fig. 2 shows that the PRC of a pulse intensity just able to drive S with 150 ms intervals just reaches the maximal advance of 190 ms at a latency of 80 ms (see Fig. 1C at 5.25 µA), approximately equal to the difference between the -1 slope line and the PRC at $\phi = 70$ ms.

Since it was found that a single stimulus of a given strength only resets the phase of the oscillation without influence on its time course after the pulse current is finished, the PRC for that stimulus may be used to describe the successive intervals of S, when S is perturbed by a train of those pulses starting at an arbitrary phase (for the exact procedure, see Appendix). We calculated the successive intervals from the PRC for 5.13 µA pulses (which is slightly below the PRC for 5.25 µA pulses in Fig. 2) and found indeed a periodic fluctuation in interval (see Fig. 1C). In addition, the PRC for 8.00 μA pulses (not shown in Fig. 2, but found to be above that one for 5.25 μA in Fig. 2) predicted a latency of 40 ms, which is consistent with the latency found at 8.00 μA in Fig. 1C. Similarly it is possible to check whether the PRC's in Fig. 2 at 2.17 and 0.62 μA are consistent with 5:3 and 2:1 entrainment, respectively. This problem is studied in detail by Scott (1979).

Since the PRC does not show phase delays with depolarizing pulses, the pacemaker cell model cannot be paced by pulse frequencies lower than the intrinsic frequency of the model pacemaker cell. The parameters of the model influencing this property can be adjusted as to introduce a delay in the PRC. The role of this pacemaker cell property will, however, be discussed below for a cardiac pacemaker cell cluster.

MUTUAL SYNCHRONIZATION

When two model pacemaker cells of different intrinsic frequencies are made to synchronize by decreasing the "nexal" resistance in small steps (Fig. 3), the same fringe and stable entrainment sequences occur (Ypey et al., 1980) as during unidirectional synchronization (cf. also VanCappelle and Durrer, 1980).

Figure 3A-C illustrates the sequential phases of 2:1, 3:2 and 1:1 entrainment. The oscillation period of the fast cell F at $R_c = \infty \Omega$, $T_{f\infty}$ (intrinsic period), is equal to 195 ms, while the intrinsic period of the slower cell (S), $T_{s\infty}$, is 440 ms. The mean period of F, $\bar{T}_f$, and that of S, $\bar{T}_s$, come closer together with decreasing nexal resistance. The significant difference with the unidirectional synchronization experiment is that both $\bar{T}_s$ and the mean period of the fast oscillator, $\bar{T}_f$ (instead of T_d), change. Periodic interval fluctuations, characteristic for fringe entrainment are now present in both T_f and T_s (Fig. 3A at $R_c = 1.07$ M and 540 k, Fig. 3B at $R_c = 210$ k and 250 k and Fig. 3C at $R_c = 140$ k). In addition, during one m:n entrainment cycle, when n action potentials of S occur per m action potentials of F, there are n action potential latencies (time periods between upstrokes of action potentials of S and the preceding action potentials of F), while F fluctuates with m different interval values or less and S with n different interval values or less. Finally, within the m:n entrainment range of R_c, the latencies between the action potentials of F and S decrease with decreasing R_c (compare in Fig. 3A $R_c = 1.05$ M and 570 k and in Fig. 3C $R_c = 134$ k and 30 k).

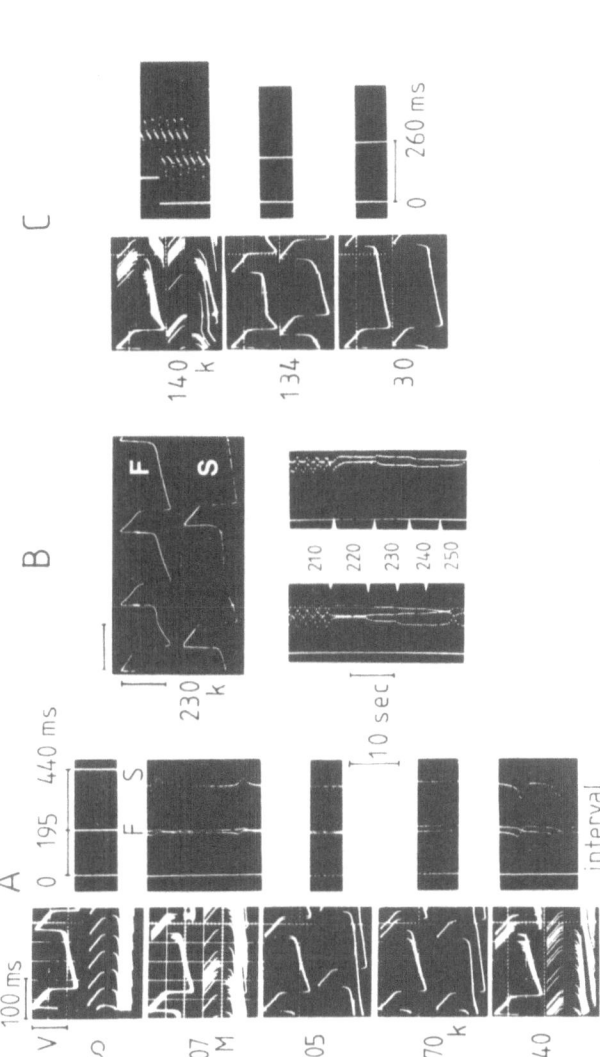

FIGURE 3 *Mutual synchronization of two model pacemaker cells of different intrinsic frequencies by a decrease in coupling resistance. Fig. 3A illustrates the development and disappearance of 2:1 entrainment, Fig. 3B of 3:2 entrainment and Fig. 3C show the development of synchrony. The left hand frames of Fig. 3A and 3C shows superimposed recordings of action potentials of the fast cell F (upper recordings in each frame) and of the slow cell S (lower recordings), triggered on the upstrokes of the action potentials of F. The upper frame of Fig. 3B shows one record of F and S, triggered on F. The right hand frames of Fig. 3A and 3C and the lower frames of Fig. 3B are recordings of action potential intervals (horizontal axis) of F and S as a function of time (vertical axis). Each white dot is one interval. The interval records of F and S have been separated in Fig. 3B, and in Fig. 3C at 140 k (shifted baseline). The action potential records illustrate the latency behaviour and the interval records the nature of the interval fluctuations during synchronization. This figure is made up, with permission, from Figs. 4, 5 and 6 of Ypey et al., J. Theor. 86, 731–755, 1980. Copyright by Academic Press Inc. (London) Ltd.*

Other differences between unidirectional and mutual synchronization concern effects of R_c on T_f at weak coupling (R_c = 1.07 M) and on T_f and T_s during subharmonic entrainment (R_c = 1.05 M to 570 k) and synchrony ($R_c \leq$ 134 k). T_f < $T_{f\infty}$ at R_c = 1.07 M, 1.05 M and 134 k, though F is connected to the slower os- cillator S. Further, this accelerating effect of S on F disappears with better coupling (compare intervals at R_c = 1.05 with those at 570 k and at R_c = 134k with those at 30k).

We conclude from these effects that at weak coupling the interaction of F and S through effects of their action potentials on each others pacemaker poten- tials is stronger than through pacemaker potential interactions. For depolariz- ing current pulses, as flowing during action potentials in F or S, can only ac- celerate the pacemaker potential of the not-firing cell (see the PRC, Fig. 2) while pacemaker potential interactions can only decelerate F. Thus, at weak coupling the action potential is a stronger synchronizer and rate determining factor than the pacemaker potential. During 2:1 entrainment and synchrony part of this rate determining effect disappears with decreasing R_c, for the latency declines causing less overlap of the action potential of S with the pacemaker potential of F (compare intervals at R_c = 1.05 M to those at 570 k and intervals at 134 k to those at 30 k). Indeed, the paradoxical accelerating effect of S on F could be made even more pronounced by increasing the action potential duration of S relative to that of F. However, the fact that T_f may become longer than $T_{f\infty}$ if no action potential of S perturbs the pacemaker potential of F (as for example in Fig. 3A at 570 k) reveals that pacemaker potential interactions are effective at any degree of coupling.

The synchronized frequency of F and S at R_c = 0 Ohm, appeared intermediate between the intrinsic frequencies of F and S. The exact value of the inverse of the length of the diastolic interval T^* (= T minus the action potential duration of 50 ms) at R_c = 0 Ohm ($1/T^*_{sync0}$ = 4.75 s^{-1}) was equal to the mean value of the inverse diastolic intervals $1/T^*_s$ = 2.56 s^{-1} and $1/T^*_f$ = 7.0 s^{-1} of the un- coupled cells S and F. This value also followed directly from the relationship between the diastolic interval of the pacemaker cell and the leakage resistance (controlling the linear background current), assuming that F and S only differ in R_L (Ypey et al., 1980). The experiment of Fig. 3, therefore, provides an example in which the synchronized frequency at very low R_c simply follows from the pacemaker properties of the single cells and illustrates that the fast pacemaker cell F does not necessarily function as the "ratemaker" during synchrony with the slower pacemaker cell S. In fact, F only seems to do so (i.e. to "drive" S at its own rate) at some specific coupling strength (R_c slightly smaller than 134 k, see Fig. 3C). But even in that case, it should be kept in mind that it is not only F that determines this synchronized rate (accidentally with the intrinsic period of F), but also the reverse effect of the action potential of S on the pacemaker potential of F and the pacemaker potential interactions contribute to the synchronized rate. For the case, that only action potentials have effects on the neighbour cell, the synchronized frequency may be calculated with the method described in the appendix.

HEART CELL AGGREGATE SYNCHRONIZATION

UNIDIRECTIONAL HEART CELL AGGREGATE SYNCHRONIZATION

The Phase Response Curve (PRC) of an oscillator for a given pulse intensity may be used to describe quantitatively synchronization, m:n entrainment and periodic entrainment by a train of pulses at a given frequency if each pulse of the train causes an instantaneous shift of the oscillation. This implies, that a pulse perturbing a given cycle does not influence the next cycle and that the oscillator does not change its intrinsic frequency during the application of the pulse train. In this section we investigate whether this requirement is met by the spontaneously beating chicken embryonic heart cell aggregate and, if not, how "pacing the pacemaker" interferes with entrainment. Fig. 4B shows a PRC of an aggregate, beating spontaneously in the presence of TTX. One intracellular electrode was used to pass 1 nA/80 ms current pulses. The upper, low gain traces in Fig. 4A1 and A2 show one unperturbed oscillation cycle and, superimposed, one perturbed cycle. The phase and duration of the current pulse is marked by the square voltage drop across the micro-electrode resistance (approx. 40 MOhm). The pulse in Fig. 4A1 occurs early in the pacemaker potential ($\phi=$ 150 ms) and causes a considerable delay (> 100 ms) in the occurrence of the next action potential, though the depolarization on top of the unperturbed pacemaker potential is only approximately 1 mV (lower high gain traces Fig. 4A1).

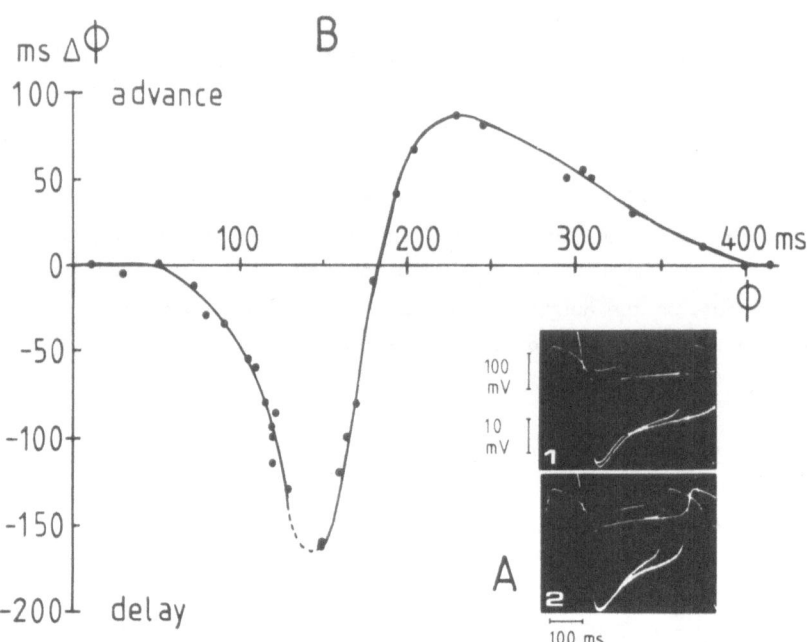

FIGURE 4 *Phase Response Curve (PRC) of an embryonic heart cell aggregate (150 μm in diameter), spontaneously beating in the presence of TTX (1.0 x 10 gr/ml). A1 and A2 show low gain (upper traces) and hight gain records (lower traces), in which one perturbed cycle is superimposed on one unperturbed cycle. The low gain records are from the electrode used to pass the 80 ms/1 nA current pulses. The square voltage deflections (voltage drop across the electrode resistance) in these records indicate the phase at which the pulses have been applied. The (lower) high gain records are from another intracellular microelectrode. In B both the phase, φ, and the change in phase, Δφ, have been plotted in ms. Note, that the PRC shows action potential delays for pulses applied just after the action potential and advances for pulses applied later in the cycle. The slow action potential upstroke indicates that the fast sodium conductance is blocked by TTX.*

If the same pulse occurs later in the cycle (φ= 215 ms, as shown in Fig. 4A2), it advances the next action potential 70 ms. The change in phase, Δφ , is plotted as a function of the phase φ in Fig. 4B. The resulting PRC exhibits both a significant delay and advance part. A similar PRC-shape has been found in control experiments without TTX, as has been reported by Scott (1979). Therefore, this shape does not critically depend on the presence of the fast sodium conductance system. In addition, it follows from the PRC that phase resetting results almost exclusively from effects of the pulses on the ionic processes underlying diastolic depolarization.

The phase changes in Fig. 4 were measured with pulses separated by approximately 10 undisturbed oscillation cycles. A plot of all successive intervals in the experiment of Fig. 4 showed that the intervals immediately following the perturbed oscillation cycle were not significantly different in length from the mean undisturbed cycle length.

The aggregate, characterized by the PRC of Fig. 4, was driven by pulse trains at different frequencies near the intrinsic frequency in order to determine the frequency limits of entrainment. Fig. 5 gives the interval records for each frequency (Fig. 5a1 to g1) and some corresponding action potential records (Fig. 5a2, b2, c2, e2 and f2).

As expected from the PRC, the aggregate can be accelerated (Fig. 5a, b) by a pulse train faster than its intrinsic frequency and decerelated (Fig. 5f) by a train of lower frequency. During accelerated synchrony the pulse immediately precedes the action potential (Fig. 5a2 to c2). During decelerated synchrony, which was impossible in the model pacemaker cell, the action potential precedes the pulse (Fig. 5e2, f2).

Significant time dependent effects appear near the limits of entrainment (fig. 5c, d, f, g). When the limits of synchrony are determined from the records in which synchrony immediately after the fast transient following the onset of the train just does not occur anymore, one finds an entrainment range of frequencies of 2.1 to 3.1 Hz, corresponding to an interval range of 320 to 480 ms. This is in rather good agreement with the range of 330 to 480 ms, predicted from the PRC (Fig. 4), taking in consideration the stability criterion (Pavlidis, 1973, pp. 88), that the pacemaker only synchronized to the pulse train at pulse phases for which the PRC has a slope s, $-2 < s < 0$. The small difference in observation and prediction is thought to be due to the scatter in the data points in the PRC and to a small drift in intrinsic interval of the aggregate from 415 to 400 ms during the experiment.

The time dependent effects, however, are such that the actual limits of synchrony during steady state driving are smaller than those just after the onset of the train. For example, in Fig. 5c and f the aggregate first seems perfectly entrained, but after about 0.5 min periodic entrainment starts to

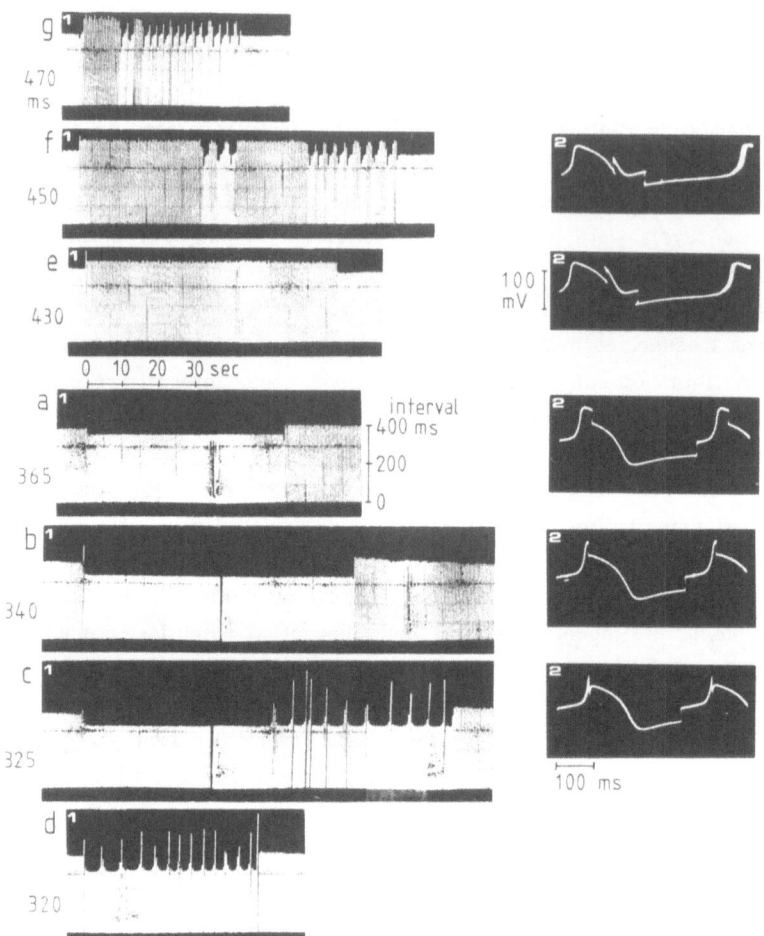

FIGURE 5 *Unidirectional synchronization of the heart cell aggregate by current pulses at frequencies around the intrinsic frequency of the aggregate. Same aggregate, conditions, pulse duration and intensity as in Fig. 4. The left hand interval records have been taken in the order a1 to g1. The right hand interval records of a few superimposed action potentials have been made within 20 s after the initial fast transient of a few pulses. The square current pulse artifacts on the action potential recordings indicate the phase relationship at each driving frequency. The intervals at which the aggregate has been driven are indicated left of the records a1 to g1. Driving starts at t = 0 s and stops after 45 to 100 s. Driving at too short (c1 and d1) or too long intervals (f1 and g1) results in a loss of synchrony characterized by periodic interval fluctuations.*

occur. Inspection of records b1 and c1 shows that the intrinsic interval of the aggregate is transiently increased after driving at a faster rate. This pheno- menon is known as overdrive suppression (Lange, 1965) and is probably due to changes in potassium concentration in the extracellular space (Boyett and Jewell, 1980). Apparently, overdrive suppression interferes with synchroniza- tion making synchronization of a slow pacemaker by a dominant faster pacemaker more difficult instead of more easy (Vassalle, 1971). This is consistent with reports (Ypey et al.,, 1980; Pavlidis, 1973) that two pacemakers require a greater degree of coupling (i.e. stronger pulses) to become synchronized, the more they differ in intrinsic frequency.

The behavior of the oscillator near the limits of entrainment appears to be a sensitive monitor of the process of overdrive suppression, since this process is also reflected in a lengthening of the latency even within the frequency range of stable steady state entrainment (for example in record Fig. 5b). Even after the establishment of periodic entrainment, time dependent effects may still be visible in the period of periodic escape from entrainment (Fig. 5c, d, f, g).

If acceleration slows the intrinsic rate of a pacemaker, one may expect that deceleration would act in an opposite way to increase the endogenous pace- maker rate. Fig. 5e1 and f1 show that this is the case. Immediately after the end of the train the action potential interval is shorter than just before the train. This accelerating effect of decelerating entrainment also opposes entra- inment, as is apparent from Fig. 5f1 and g1. Again, the difference between the entraining pulse frequency and the intrinsic pacemaker frequency becomes greater during entrainment and time dependent effects are visible in the interval re- cords. This phenomenon could be called "underdrive acceleration", in contrast to overdrive suppression.

Similar time dependent effects have been observed without TTX and during experiments in which the frequency range was determined for 2:1 and 4:3 entrain- ment. Therefore, we conclude that entrainment of the heart cell aggregate to- wards higher or lower frequencies changes the intrinsic oscillator properties, so that the PRC cannot be used to exactly predict steady state entrainment char- acteristics, unless some type of correction is applied. However, entrainment just after the onset of the train is well accounted for by the PRC.

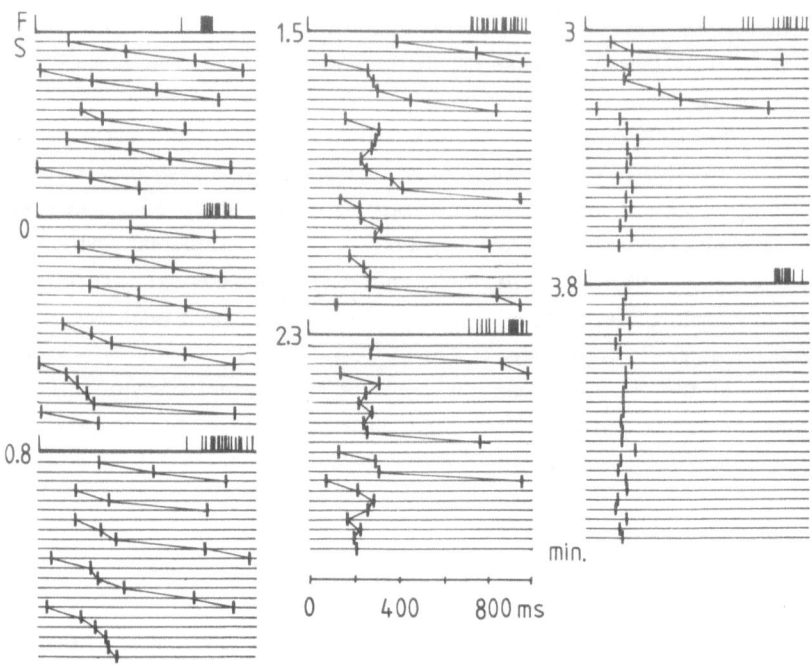

FIGURE 6 *Development of synchrony between two spontaneously beating aggregates F (faster aggregate) and S (slower aggregate) with close intrinsic frequencies. The electrical activity of both aggregates was recorded continuously by extracellular electrodes inside the suction pipets, holding the aggregates. The spike recordings of F were superimposed to illustrate changes in the interval (upper trace in each frame). The spike recordings of S were displayed as successive single sweeps triggered by the spikes of F. The recordings in the upper left frame have been made 6 min before bringing the aggregates into contact at t = 0 min. Numbers left to each frame indicate times in min after contact. To illustrate the latency behaviour of S, the spikes of S in successive records have been connected by lines. Cytochalasin B (0.33 µg/ml) was used to block mechanical contractions. In this preparation no TTX was present. The aggregates were approximately 160 µm in diameter. The spikes, drawn schematically in this figure, were approximately 1 ms in duration and a few mV in amplitude.*

MUTUAL HEART CELL AGGREGATE SYNCHRONIZATION

The entrainment phenomena described in the previous sections for unidirectional synchronization may be recognized when two aggregates mutually synchronize as a result of the development of electrical coupling (Ypey et al., 1979; Scott, 1979). Recognition may, however, be more difficult, because of the continuous decrease in coupling resistance and due to intrinsic spontaneous fluctuations in the length of the oscillation cycle.

Fig. 6 shows an example of periodic entrainment during the development of synchrony between two aggregates F and S which did not differ much in their mean intrinsic periods ($\bar{T}_s \simeq 860$ ms, $\bar{T}_f \simeq 800$ ms). The extracellular records of F and S are displayed on the screen of a scope while triggering the sweeps on the spikes of F and moving the trace of S downward in steps after each sweep. The uppermost trace in each frame displays the superimposed records from F.

Before contact (Fig. 6, upper left frame) the latency between F and S is not constant, but increases with constant mean increments equal to the difference in the mean intervals of S and F, $\bar{T}_s - \bar{T}_f$. Since the scope is triggered by each second spike of F, the records show increments of 2 $(\bar{T}_s - \bar{T}_f)$. In addition, interval fluctuations are visible in the superimposed sweeps of F. Part of these fluctuations must be present in the fluctuations visible in the phase difference increment per two cycles of F.

Already 1.5 min after contact interactions between F and S begin in that the latencies of successive intervals of S start to cluster in groups near a value of 150 ms. This phenomenon, termed "partial synchrony" by DeHaan and Hirakow (1972), becomes more pronounced until synchrony is established at a seemingly constant mean latency of about 200 ms, 3.5 min after initial contact. During partial synchrony, interval fluctuations in F are increased. After synchrony is achieved, this excess fluctuation disappears and the aggregates beat with an interval approximately equal to that of S before contact. During the subsequent 30 - 60 min, the mean latency declines slowly to < 1 ms (Ypey et al., 1979; Clapham et al., 1980).

The phenomenon of partial synchrony may now be identified with periodic entrainment as described in the previous section and in other papers on coupling of oscillators. In experiments like illustrated in Fig. 6, periodic entrainment was not obvious from the interval recordings (as in Fig. 3) because of the spontaneous fluctuations in the oscillation cycle of both aggregates.

Fig. 7 gives another example of mutual aggregate synchronization in which periodic interval fluctuations associated with entrainment were difficult to separate from randomly looking fluctuations. In this case, the intrinsic periods of the two aggregates seemed to differ more than a factor of five, the slow aggregate being very irregular. The records show that S becomes faster during

sec Interval

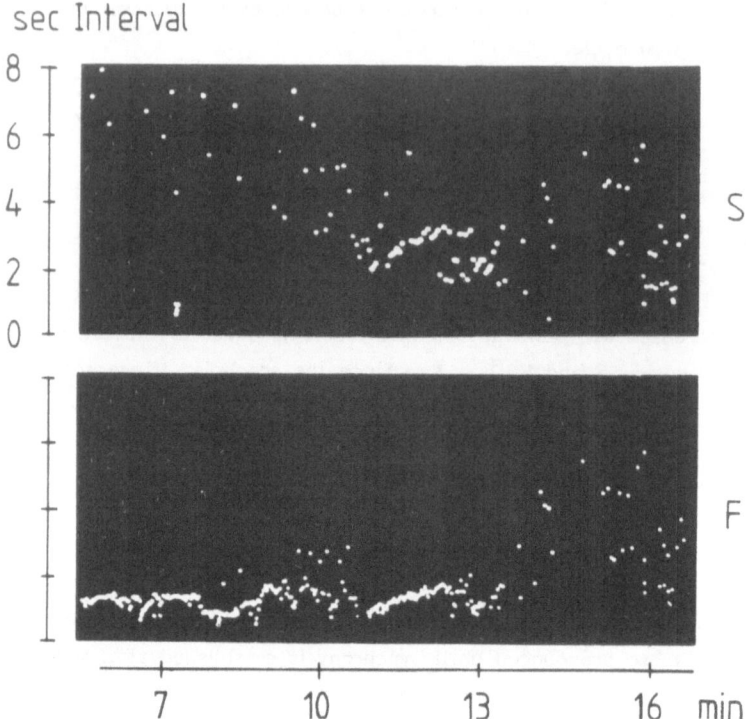

FIGURE 7 Development of synchrony between two spontaneously aggregates F (faster aggregate) and S (slower aggregate) with widely different intrinsic frequencies. At t = 0 min, the aggregates were pushed together. Within about 5 min
after contact each aggregate was impaled by an intracellular electrode. Both
frames are records of successive intervals of S (upper frame) and F (lower
frame). Each white dot represents one interval. After about 13.5 min the dot
patterns of F and S are identical (apart from a few missed intervals), indicating synchrony. Note the changes in the interval fluctuations and in the mean
interval during synchronization. Cytolchalasin B (0.33 µg/ml) was used to suppress contractions. S was 180 µm and F 150 µm in diameter.

the development of coupling. Only the 2:1 entrainment phase is clearly recog-
nizable in the period 11-12.5 min. In this phase the increase in coupling is
accompanied by an increase in the mean interval of F and S, as observed in the
model pacemaker cell coupling experiment. This increase cannot be due to the
disappearance of the accelerating feedback effect of the S spike on the diastolic depolarization of F (as assumed in model cell coupling), since the PRC of ag-

gregates has a phase delay part in the early phase of the pacemaker potential. Therefore, the increase in mean interval during this subharmonic entrainment phase may be due to increased pacemaker potential interactions and/or to a change in phase of the action potential of F, which is not closely followed by an action potential of S.

After synchrony at t = 13.5 min, while the latency between the action potentials of F and S is decreasing (Ypey et al., 1979) the mean interval is between that of F and S at the beginning of the records. However, the pair also has become very irregular. Therefore, it seems that S not only influences the synchronized rate of the pair, but also imposes its irregularity on the pair. Other examples of this were shown by DeHaan and Hirakow (1972) in the entrainment of pairs of single cells.

DISCUSSION

The entrainment phenomena observed during model pacemaker cell synchronization, i.e. the successive occurrence of periodic entrainment and m:n entrainment phases, have also been found in the unidirectional and mutual synchronization experiments on the heart cell aggregates despite the differences between these model systems in PRC and pacemaker mechanism. Apparently, these phenomena do not require a specific type of Hodgkin-Huxley model. On the other hand, we even observed that two pacemaker model cells of different pacemaker mechanisms may synchronize and simply skip the entrainment phases preceding synchrony (unpublished results). Still, the recognition of these phenomena in clinical conditions or physiological experiments is of importance since they signal changes in coupling strength between pacemakers or pacemaker areas. If under certain conditions the value of the coupling conductance between two pacemakers would remain constant, but the pacemakers would change their properties or increase the differences in their intrinsic rates, one may even expect these phenomena in the reverse direction as seen in our experiments, since the original coupling conductance may become insufficient for synchrony. In such cases "relative coupling strength" is changing. The periodic variations in interval length between

SA-nodal discharges found by Schaer (1968) in low Ca^{++} concentrations, which were not understood at that time, may be explained by changes in the relative coupling between two pacemaker areas within the SA-node. Clinical conditions for the occurrence of many of the entrainment phenomena described are well known as AV-blocks of different degrees.

DeHaan and Hirakow (1972) demonstrated that a fast pacemaker cell does not necessarily impose its rate on a slow cell, that is, pacemaker cells undergo mutual synchronization. Similarly, the synchronization of the pacemaker structures within the intact embryonic heart is also interactive (DeHaan, this volume). In the adult human heart, the SA-node rate dominates the AV-node rate. Thus, on must conclude that the coupling structure between the SA- and the AV-node (which includes the atrium) is such, that synchronization between these pacemakers is unidirectional. However, the SA nodal rate may be under influence of the surrounding atrial tissue. Within the SA-node interaction between pacemaker cells may be recognized as mutual synchronization (Sano et al., 1978).

From the experiments discussed it seems useful to discriminate two main types of pacemaker cell interactions during synchronization: 1) effects of action potentials of one cell on the cycle of the other cell and 2) pacemaker potential (or diastolic) interactions between the cells. Interactions between the action potentials of two cells and effects of the pacemaker potential of one cell on the shape of the action potential of the other cell, do also exist but are not likely to have significant influences on the rate of discharge of the two coupled cells.

If interaction type 1 dominates, the complete behavior of two coupling oscillators, including the synchronized rate of discharge, follows from the PRC's of both oscillators for any degree of coupling (see Appendix). In that case a PRC of a pacemaker cell is a curve of the phase resetting effect of an action potential-like pulse from another pacemaker cell, the intensity of which is determined by the coupling conductance. Depending on the amplitude of the phase delay and phase advance part of the PRC, one may expect any of the three possibilities observed by DeHaan and Hirakow (1972): The synchronized rate may be faster than that of the fast cell, it may be slower than that of the slow cell, or it may be intermediate between that of the fast and the slow cell.

The stronger the phase resetting effects of the action potentials of two coupled cells are on each others pacemaker potentials at a given degree of cou-

pling, the more this type (1) of interaction will dominate the pacemaker potential (type 2) interaction. However,after synchrony has been established, type 2
interaction comes more and more into play with stronger coupling.   In the extreme case, when coupling resistance falls to a value which is very small relative to membrane resistance, two oscillators fuse to a new single oscillator and
pacemaker potential interactions seem dominant in controlling the synchronized
frequency. For the simple case of the model pacemaker cell synchronization, in
which a linear background current was used to control pacemaker rate, the synchronized frequency at zero coupling resistance was intermediate between the
frequencies of the single cells and followed from the relationship between the
leakage resistance and the intrinsic rate of the single cell. This relationship
was identical for both cells.

In the unidirectional synchronization experiment on the model cell it was
found that certain m:n entrainment phases were stable over a larger range of
pulse intensities than others. This property of the cell results from the shape
and amplitude of the PRC (see Appendix). How this entrainment property exactly
relates to the PRC is an open question, which may have functional implications
for the entrainment properties of the AV-node of the heart.

The role of overdrive suppression in mutual synchronization may be viewed
as follows: suppose that two pacemaker cells synchronize by way of action potential interactions towards an intermediate frequency. Since, in that case the
slow cell S will fire at an increased rate, it is subject to overdrive suppression and decreases its intrinsic rate. The fast cell F is slowed by the interaction, develops underdrive acceleration, and increases its intrinsic rate.
This means that the difference between the intrinsic rates increases during synchronization, requiring a greater degree of coupling than would be predicted by
the original rates to maintain synchrony (Ypey et al., 1980). Thus, the development of overdrive suppression reduces the "safety factor" of synchronization. This is contrary to the view of Vassalle (1971).

CONCLUSIONS

(1) When two pacemaker cells develop nexal junctions one may expect the successive development of a series of periodic entrainment phases and m:n entrainment
phases before synchrony establishes. (2) These phases - at least partly - result from phase resetting effects of the action potentials of the cells on each
others pacemaker potentials, since these phases do also occur during unidirectional synchronization of a single pacemaker cell to a pulse train of a given
(higher) frequency, if the pulse intensity is gradually increased. Therefore
(3), the PRC technique is an useful aid in the interpretation of the resulting
entrainment phenomena. (4) During mutal synchronization, however, one observes
changes in the mean frequency of both oscillators. Part of these rate changes
are due to pacemaker potential interactions. (5) Overdrive suppression appeared
to "counteract" synchronization.

APPENDIX by W.P.M. VanMeerwijk

THE PHASE RESPONSE CURVE AND SYNCHRONIZATION
Consider a spontaneously firing cell, with period P. Suppose the only effect of
a short current pulse at phase ϕ is to advance or delay the next coming action
potential without any influence upon subsequent intervals, thus "shifting the
whole spike train". Then we may say that the pulse "renewed" the phase of the
oscillator:

$$\phi_{new} = f(\phi) = \phi + \Delta(\phi) \tag{1}$$

A plot of $\Delta(\phi)$ as a function of ϕ is called a phase response curve (PRC). If we
apply pulses with a fixed interval T and look for 1/1 synchrony, we will obtain
a recurrence relation for the phases at which two subsequent pulses fall (Fig.
8A). After the n-th action potential, a pulse at phase ϕ_n resets the phase to
$f(\phi_n)$. When the next pulse arrives T ms later, it should fall in a subsequent
interval, at ϕ_{n+1}. To establish a relation between ϕ_n and ϕ_{n+1}, we note:

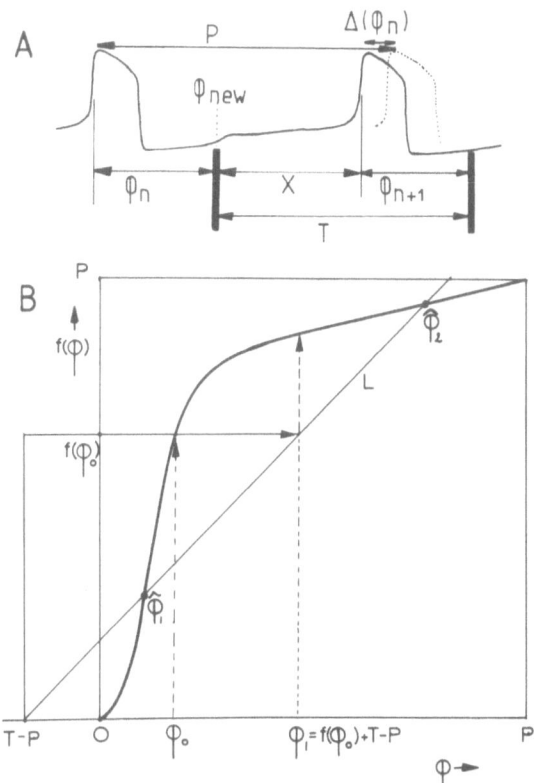

FIGURE 8 A. *Action potentials number n and n+1 of a regularly firing (model) cell. The dotted action potential would have been recorded if no current pulse was given at phase ϕ_n. This pulse changes the phase with $\Delta(\phi_n)$. After this change, the oscillator behaves as if it was in the new phase ϕ_{new}, so that the latency x until the next action potential is equal to the difference between the intrinsic period P and ϕ_{new}. B. Plot of the new phase $\phi_{new} = f(\phi)$ versus the old phase ϕ, as measured from the model pacemaker cell for a given current pulse intensity. L is a line with unity slope and horizontal intercept T-P (negative in this case!). Further explanations in the text.*

$$T = x + \phi_{n+1}$$

in which x is the latency between the pulse and the first coming action potential; x is also equal to:

$$x = P - \phi_{new}$$

Hence

$$\phi_{n+1} = T - P + f(\phi_n) \tag{2}$$

The properties of (2) determine whether we actually will see entrainment. This can be graphically illustrated with the aid of Fig. 8B. It consists of the graph of f and a line L through $\phi = T - P$ with slope unity. Starting at a phase ϕ_o one finds a function value $f(\phi_o)$. If we now construct a square with sides $f(\phi_o)$ and diagonal L, we find that the lower right corner has abscissa $f(\phi_o) + T - P$, or ϕ_{o+1}. (Note that T-P is negative in Fig. 8). This gives the following recipe for finding the successive phase at which a next pulse comes in: go vertically to the graph of f, thence horizontally to L. The abscissa of this point is the next ϕ. It is easy to see in Fig. 8B, that if we start anywhere right from $\hat{\phi}_1$, we arrive in $\hat{\phi}_2$ and stay there: a fixed phase relationship between the cell and pulse generator is established, i.e. they are synchronized. The analytical formulation of this so called stability criterion can be found in Guckenheimer et al. (1977). An initial value left of $\hat{\phi}_1$ leads to a negative next phase, i.e. a second pulse in the same interval, so we enter the graph again from the right.

It is the form of f that determines whether we will actually see entrainment. When f does not intersect L, we cannot drive the cell with this period T. We can perhaps if we use a higher pulse intensity to give the PRC sufficiently more amplitude.

A similar reasoning can be used to describe mutual synchronization of two pacemaker cells (Fig. 9A). In the upper trace a cell is influenced between its two spikes, number n and n+1, at phase ϕ_n by his neighbour. The lower trace is of the other cell, showing his spike number n+1, being reset before and after it by the upper cell at respective phases ψ_n and ψ_{n+1}. We see, that:

$$\psi_{n+1} = P1 - f(\phi_n)$$

and:

$$\phi_n = P2 - g(\psi_n)$$

with f resp. g the renewed phase function of cell 1, resp. 2. Substitution gives:

$$\psi_{n+1} = P1 - f(P2 - g(\psi_n)) \tag{3}$$

So, we have again a first order recurrence relation, now depending upon both the PRC of cell 1 and cell 2 and allowing for asymmetric influence of the partners upon each other. Again it is possible to illustrate graphically the sequence of events: Fig. 9B.

Along the vertical axis the function P2 - g (.) is plotted against a horizontal argument, the continuous curve. So for a given ψ we find vertically above it the function value P2 - $g(\psi)$. Because this number is in eq. (3) used as the argument of another function, P1 - f(.), it is possible to find this second function value in the same figure by simply plotting the graph of P1 - f(.) along the horizontal axis for a vertically increasing argument. This is the dotted curve in Fig. 9B. Combining the two graphs gives the following recipe for iterating (3):

For an initial phase difference between cell 1 and cell 2, say cell 2 is in advance by an amount ψ_o, start at this point at the horizontal axis. Find the effect of the spike of cell 1 upon cell 2 as the function value P2 - $g(\psi_0)$. This is the phase at which cell 1 in his turn is affected, thus leading to an effect which is found by moving horizontally to the other graph (the inverse of P1 - f(.)). This point is thus our next $\psi:\psi_1$. The stability criterion is easily derived from the angle of intersection of the two graphs.

We can derive a general recursion relation for the description of a driving experiment. Consider an oscillator that is producing an continuous file of substance called "phase" (ϕ), starting from time zero. A stimulus causes it to instantaneously change the amount hitherto produced by an amount D, dependent upon the amount produced already:

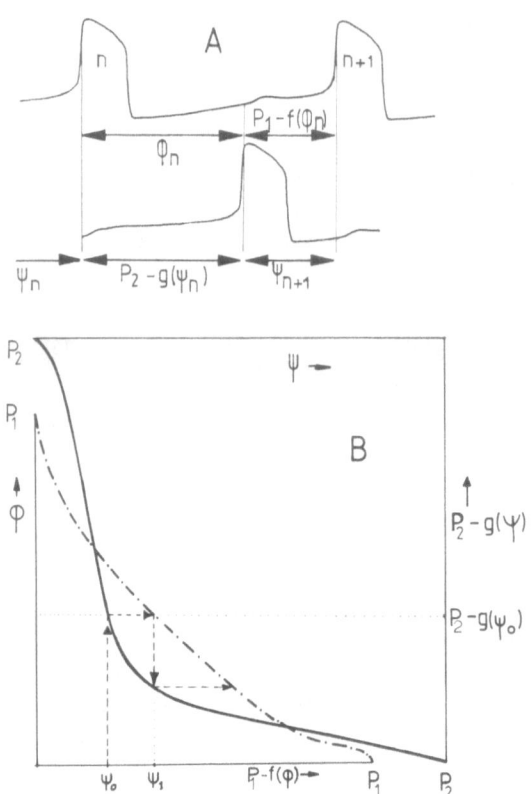

FIGURE 9 A. *Mutual synchronization of two pacemaker cells. When the lower cell is in phase* Ψ_n, *the upper cell fires and resets the phase of the lower to* $g(\Psi_n)$. *After a latency of* $P_2 - g(\Psi_n)$ *the lower cell fires and resets the phase of the upper one from* ϕ_n *to* $f(\phi_n)$. *B. The continous line is the graph of* $P_2 - g(\Psi)$ *versus* Ψ, *as indicated on the right and upper side of the graph. The dotted curve is* $P_1 - f(\phi)$ *in mirror image, with* ϕ *vertically and* $P_1 - f(\phi)$ *horizontally (see left and lower axis respectively). Further explanations in the text.*

$$D = D(\phi) = \Delta\,(\phi(\text{mod } P))$$

If we now stimulate the process repetitively with a constant interval T and number our successive stimuli, we get a recursion relation for the phase at the arrival of the next stimulus, as a function of the phase its predecessor saw:

$$\phi_{n+1} = \phi_n(\text{new}) + T = f(\phi_n) + T \overset{\text{def}}{=} F(\phi_n)$$

The graph of F is simply the old phase-new phase curve endlessly repeated along the main diagonal against ϕ, (Fig. 10; the example is the curve of the elec- tronic model). The question "Is there for every pulse intensity only one entra- inment ratio m:k (for fixed duration of the pulse)?" is equivalent to the graph- ical problem:

"Is there an m, such that after m squares in Fig. 10, the next phase (mo- dulo P) equals the initial phase, because of the accumulated effect of k equi- distant stimuli?"

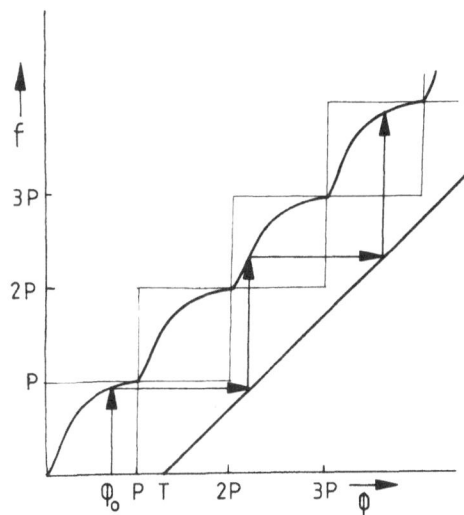

FIGURE 10 General representation of a driving experiment. Each square con- tains an exact copy of the old phase – new phase curve of fig. 8B. The thick line parallels the main diagonal at hor- izontal distance T. The phase in which each next pulse falls (vertical arrow) is found from $\phi_{n+1} = f(\phi_n) + T$, in a similar way as illustrated in Fig. 8B.

In formula:

$$\phi_{n+k} = mP + \phi_n$$

If so, then the time required to do this is:

$$kT = mP - \sum_{i=1}^{k} \Delta(\Omega_i)$$

Ω_i being the phase (mod P) of the i-th stimulus. This defines a mean period $\bar{P}$ for the driven oscillator:

$$kT = m\bar{P}$$

The general problem of one-sided synchronization is: Under what conditions upon the PRC is there an unique solution for k, m and a vector of k different ϕ's in the problem

$$F^{(k)}(\phi) = \phi + mP$$

$$kT = mP - \sum_{i=1}^{k} \Delta(\Omega_i)$$

$$\Delta(\Omega_i) = (F(\phi_{i-1}) - \phi_{i-1})(\text{mod } P)$$

Now we may ask what happens if we change the stimulus intensity, i.e. the form of F?   Can we expect the synchronization phenomena as described in Ypey et al. (1980), or are these phenomena only properties of the special type of PRC.   It seems natural to expect a deviation from the monotony properties found there in case of a PRC with a phase delay part.

The general problem of mutual synchronization of two pacemakers remains to be formulated.   However, its solution will probably not be easy to find if at all. The first papers on the PRC to describe synchronization in a different context were by Moore et al. (1963) and Perkel et al. (1964). Formulas (2) and (3) can also be found in Pavlidis (1973; 1978). Some mathematical properties of difference (or recurrence) relations can be found in Guckenheimer et al. (1977). It will be interesting to compare the bifurcation of behaviour with increasing stimulus intensity with results in theoretical population biology. For a review see May (1976).

ACKNOWLEDGEMENT

We are very grateful to Drs. D.E. Clapham (Dept. Anat., Emory University, Atlanta), G. Groos and C. Ince (Dept. Physiol., Univ. of Leiden) for their cooperation in parts of the work, reviewed in this paper.

REFERENCES

Bleeker, W.K., Mackaay, A.J.C., Masson-Pevet, Bouman, L.N. and Becker, A.E.: Functional organization of the rabbit sinus node. Circ. Res., 46: 11-22, 1980.

Boyet, M.R. and Jewell, B.R.: Analysis of the effects of changes in rate and rhythm upon electrical activity in the heart. Progr. Biophys. Mol. Biol., 36: 1-52, 1980.

Capelle, F.J.L. van, and Durrer, D.: Computer simulation of arrhythmias in a network of coupled excitable elements. Circ. Res., 47: 454-466, 1980.

Clapham, D.E., Shrier, A. and DeHaan, R.L.: Junctional resistance and action potential delay between embryonic heart cell aggregates. J. Gen. Physiol., 75: 633-654, 1980.

Clay, J.R., DeFelice, L.J. and DeHaan, R.L.: Current noise parameters of current noise derived from voltage noise and impedance of chick embryonic heart cell aggregates. Biophys. J., 28: 169-184, 1979.

DeHaan, R.L. and Hirakow, R.: Synchronization of pulsation rates in isolated cardiac myocytes. Exp. Cell Res., 70: 214-220, 1972.

DeHaan, R.L. and Fozzard, H.A.: Membrane response to current pulses in spheroidal aggregates of embryonic heart cells. J. Gen. Physiol., 65: 207-222, 1975.

Guckenheimer, J., Oster, G. and Ipaktchi, A.: The dynamics of density dependent population models. J. Math. Biol., 4: 101-147, 1977.

Jalife, J. and Antzelevitch, C.: Phase resetting and annihilation of pacemaker activity in cardiac tissue. Science, 206: 695-697, 1979.

Jalife, J. and Moe, G.K.: Effect of electrotonic potentials on pacemaker activity of canine Purkinje fibers in relation to parasystole. Circ. Res., 39: 801-808, 1976.

Jongsma, H.J., Masson-Pevet, M., Hollander, C.C. and DeBruijne, J.: Synchronization of the beating frequency of cultured rat heart cells. In: Developmental and Physiological Correlates of Cardiac Muscle. Lieberman, M. and Sano T., eds., Raven Press, New York, pp. 185-196, 1975.

Lange, G.: Action of driving stimuli from intrinsic and extrinsic sources on in situ cardiac pacemaker tissues. Circ. Res., 17: 449-459, 1965.

Linkens, D.A.: Theoretical analysis of beating and modulation phenomena in weakly inter-coupled Van der Pol oscillator systems for biological modeling. J. Theor. Biol., 79: 31-54, 1979.

Lu, H., Lange, G. and Brooks, C.C.: Factors controlling pacemaker action in cells of the sinoatrial node. Circ. Res., 17: 460-471, 1965.

Mackaay, A.J.C., Op 't Hof, T., Bleeker, W.K., Jongsma, H.J. and Bouman, L.N.: Interaction of adrenaline and acetylcholine on cardiac pacemaker function. Functional inhomogeneity of the rabbit sinus node. J. Pharmac. Exp. Ther., 214: 417-422, 1980.

May, R.: Simple mathematical models with very complicated dynamics. Nature, 261: 459, (erratum: Nature, 262: 236), 1978.

Moore, G.P., Perkel, D.H. and Segundo, J.P.: Stability patterns in interneuronal pacemaker regulation. In: Proc. San Diego Symp. Biomed. Eng., Paul A., ed., La Jolla, California, 1963.

Pavlidis, T.: Biological Oscillators: Their mathematical analysis. Academic Press, New York and London, 1973.

Pavlidis, T.: Qualitative similarities between the behavior of coupled oscillators and circadian rhythms. Bull. Math. Biol., 40: 675-692, 1978.

Perkel, D.H., Schulman, J.H., Bullock, T.H., Moore, G.P. and Segundo, J.P.: Pacemaker neurons: Effects of regularly spaced synaptic input. Science, 145: 61-63, 1964.

Sachs, H.G. and DeHaan, R.L.: Embryonic myocardial cell aggregates: volume and pulsation rate. Devel. Biol., 30: 233-240, 1973.

Sano, T., Sawanobori, T. and Adaniya, H.: Mechanism of rhythm determination among pacemaker cells of the mammalian sinus node. Am. J. Physiol., 235: H379-H384, 1978.

Schaer, H.: Antagonistische Wirkungen von Magnesium-, Calcium- und Natriumionen auf die Impulsbildung im Sinusknoten des Meerschweinchenherzens. Pfluegers Arch., 298: 359-371, 1968.

Scott, S.: Stimulation simulations of young yet cultured beating hearts. Ph. D. Thesis, State University of New York, Buffalo, 1979.

Vassalle, M.: Automaticity and automatic rhythms. Am. J. Cardiol., 28: 245-252, 1971.

Von Holst, E.: Entwurf eines systems der lokomotorischen Periodenbildungen bei Fischen. Zeitschr. f. Vergl. Physiologie, 26: 481-528, 1939.

Wever, R.: Virtual synchronization towards the limits of the range of entrainment. J. Theor. Biol., 36: 119-132, 1972.

Winfree, A.T.: Phase control of neural pacemakers. Science, 197: 761-763, 1977.

Ypey, D.L., Clapham, D.E., DeHaan, R.L.: Development of electrical coupling and action potential synchrony between paired aggregates of embryonic heart cells. J. Memb. Biol., 51: 75-96, 1979.

Ypey, D.L., VanMeerwijk, W.P.M., Ince, C. and Groos, G.: Mutual entrainment of two pacemaker cells. A study with an electronic parallel conductance model. J. Theor. Biol., 86: 731-755, 1980.

FACTORS INFLUENCING REGULARITY AND SYNCHRONISATION OF BEATING

OF TISSUE CULTURED HEART CELLS

Habo J. Jongsma and Larisa Tsjernina

INTRODUCTION

It is generally assumed that the free running pacemaker of the heart, located in the wall of the right atrium between the orifice of the Vena Cava Superior and the Vena Cava Inferior, generates impulses in a very regular rhythm. Indeed when one excises the tissue region known as the sinus (SA) node, superfuses it in a tissue bath and records electrical activity, a very regular rhythm is observed (fig. 1). The sino-atrial primary pacemaker has been shown to consist of a few thousand virtually simultaneous discharging cells (Bleeker et al., 1980), which are electrically coupled (Bonke, 1973; Bukauskas et al., 1977) and between which nexuses are present (Masson-Pevet et al., 1979).

Single isolated pacemaker cells on the other hand vary their interval duration almost at random (Jongsma et al., 1975), thus the cellular pacemaker concept as discussed by DeHaan (this volume) does not hold true. Consequently the question arises which mechanism is responsible for the very regular firing rhythm of the ensemble of interconnected pacemaker cells which together form the sino-atrial primary pacemaker.

Earlier we have presented evidence that coupling between cells is necessary both for synchronization of the beating rate of individual pacemaker cells and for obtaining a regular common firing rhythm (Jongsma et al., 1975).

In this paper we want to adress two questions:
1. Which factors cause single isolated pacemaker cells to discharge irregular?
2. Does the irregularity of discharge decrease upon increasing the number of interconnected cells, i.e. is there a lower limit for the number of interconnected cells in a pacemaker group to exhibit a regular firing pattern?

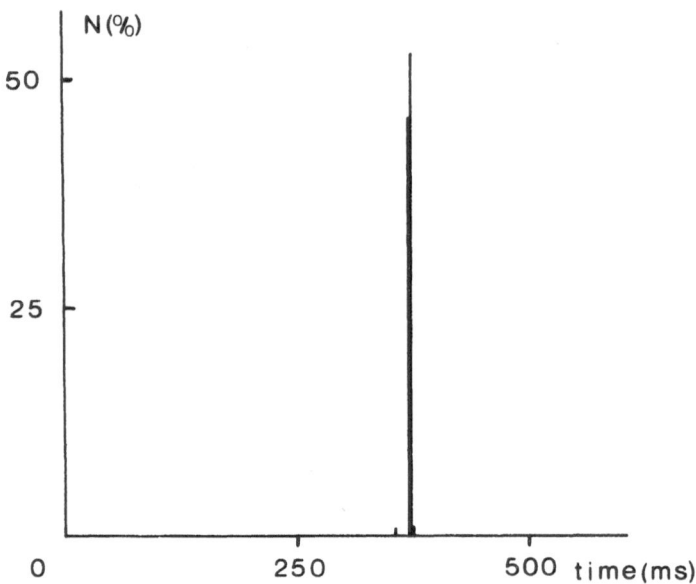

FIGURE 1 *Interval histogram of free running isolated rabbit sinus node.* $\bar{I}$ = *371 ms; C = 0,4 %; N total = 300; binwidth 4 ms*

METHODS

CULTURES

Suspensions of neonatal rat heart cells were prepared as described previously (de Bruijne and Jongsma, 1980). Cells were plated in various densities and different geometries in plastic Petri dishes (Falcon $\emptyset$ 5 cm) and incubated in growth medium consisting of Ham's F 10 (Flow) supplemented with 10 % fetal bovine serum (Flow) and 10 % Horse serum (Flow). No antibiotics and/or fungicides were added. The electrolyte composition of the growth medium was (in mM): NaCl 129, KCl 4.4, $CaCl_2$ 1.0, $MgSO_4$ 0.6, $NaHCO_3$ 14. The cultures were placed in a pH, temperature and humidity controlled incubator and kept at 37 $^{\circ}$C and pH 7.2-7.4. Every 24 hours and two hours prior to experimentation the medium was refreshed.

The number of cells per unit area of culture dish was asessed by counting the number of nuclei in fixed and stained preparations,and allowing for 20 % binucleated cells (Anversa et al., 1980).

MEASUREMENT OF SPONTANEOUS BEATING

The cell cultures were placed on the stage of an inverted microscope (Reichert Biovert) provided with an optically clear heating plate (Schreurs et al., 1981) the temperature of which could be controlled to within 0.1 $^{\circ}$C. Temperature was monitored continuously with a thermistor. Evaporation was checked by layering a little mineral oil (Merck; Paraffin Uvasol) on top of the culture medium (DeHaan and Gottlieb, 1968). Contractions were recorded either with a photomultiplier attachment to the microscope (Leitz MPV) or with light sensitive resistors placed on the screen of a TV monitor which displayed the field of view recorded with a TV camera attached to the microscope. In both cases the moving edges of cells were detected. The resulting voltage deflections were filtered, (Kronhite 3321, in low pass mode; cut off frequency 30 Hz), and fed into a pulse shaping circuit. The 1 V 15 ms pulses from the pulse shaper were recorded on magnetic tape (Ampex FR 1300) for off line data processing, or fed directly into a PDP 11/10 computer (Digital) via an analog input device (LPS; Digital). The time intervals between the pulses were measured with a resolution of 0.1 ms. From series of 300 to 750 interval (depending on the interval length itself) time-interval histograms were constructed. The mean interval (I) and coefficient of variation (C = 100 * SD/I) were calculated. C was used as a measure of regularity (but see Jongsma et al., 1981).

RESULTS AND DISCUSSION

IRREGULARITY OF SINGLE CELLS

To verify that irregularity is an intrinsic property of single isolated pacemaker cells we prepared very sparse cultures (plating density 0.5×10^{5} cells/ml). In these cultures the majority of cells were isolated just after plating; many of them exhibited an irregular beating pattern. Up to about 90 hours after plating single isolated cells could be found in the cultures. Fig. 2 shows the interval histogram of a 73 hour old single isolated cell. I = 1292 ms and C = 39.6 %; apparently the irregularity of the beating pattern is caused by the fact that the cell is isolated, because a confluent monolayer of the same age is always very

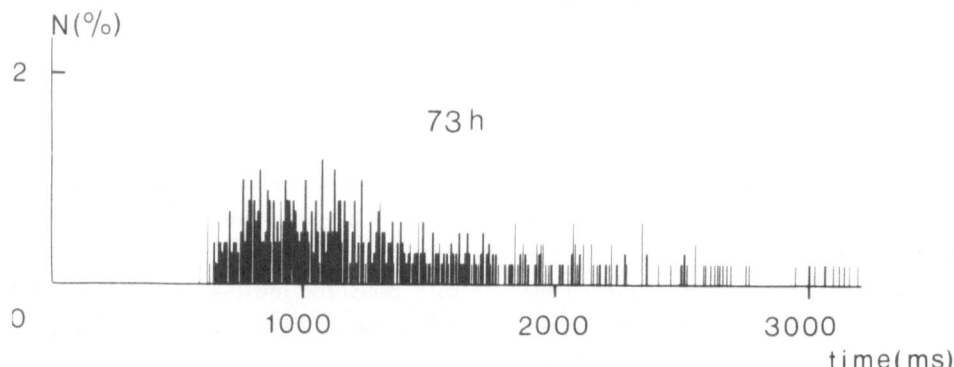

FIGURE 2 *Interval histogram of a single isolated heart cell after 73 hr in cul-ture.* $\bar{I}$ = 1292 ms; C = 39,6 %; N total = 500; binwidth 4 ms

regular and most often very fast beating. Moreover Masson-Pevet et al. (1976) have shown that enzyme-dissociation induced damage is, from an ultrastructural point of view, overcome completely after 48 hours in culture.

It seems warranted therefore to conclude that the irregularity of beating of single isolated cells is not caused by the isolation procedure nor by the lack of conditioning factors in the medium (also see Jongsma et al., 1981).

Individual single cells however differ very much in their mean beating rate ($\bar{I}$) and in their beating regularity (C). This is evidenced by the histograms of fig. 3, where $\bar{I}$ and C are grouped in classes of 100 ms and 5 % respectively. $\bar{I}$ varies from small values comparable to those of cells in confluent and com-pletely synchronized monolayers to very large ones. Although we did not perform a rigid statistical analysis it seems safe to conclude that there is a group of cells with a mean beating interval of around 500 ms and a group with a mean in-terval duration of about 1000 ms or more. This is seen also with regard to regu-larity: there seem to be at least two populations of cells, one group with a C ranging between 5 and 15 % and a group with a C of 20 % ore more.

According to Norwood et al. (1980) there are several different types of cells present in rat heart cell cultures;they can be distinguished by their mor-phology and by their apparent beating rate. Atrium cells are spindle shaped

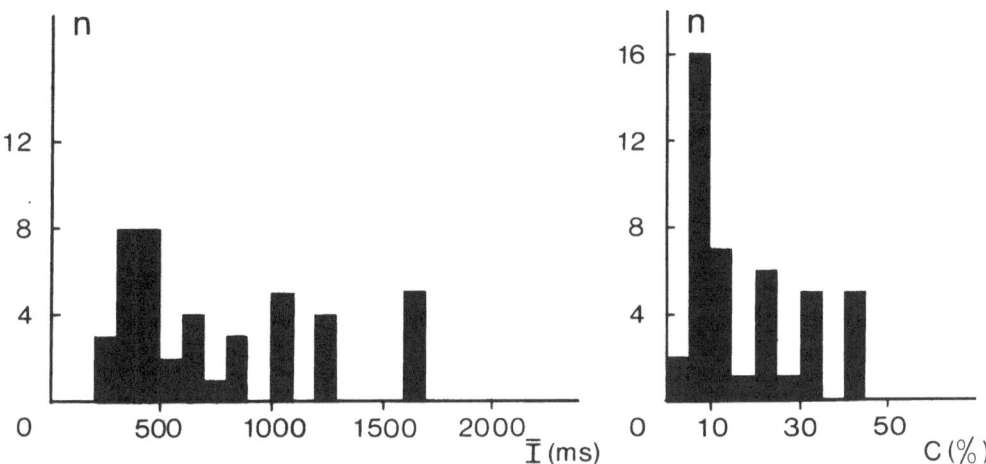

FIGURE 3 *Distribution of $\bar{I}$ and C of 43 single isolated cells. n = number of cells in each bin; binwidth intervals: 100 ms; binwidth coefficient of variation: 5%.*

densely opaque cells exhibiting a fast rising twitch. They beat faster than ventricular cells. These ventricular cells are much more spread out over the bottom of the dish and are therefore more translucent. They have various shapes varying from almost round to irregular with may processes. Perhaps the best criterium is that they are definitely not spindle shaped.

To corroborate this finding and to see whether there existed also differences in beating regularity, we prepared sparse cultures of atria and ventricles separately, and measured beating rate and regularity of cells in both cultures. We selected the cells following the above mentioned criteria. Table I shows the result. It can be seen that C of ventricular cells is significantly larger than that of atrial cells, and, in accordance with the results of Norwood et al. (1980), that the mean beating interval duration of ventricular cells is significantly larger that that of atrial cells. It seems therefore that the large variation in beating rate and regularity of single cells that we reported before (Jongsma et al., 1975) is at least partly due to differences in cell type in

TABLE I

MEAN BEATING INTERVAL (I) AND REGULARITY (C)
OF SINGLE ISOLATED ATRIUM AND VENTRICLE CELLS

Atrium		Ventricle	
I̅(ms)	C(%)	I̅(ms)	C(%)
252	7.7	680	21.2
324	11.0	826	69.3
334	9.0	880	58.1
396	9.4	1282	20.6
418	6.6	1650	68.2
441	13.3	1726	44.7
478	5.8	2141	46.8
1072	5.6		

1312	207	47	7.6	464	90	8.6	0.9
	(sem)						

Each individual value of I̅ is the mean of 500 interval durations.

the whole heart cultures that we used in that study.

The finding that the faster beating atrial cells have a smaller coefficient of variation than the slower beating ventricular cells suggests that C might be dependent on the beating interval length. We tested this supposition by applying interventions that change the beating interval of heart cells. In the first instance we choose temperature decrease as a simple means to increase the cycle length of already confluent monolayers. Fig. 4 gives the relation between mean cycle length and temperature for three monolayers. Cycle length increases with decreasing temperature; the Q_{10} for the preparations is 1.6 which is slightly lower than that of the isolated rat SA node and in agreement with the value given by McCall (1976) taking into account the biphasic relation between contraction frequency and temperature reported by this author. Table II gives the values of C at the different temperatures for the three preparations. There is no relation between coefficient of variation and temperature in these experiments. This can mean several things. First it might be that C is independent of cycle length indeed. Another possibility is that the synchronization process that has occurred in confluent monolayers makes their beating rhythm virtually insensitive

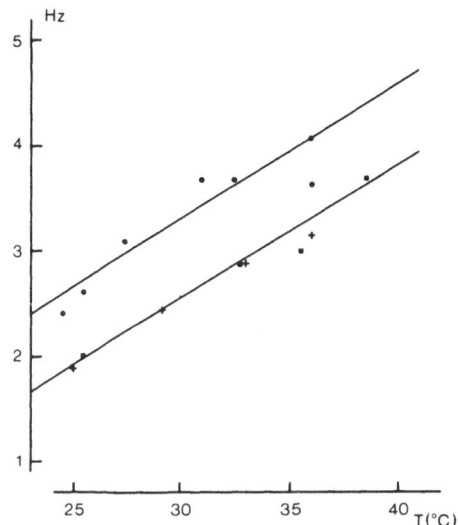

FIGURE 4 *Mean frequency as a function of temperature for three confluent mono-*
layers. Regression lines:
(●) *a:* $F = 0.12 \ (^{\circ}C) - 0.39; \quad r = 0.93$
(✚) *b:* $F = 0.11 \ (^{\circ}C) - 0.93; \quad r = 0.99$
(■) *c:* $F = 0.12 \ (^{\circ}C) - 1.09; \quad r = 0.98$
the lines for and are virtually identical.

TABLE II

COEFFICIENT OF VARIATION FOR THREE
CONFLUENT MONOLAYERS AT DIFFERENT
TEMPERATURES (SEE FIG. 4)

Temperature	Coefficient of Variation		
	●	■	✚
38.5			6.1
36	2.0	5.5	
35.5	2.9		5.8
33		3.0	
32.5	1.6		3.3
31	2.5		
29.0		2.0	
27.5	2.7		
25.5	2.7		8.0
25		1.7	
24.5	3.3		

to changes in cycle length. Finally it might be that the range over which mean cycle length can be shifted by temperature changes is so small that significant changes in regularity cannot be observed. To test this last possibility we applied adrenalin to isolated heart cells of both ventricular and atrial origin in a dose sufficient to obtain maximal acceleration in intact rat hearts. Fig. 5 shows the result of application of $6 * 10^{-7}$ M Adrenalin to respectively a single isolated atrial and ventricular cell.In both instances cycle length is decreased, but much more so in the ventricular cell than in the atrial cell. The coefficient of variation also decreases in both cells but again much more in the ventricular cell than in the atrial cell. As the mean cycle length and the coefficient of variation of ventricular cells is much larger than those of the atrial cell this observation appears to sustain the idea that regularity of beating is dependent on the cycle length itself.

The reason for slow beating isolated cells to do so irregularly is not clear. Clay and DeHaan (1979) presented evidence that irregular beating is brought about by membrane voltage fluctuations during diastolic depolarization. When we suppose that the frequency spectrum is the same in slow and fast firing cells, the rate dependence of irregularity can be explained as follows. (See figure 6). The slow firing cells have a low rate of diastolic depolarization and their membrane potential is therefore relatively long in the neighbourhood of the firing level; random jumps in membrane potential can bring these cells during this period just over the firing level or keep it away from it. Actual firing can occur thus over a long range of time:a large coefficient of variation is the result. Fast firing cells have a much steeper diastolic depolarization and the same jumps in membrane potential are during a shorter time instrumental in delaying or advancing the moment of activation. Small fluctuations in beating interval and a small coefficient of variation will be the result. The only function of adrenalin in the experiment described would be a decrease of cycle length by increasing the rate of diastolic depolarization. This function of adrenalin brought about by a shift of the i_{K2} - activation curve in the depolarizing direction is well known (see e.g. Noble, 1979).

Adrenalin is also known to increase slow inward current (Brown and Noble, 1974; Brown et al., 1979); this current is among other things responsible for subthreshold oscillations seen in several cardiac preparations (Cranefield, 1977). If these subthreshold oscillations are also present in our rat heart

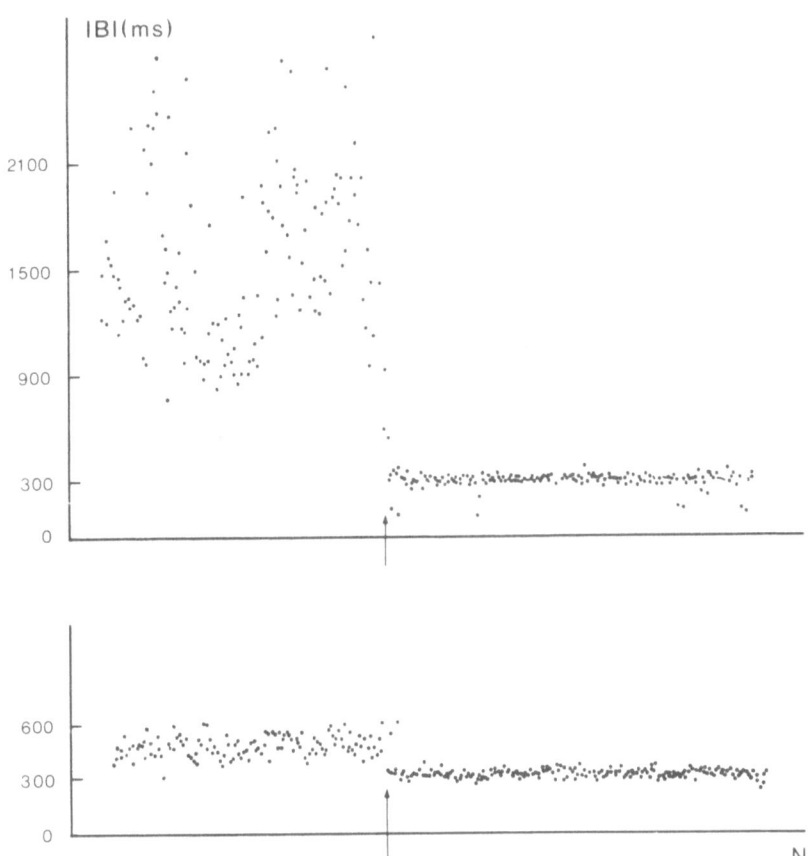

FIGURE 5 *Sequential plot of interval lengthes for a ventricular cell (upper panel) and an atrium cell (lower panel). At the arrow adrenaline (Adr) was added to a final concentration of 6 x 10⁻⁷ m.*

	before Adr.		after Adr.	
	$\bar{I}(ms)$	C(%)	$\bar{I}(ms)$	C(%)
atrium cell	487	10.5	314	6.8
ventricle cell	1492	33.7	293	5.5

N = 300

cells, then adrenalin could act by increasing the amplitude of them. Ventricular cells would speed up their rate of beating considerably because many subthreshold oscillations occur during diastolic depolarization which upon addition of adrenalin would increase so much in magnitude that virtually every oscillation crosses the firing level, while in atrial cells this already in the absence of adrenaline happens. Several observations sustain this idea:

1. quiescent cells can be induced to spontaneous activity by adrenalin (Gough et al., 1977; Jongsma, unpublished observations).

2. Single isolated atrial and ventricular cells attain about the same firing interval (with about the same coefficient of variation) after adrenalin application (see legend to fig. 5).

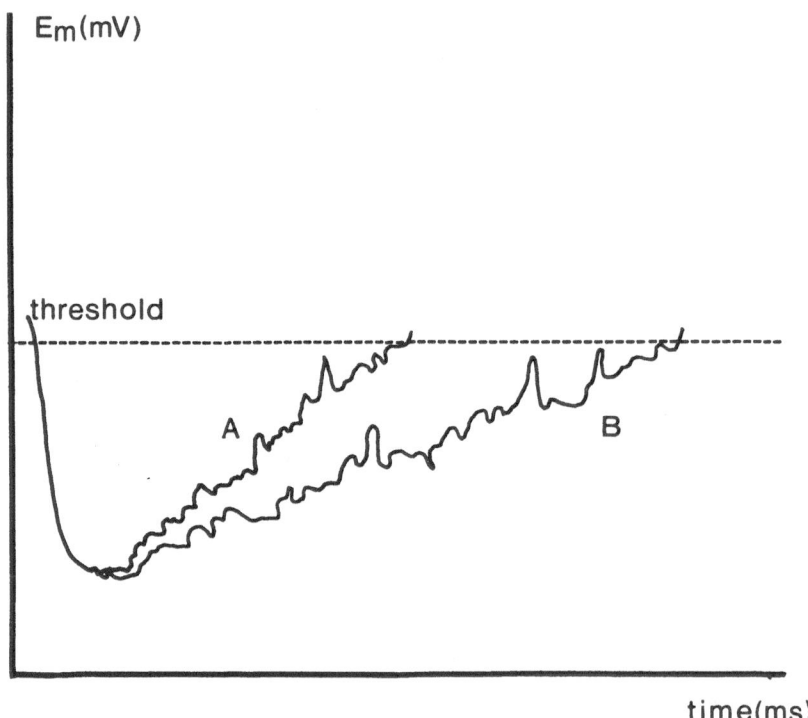

FIGURE 6 *Schematic drawing of noisy diastolic depolarization of (B) a slow firing cell and (A) a fast firing cell. For further explanation: see text.*

3. In isolated rabbit sinus nodes the effect of adrenalin is dependent   on   the
basic cycle length.   Nodes with a long basic cycle length speed up more than
nodes with a short one. (Op 't Hof, personal communication)

   An alternative explanation for the different   reaction   of   ventricular   and
atrial   cells to adrenalin addition might be that both types of cell have a different sensitivity towards the drug either because they contain different numbers
of the same receptor molecule per unit area in their membranes or because the receptor molecules themselves are different. This problem is currently   under   investigation.

   In conclusion then we have shown that single isolated heart cells have an
irregular beating rhythm, that the mean beating interval is dependent on the type
of cell and that regularity of beating is rate dependent.

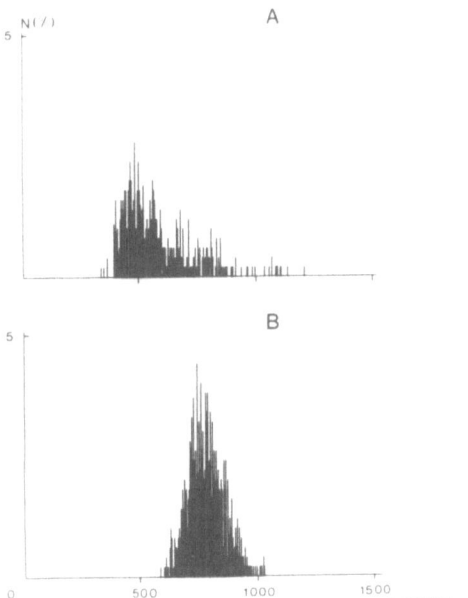

FIGURE 7 *Interval histogram of two small groups of interconnected cells.*
A: 5 cells; $\bar{I}$ = 578 ms;   C = 26%;
N total = 500
B: 14 cells; $\bar{I}$ = 781 ms;   C = 10%;
N total = 700
binwidth = 4 ms

DEVELOPMENT OF REGULARITY IN POPULATIONS
OF INTERCONNECTED HEART CELLS

The coefficient of variation of beating observed in single isolated heart cells never is smaller than 5%, whereas confluent monolayers or the isolated sinus node easily fire with a 1% coefficient of variation. It seems therefore that inter- connection of pacemaker cells renders them less sensitive to rate disturbing in- fluences. An obvious way to investigate this possibility is to study the rela- tion between the number of interconnected cells and the regularity of beating. Clay and DeHaan (1979) showed that the coefficient of variation of their embryon- ic chick heart cells decreased upon increasing the number of cells in an aggre- gate from 1 to 125, whereafter no further increase in regularity could be ob- served. Jongsma et al. (1975, 1981) showed that there is a strong correlation between the increase in number of interconnected cells (represented by the time the culture was allowed to develop) and the increase of regularity.

Pacemaker cells may be considered as oscillators which, on coupling to each other, synchronize their beating rate. The degree of synchronization is depen- dent on the strength of the coupling (Ypey et al., 1979), the difference in be- ating rate of the individual cells (see Winfree, 1980, for an extensive discus- sion) and on the magnitude of the synchronizing agent (in this case current flow either during diastole or during an action potential). The electrotonic interac- tion between cells also may be responsible for a decrease of irregularity on cou- pling. Although no mathematical model exists which describes the behaviour of "irregular oscillators" upon coupling, it has been argued that "an enhancement of precision" is to be expected in this case (Winfree, 1980).

In order to gain some insight in this problem, we tried to correlate the number of interconnected pacemaker cells in monolayer cultures with the coeffi- cient of variation by allowing a known number of cells to interconnect to each other whereafter the beating rate and regularity of these cell groups were meas- ured. In figure 7 intervals histograms of a group of 5 and 14 cells respectively are depicted while figure 8 shows a interval histogram of a group of 7000 cells. Although from figure 7 it may be deduced that C decreases upon increasing the number of interconnected cells, the data from figure 8 indicate that a 500 fold increase in number of interconnected cells does not result in a further decrease in C. Table III extends these observations; here I and C of different sized groups are tabulated. It is clear that no relation exists between the number of

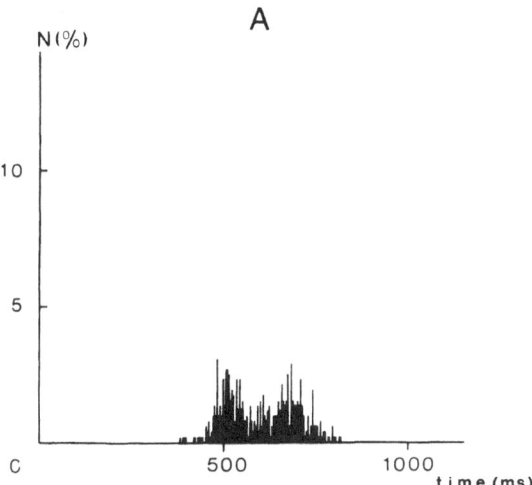

FIGURE 8 *Interval histogram of a group of 7000 interconnected cells. $\bar{I}$ = 598 ms;*
C = 15.6%; N total = 500; binwidth 4 ms

TABLE III

MEAN INTERVAL LENGTH ($\bar{I}$) AND COEFFICIENT OF VARIATION (C) OF GROUPS
OF VARIOUS NUMBERS OF INTERCONNECTED CELLS

		Number of interconnected cells					
200		900 - 1500		7000		15000	
I(ms)	C(%)	I(ms)	C(%)	I(ms)	C(%)	I(ms)	C(%)
967	9.6	674	10.5	600	8.0	1344	35.0
673	9.0	733	11.1	527	9.4	1076	26.0
799	7.8	747	23.0	912	7.6	898	14.0
				809	24.0	558	11.0
				713	17.3		
				684	9.6		

Each value of $\bar{I}$ is the mean duration 500 intervals

interconnected cells and the coefficient of variation. The very large coeffi-
cients of variation observed in ventricular cells are not present however. It
appears that interconnection of cells decreases the irregularity to a certain extent but that even in groups of 15.000 interconnected cells regularity of beating
comparable to that of confluent monolayers is not attained.

As stated before the mechanism of synchronization of the beating rate of pacemaker heart cells depends on current flow between the cells (Jongsma et al.,
1975, 1981; Clay and DeHaan, 1979; DeHaan and Hirakow, 1972; Ypey et al.,
1979).

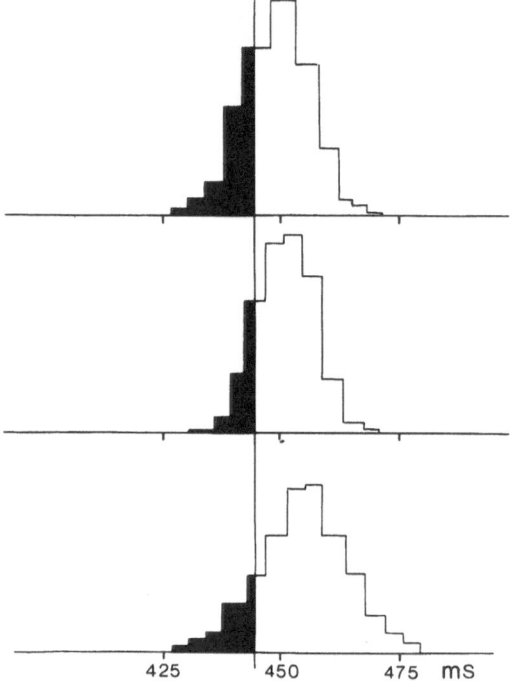

FIGURE 9 *Schematic drawing of interval histograms of three pacemaker cell groups. For explanation: see text.*

Both in the isolated rabbit sinus node and in monolayers of neonatal rat
heart cells, electrical interaction is possible to a limited extent only due to
the relative shortness of the space constant compared to the dimensions of the

preparations (Bonke, 1973; Bukauskas et al., 1977; Jongsma and van Rijn, 1972; Hyde et al., 1969; Bleeker et al., 1980; Masson-Pevet et al., 1979). It seems therefore that mutual synchronization of action potential generation due to electrotonic interaction is limited to small groups of cells. In a confluent monolayer there will be several of these small, synchronized groups of pacemaker cells with a more or less regular beating pattern. When it is supposed that once one of these groups fires all other groups are activated by the propagated action potential from it, a fast and regular beating monolayer can be the result. Figure 9 graphically explains this hypothesis, which is based on the statistics of extremes (Gumbel, 1963). The histograms of three groups of cells are depicted. There is a small but finite chance that one of them fires after a short interval (lying in the black part of one of the histograms). Once this group fires, its action potential is propagated to all other groups which, if not forming part of the ensemble, would have fired after a longer interval. The next beat will be initiated by the group which at that moment tends to fire after a short interval. In this way only short intervals will be produced and long intervals (in the white part of the histograms) will not occur any more. The result is that the mean beating rate of the population of cells increases while the coefficient of variation decreases. This mechanism will only work when so many pacemaker cell groups are present in the population that there is a 100 % chance that at every beat at least one group will fire with a short interval. On the other hand the pacemaker cell groups must lie so near each other that the action potential of the first firing cell group reaches most other groups before they discharge themselves (most likely after their mean beating interval). As the number of pacemaker cell groups increases, beating rate and regularity would increase further until the distance between the groups becomes so large that action potentials from one group could not reach most others fast enough to prevent them firing themselves. A decrease of regularity would be the result! A corollary of the hypothesis is that interventions which decrease conduction velocity (e.g. hypoxia or increase in the number of non-excitable but conducting cells like fibroblasts (Goshima, 1970)) will result in a decrease of regularity.

While several of the prerequisites for the hypothesis are met both in monolayer cultures of heart cells and in the isolated sinus node (Bleeker et al., 1980, James et al., 1966), it remains to be proved that the mechanism proposed is in operation indeed.

REFERENCES

Anversa, P., Olivetti, G. and Loud, A.V.: Morphometric study of early postnatal development in the left and right ventricular myocardium of the rat. Circ. Res., 46: 495-502, 1980.

Bleeker, W.K., Mackaay, A.J.C., Masson-Pevet, M., Bouman, L.N. and Becker, A.E.: Functional and morphological organization of the rabbit sinus node. Circ. Res., 46: 11-22, 1980.

Bonke, F.I.M.: Electrotonic spread in the sinoatrial node of the rabbit. Pfluegers Arch., 339: 17-23, 1973.

Brown H.F. and Noble, S.J.: Effects of adrenaline on membrane currents underlying pacemaker activity in frog atrial muscle. J. Physiol. (London), 238: 51P-53P, 1974.

Brown, H.F., DiFrancesco, D. and Noble, S.J.: Adrenaline action on rabbit sino-atrial node. J. Physiol. (London), 290: 31P-32P, 1979.

Bruijne, J. de and Jongsma, H.J.: Membrane properties of aggregates of collage-nase-dissociated rat heart cells. In: Advances in Myocardiology, Vol. I, Tajudding, M., Das, P.K., Tariq, M. and Dhalla, N.S., eds., University Park Press, Baltimore, pp. 231-242, 1980.

Bukauskas, F.F., Veteikis, R.P., Gutman, A.M. and Mutskus, K.S.: Intracellular coupling in the sinus node of the rabbit heart. Biofyzica 22: 108-112, 1977.

Clay, J.R. and DeHaan, R.L.: Fluctuations in interbeat interval in rhythmic heart cell clusters. Biophys. J., 28: 377-390, 1979.

Cranefield, P.F.: Action potentials, afterpotentials and arrhythmias. Circ. Res., 41: 415-423, 1977.

DeHaan, R.L. and Gottlieb, S.H.: The electrical activity of embryonic chick heart cells isolated in tissue culture singly or in interconnected cell sheets. J. Gen. Physiol., 52: 643-665, 1968.

DeHaan, R.L. and Hirakow, R.: Synchronization of pulsation rates in isolated cardiac myocytes. Exp. Cell Res., 70: 214-220, 1972.

Goshima, K.: Formation of nexuses and electrical transmission between myocardial and FL cells in monolayer culture. Exp. Cell Res., 63: 124-130, 1970.

Gough, W.B., Angelakos, E.T. and Morad, M.: Dependence of pacemaker activity on tissue epinephrine content and $(Ca^2)_o$. Proc. Int. Union Physiol. Sci., vol XIII, 277, 1977.

Gumbel, E.J.: The statistics of extremes. Columbia University Press, New York, 1958.

Hyde, A., Blondel, B., Matter, A., Cheneval, J.P., Filloux, B. and Girardier, L.: Homo and heterocellular junctions in cell cultures. In: Progress in Brain Res., Vol. 31, Akert, K. and Waser, P.G., eds., Elsevier, Amsterdam, pp. 283-311, 1969.

James, T.N., Sherf, L., Fine, G. and Morales, A.R.: Comparative ultrastructure of the sinus node in man and dog. Circulation, 24: 139-163, 1966.

Jongsma, H.J. and van Rijn, H.E.: Electrotonic spread of current in monolayer cultures of neonatal rat heart cells. J. Memb. Biol., 9: 341-360, 1972.

Jongsma, H.J., Tsjernina, L. and de Bruijne, J.: The establishment of regular beating in populations of pacemaker heart cells. Submitted, 1981.

Jongsma, H.J., Masson-Pevet, M., Hollander, C.C. and de Bruijne, J.: Synchronization of the beating frequency of cultured rat heart cells. In: Developmental and Physiological Correlates of Cardiac Muscle. Lieberman, M. and Sano, T., eds., Raven Press, New York, pp. 185-196, 1975.

Masson-Pevet, M., Jongsma, H.J. and de Bruijne, J.: Collagenase and Trypsin dissociated heart cells: a comparative ultrastructural study. J. Mol. Cell. Cardiol., 8: 747-757, 1976.

Masson-Pevet, M., Bleeker, W.K. and Gros, D.: The plasma membrane of leading pacemaker cells in the rabbit sinus node. Circ. Res., 45: 621-629, 1979.

McCall, D.: Effect of quinidine and temperature on sodium uptake and contraction frequency of cultured rat myocardial cells. Circ. Res., 39: 730-735, 1976.

Noble, D.: The Initiation of the Heartbeat. Oxford University Press, Oxford, pp. 109-118, 1979.

Norwood, C.R., Castaneda, A.R. and Norwood, W.I.: Heterogeneity of rat cardiac cells of defined origin in single cell culture. J. Mol. Cell. Cardiol., 12: 201-210, 1980.

Schreurs, W., van Leeuwen, J.R. and Jongsma, H.J.: An optically clear heating plate for tissue culture experiments. Submitted, 1981.

Winfree, A.T.: The geometry of biological time, Springer Verlag, Berlin, 1980.

Ypey, D.L., Clapham, D.E. and DeHaan, R.L.: The development of electrical coupling and action potential synchrony between paired aggregates of embryonic heart cells. J. Memb. Biol., 51: 75-96, 1979.

SYNCHRONIZATION OF HODGKIN-HUXLEY-TYPE

AND RELATED OSCILLATORS

Derek A. Linkens

INTRODUCTION

It should be noted that the experimental investigation into oscillator synchronization described here has been motivated by an interest in pacing experiments
on the gastro-intestinal tract. Of particular importance have been phenomena
such as the ability to pace at frequencies below and above the natural frequency
of the model, and phase-shift induced along a synchronized chain under external
stimulation. It is hoped that the results obtained will prove useful in the
closely-related field of cardiac synchronization.

The type of pacing referred to in this work comprises pulse waveforms,
since this is the type that has been used in physiological studies in the gut.
The reason for this is that pulse stimulators are commonly available, and also
the fact that narrow pulse stimulation allows artefacts caused by the stimulus
to die away between pulses, which thus enables the pacemaker rhythm to become
apparent in the recordings.

Successful pacing experiments have been performed on both the canine stomach and small-intestine in vivo. Kelly and Laforce (1972) performed pacing
experiments on the intact canine stomach using both encircling and point electrodes. Pulses with an amplitude of 4 mA and 0.5 s width (about 4% of stimulus
period) were used, and the normal rhythm of 0.083 Hz was driven down to a minimum of 0.07 Hz, and up to a maximum of 0.133 Hz. The extremes of driving frequency were thus asymmetrically disposed about the normal undriven frequency.
They reported that there was no change in phase shift along the organ as the
pacing frequency was increased. This is in contrast to the experiments on ana-
esthetized dogs by Sarna and Daniel (1973) who reported an increase in phase-lag

over the whole corpus and antrum as driving frequency increased.   Their   upper
limit of pacing was 0.11 Hz, but they used a stricter definition of entrainment
than Kelly and Laforce. A further finding was that the minimum pulse   amplitude
necessary for synchronization increased as the pacing frequency increased.   No
results were reported for pacing the stomach at frequencies lower than the   normal value.

Pacing   experiments   have   also   been   performed   on   the   intact   canine
small-intestine both in the conscious state (Akwari et al., 1975) and an ana-
esthetized condition (Sarna et al. 1975). Kelly   and   his   coworkers   used   a
pulse stimulus of 8 mA and 50 ms width (equivalent to about 1.5% of the normal
period), and applied the stimulus at several places along the intestine. Pacing
at   the   upper   end   of   the duodenum gave a maximum driving frequency of 20-25%
above the normal value. Pacing in the jejunum caused a   change   in   the   phase
shift from lagging to leading down the duodenum. In this work they reported an
increase in phase lag as the driving frequency was increased.   These   results
agree with the findings of Sarna and Daniel using very similar techniques on an-
aesthetized dogs.

PACEMAKER MODELS USED FOR SYNCHRONIZATION STUDIES

A commonly accepted mathematical model for the myoelectrical activity of the gut
comprises   a   set   of linked non-linear oscillators. This basic model structure
has been used in one-dimensional chain form for modelling   the   small-intestine
(Sarna et al., 1971; Robertson-Dunn and Linkens, 1974) and in two-dimensional
form for the stomach (Sarna et al., 1975). In these studies   the   model   has
usually been simulated on either analog or digital computers using a non-linear
oscillator dynamic based on the well-known van der Pol equation. More recently,
attention has been focussed on the electrical equivalent circuit representation
of the model so that different structures of inter-coupling can   be   quantified
(Linkens,   1977).   For example, it has been shown that reactive coupling of oscillators could account for the dual frequency   phenomenon   recorded   from   the
human colon (Linkens et al., 1976).

In the work reported here the synchronization experiments were carried out on three electronic hardware models rather than on a computer simulation. The first model comprises an electronic implementation approximating to van der Pol's equation which is given by $\ddot{x} - \varepsilon(a^2 - x^2)\dot{x} + w^2x = 0$, where the degree of non-linearity is determined by the parameter "ε". The circuit uses a tuned LC circuit together with a non-linear shunt conductance implemented via an operational amplifier (Datardina and Linkens, 1978). The normal frequency of this model is about 5 KHz. The model is presently constructed as a 16 oscillator structure capable of chain, matrix and tubular interconnection, with resistive, capacitive and inductive coupling components.

The second hardware model comprises a simplified electronic equivalent of the Hodgkin-Huxley equations for nerve axon electrical behaviour. Computer simulations have shown, that if the Hodgkin-Huxley dynamics are made auto-rhythmic, and then used as the basic oscillator in a coupled intestinal model the phenomena of frequency entrainment and modulation efects can be observed (Linkens and Datardina, 1977). Such computer simulations are very slow and difficult numerically, and it would have been prohibitive to have performed the pulse synchronization experiments described in this paper using digital techniques. Using FET devices as variable conductances a simple electronic approximation to Hodgkin-Huxley dynamics has been implemented and shown also to give phenomena recorded in the gut and simulated by the van der Pol computer models (Patton and Linkens, 1978). In this model each oscillator has five potentiometers which determine the waveshape and frequency of the oscillations. Typically the frequency from uncoupled oscillators in this model is about 150 Hz. The relatively high speed of solution and the parallel operation of the coupled oscillators enabled synchronization bands to be determined quickly using this hardware analog implementation.

The third model uses relaxation oscillators with operational amplifiers acting as threshold switches (Brown et al., 1975). Instead of a conventional RC switching waveform this oscillator has a charging waveform with a rising positive exponential waveshape. The reason for choosing this waveform was that oscillators of this type when coupled together resistively give a rise in entrained frequency above their uncoupled value, and this is a requisite when modelling the small intestine. Also, the waveshape has some resemblance to the classical van der Pol dynamic. A chain of 64 oscillators of this type has been con-

structed as a small-intestinal model and shown to reproduce the major physiological features of the electrical activity (Brown et al., 1975). The frequencies of these oscillators are not intended to represent actual biomedical
rhythms.   One advantage of using a faster time-scale for modelling studies is
that fast experimentation is possible. It is obvious that simulations run at
realtime would not only be very lengthy, but also very difficult for determining
synchronization boundaries. The van der Pol oscillators operate at high frequency to give suitable component values, particularly for the internal induc-
tors required for this type of electronic implementation.   The Hodgkin-Huxley
and relaxation-type models also give convenient component values at their frequencies, together with relative ease in visual detection of non-synchronization
conditions via an oscilloscope.   This would not have been easily feasible at
lower frequencies. Circuit diagrams for the oscillators can be found in references already cited.

EXPERIMENTAL METHODS

Each of the three models is available as an electronic hardware implementation
comprising four oscillators per card. The intrinsic frequencies with zero coupling were set up in each case to be equal along the chain (i.e. no frequency
gradient). Coupling between oscillators was via potentiometers which were calibrated in each case. In the Hodgkin-Huxley model, capacitive coupling was possible, and for the van der Pol model both capacitive and inductive coupling were
also available. The waveshape of individual units could be changed from nearly
sinusoidal to a highly non-linear shape for both the van der Pol and
Hodgkin-Huxley type models by adjustment of potentiometers.   The waveshape of
the relaxation oscillators was fixed and had a fairly non-linear form.

In each experiment the models were paced from a pulse generator via a fixed
resistor into one only of the oscillators. In most cases stimulation was via
the end oscillator in a chain, although sometimes a ring connection was also
used.   Similar stimulation pulse amplitudes were used for the three models, but
the resistance was varied since the output amplitudes of the models were very

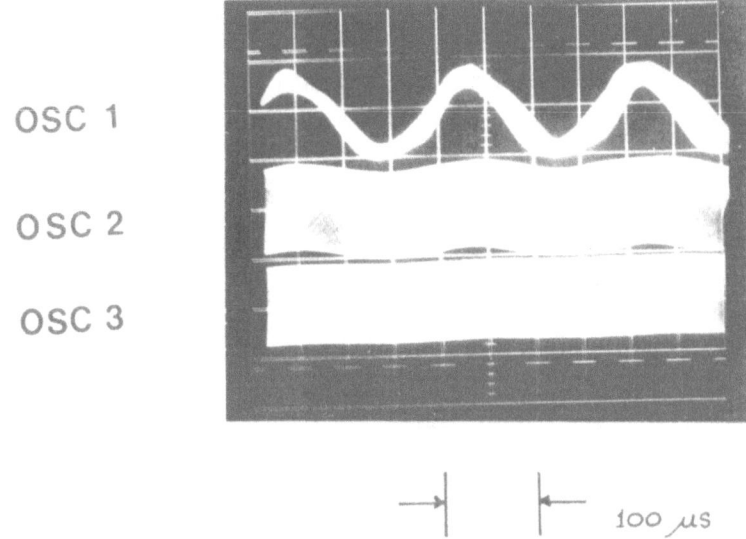

FIGURE 1 *Three paced non-linear van der Pol oscillators under desynchronised conditions. Display triggering on oscillator 1.*

different. The van der Pol model had a normal amplitude of about 10 V peak, the Hodgkin-Huxley model was about 100 mV, and the relaxation model about 1 V. Indication of synchronization was made visually from an oscilloscope using two adjacent oscillator outputs as the display. Under synchronised conditions the waveforms were steady, while outside the synchronisation range the waveforms became disorganised with both amplitude and frequency fluctuations. An example of this disorganisation can be seen in Fig. 1 which is for the van der Pol model. In this figure oscillator 1 was used to trigger the oscilloscope and the apparent blurred trace is due to non-synchronised amplitude and frequency fluctuations. The other oscillators were non-entrained and gave a "slipping" display.

The protocol to determine the synchronisation range in each experiment was as follows. The pulse generator frequency was increased within the synchronised region until the beginning of disorganisation was reached. The period of oscillations was then noted using a Counter/Timer attached to the oscillator adjacent to the one being stimulated. This was done to avoid spurious period measurements that could sometimes occur when the stimulating pulse caused large distortions in the oscillator nearest to the stimulation.   The   pulse   frequency   was then reduced until the opposite limit of synchronisation was reached and the period again measured. Detailed measurements of phase shift were not made, but general observations were noted and will be referred to in the following section.

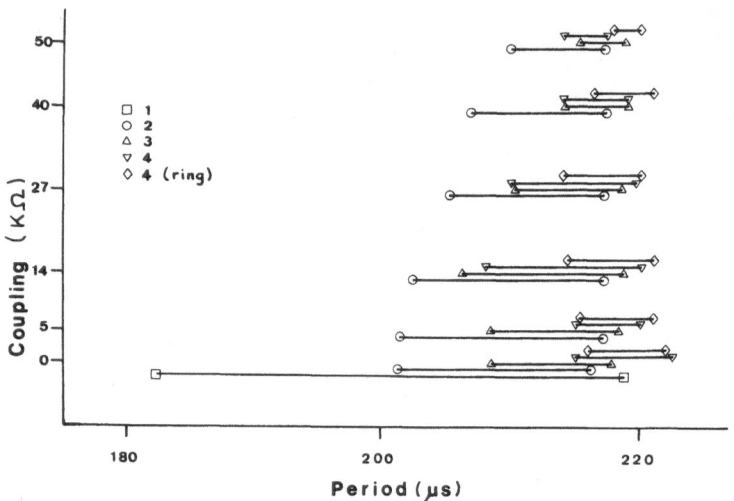

FIGURE 2 *Synchronisation bands for different numbers of van der Pol oscillators under varying coupling conditions.   Horizontal lines denote the width of the synchronisation range. Stimulus of 20 V; 20 µs width for waveshape factor ε ≈ 1.*

RESULTS AND DISCUSSIONS

The results of the various experiments have been grouped together in this section so that the three models can be compared together for a particular parameter variation. The order of presentation will be van der Pol, Hodgkin-Huxley, followed by the relaxation model. In all the figures the coupling between oscillators is resistive in nature, unless otherwise stated.

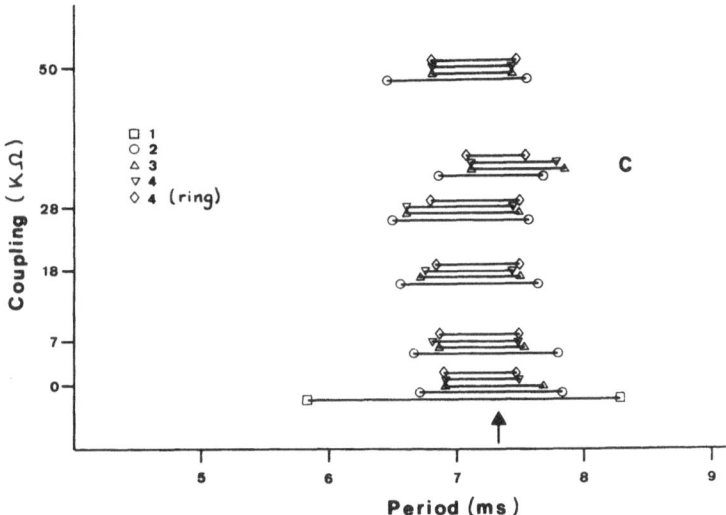

FIGURE 3 *Synchronisation bands for different numbers of Hodgkin-Huxley type oscillators under varying coupling conditions. Stimulus of 20 V; 375 μs width for waveshape factor ε ≈ 10. "C" denotes capacitive coupling.*
NOTE: In following figures the solid arrows denote the unpaced coupled frequency.

CHANGES IN THE NUMBER OF OSCILLATORS

Fig. 2 shows the synchronisation ranges for the van der Pol model for changes in the number of oscillators and the strength of coupling. The range is indicated by a horizontal line with symbol terminators to show the different conditions. This convention will be followed in the succeeding figures. The decrease in the range was very marked going from one to two oscillators, for all values of resistive coupling. The change from two oscillators to three oscillators was smaller, while very little change in the synchronisation range was observed when increasing the number of oscillators from three to four. It can

also be seen that there was only a small change in the synchronisation range
when changing from a 4-oscillator chain to a 4-oscillator ring. It should be
noted that in this experiment there was a frequency gradient along the chain and
hence the range lines are displaced with respect to each other as the number of
oscillators increased. In all the following results there was no frequency gradient.   The range for a single forced oscillator relative to its intrinsic frequency was 17.7%. The pulse width was about 10% in this experiment.

The results for a similar experiment on the Hodgkin-Huxley model are shown
in Fig.   3.   The synchronisation band for a single oscillator was 34.2%, indicating a stronger stimulating pulse than in the previous figure. The narrowing
in range going from one to two oscillators was approximately 45% for most values
of coupling. The narrowing caused by going from two to three, and three to
four, were respectively 60% and 100%. Similarly, there was very little difference in range when going from a chain to a ring connection.   Also included in
Fig. 3 are the results obtained using capacitive coupling having a reactance of
33 KOhm at the unpaced frequency of the model. In this case very little change
in synchronisation range was observed as the number of oscillators was changed.
In this experiment the pulse width of the stimulus was 5% of the repetition period.   The equivalent waveshape factor was about 10, in contrast to the previous
results which represented a van der Pol oscillator with $\varepsilon \simeq 1.0$.   It should be
noted that estimates of waveshape factor have been made by visual examination of
oscilloscope displays.

Similar results were obtained for the relaxation switching model, in that a
large change in synchronisation range occurred when increasing from one to two
oscillators. Changing from two to three oscillators gave a very small change in
range.   In this case the waveshape factor was fixed and the waveform has some
resemblance to the classic van der Pol dynamic for $\varepsilon = 10$.

From these observations it was apparent that a three oscillator chain was a
sufficient structure for investigation of synchronisation effects. Accordingly,
for further experiments involving other parameter changes the chain length was
usually kept to three oscillators. It is also evident that pacing a single oscillator is not a sufficient structure for investigation of the pacing effects
on coupled oscillators.

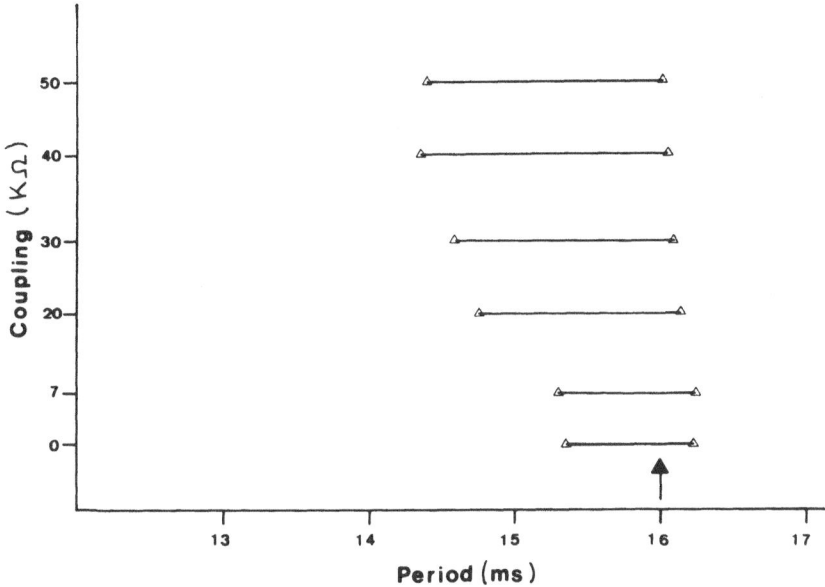

FIGURE 4 *Synchronisation bands for switching oscillators under varying coupling conditions.*

CHANGES IN COUPLING STRENGTH

The effect of coupling strength on synchronisation range is indicated in Figs. 2 and 3 for the van der Pol and Hodgkin-Huxley model respectively. For the van der Pol oscillators with a waveform that was fairly sinusoidal (i.e. $\varepsilon \simeq 1.0$) the range decreased as the coupling strength decreased from 14 KOhm (fig. 2). The decreased range was of the order of 30% depending on the number of oscillators in the chain. For tighter coupling than 14 KOhm, there was a small decrease in the synchronisation range.

For the Hodgkin-Huxley model Fig. 3 shows that there was very little change in the range for varying coupling strength for any number of oscillators considered. The effect of coupling on the relaxation model is shown in Fig. 4, which indicates a reverse trend, in that stronger coupling gave a narrower range. Thus for this model it is easier to stimulate a weakly coupled system.

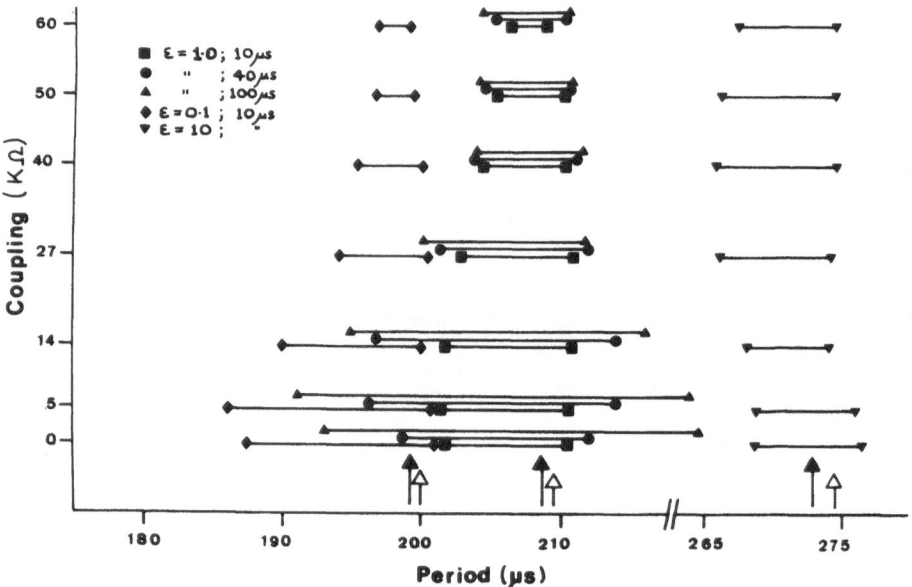

FIGURE 5 *Effect of waveshape and stimulus width on synchronisation band for 3 van der Pol oscillators. Open arrows denote the uncoupled frequencies.*

CHANGES IN WAVESHAPE

The difference in the effect of coupling for the three models suggest that waveshape may be a factor of importance in the case of synchronisation. Accordingly, three different waveshape factors were investigated for the van der Pol model. For ε of 0.1, 1.0 and 10.0 the effect of coupling strength is shown in Fig. 5, keeping the stimulating parameters constant. The effect of coupling on range clearly decreased as the waveforms became more non-linear. For almost-sinusoidal waveshape (ε = 0.1) the decreased range as coupling was weakened was very marked at 17%. For ε = 1.0 the decreased range was 27% while for ε = 10.0 there was no clear change in the range at all. A similar result was obtained for the Hodgkin-Huxley model when the waveshape was modified from nearly sinusoidal to very non-linear. It should be noted, however, that the reverse effect of easier pacing of weakly coupled systems as found in the switching model was not observed for any waveshape factor for the other two models.

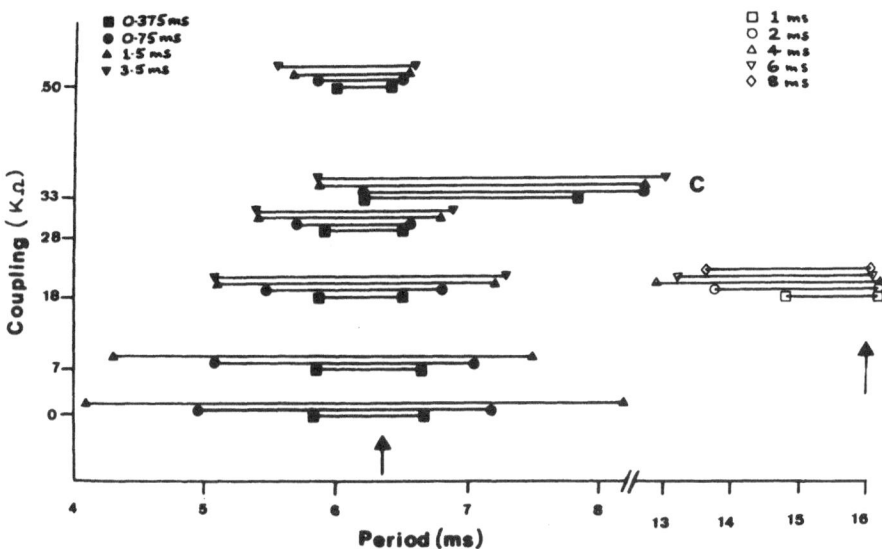

FIGURE 6 *Effect of stimulus width on synchronisation band for 3 Hodgkin-Huxley type oscillators with waveshape factor of ε ≈ 1. "C" denotes capacitive coupling. Open symbols indicate bands for 3 switching oscillators for varying stimulus width.*

CHANGES IN PULSE WIDTH

The synchronisation range was considerably affected by the pulse width of the stimulation for the van der Pol model set to ε = 1.0, (Fig. 5). For all values of coupling the range increased for increasing pulse width. Thus, changing from a 5% pulse width (10 μs) to a 50% width with a mark: space ratio of almost 1.0 (100 μs) gave an increased range of about 250%.

Similar results were obtained from the Hodgkin-Huxley model for ε ≈ 1, giving increased ranges of about 300% for pulse widths increasing from 5% to 50% (Fig. 6). The equivalent results for ε = 10.0 are shown in Fig. 7, which also indicates that large pulse widths gave easier pacing for weak coupling. The increased range caused by going from 5% to 50% pulse width was considerably less than for ε = 1.0. The result of a similar experiment on the relaxation model for one value of coupling (18 KOhm) is superimposed in Fig. 6. Again, a reverse trend is observable in that as pulse width was increased from 5% to 50% the synchronisation range first increased and then decreased.

CHANGES IN PULSE AMPLITUDE

It would be expected that an increasing pulse height would give increased synchronisation ranges and this was verified for the Hodgkin-Huxley and relaxation
models. Similar results were obtained for the three experiments as shown in
Fig. 8. Neither waveshape nor model structure seemed to affect the relative
change in range greatly, and the decreased range was about 5% for an amplitude
reduction of 80 times. A different phenomenon is, however, observable from Fig.
8 for the relaxation model. This relates to the position of the synchronisation
band relative to the unpaced frequency. For small pulse amplitudes the relaxation model range had periods entirely below the unpaced model period. Thus, the
model was being paced at frequencies above the normal value, and could not be
paced at frequencies below the unstimulated value. This phenomenon is related
to the question of phase shift along a chain and will be referred to in the next
section. In contrast, the other two models showed synchronisation bands which
straddle the unpaced periods. In all cases, however, there was a marked asymmetry in the location of the band relative to the normal period. Thus, it can be
seen from Figs. 6, 7 and 8 that the models were easier to pace at lower periods
(i.e. higher frequencies) than normal, for most conditions of coupling, pulse
width and amplitude. Fig. 5 suggests that the asymmetry is more marked for
more sinusoidal waveforms for the van der Pol model and this agrees with the
Hodgkin-Huxley results in Figs. 6 and 7. It also appears that smaller pulse
amplitude gave increased asymmetry as can be seen in Fig. 8 for the
Hodgkin-Huxley model. It can also be seen that the asymmetry was more marked
for narrow pulses or low amplitude pulses for both van der Pol and
Hodgkin-Huxley models. Also, in general the asymmetry was greater for weak coupling than for strong coupling. Although there were considerable variations in
the degree of asymmetry the ratio of synchronisation band below the unpaced period to that above was between 4:1 and 1:1. It should be noted that for the relaxation model the pulse amplitude had a major effect on the movement of the
synchronisation range relative to the unpaced period, while pulse width and coupling had relatively little effect.

PHASE SHIFTS ALONG A CHAIN

Phase shifts along a model comprising entrained non-linear oscillators is of
major interest, since phase lag is indicative of propagation in the direction of

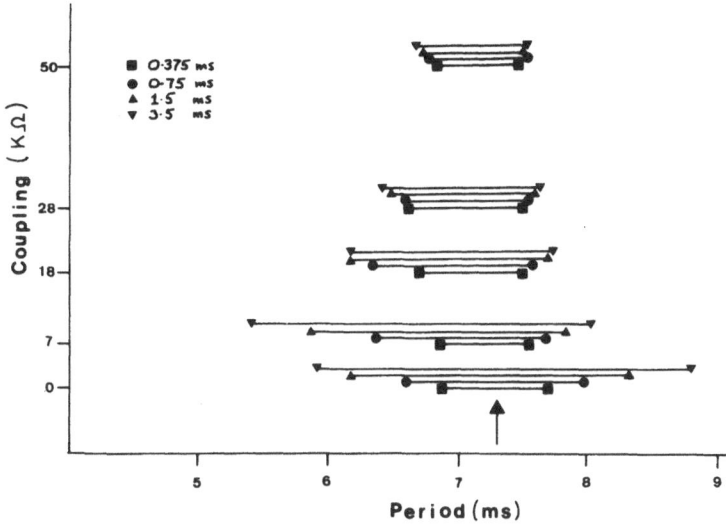

FIGURE 7 *Effect of stimulus width for 3 Hodgkin-Huxley type oscillators with waveshape factor of ε ≈ 10.*

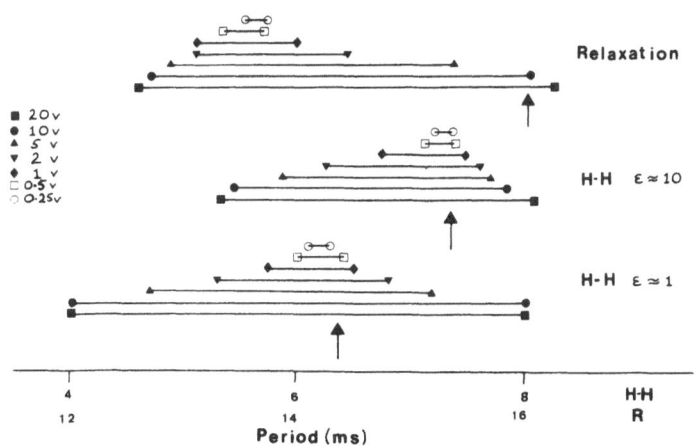

FIGURE 8 *Effect of stimulus amplitude on synchronisation bands for switching (relaxation) oscillators and Hodgkin-Huxley type oscillators.*

the lag, whereas phase lead indicates propagation in the opposite direction.

In the majority of experiments reported here there was   no   intrinsic   frequency   gradient   along the chain, and hence the normal condition under entrainment gave zero phase shift along the chain. Phase shifts were, however, induced under   pacing conditions. Although detailed measurements were not made on phase shifts, a number of qualitative effects were observed. In general, it was noted that   phase shifts were greater for weakly coupled chains, and that phase shifts increased near the edges of the synchronisation band. For strong   coupling   the phase shift never approached 90° per oscillator even at the edge of synchronisation. For the van der Pol and Hodgkin-Huxley oscillators   under   weak   coupling 90° phase   shift   per   oscillator was approached at the edge of synchronisation particularly for low waveshape factors. With pacing frequencies higher than the normal   frequency a phase lag was induced along the chain and, in general, phase lags of nearly 90° were common. Pacing at a lower frequency   than   normal   gave phase   lead   along the chain and generally it was difficult to achieve more than 60° per oscillator. This phenomenon is probably related to the asymmetry of the synchronisation bands which mostly favoured the higher frequency forcing (i.e. phase lag along the chain). An example of the waveforms obtained   for   the   van der   Pol   model   is   shown in Fig. 9 which represents conditions at the extreme ends of synchronisation. Fig. 9a shows a phase lag approaching 90° per oscillator, while a correspondingly smaller phase lead is indicated in Fig. 9b for a stimulating frequency lower than the unpaced value. Examination of   the   top trace   in   each   of   these photographs indicates the position of the stimulating pulse (aproximately 0.5 division wide) and shows that the   phase   shift   between the   stimulating   pulse   and   the first oscillator output approached 90° lag and lead respectively.

Phase shifts for the relaxation model   were   entirely   different,   in   that phase   leads   were   not   observed. A typical condition is shown in Fig. 10 for three oscillators. In Fig. 10a the stimulating frequency was above the   normal value   and on the verge of desynchronisation. A phase lag of 90° per oscillator is evident and the top trace indicates that the pulse was located at the   bottom of   the   first   oscillator   output i.e. almost 180° phase lag (note that all pulses were positive going in all the   experiments).   In   contrast,   the   model could not be paced at a frequency lower than normal. Fig. 10b shows the condition at the low frequency end of the synchronisation band, when the phase   shift

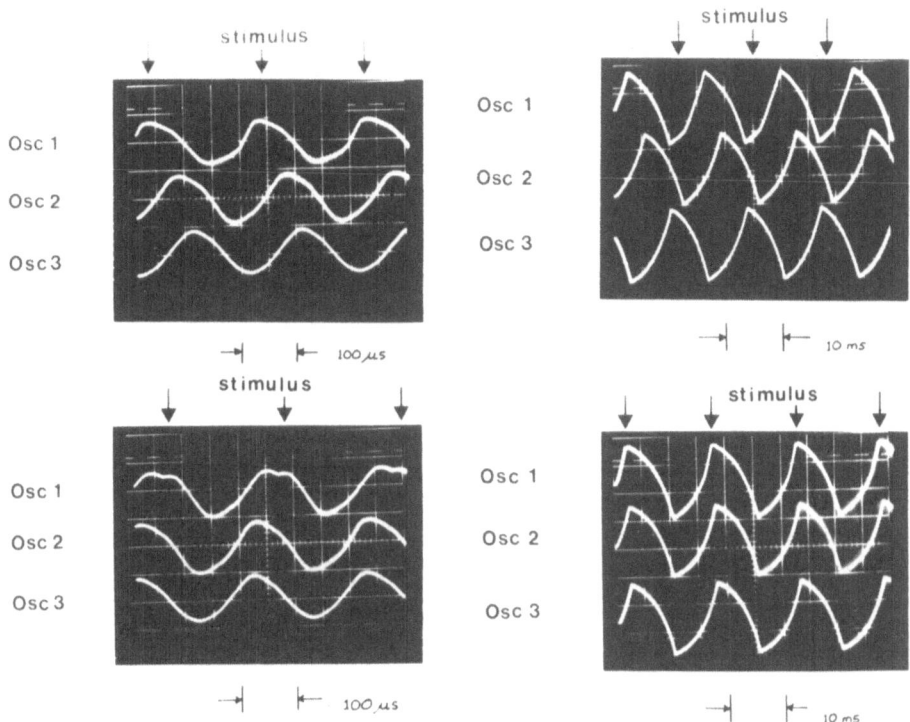

FIGURE 9 *Pulse synchronisation of 3 coupled van der Pol oscillators with pacing into oscillator 1.*
a) Stimulus frequency greater than unpaced frequency, giving phase lag, or velocity away from the stimulus.
b) Stimulus frequency less than unpaced frequency, giving a phase lead, or velocity towards the stimulus.

FIGURE 10 *Waveforms for 3 coupled relaxation oscillators at edge of synchronisation band with pacing into oscillator 1.*
a) Stimulus frequency greater than unpaced frequency giving phase lag of about 90° per oscillator.
b) Stimulus frequency less than unpaced frequency giving almost zero phase shift along the chain.

was almost zero. The top trace shows the stimulating pulse straddling the top
of the first oscillator output indicating zero phase between the stimulus and
the model.

CONCLUSIONS

From the results in the previous section it is clear that there is a considerable difference between the relaxation model and the other models under pulse
synchronisation conditions. The major difference is that the relaxation model
was very difficult to pace at a lower frequency that its normal condition, with
the associated fact that phase lead along the chain could not be induced. This
is a serious disadvantage for its use as an intestinal model since phase leads
have been achieved in animal experiments in vivo. There is, in fact, a gener-
ic difference in this model from the others in that its operation is based on
threshold switching of active amplifiers. In contrast, the other two models can
be represented in equivalent circuit form as having non-linear conductance elements without discrete switching. It is interesting to note that van der Pol
originally formulated his equation to explain thyratron relaxation switching oscillations. It has, however, been recognised that his equation does not really
match such switching type circuit behaviour (Alexander, 1976).
    A further difference between the relaxation model and the others is that it
was harder to pace under strongly coupled conditions than when weakly coupled.
This also appears to be contrary to physiological experiments in that both stomach and small-intestine pacing have been readily achieved, whereas canine colonic pacing has produced greater disorganisation rather than synchronisation
(Linkens, 1978). It is also considered that the colon is much more weakly coupled than the stomach and small-intestine which show well co-ordinated entrainment conditions (Shearin et al., 1978) and hence the switching model appears
to show the wrong pulse synchronisation behaviour.
    The van der Pol and Hodgkin-Huxley models showed a similar behaviour under
pacing conditions, and gave results which are consistent with known physiological in vivo experiments. The behavioural pattern can be summarised as fol-

lows.   Increasing   the   chain beyond three oscillators had comparatively little
effect on synchronisation width.   In general, weakly coupled models were   harder
to   pace   than   strongly   coupled ones, with this effect being greater for small
non-linear waveshape factor ε (i.e. waveforms nearly sinusoidal).   The   effect
of   changing the strength of the forcing pulse was predictable, in that both increasing amplitude and pulse width gave a larger synchronisation range.   An   asymmetry   occurred, howevver, in the synchronisation band so that its range above
the normal unpaced frequency was higher than that below.   This was true for most
conditions   of   pacing and agrees with the pacing experiments on the canine stomach in which the normal rhythm of 0.084 Hz could be driven upwards to 0.133 Hz,
but   downwards   to   only   0.07 Hz (Kelly and Laforce, 1972).   The relative phase
shift along the chain depended on whether the stimulating frequency was above or
below the unpaced model frequency.   Phase lags of nearly $90°$ could be induced by
higher pacing frequencies, and phase leads of about $60°$ could   be   induced   by
lower   pacing   frequencies.   The phase lag corresponds to a downwards travelling
wave   in   the   gut   which   is   the   normal   direction   in   the   stomach   and
small-intestine.   The phase lead corresponds to an upwards travelling wave which
was slightly more difficult to produce with pacing, but which has also been   observed in physiological pacing experiments.

It is interesting to note that the   coupling   impedances   representing   the
normal   coupling   range   for each of the oscillators were very similar (between 5
KOhm and 50 KOhm) in spite of the large differences in   the   model   frequencies.
It was also observed that similar synchronisation bands were obtained when using
capacitive rather than resistive coupling.   In this case similar   reactances   to
the resistance range shown in Figs.   2-7 were used, giving coupling capacitances
much less than the internal capacitances of the oscillators.   Thus,   intercellular   capacitances   less   than membrane capacitances would be sufficient to cause
significant coupling between oscillating units.

In comparing the results with the physiological pacing   experiments   it   is
seen   that   the van der Pol and Hodgkin-Huxley type models gave the same type of
phenomena under pacing.   It thus appears that pacing experiments have   distinguished   a   difference   in   the class of models which did not appear in studies on
frequency entrainment, frequency gradient and frequency modulation   conditions,
and that a major disadvantage in the relaxation switching model exists.

REFERENCES

Akwari, O.E., Kelly, K.A., Steinbach, J.H. and Code, C.F.: Electric pacing of intact and transected canine small-intestine and its computer model. Am. J. Physiol., 229: 1188-1197, 1975.

Alexander, J.W.: On the doubtful validity of van der Pol's theory on relaxation oscillators. J. App. Sci. and Eng. Section A., 237-243, 1976.

Brown, B.H., Duthie, H.L., Horn, A.R. and Smallwood, R.H.: A linked oscillator model of electrical activity of human small-intestine. Am. J. Physiol., 229: 384-388, 1975.

Datardina, S.P. and Linkens, D.A.: Multimode oscillations in mutually coupled van der Pol type oscillators with fifth power non-linear characteristics. IEEE Trans. Cct. and Sys. CAS-25, 308-315, 1978.

Kelly, K.A. and Laforce, R.C.: Pacing the canine stomach with electric stimulation. Am. J. Physiol., 222: 588-594, 1972.

Linkens, D.A.: The stability of entrainment conditions for RLC coupled van der Pol oscillators. Bull. Math. Biol., 39: 359-372, 1977.

Linkens, D.A.: Canine colonic pacing and coupled oscillator synchronisation. J. Physiol. (London), 278, 26P, 1978.

Linkens, D.A. and Datardina, S.P.: Frequency entrainment of coupled Hodgkin-Huxley type oscillators for modelling gastrointestinal electrical activity. IEEE Trans. Bio. Med. Eng., BME 24, 4: 362-365, 1977.

Linkens, D.A., Taylor, I. and Duthie, H.L.: Mathematical Modelling of the colorectal myoelectrical activity in humans. IEEE Trans. Bio. Med. Eng., BME 23, 101-110, 1976.

Patton, R.J. and Linkens, D.A.: Hodgkin-Huxley type electronic modelling of gastrointestinal electrical activity. Med. and Biol. Eng. and Comp., 16: 195-202, 1978.

Robertson-Dunn, B. and Linkens, D.A.: A mathematical model of the slow-wave electrical activity of the human small-intestine. Med. and Biol. Eng., 750-758, 1974.

Sarna, S.K., Daniel, E.E. and Kingma, Y.J.: Simulation of slow-wave electrical activity of small-intestine. Am. J. Physiol., 221: 166-175, 1971.

Sarna, S.K., Daniel, E.E. and Kingma, Y.J.: Simulation of the electrical control activity of the stomach by an array of relaxation oscillators. Am.

J. Dig. Dis., 17: 299-310, 1972.

Sarna, S.K. and Daniel, E.E.: Electrical stimulation of gastric electrical control activity. Am. J. Physiol., 225: 125-131, 1973.

Sarna, S.K. and Daniel, E.E.: Electrical stimulation of small intestinal electrical control activity. Gastroenterol., 69: 660-667, 1975.

Shearin, N.L., Bowes, K.L., Kingma, Y.J. and Koles, Z.T.: Frequency analysis of electrical activity in dog colon. 6th Inst. Symp. on G.I. Motility, Edinburgh, 1977.

DYNAMIC PROPERTIES OF ELECTRICALLY

INTERACTING EXCITABLE CELLS

Vincent Torre

INTRODUCTION

Interaction between nerve cells mediated by electrical coupling is a common feature of the nervous system (for a review see Bennett, 1977). This interaction
may be specific to a restricted number of cells, or even to part of a cell as in
the case of the electrical inhibition in the initial segment of the Mauthner
fibre (Korn and Faber, 1975).

In other cases electrical interaction may occur within an entire population
of similar neurones. In this case the dynamic behaviour of individual cells is
influenced and shaped by the entire network of cells.

In the vertebrate retina photoreceptors are commonly coupled to each other
through gap junctions. This electrical interaction has been shown between cones
in the turtle retina (Baylor et al., 1971), between rods in the turtle retina
(Copenhagen and Owen, 1976) and in the retina of toads, tiger salamanders and
bullfrogs. This interaction is essentially electrical and selective, that is
rods interact only with rods and cones interact only with cones of the same co-
lour (Detwiler and Hodgkin, 1979). The electrotonic space constant is 20 - 70
μm.

Horizontal cells in the fish retina (Kaneko, 1971) and in the turtle retina
(Simon, 1973) are electrically coupled; the activity of a single cell can
spread to the successive four or five cells, covering a distance of 400-700 μm.
Chemical interactions may also be involved (Lasansky and Vallerga, 1975).

The electrical coupling between smooth muscle cells can be strong. The excitation can spread over 1-4 mm through several cells (Bennett, 1972; Holman
and Hirst, 1977).

Heart muscle cells too form an electrical syncitium (Weidmann, 1952; Noble, 1979). In the sino-atrial node pacemaker cells are 15-20 μm long and 2-8 μm wide with an electrotonic space constant of 460 μm (Bonke, 1973). This interaction is of fundamental importance to the setting of the heart beat.

The electrical interaction between a population of almost homogenous excitable cells may produce completely different patterns of activity in the network. In the sino atrial node electrical interaction produces synchronization. In the retina the same mechanism can produce between rods a kind of "negative velocity" first described by Detwiler et al. (1978) in the turtle retina.

In what follows I will present a review of analytical results already published (Torre, 1976; Grattarola and Torre, 1977) and recently obtained in Cambridge during an electrophysiological analysis of the network of toad rods in collaboration with Dr. W.G. Owen under the supervision of Sir Alan Hodgkin.

Electrical interaction occurs generally through specialized patches of cell membrane called gap junctions. These structures are regions of low resistance between neighbouring cells and may be represented by the electrical equivalent of a resistance R_s. The capacitance of gap junctions is rather low and can be neglected. In some electrical synapses there is a leakage out of the edges of the junction. In this case the electrical equivalent of the junction is a T structure of resistance. The coupling resistance R_s in most cases is constant over a range of ± 25 mV (egg cells, septate axon - see Bennett, 1977). In other cases the electrical synapses seem to rectify as in the giant motor synapse of the crayfish (Furshpan and Potter, 1959), and the giant fibre synapses on motor neurones of the hatchfish (Auerbach and Bennett, 1969).

Fig. 1A shows the electrical equivalent circuit of a one dimensional array of identical cells interacting electrically through shunting resistances R_s. In Fig. 2A a two dimensional model is represented. The electrical properties of the cell membrane are represented by a generalized impedance Z_m.

The dynamic behaviour of the network depends critically on the properties of Z_m. If the membrane impedance can be linearized to a satisfactory approximation, then this "phenomenological" impedance characterizes the dynamics of the network. In this case the strength of the coupling, that is the magnitude of R_s cannot change the qualitative behaviour.

On the contrary if the membrane impedance has regions of negative resistance for physiological membrane potentials then the qualitative dynamic behavi-

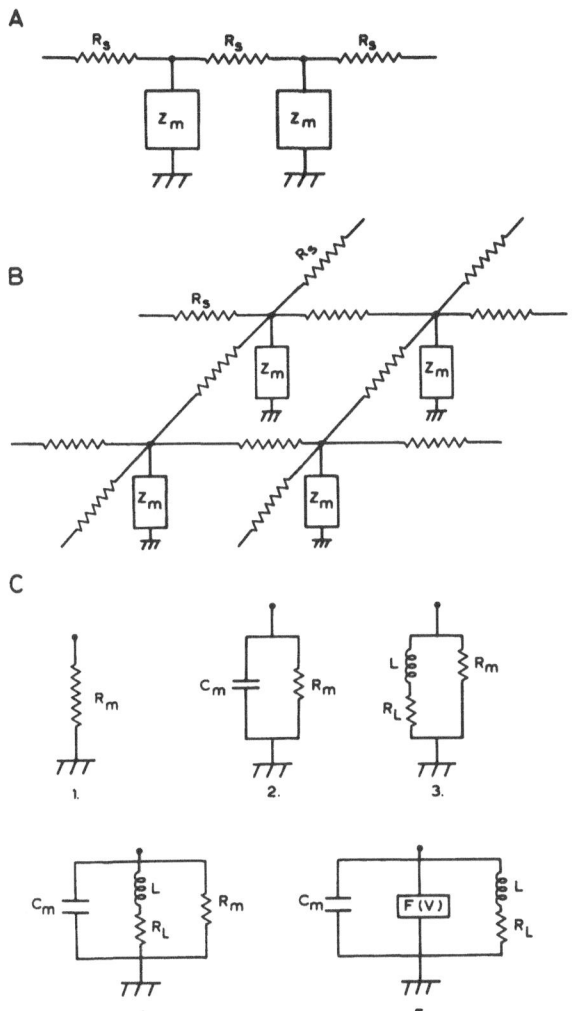

FIGURE 1 A. *Electrical equivalent of a unidimensional network of electrically coupled cells. R_s is the coupling resistance and Z_m is the membrane impedance of the cells. B. Electrical equivalent of a two-dimensional network of electrically coupled cells. C. Types of membrane impedance: 1, purely resistive (R_M = membrane resistance); 2, low pass (C_M = membrane capacitance); 3, high pass (L = phenomenological membrane inductance. R_L = phenomenological associated membrane resistance); 4, band pass; 5, non-linear impedance ($F(V)$) represents the I,V relation of the cell membrane).*

our of the network depends not only on Z_m but also on R_s.

LINEAR IMPEDANCE

When the membrane impedance Z_m can be linearized, that is when the linear approximation is satisfactory over the range of voltages under analysis, the properties of the network can be almost fully described in terms of the linear phenomenological impedance $Z_m(\omega)$.

UNIDIMENSIONAL NETWORK

OHMIC   In the simplest case of purely ohmic impedance, we have $Z_m(\omega) = R_M$ (Fig. 1C1).   Some features of this case have already been solved (see Lamb and Simon, 1976; Detwiler and Hodgkin, 1979). If a current $I_1(t)$ is injected in cell 1 in a unidimensional array of n cells, the voltage in cell k when n $\gg$ k is

$$V_k(t) = \frac{R_s \alpha^2}{\alpha^2 - 1} \left(\frac{1}{\alpha} \right)^k \tag{1}$$

where

$$\alpha = \frac{a}{2} + \frac{\sqrt{a^2 - 4}}{2} \qquad a = \left(\frac{R_s}{R_M} + 2 \right)$$

if the spacing between cells is D, the electrotonic space constant is

$$\lambda = \frac{D}{\ln\left(1 + \dfrac{\gamma^2 + \sqrt{\gamma^2 + 4\gamma}}{2} \right)} \qquad \gamma = \frac{R_s}{R_M} \tag{2}$$

NON OHMIC   An explicit analytical solution can be obtained in   all   cases   when
the   poles of $Z_m(\omega)$ are known (Owen and Torre, in preparation).   This analytical
solution may be rather complex but it is possible to understand, at least qualitatively, the behaviour of the network from simpler considerations.   The attenuation of the network is a function of frequency and for sinusoidal   currents   we
have

$$\lambda(\omega) = \frac{D}{\ln\left(1 + \dfrac{\gamma^2(\omega) + \sqrt{\gamma^2(\omega) + 4\gamma(\omega)}}{2}\right)} \tag{3}$$

where

$$\gamma(\omega) = \frac{R_s}{|Z_m(\omega)|}$$

From eqn. (3) we can easily understand the qualitative behaviour   of   the   network.   If   the membrane impedance $Z_m(\omega)$ is a simple RC, the network will behave
as a low pass system (Fig. 1C2).

In the toad retina, as in the turtle retina (Detwiler et al., 1980), when
a narrow slit of light (width 11 μm) is briefly shown over the rod whose electrical activity is recorded, a slow hyperpolarizing wave is induced with a time to
peak of around 600-900 ms.
In Fig. 2A the result of an experiment is shown in which the slit of light   was
displaced   by   steps   of 10 μm from the impaled rod.   When the slit is moved the
voltage recorded is smaller but, surprisingly, has a shorter time to peak.   This
is   paradoxical   if   the   current   has   spread   from neighbouring rods through a
cable-like structure with resistive and capacitative elements.   To explain   this
surprising   property   Detwiler   et al. (1980) suggested that the rod membrane
might have the electrical equivalent of an inductance.

We have collected some evidence that for small signals (less than   5-8   mV)
the rod membrane has a voltage and time dependent K^+ conductance that mimics the

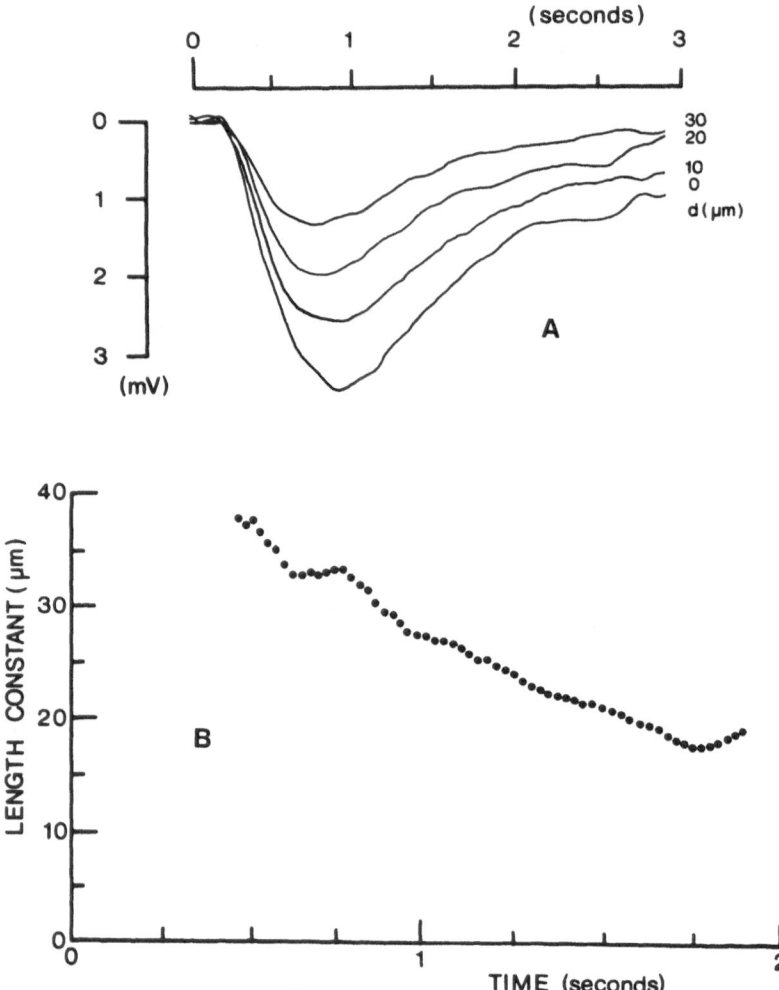

FIGURE 2 A. Responses recorded intracellularly from a rod bathed in Ringer solution containing: 132 mM Na$^+$, 2.6 mM K$^+$, 120.6 mM Cl$^-$, 2 mM Ca^{++}, 2 mM Mg^{++}, 5 mM glucose, buffered with bicarbonate-CO$_2$ to pH 7.8. Rods were stimulated from above by projecting onto the retina the sharply focused, reduced image of a long narrow slit. Stimuli were of wavelength 498 nm, 50 ms duration and produced on average 13.5 photoisomerizations (Rh) per rod. Four responses were recorded at each stimulus position and were subsequently averaged. B. The length constant of the rod network computed from the responses of 2A at 20 ms interval and plotted as a function of the time following stimulus presentation.

behaviour of an inductance. Therefore the phenomenological impedance of the rod membrane $Z_m(\omega)$ has an equivalent inductance (Fig. 1C3) that is responsible for the high pass filtering properties of the rod network.

In the rod network (as in any other network), if $Z_m(\omega)$ has high pass characteristics so will the network. In this case it is important to recall that the electrotonic space constant will be a function of the input signals and will change with time when the input is not sinusoidal.

Fig. 2B shows the dependance of λ on time for the experiment of Fig. 2A. λ initially has a high value of around 35 μm and falls to 17 μm after 1-2 seconds. In an inductive network we have an initial high spread of excitation followed by a contraction. If the cell membrane phenomenological impedance $Z_m(\omega)$ is band-limited (Fig. 1C4) the network will have band-limited characteristics, that will closely follow those of $Z_m(\omega)$.

TWO DIMENSIONAL NETWORK

OHMIC CASE   The two dimensional case is analytically more complicated, but has essentially the same behaviour (Owen and Torre, in preparation). In a purely resistive network of $(2n + 1) \times (2n + 1)$ cells, injection of current $I_{o,o}(t)$ into cell n+1,n+1 at the centre of the two dimensional network will give rise to a voltage at cell h,k of

$$V_{h,k} = R_s \left(\sum_{i}^{2n+1} \sum_{j}^{2n+1} b_{ijhk} \right) I_{o,o}(t) \qquad (4)$$

where

$$b_{ijhk} = \frac{a_{hi} a_{kj} a_{n+1,i} a_{n+1,j}}{4 + \dfrac{R_s}{R_M} + 2\cos \dfrac{i\pi}{2n+2} + 2\cos \dfrac{j\pi}{2n+2}} \qquad (5)$$

$$a_{ih} = \frac{(-1)^{i-1}\sin\frac{ih\pi}{2n+2}}{\sqrt{n + \frac{1}{2} - (-1)^h \frac{\sin\frac{2n+1}{2n+2}h\pi}{2\sin\frac{h\pi}{2n+2}}}} \tag{6}$$

NON-OHMIC CASE   Also in the two dimensional case an explicit analytical solution can be obtained when the poles of $Z_m(\omega)$ are known, following a method obtained by Owen and Torre (in preparation). The frequency attenuation can easily
be analysed by substituting R_M by $|Z_m(\omega)|$ in Eqn. (5). As in the one dimension-
al case the frequency properties of the network are very similar to the spectrum
of $Z_m(\omega)$.

NON-LINEAR IMPEDANCE

If Z_m is not linearizable and the cell membrane I,V characteristics have a region of negative resistance a completely different dynamical pattern may appear.

      If the equilibrium position of the membrane potential is unstable, that is
if the membrane potential is steadily oscillating (or pacing), the electrical
coupling may be the synchronizing mechanism. For simplicity let us assume that
the electrical properties of cell membranes are represented by the circuit of
Fig. 1C5, where F(V) represents the I,V relation of the cell membrane and may
be n-shaped. That is with $\lim\limits_{V \to \pm \infty} F(V) = \pm \infty$, and for some $\bar{V}$, $F(\bar{V}) = 0$. If
the membrane potential is unstable and the cell is pacing we must have an unst-
able equilibrium potential for some $\tilde{V}$. Setting $\tilde{V}$ equal to 0 we have $F(0) = 0$.

      It can be shown (Torre, 1976) that if R_s is sufficiently small, that is if
the electrical coupling is sufficiently strong, the cells will tend to synchronize their pacing phase and will tend to oscillate in a synchronized pattern. In
this case the one-dimensional and the two-dimensional networks are not essentially different. The main difference is that in the two dimensional network
synchronization can be reached for values of R_s higher than those required in
the one-dimensional case (see Theorem 3, Torre 1976).

An interesting property of a population of non-linear synchronized oscillators is that they have a "robust" dynamic behaviour. That is, if the network is
slightly perturbed (e.g. the characteristics of one or more oscillators are
changed) the dynamics are not greatly influenced, the period is only slightly
changed. On the other side a population of linear synchronized oscillators
(harmonic oscillators) is not robust in the same sense. An arbitrary small perturbation will drastically affect the period and possibly destroy the phase synchronization. This different behaviour is due to the fact that only non-linear
systems can have structurally stable periodic solutions (Abraham and Robbin,
1967). It is not, therefore surprising that biological oscillators, to fulfil
the requirement of "robustness", are represented by a set of non-linear differential equations.

In Torre (1976) it is proved analytically that synchronization will occur
between pacing cells whose electrical membrane properties can be described by
the circuit of Fig. 1C5. Slightly more general conditions have been presented
in Grattarola and Torre (1977) but I think that the set of non-linear structurally stable oscillators for which a sufficiently strong electrical coupling is a
synchronizing mechanism is much wider.

If the set of non-linear differential equations describing the oscillator
has only one stable trajectory, and all other singular points are unstable, it
is likely that electrical coupling synchronizes the oscillators. In general oscillators describing electrical repetitive activity in excitable membranes, like
the Hodgkin-Huxley model or the Noble model, have a more complex configuration
in phase space. Cooley et al. (1965) have shown that in the Hodgkin-Huxley
model for some current steps there is a stable singular point and a stable limit
cycle; in this case the system could switch from the stable singular point to
the stable limit cycle in response to suitable shocks, and then it is possible
that electrical coupling may not synchronize the oscillators.

If the membrane potential of the cells is not pacing, then a signal sufficiently small, that will not reach the region in the I,V curves of negative resistance, will spread in the network approximately as described in the previous
case.

In some cases the signal may reach the region of negative resistance and
may be transmitted along the network across distances longer than those compatible with passive cable properties. For instance when the toads retina is per-

fused with a Ringer medium containing 15 mM of TEA and 200 μM of Co^{++}, the electrotonic space constant λ in rods may increase 2-4 times (Owen and Torre, in preparation). This increase in λ cannot be simply explained by an increase of membrane resistance due to the TEA and Co^{++} action and has to be explained by active membrane properties.

When R_s is sufficiently small and the regenerative response can be fully activated in a neighbouring cell, the signal will be perfectly transmitted through the network without attenuation. This is the classical case of active propagation already fully analysed and discussed (Jack et al., 1975).

ACKNOWLEDGEMENT

I would like to thank Drs. P.A. McNaughton and T.D. Lamb for reading the manuscript. The work was carried out with the support of an EMBO Long-term Fellowship.

REFERENCES

Abraham, R. and Robbin, J.: Transversal mapping and flows. Benjamin, New York, 1967.

Auerbach, A.A. and Bennett, M.V.L.: A rectifying synapse in the central nervous system of a vertebrate. J. Gen. Physiol., 53: 211-237, 1969.

Baylor, D.A., Fuortes, M.G.F. and O'Bryan, P.M.: Receptive fields of single cones in the retina of the turtle. J. Physiol. (London), 207: 77-92, 1971.

Bennett, M.R.: Autonomic neuromuscular transmission. Cambridge University Press, Cambridge, (Monograph of Physiological Society), 1972.

Bennett, M.V.L.: Electrical transmission: a functional analysis and comparison to chemical transmission. In: Handbook of Physiology. American Physiological Society, Bethesda, Maryland, 1977.

Bonke, F.I.M.: Electrotonic spread in the sino atrial node of the rabbit heart. Pfluegers Arch., 339: 17-23, 1973.

Cooley, J., Dodge, F. and Cohen, H.: Digital computer solutions for excitable membrane models. J. Cell. Comp. Physiol., 66, 99-108, 1965.

Copenhagen, D.R. and Owen, W.G.: Functional characteristics of lateral inter- actions between rods in the retina of snapping turtle. J. Physiol. (London), 259: 251-282, 1976.

Detwiler, P.B., Hodgkin, A.L. and McNaughton, P.M.: A surprising property of electrical spread in the network of rods in the turtle's retina. Nature, 274: 562-565, 1978.

Detwiler, P.B. and Hodgkin, A.L.: Electrical coupling between cones in the turtle retina. J. Physiol. (London), 291, 75-100, 1979.

Detwiler, P.B., Hodgkin, A.L. and McNaughton, P.A.: Temporal and spatial char- acteristics of the voltage response of rods in the retina of the snapping turtle. J. Physiol. (London), 300: 213-250, 1980.

Furshpan, E.G., Potter, D.D.: Transmission at the giant motor synapses of the crayfish. J. Physiol. (London), 145: 289-325, 1959.

Grattarola, M. and Torre, V.: Necessary and sufficient conditions for syn- chronization of non-linear oscillators with a given class of coupling. IEEE Trans., 24: 209-215, 1977.

Holman, M.E. and Hirst, G.D.S.: Junctional transmission in smooth muscle and the autonomic nervous system. In: Handbook of Physiology, American Physi- ological Society, Bethesda, Maryland, 1977.

Jack, J.J.B., Noble, D. and Tsien, R.W.: Electric current flow in excitable cells. Clarendon Press, Oxford, 1973.

Kaneko, A.: Electrical connexions between horizontal cells in the dogfish reti- na. J. Physiol. (London), 213: 95-105, 1976.

Korn, H. and Faber, D.S.: An electrically mediated inhibition in goldfish me- dulla. J. Neurophysiol., 38: 430-451, 1975.

Lamb, T.D. and Simon, E.J.: The relation between intercellular coupling and electrical noise in turtle photoreceptors. J. Physiol. (London), 263, 257-286, 1976.

Lasansky, A. and Vallerga, S.: Horizontal cell responses in the retina of the larval tiger salamander. J. Physiol. (London), 236: 171-191, 1975.

Noble, D.:   The Initiation of the Heart Beat, Clarendon Press, Oxford, 1979.

Simon, E.J.:   Two types of luminosity horizontal cells in the retina of the turtle.   J.   Physiol.   (London), 230:   199-211, 1973.

Torre, V.:   A theory of synchronization of heart pacemaker   cells.   J.   Theor.
Biol., 61:   55-71, 1976.

Weidmann, S.:   The   electrical   constants   of   Purkinje   fibres.   J.   Physiol.
(London), 118:   348-360, 1952.

FIBRILLATION AS A CONSEQUENCE OF PACEMAKER PHASE-RESETTING

Arthur T. Winfree

INTRODUCTION

The abundant variety of spontaneously rhythmic neurons have certain simple properties in common.   Some of the most intriguing among these common properties
concern the manner of reaction to a single stimulus. The stimulus is   typically
followed by transient hyperpolarization or depolarization and a derangement of
normal rhythmicity which may persist as long as several cycles. But when these
transients are past, the neuron typically reasserts its prior waveform and period. The only lasting consequence of the stimulus is a residual offset of the
pacemaker's timing: it now fires between firings of an unperturbed replicate
control, or between the rhythmically extrapolated projections of its own
pre-stimulus firings.   The amount of this rescheduling depends, of course, on
the nature and magnitude of the stimulus. It also typically depends on the timing of stimulus onset within the pacemaker cycle.

   Within the past several years, there have appeared dozens of careful measurements of this dependence, using a wide variety of spontaneously rhythmic preparations. Parallel studies have been undertaken on theoretical models of such
pacemakers. From all these investigations there emerge three conspicuous generalizations which, to my mind, deserve special attention. The third of these has
come into focus only within the last three years. It has some rather surprising
implications. So far as they have been tested up to now, these implications
seem to include experimentally reproducible events of a curious nature. The
purpose of this paper is to review them and to draw your attention to further
testable implications that may have a bearing on the complex phenomena of
flutter and fibrillation. I will attempt to draw these out in a way that is as
nearly mathematics-free and model-independent as possible by starting from the
aforementioned three empirical generalizations.

SPACE-INDEPENDENT PREPARATIONS

Before reminding you of those three main results, I ask you to bear with me through a short digression to clarify the format I find most convenient for plotting them. This turns out to be important: the third and most critical generalization seems to have escaped notice in other plotting formats.

The main peculiarities of this format are:

1) that I plot the data directly without the subtractions or comparisons implicit in describing results as "phase advances" or "phase delays", and

2) that I take no interest in the transient aftermath of perturbation, prior to resumption of the normal pacemaker rhythm. Only by attending these transients, of course, can one interpret the rescheduling as "advance" or "delay". The attempt to impose this distinction on experimental results commonly leads to paradoxical contradictions (Winfree, 1980 a,b). For my purposes it is sufficient to evade this "problem" by abjuring the terminology of advances and delays and ignoring transients.

The next few paragraphs lay out this plotting format in terms of a simple-minded idealization: rescheduling a perfectly periodic heartbeat by a single stimulus to the sino-atrial node.

In Fig. 1 you see a dashed horizontal line along which time increases from right to left. Once per second a heartbeat occurs, indicated by a dot. At point S a stimulus is applied. Heartbeats after this stimulus are plotted along the same time axis but now bent upwards. By bending the time axis upward at the moment of shock we can now plot on one page the timing of the heartbeat after a shock given at any time between beats (along the fainter vertical lines). To use the graph, follow the horizontal line leftward to where you want to give a stimulus then continue upward to see its effect on the timing of subsequent beats. They come at regular intervals (after the omitted transients), so we see beat after beat vertically on each line. Giving a stimulus at point S is the same as giving it at point S' (the same stage of the prior cycle) so we expect the subsequent beats to come at the same times after the stimulus: the vertical line above S' is an exact copy of the one above S. In fact the whole diagram is periodic both vertically and horizontally, like a piece of wallpaper.

Note that I described the layout of this peculiar graph in terms of a time axis running backward from right to left, then upward after the stimulus. It

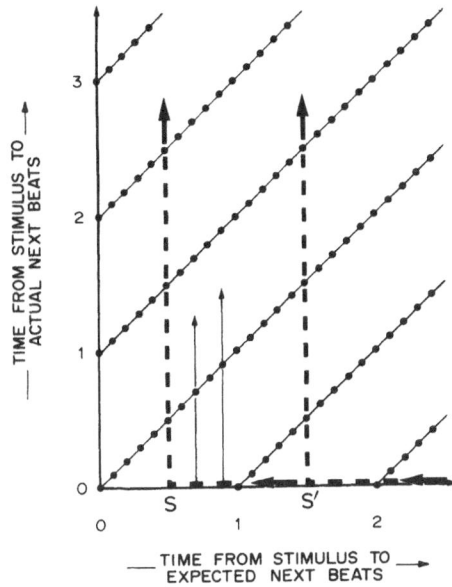

FIGURE 1 *An idealized latency diagram for any spontaneously rhythmic neuron. Each dot represents by its horizontal position the time in the pacemaker cycle when a stimulus is given, and by its vertical position above the axis, the subsequent time after the stimulus until the next beat (and the next ...). The diagonal lines correspond to a completely ineffectual control stimulus.*

would be equivalent to say that we are plotting vertically the ACTUAL intervals (latencies) from stimulus to heartbeats and horizontally the EXPECTED (pre-stimulus) intervals (latencies) from stimulus to heartbeats: time being measured from the right, the distance remaining to the left edge of the graph is the time remaining to an anticipated heartbeat.

Now why do the beats line up along a 45-degree slope? Fig. 1 plots an extreme case, the case of a stimulus so faint that it has no noticeable effect. (Suppose for example that we accidentally left the stimulator unplugged.) So the time from the (negligible) stimulus to the next beat (the vertical position of the beat) is exactly the same as the time to the EXPECTED next beat (the horizontal position of the beat). Or to put it another way, the next beat will come practically a full cycle after a "stimulus" given right after a beat, or 2/3 cycle after a "stimulus" given 1/3 cycle after a beat (2/3 cycle before the expected next beat), or immediately after a "stimulus" given right at the end of a cycle, just before the next beat. Those points (and all intermediates) comprise the fine rising diagonal line in Fig. 1.

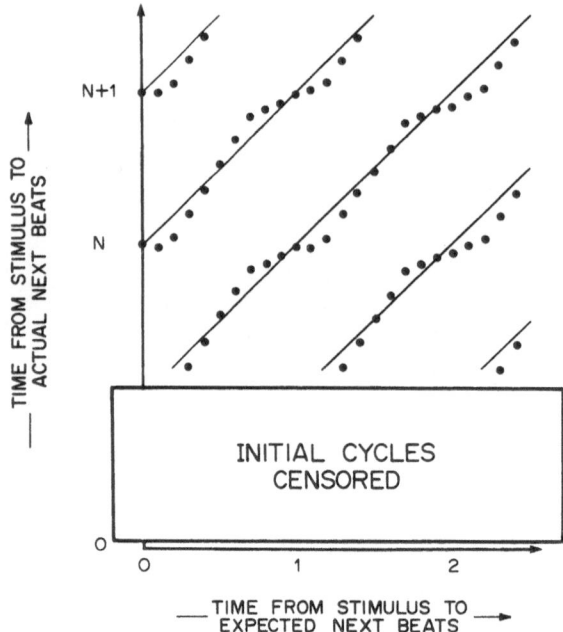

FIGURE 2 *As in Fig. 1 but with a stimulus big enough to cause some small advances and delays. This is type 1 resetting (so is fig. 1). The omitted region is supposed to represent an interval after stimulation and prior to resumption of normal rhythmicity.*

If we remember to plug in the stimulator, but use it gently, things are not much different (Fig. 2). At some phases of the cycle the stimulus has a little advancing effect (beats come sooner than expected: beats below the fine line), and at other phases it may have a little delaying effect (beats come a bit later: beats just above the fine diagonal line). In real experiments the beats stray systematically in this way above and below the fine idealized line, like beads on a necklace that snakes up the 45-degree slope. Progressive change in stimulus timing causes progressive changes in the timing of subsequent beats, and in order to satisfy the necessary periodicity of the wallpaper the curve must rise a full cycle as it goes full cycle to the right. This is called "type 1 resetting" because the curve necessarily rises with average slope = 1 exactly.

The format of this plot is exactly as used throughout Winfree (1980a) and prior papers, but for a 180-degree rotation of the whole diagram to bring the direction of the axes into conformity with convention in this literature.

This ends the hypothetical digression. We now return to the real world and the three main results of neurophysiological phase-resetting experiments reported in the last few years.

EMPIRICAL GENERALIZATION 1 (obvious): All pacemaker neurons exhibit type 1 resetting in response to sufficiently delicate stimuli.

EMPIRICAL GENERALIZATION 2 (surprise): Stimuli stronger than required to elicit type 1 but not yet strong enough to elicit type 0 resetting (see below) commonly elicit a discontinuity of about 1/2 cycle in the resetting curve.   In the case of hyperpolarizing stimuli the discontinuity usually appears about 0.1 cycle after the upstroke of the action potential; depolarizing stimuli commonly show it at the opposite phase, about 0.6 cycle after upstroke. Examples are tabulated in Winfree (1980a page 172, 1980b) (NOTA BENE: it is essential to   distinguish this real physiological discontinuity of about 1/2 cycle from an artifactual discontinuity of exactly 1 cycle which appears in many published plots simply because large advances are conventionally reinterpreted as complementary delays.)

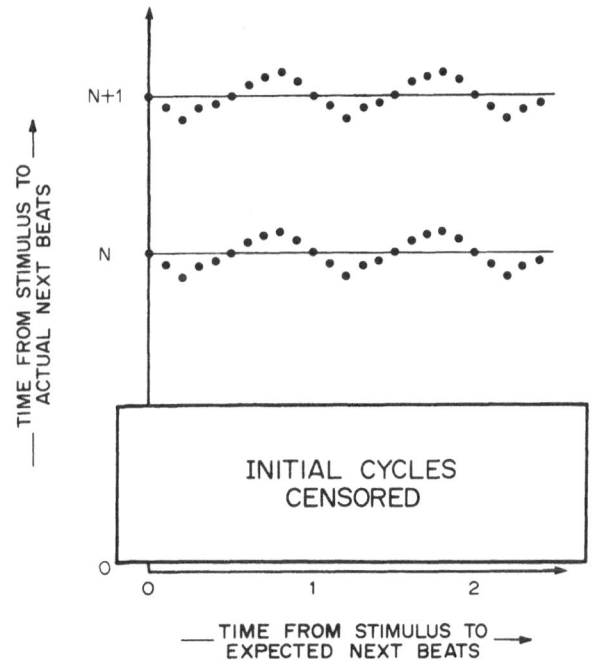

TIME FROM STIMULUS TO ACTUAL NEXT BEATS

N+1

N

INITIAL CYCLES
CENSORED

0   1   2

TIME FROM STIMULUS TO
EXPECTED NEXT BEATS

FIGURE 3 *As in Fig.   2 but the stimulus is still bigger. The horizontal lines correspond to the idealized limiting case of a stimulus strong enough to so completely reset the pacemaker that its latency to next firing scarcely varies. This is type 0 resetting.*

EMPIRICAL GENERALIZATION 3 (anticipated from theoretical considerations not here belabored;   see Winfree (1977, 1980a)): Something different happens when you give a substantial shock. Fig. 3 shows the general layout of beat timing after a big stimulus.   I drew the extreme case of a really big stimulus as a fine horizontal line: beats recur at the same latency after the stimulus no matter when it was given; it simply resets the heartbeat to zero phase, regardless. That is an idealization. In real experiments beats stray systematically above and below the fine line, just as they did in Fig. 2; but here they stray about a HORIZONTAL line. This is called "type 0 resetting" because the curve's average slope is necessarily exactly zero.

COMMENT: It turns out that we get into a bit of a crisis when we   try to sketch curves that might be found at intermediate stimulus strengths, because there is no way to smoothly deform a set of curves like Fig. 2 into a set of curves like Fig. 3. Try it. Think of the necklaces as though they were strung on rubber bands, and deform them as you imagine stronger and stronger stimuli starting from Fig. 2, or weaker and weaker, starting from Fig. 3. You'll see that at some stimulus strength you will have to cut the rubber bands to change them over to the other format. At that cut you can not say when the next beats will come: the curve is interrupted there; it doesn't exist. Type 0 resetting is diagnostic for this effect.

What is going on? This trivial topological dilemma is telling us that something physiologically very irregular HAS TO occur when a stimulus of some intermediate strength arrives at some special phase in the heartbeat... something so irregular that no one, no matter how clever, will ever be able to predict the timing (the phase shift or the latency) of the subsequent heartbeats. What could such a singular event be? Mathematicians call it a "phase singularity", but what does it amount to physiologically? Is it too much to imagine that the heart might be as indecisive as we are and simply not beat again? We return to this later.

Type 0 resetting apparently occurs in quite a few preparations in response to sufficiently strong stimuli.   Examples, including spontaneously rhythmic cells of the mammalian heart, are tabulated in Winfree (1977, 1980a page 111, 1980b).   Jalife (unpublished personal communication) has also encountered what appears to be type 0 resetting of the SA node by a vagal volley. Another intriguing case is reported by Jalife et al. (1980): with further increased stimu-

lation type 0 resetting reverts to type 1! So the indeterminacy   crisis   recurs
at this additional stimulus magnitude.

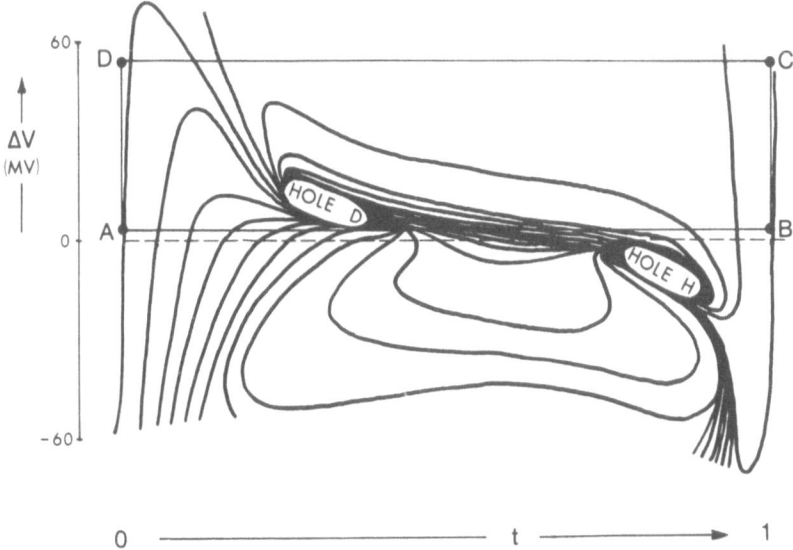

FIGURE 4. *A tracing from Best (1979) Fig.   12 with biasing current $I = -6\,\mu A/cm^2$
and $[Ca^{++}] = 28$ mM.   Isochron contour lines are sketched through the original ta-
bular data arranged according to stimulus magnitude DV (vertically   in   millivolts, depolarization upward) and time t of stimulus onset after a previous firing (horizontally, in units of 1 pacemaker cycle).   Each isochron threads   equal
values of computed latency from the stimulus to the Nth subsequent firing, modu-
lo 1, for big N.   (Practically N = 1 or 2, as there were virtually no transients
except   near   the   black holes).   Contours are identified by their t values at
DV=0.   Regions of annihilating stimuli are indicated by D for access   via   depolarization and H for access via hyperpolarization.   For Box ABCD, see text.*

BLACK HOLES OF THE HEARTBEAT

These observations can be put together in a single diagram. Fig. 4 shows an
example, calculated for the   sake   of   concreteness, from the Hodgkin-Huxley
space-clamped equation for squid axon.   The extracellular calcium and   transmembrane biasing current are arranged to elicit regular spiking.   The contour lines
depict combinations of stimulus timing and magnitude that   equivalently   resche-
dule pacemaker   firings.   By "equivalently" I mean that firings recur (after

transients, if any) at the same times after the stimulus.   These contours are
called "isochrons" ("same-time").   Fig.   4 distinguishes 20 isochrons spaced
1/20 cycle apart.   The one that goes through point A consists of stimuli that
result in firing at integer multiples of one cycle after the stimulus. On the
next contour beneath it and to the right firings occur 1/20 cycle earlier, and
so forth.   The horizontal coordinate depicts stimulus timing, measured from the
peak of the action potential at t=0 (and points A and D) through one full cycle
to   the   next action potential peak at t=1 (and points B and C). The vertical
coordinate depicts stimulus magnitude in millivolts displacement from the instantaneous   membrane potential. Depolarization is plotted upward, hyperpolarization downward.   Along the midline DV=0 we encounter all 20 isochrons disposed
at equal intervals as they should be: action potentials occur 1/20 cycle sooner
after a negligible stimulus given 1/20 cycle later.

It takes a few minutes of puzzling over this diagram to absorb its meaning
in terms of the familiar properties of pacemaker neurons. A discussion along
these lines is given in Winfree (1980b). For present purposes I draw your attention only to the few features that may prove pertinent to irregularities of
the heartbeat.

Along locus AB we see the consequences of small depolarizing stimuli in-
flicted at all stages of the cycle. The contour lines are not evenly spaced
along this locus, indicating that there are slight displacements of timing. For
example the stimulus at the third contour to the right of A reschedules firings
to the same latencies as though the membrane had been somewhat earlier in its
cycle and received no stimulus (follow the contour down to DV=0). But all contours are still encountered in order as we scan the cycle from A to B. This is
type 1 resetting.

At the action potential's peak (phase 0 or 1, loci BC or DA) the isochron
is nearly vertical, indicating that at this phase in the cycle the stimulus magnitude has very little influence on timing. Along locus DC (big depolarizations) we find ourselves above many contour lines which do not reach so high.
Those that do are encountered twice along DC, once in an increasing direction
then again in a decreasing direction. This is the qualitatively different type
0 resetting.

A full set of contour lines enter box ABCDA along locus AB. None exit DC
without re-entering, so we have a problem: a full set of contour lines must end

somewhere inside the box. This happens along the boundary of the conspicious BLACK HOLE. A similar box might have been drawn for hyperpolarizing (inhibitory) stimuli below the DV=0 axis, where you see another BLACK HOLE about 1/2 cycle later. What happens after stimuli in these areas? There are no contour lines in the BLACK HOLE: no timing is indicated for the subsequent action potentials. In fact none did follow: in the Hodgkin-Huxley calculations, membrane potential simply reverted to a steady equilibrium. The pacemaker was switched off.

The recent experimental measurements of Guttman et al. (1980) tested this calculation in real squid axon, biased to spontaneous rhythmicity. Both BLACK HOLES were found.

Please note that the existence of a BLACK HOLE follows from the observation of type 0 resetting. The Hodgkin-Huxley calculation only gives an example. Any other pacemaker exhibiting type 0 resetting must also have a stimulus or locus of stimuli at which the rescheduling is indeterminate because the contour lines must converge somewhere to terminate. This might correspond to annihilation of rhythmicity or just to an unpredictable interruption followed by recovery at arbitrary phase. Both results were observed in the corresponding experiments of Jalife and Antzelevitch (1979, 1980) using mammalian Purkinje fibers and sino-atrial node tissue. The earlier experiments of Wit and Cranefield (1976) using a somewhat different protocol also encountered annihilation of rhythmicity in monkey mitral valve fibers following a single impulse: it is not yet clear whether this corresponds to the BLACK HOLE required by type 0 resetting.

Returning to the contour map, it is evident that curves such as in Fig. 1, 2, and 3 may be taken from the contour map by crossing it as a fixed level of stimulus magnitude, DV. At levels of DV that penetrate the BLACK HOLES such curves must be ruptured by two discontinuities delimiting a gap in which the curve does not exist. This gap is the BLACK HOLE, the range of stimulus latencies that result in switching off the pacemaker. The discontinuities are the boundaries of the BLACK HOLE where the contour lines swirl together to theoretically infinite closeness, so that firing latency becomes arbitrarily sensitive to stimulus latency near those boundary points.

This gap comprises a measurable range of phases in the example computed here, but it need not in general. In fact the Hodgkin-Huxley parameters had to be adjusted with some care to make the BLACK HOLE big enough for easy detection when we were not sure whether all this was a fantasy or not. This was done by making the resting potential STABLE and at the same time making spontaneous cycling stable. In the more usual case the resting potential is unstable and the BLACK HOLE is only a point at which all contours converge. Every stimulus then corresponds to SOME reset timing, but near the singular point the contours are packed so close together that the slightest change of stimulus timing or magnitude (or membrane parameters) results in a substantial and unpredictable rescheduling of subsequent firings. In such cases rhythmicity DOES recover, usually through a prolonged train of growing subthreshold oscillations.

In either case - finite or punctate BLACK HOLE - it seems that the BLACK HOLE commonly has a "gullet": about half of the isochrons are packed very close together in a bundle funnelling into the singularity point or boundary of the hole. This bundle corresponds to EMPIRICAL GENERALIZATION 2 and to the separatrix characteristic of excitable kinetics. Stimuli that move the pacemaker to one side of the separatrix result in firing latencies distinctly different from those of stimuli that move it to the other side. The difference, typically about 1/2 cycle, is mediated continously but over a very narrow range of stimulus magnitudes and timings. Any resetting curve (or latency diagram as we might call it: such as in Fig. 1, 2, or 3) taken at a DV level that cuts through this bundle of contours will show this abrupt jump, practically indistinguishable from a discontinuity. Scott (1979) has made marvelous measurements of this phenomenon in cultured chick pacemaker cells.

SPATIALLY-DISTRIBUTED PACEMAKERS AND
SPATIALLY-DISTRIBUTED STIMULI

All the foregoing requires space-clamped preparations and is presented here mainly by way of introduction. A fuller discussion is given in Winfree (1980b). My main purpose in this paper is to try now to expand the foregoing to encompass the more realistic and practical situation encountered in spatially distributed

In Fig. 4 it is more conspicuous near H than D

pacemakers (e.g. real myocardium in situ) subjected to spatiallly distributed stimuli (e.g. currents surrounding an extracellular electrode, vagal arbor-
ization, or irritable focus).

The essence of this expansion is the observation that any slight departure
from the range of annihilating stimuli (the BLACK HOLE) has quite a different
effect. Instead of turning off the cell's clock it just resets its timing as
discussed above.   So if you shock a big piece of periodically pulsing tissue,
you turn off only a small patch of fibers while all around that patch your stimulus was a little too strong or too weak or your timing was a millisecond too
early or too late. It is a consequence of theory not here belabored, and of
Fig.   4, that the pattern of reset timing around a phase singularity has an inevitable vorticity to it: excitation thereafter CIRCULATES around the quiescent
patch.   This sounds something like the pernicious "circus wave" long sought by
cardiologists as a wreaker of havoc in the otherwise-synchronous heartbeat.   It
might therefore be worthwhile to consider the matter in a little more detail,
still remaining as model-independent as possible, to see whether it is really
pertinent.

NEIGHBORHOOD TIMING RELATIONS

Once again, I invite you to idealize excessively. Think of a tissue composed of
pacemaker cells, e.g. Purkinje fibers. (Actually it doesn't much matter;
even an excitable-but-not spontaneous membrane will serve the purpose).   Let
there be waves of excitation coursing across this tissue. Apply a grossly distributed stimulus, as from a defibrillating electrode or vagal volley.
Different   places will experience different amounts of depolarizing and hyperpolarizing stimulus and they will encounter these stimuli at different stages of
relaxation after recent passage of an action potential. Now in imagination take
each little fiber and draw it on Fig. 4 at the coordinates of its instantaneous
phase in the cycle (t) and the stimulus intensity it feels (DV). When you have
done this for all fibers in the heart you will have assembled a distorted image
of the whole heart on Fig. 4. It may be grossly stretched and repeatedly fold-

ed, but it will be continous and smooth (Fig. 5).

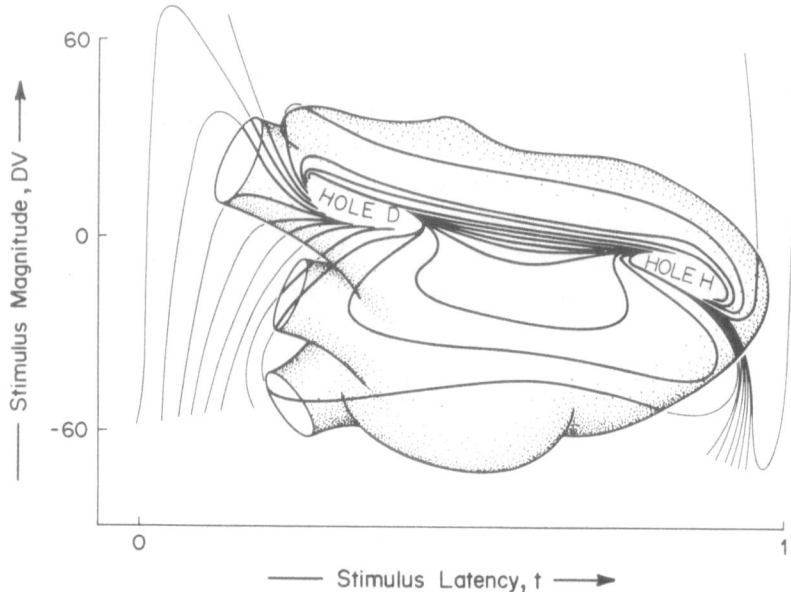

FIGURE 5 *Fig. 4 is repeated with a heart mapped on to it, point by point according to local stimulus magnitude and timing relative to the local spontaneous
cycle initiated by the previous local excitation. Isochrons on the heart are
drawn solid.   These will be the wavefront positions initially. (Labelling is
omitted to minimize clutter).*

Notice where the isochrons lie on this image of the heart. Those are the
loci on the heart that get reset to the same latencies. If they were not
electrically coupled by gap junctions, etc. and if their spontaneous firing
rates were exactly equal, then those loci would fire synchronously one after the
other, repeatedly, forever. If and only if the image of the heart overlaps either of the BLACK HOLES, these loci of synchronous firing will be found to circulate around patches of quiescence or irregularity. Inasmuch as the image is
most likely severely distorted and folded, there will be multiple representa-
tions of both BLACK HOLES with a complicated tangle of clockwise and
counter-clockwise wavelets connecting them. The scene would resemble turbulence
and might correspond to one kind of aggravated flutter or even fibrillation.
Note that no hole or lesion in the physical tissue is required around which to

circulate: Hodgkin-Huxley-like models, such as the McAllister-Noble-Tsien (MNT) (1975) formalism, or indeed any mechanisms allowing type 0 resetting, implicitly contain the equivalent of a portable lesion in the guise of a BLACK HOLE or (if it be vanishingly small) a pivot point for the full set of terminating isochrons. It is nothing short of astonishing that mathematicians overlooked this feature of the HH formalism for over a quarter century.

Of course, I have also swept under the rug some essential realities of cardiac physiology. Besides the realities that I don't even know about, there is the critical fact that the fibers comprising ventricular myocardium ARE electrically coupled. This is an awkward mattter to approach mathematically; I resorted to numerical simulations in a digital computer. From such computations as I have attempted with greatly simplified models it appears that the effect of coupling is mainly:

1) to make the waves propagate at a standard speed determined by the electrical space constant, rather than at the essentially arbitrary speeds initially determined by timing relationships alone; and

2) to make the "rotor", as I call it, spin at a rate proportional to that standard speed rather than at the frequency of spontaneous discharge of the underlying cells; and

3) to eliminate counter-rotating pairs of rotors that happen to lie too close together. How close is too close? I don't know. The answer will require expensive computations with the complete MNT equations. But it may be important if it has something to do with the critical mass required for persistent fibrillation.

A second conspicuous deficiency of my argument is that the fibers comprising the myocardium do not all follow the same kinetics. Any simplification that ignores the heterogeneity of real heart muscle must be regarded with suspicion if it be regarded at all. This complication is not only intractable to mathematics, but it presents substantial practical problems for simulation too. Diverse attacks on these challenging problems are summarized in Ivanitskii et al. (1978). I have not attempted such simulations but I feel sure that they would have a very different outcome in the idealized case of uncoupled fibers considered above.

I also feel pretty sure that introduction of realistic electrical coupling in this case will virtually remove the complicating effect of heterogeneity!

This helpful accident stems from a peculiarity of electrically excitable membranes: that they spend a lot of time loitering near their equilibrium voltage,
whether this time be limited by the slow generator potential of spontaneously
active cells, or be potentially infinite as in merely excitable cells with a
stable resting potential. The effect of electrical coupling is to "blur over"
this tiny region of state space near equilibrium and thus to blur over the distinctions between cells whose spontaneous periods are short, long, or infinite.
What seems to matter most for the kinetics of COUPLED cells is that they loiter
long near equilibrium, and then, when they have prematurely escaped the neigh-
borhood of equilibrium with the help of currents from adjacent cells, they fire
an action potential and return to the slow, near-equilibrium changes that are so
easily over-ridden by currents from outside. In these respects the diverse
fibers of heterogeneous heart muscle behave quite similarly.   The differences
among their residence times near equilibrium will surely affect the detailed
pathways followed by circulating wavelets during fibrillation, and fibrillation
may be difficult to study in such detail. But I think its EXISTENCE and origin
can be appreciated without invoking heterogeneity as an essential part of the
cause.

OF HISTORICAL INTEREST

In emphasizing continuity and homogeneity the arguments presented here differ
from the pioneering insights of Moe and Abildskov (1959), Moe (1962), and Moe
et al. (1964) and of Krinskii (1966, 1968, 1978) which emphasized heterogeneity and discontinuities. I believe that turbulence is implicit even in the equations of voltage and permeability for membranes of smoothly-graded properties.
Moe et al. (op. cit.) implicitly argued along these lines by comparing fibrillation to hydrodynamic turbulence, even writing a mathematical expression
analogous to the Reynolds' number.

      Rozenstraukh et al. (1970) make an argument of this sort using vagal
stimulation of the atrium to introduce a TEMPORARY inhomogeneity, much as we
here use a graded stimulus. Gulko and Petrov (1972) also computed a stable

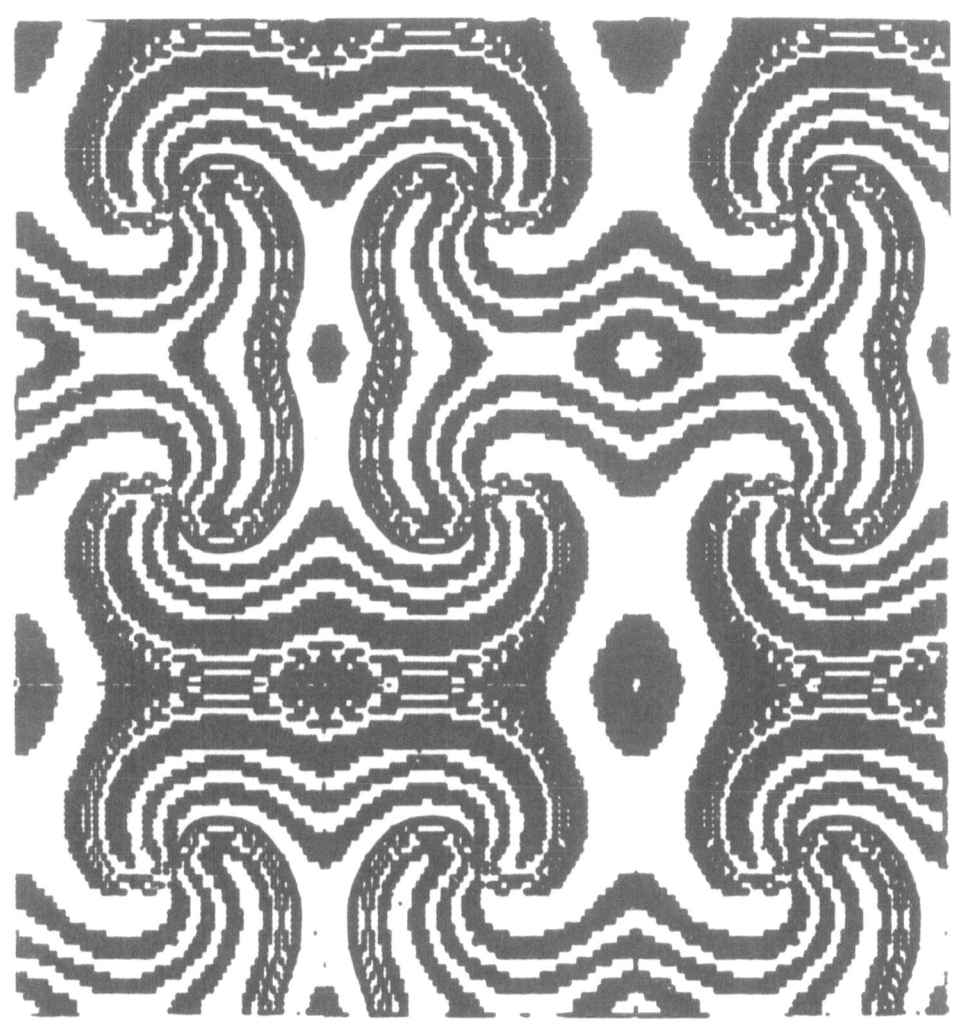

FIGURE 6 *This checkerboard pattern is composed of 9 mirror-image squares, each of 75 x 75 simulated cells. A cable equation couples all these cells. Each cell is excitable. Its state of excitation (membrane voltage) is digitized into the 7 levels for printout only. Levels are printed alternately black and white. In each of the 9 squares excitation is rotating around a central pivot where voltage and refractoriness remain intermediate between the conventionally-named states. Waves collide and annihilate one another along the boundaries of squares.*

rotor in a homogeneous Hodgkin-Huxley-like medium. The rotor computed by
Shcherbunov et al. (1973) was among the first using continuous media described
by continuous partial differential equation (the Noble equation), but the computation included a parameter gradient and the rotor proved quickly unstable.

Fig. 6 shows my own (vintage 1973) snapshot of this kind of turbulence in
an excitable medium described by a gross simplification of excitable membrane
kinetics. The simplification states only that there is a resting potential and
a threshold not far away, beyond which an excitation variable and a recovery
variable smoothly rise one after the other and fall back again. In this particular computation cells were coupled through both quantities but the results are
scarcely different when they are coupled more realistically through only the excitation variable (voltage). A spatially graded stimulus created the symmetrical initial conditions from which this checkerboard pattern of alternating vortices emerged and persisted through more than 50 rotations with no sign of instability. In this simple-minded computation all vortices turn out to rotate at
exactly the same rate, but in real myocardium their symmetric layout and exact
synchrony would not long persist.

A recent report by Herbschleb et al. (1980) in fact shows extraordinarily
persistent local periodism in fibrillating heart at a frequency comparable to
that of Allessie's rotors. Rotors in continuous simply-connected excitable
media with continuous kinetics have also been computed by Reshodko and Bures
(1975) and by Karfunkel (1975).

Fig. 7 shows analogous vorticity in an electrochemical excitable medium
constructed by Nagumo et al. (1963, but unfortunately published only in Japan-
ese until Suzuki 1976). This is essentially Lillie's iron wire preparation of a
half century ago, extended to two dimensions by replacing the single wire with a
mesh. A spatially graded stimulus was applied in the wake of a wave to initiate
a rotor. Local inhomogeneities are apparently responsible for creation of additional rotors and for their complex movements.

(As a matter of historical interest, E.E. Smith and A.C. Guyton (1961)
also attempted to discover whether vorticity and turbulence are latent even in
simple homogeneous excitable media. They chose to remain more faithful to the
surface topology of the heart by lowering a large iron SPHERE into a vat of nitric acid: such an unlikely scene in a medical school that they took the trou-
ble to film it. The spherical surface eliminated the edge effects inevitable to

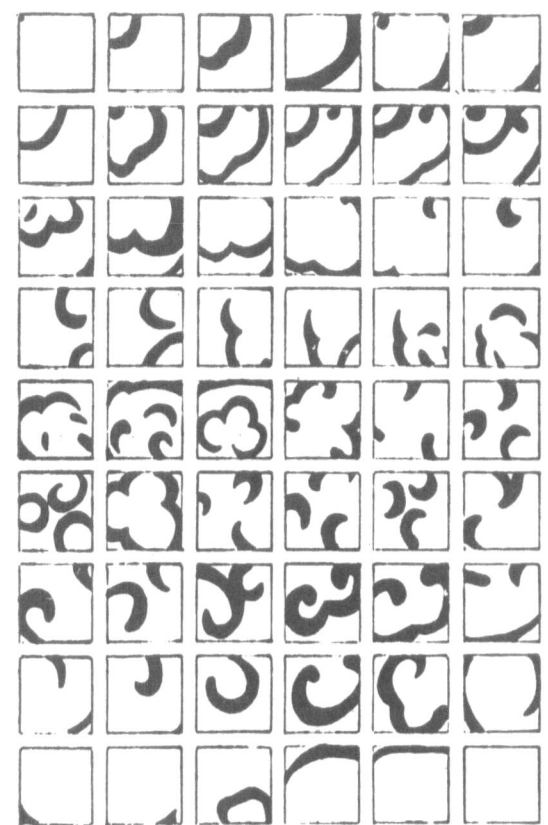

FIGURE 7 *Pencil tracings at 1/8 second intervals (left to right, then down a row) from photographs of a 30 cm x 30 cm grid of 26 x 26 iron wires in nitric acid. Stimuli are introduced near the upper left corner in frames 1,5,8,11. Spontaneous activity persists for a while in the form of waves irregularly pivoting about wandering endpoints. (From Nagumo et al., 1963 Fig. 15).*

Nagumo's independent experiment with a flat iron gridwork, and admitted the possibility of "circus waves" along closed great-circle paths. The movies, kindly loaned to me by Prof. Guyton, show much disorganized wave motion but I believe it consists mostly of simple waves from a point origin complicated by convection and bubbling of the nitric acid. The experiment would have to be tried again under gravity-free conditions to serve its intended purpose.

A more convenient chemical analog of excitable media was invented by Zaikin and Zhabotinsky in 1970. The remarkable similarity of its kinetics to the Hodgkin-Huxley kinetics has become the subject of many technical papers by mathematicians and physical chemists (Winfree, 1974, 1978, 1980a; Tyson, 1976; Troy, 1978; Field and Troy, 1979).

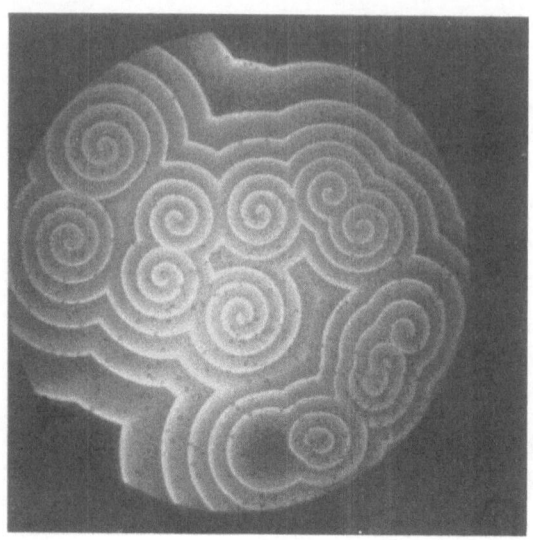

FIGURE 8 *Rotating waves of oxidative excitation in a motionless 1 1/2 mm depth of Zhabotinsky's reagent, viewed by transmitted light. The tiny dots are bubbles of CO_2, a reaction end product.*

Fig. 8 shows a rather coarse mode of multiple vorticity in a thin layer of this reagent. Each spiral is a wave radiating outward from a vortex-like origin where its endpoint rotates about a tiny circle. There is no chemical inhomogeneity at that origin; the positions of the origins were simply determined by a spatially graded stimulus applied to circular waves emanating from the points at which an earlier stimulus was applied. A more complicatedly-graded stimulus would have produced a greater profusion of close-packed rotors. In somewhat deeper films of this reagent, 3-dimensional modes of vorticity are stable, giving rise to still more complicated turbulence. None of this depends on inhomogeneities or discontinuities.

Krinskii (1966, 1968) came very close to anticipating these rotating excitations on purely theoretical grounds. It is perhaps hair-splitting for me to refer to them as "rotors" rather than by his much earlier term "reverberators". I do so only to emphasize that rotors can be understood in the continuous terms of kinetics and diffusion whereas the original reverberator was specifically a consequence of discontinuity and inhomogeneity both in the physical medium and in the time-course of its excitation at any point. The lifetime of a reverberator and its prospects of multiplying were determined by those factors. Discontinuity and inhomogeneity are real properties of myocardium and undoubtedly do much to condition the detailed development of vorticity. But the point I wish to emphasize here is that they are not the essential causes of vorticity: the rotor can be induced and is stable even in perfectly homogeneous media with smooth kinetics.

Now going back to the individual rotor, it is of interest to enquire about the state of the membrane near its center, about which the wave pivots. In the earliest experiments with circulating waves, (Mayer, 1908, 1914; Garrey, 1914; Mines, 1914) there was no center: circulation on a ring was ensured by punching a hole in the medium. The pulmonary vasculature plays the role of a hole in the arguments of Stibitz and Rytand (1968) about atrial flutter as a "circus wave". In the experiments of Shibata and Bures (1973, 1974) and of Martins-Ferreira et al. (1974) a wave of spreading depression rotates persistently in a sheet of neurons, but the center of the rotation is an inexcitable lesion: functionally a hole. The mathematical analysis of Wiener and Rosenblueth (1946) required a hole of a certain minimum circumference around which a normal action potential might circulate indefinitely. Balakhovskii (1965) and Krinskii (1968, 1978) argue that the hole might be replaced by a discontinuity of much smaller dimensions in the case of a more heart-like medium with a prolonged excited state. By all these subterfuges the question was evaded: "What is going on at the center of a rotating wave? Is the medium there always refractory? If so, why doesn't it recover to excitability? If not, why doesn't the wave short-circuit through the excitable center?"

Allessie et al. (1973, 1976, 1977) were the first to deliberately create and document a rotor in real myocardium (the left atrium of a rabbit) and to focus attention on its center. They observed irregular incursions of wavelets from the excitation circulating around the center, passing through the center while attenuating, and finally dying out in the still-refractory tissue on the far side. This irregularity may not be due to structural and functional inhomogeneity in the preparation. Even in ideally homogeneous and isotropic excitable media the center can behave irregularly, e.g. in the chemical reagent of Zaikin and Zhabotinsky (Winfree, 1972), in the computations of a stable Hodgkin-Huxley-like rotor by Gulko and Petrov (1972), in the computations of a stable enzyme-kinetic rotor by Rossler (1978) and Rossler and Kahlert (1979), and in mathematical analyses by Rossler (1976, 1978) and by Kuramoto (1978).

The causes of this irregularity are not yet understood, but the consequence is that the inner endpoint of the wave lashes about unpredictably and the rotor wanders around. This behavior seems to contribute to the mutual extinction of clockwise and counter-clock-wise rotors packed too close together. It may therefore be important to study in connection with recovery from fibrillation.

ACKNOWLEDGMENTS

This work was supported by the United States National Science Foundation under grant CHE-77-24649. I am indebted to Dr. Jose Jalife for sharing with me his unpublished data and for direction to pertinent literature.

REFERENCES

Allessie, M.A., Bonke, F.I.M. and Schopman, F.J.G.: Circus movement in rabbit atrial muscle as a mechanism of tachycardia. Circ. Res., 33: 54-62, 1973.

Allessie, M.A., Bonke, F.I.M. and Schopman, F.J.G.: Circus movement in rabbit atrial muscle as a mechanism of tachycardia. II. The role of non-uniform recovery of excitability of the occurrence of uni-directional block, as studied with multiple microelectrodes. Cir. Res., 39: 168-177, 1976.

Allessie, M.A., Bonke, F.I.M. and Schopman, F.J.G.: Circus movement in rabbit atrial muscle as a mechanism of tachycardia: III. The "leading circle" concept: a new model of circus movement in cardiac tissue without the involvement of an anatomical obstacle. Circ. Res., 41: 9-18, 1977.

Balakhovskii, I.S.: Several modes of excitation movement in ideal excitable tissue. Biophysics, 10: 1175-1179, 1965.

Best, E.N.: Null space in the Hodgkin-Huxley equations. Biophys. J., 27: 87-104, 1979.

Field, R.J. and Troy, W.C.: The existence of solitary travelling wave solutions of a model of the Belousov-Zhabotinskii reaction. SIAM J. Appl. Math., 37: 561-581, 1979.

Garrey, W.E.: Nature of fibrillary contraction in the heart. Am. J. Physiol., 33: 397-414, 1914.

Gulko, F.B. and Petrov, A.A.: Mechanism of formation of closed pathways of conduction in excitable media. Biofizika, 17: 261-270, 1972.

Guttman, R., Lewis, S. and Rinzel, J.: Control of repetitive firing in squid axon membrane as a model for a neuron oscillator. J. Physiol. (London), 305: 377-395, 1980.

Herbschleb, J.N., Heethaar, R.M., Van der Tweel, I., Zimmerman, A.N.E. and Meijler, F.L.: Signal analysis of ventricular fibrillation. Computers in Cardiology, 49-53, 1980.

Ivanitskii, G.P., Krinskii, V.I. and Selkov, E.E.: The Mathematical Biophysics of Cells, Science Publishers, Moscow, 1978.

Jalife, J. and Antzelevitch, C.: Phase resetting and annihilation of pacemaker activity in cardiac tissues. Science, 206: 695-697, 1979.

Jalife, J. and Antzelevitch, C.: Pacemaker annihilation: diagnostic and therapeutic implications. Am. Heart J., 100: 128-130, 1980.

Jalife, J., Hamilton, A.J., Lamanna, V.R. and Moe, G.K.: Effects of current flow on pacemaker activity of the isolated kitten SA node. Am. J. Physiol., 238: 307-316, 1980.

Jalife, J. and Moe, G.K.: Phasic effects of vagal stimulation on pacemaker activity of the isolated sinus node of the young cat. Circ. Res., 45: 595-607, 1979.

Karfunkel, H.R.: Zur Theorie der Anregbarkeit und Ausbreitung von Erregungswellen in chemischen Reaktionssystemen. Dissertation, Universitaet zu Tubingen, 1975.

Krinskii, V.I.: Spread of excitation in an inhomogeneous medium. Biofizika, 11: 676-683, 1966.

Krinskii, V.I.: Fibrillation in excitable media. Prob. Kibernetiki, 20: 59-80, 1968.

Krinskii, V.I.: Mathematical models of cardiac arrhythmias (spiral waves). Pharmac. Ther. B., 3: 539-555, 1978.

Kuramoto Y.: Diffusion-induced chaos in reaction system. Prog. Theor. Phys., 64: (supplement), 346-367, 1978.

Martins-Ferreira, H., de Oliveiro Castro, G., Struchinea, C.J.   and Rodriques,
    P.S.:   Circling   spreading   depression   in   isolated   chicken   retina.   J.
    Neurophys., 37: 773-784, 1974.

Mayer, A.G.: Rhythmical pulsation in scyphomedusae.   Papers   of   the   Tortugas
    Lab. of the Carnegie Inst. of Wash., 1: 115-131, 1908.

Mayer, A.G.: The relation between degree of concentration of one electrolytes
    of seawater and rate of nerve conduction in Cassiope. Papers of the Tortu-
    gas Lab. of Carnegie Inst. of Wash. 6: 25-54, 1914.

McAllister, R.E., Noble, D. and Tsien, R.W.: Reconstruction of the electrical
    activity of cardiac Purkinje fibres. J. Physiol. (London), 251: 1-59,
    1975.

Mines, G.R.: On circulating excitations on heart muscles and their possible re-
    lation to tachycardia and fibrillation. Trans. R. Soc. Can., 4: 43-53,
    1914.

Moe, G.K.: On the multiple wavelet hypothesis of atrial fibrillation.   Arch.
    Int. Pharmacodyn., 140: 183-188, 1962.

Moe, G.K. and Abildskov, J.A.: Atrial fibrillation as a selfsustaining ar-
    rhythmia independent of focal discharge. Am. Heart J., 58: 59-70, 1959.

Moe, G.K., Rheinboldt, W.C. and Abildskov, J.A.: A computer model of atrial
    fibrillation. Am. Heart J., 67: 200-220, 1964.

Nagumo, J., Suzuki R. and Sato, S.: Electrochemical Active Network. Notes of
    Professional Group on Nonlinear Theory of IECE (Japan), Feb. 26, 1963.

Reshodko, L.V. and Bures, J.: Computer simulation of reverberating spreading
    depression in a network of cell automata. Biol. Cyb., 18: 181-189, 1975.

Rössler, O.E.: Chemical turbulence; chaos in a simple reaction-diffusion sys-
    tem. Zeit. Naturforsch., 31a: 1168-1172, 1976.

Rössler, O.E.: Chemical turbulence - a synopsis. In Synergetics, H.   Haken,
    Ed. Lecture Notes in Physics, Springer-Verlag, Berlin, 1978.

Rössler, O.E. and Kahlert, C.: Winfree meandering in a   2-dimensional
    2-variable excitable medium. Z. Naturforsch., 34a: 565-570, 1979.

Rozenshtraukh, L.V., Kholopov, A.V. and Yushmanova, A.V.:   Vagus
    inhibition-cause of formation of closed pathways of conduction of excita-
    tion in the auricles. Biofizika, 15: 690-700, 1970.

Scott, S.W.: Stimulation simulations of young yet cultured beating hearts. Ph.
    D. Thesis, State Univ. of N.Y. at Buffalo, 1979.

Shcherbunov, A.I., Kukushkin, N.I. and Saxon, M.E.: Reverberator in a system of interrelated fibers described by the Noble equation. Biofizika, 18: 519-525, 1973.

Shibata, M. and Bures, J.: Reverberation of cortical spreading depression along closed-loop pathways in rat cerebral cortex. J. Neurophys., 35: 381-388, 1973.

Shibata, M. and Bures, J.: Optimum topographical conditions for reverberating cortical spreading depression in rats. J. Neurobiol., 5: 107-118, 1974.

Smith, E.E. and Guyton, A.C.: An iron heart model for study of cardiac impulse transmission. Physiologist, 4: 112, 1961.

Stibitz, G.R. and Rytand, D.A.: On the path of the excitation wave in atrial flutter. Circulation, 37: 75-81, 1968.

Suzuki, R.: Electrochemical neuron model. Adv. Biophys., 9: 115-156, 1976.

Troy, W.C.: Mathematical modeling of excitable media in neurobiology and chemistry. Theoretical Chemistry, 4, Eyring, H. and Henderson, D., eds., Academis Press, New York, pp. 133-157, 1978.

Tyson, J.J.: The Belousov-Zhabotinskii Reaction, Lecture Notes in Biomathematics, vol. 10, Levin, S., ed., Springer-Verlag, Berlin, 1976.

Wiener, N. and Rosenblueth, A.: The mathematical formulation of the problem of conduction of impulses in a network of connected excitable elements, specifically in cardiac muscle. Arch. Inst. Cardiologia de Mexico, 16: 205-265, 1946.

Winfree, A.T.: Spiral waves of chemical activity. Science, 175: 634-636, 1972.

Winfree, A.T.: Wavelike activity in biological and biochemical media. In: Lecture Notes in Biomathematics, 2, Van den Driessche, P., ed., Springer-Verlag, Berlin, pp. 243-260, 1974.

Winfree, A.T.: Phase control of neural pacemakers. Science, 197: 761-762, 1977.

Winfree, A.T.: Stable rotating patterns of reaction and diffusion. In: Theoretical Chemistry, 4, Eyring, H. and Henderson, D., eds., Academic Press, New York, pp. 1-51, 1978.

Winfree, A.T.: The Geometry of Biological Time. Springer-Verlag, N.Y., 1980a.

Winfree, A.T.: Peculiarities in the impulse response of pacemaker neurons. In: Mathematical Aspects of Physiology, Lectures in Applied Mathematics 19,

Hoppensteadt, F., ed., Amer. Math. Soc., Providence, pp. 265-279, 1981.

Wit, A.L. and Cranefield, P.F.: Triggered activity in cardiac muscle fibers of the simian mitral valve. Circ. Res., 38: 85-98, 1976.

Zaikin, A.N. and Zhabotinsky, A.M.: Concentration wave propagation in two-dimensional liquid-phase self-oscillating systems. Nature, 225: 535-537, 1970.

SECTION FOUR

NEURAL CONTROL OF RATE AND RHYTHM

ON THE INTRINSIC CARDIAC RHYTHM

Lennart N. Bouman, Tobias Op 't Hof, Albert J.C. Mackaay,
Wim K. Bleeker and Habo J. Jongsma

Among writers of physiology text books it is common use to present a conceptual
model to explain the mode of action of the two divisions of the autonomic nervous system in their control of heart rate. This model states that there is an
intrinsic heart rate being the frequency of the undisturbed sinus node; an increase of frequency above this intrinsic rate will be the consequence of adrenergic activity; a fall in heart rate below the intrinsic value will be caused
by cholinergic action on the sinus node.

In man the intrinsic heart rate can be established by the simultaneous injection of propranolol (0,2 mg/kg) and atropine sulphate (0.04 mg/kg) (Jose and
Collison, 1970), under which conditions a constant heart rate is established in
a range between 78 and 126 beats/min, averaging 103.6 beats/min. This wide
range could be narrowed by taking into account a relation with the age of the
individual, older persons having lower intrinsic rates than young persons.
Furthermore time of day and foregoing periods of exercise appeared to influence
the measured rate, but after taking this into account still there is a rather
strong difference between different subjects.

Because in man, as demonstrated also by Jose and coworkers, there may be
uncontrollable variables disturbing the intrinsic activity of the cardiac pacemaker, we studied the spontaneous rhythm of the isolated rabbit heart, assuming
that these hearts show the intrinsic rhythm. When cardiac cycle length is monitored during a certain time in the awake undisturbed rabbit, a large variability
in cycle length is observed. Fig. 1 shows a registration made by our colleagues Borst and Karemaker (unpublished); during a 12 hour period every second the
RR-interval duration was sampled, and put into the histogram (Fig. 1 right);
the total number of data in this histogram is 43.200. The occurrence of very
short intervals is coupled to movements of the animal. The day after this

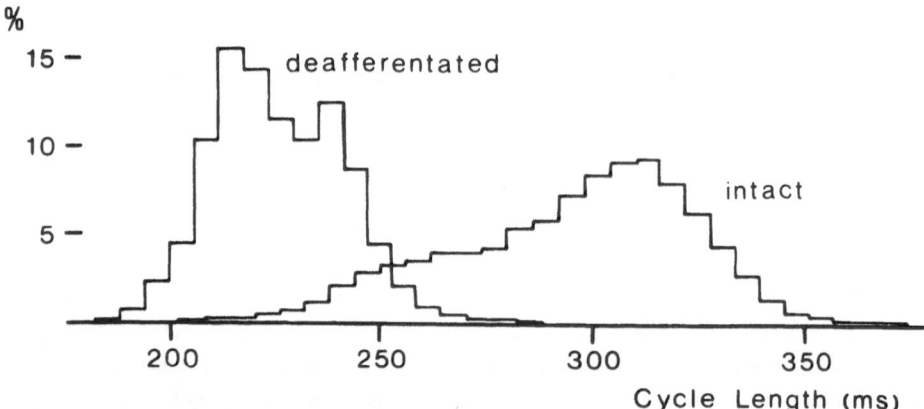

FIGURE 1 *12 hour registration of the RR-cycle length in an awake, freely moving rabbit. The right sided histogram depicts the cycle length variability in a normal rabbit; the left-sided histogram shows the cycle length distribution in the same animal after sino-aortic deafferentiation. (Courtesy Borst and Kare-maker).*

registration had been made, both the carotid and aortic baroreceptors were deaf-ferentiated causing a decrease in vagal activity. Eighteen days later, again a 12 hour recording of the cycle length was made, shown in the left-side histogram in Fig. 1. The mean cycle length is shortened by 100 ms; the range seems to be diminished too, but the ratio between the total range and the mean cycle length falls only from 0.6 to 0.5, suggesting that the main effect of the with-drawal of vagal activity is an increase of heart rate (see also Jongsma and Tsjernina, this volume).

When all nervous and humoral factors are excluded, as is the case when the heart is isolated, in general a slower and more regular heart rate is recorded than in the intact and awake rabbit. Fig. 2 shows results from Bonke (1968) who measured the length of 6000 subsequent cycles of an isolated right atrium. In A the total histogram is shown, in B and C the first and the second half of the total number of intervals separately. This was done because the isolated superfused rabbit atrium cycle length increases 10-20 ms/hr continuously during the whole experiment; when the cycle length is measured over a short time the variability in cycle length is very small and substantially less than in the in-tact animal, where no slow change in the mean cycle length is present. Bonke

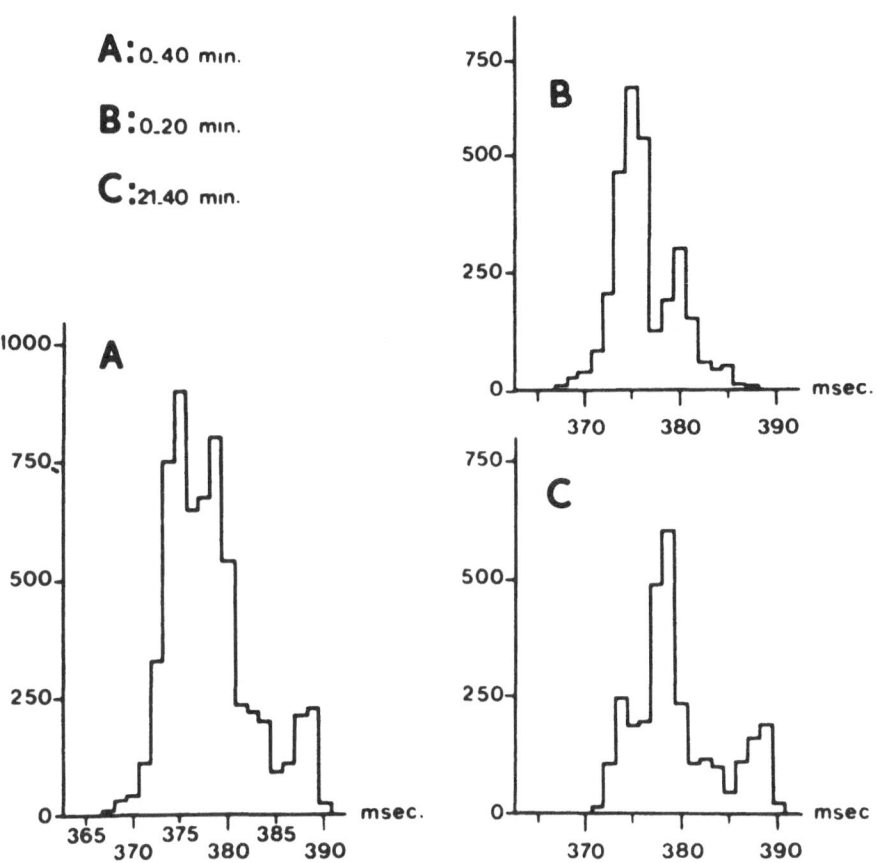

FIGURE 2 A. *Interval histogram of 6000 subsequent beats of an isolated right atrium preparation of the rabbit. B. Interval histogram of the first 3000 beats. C. Interval histogram of the last 3000 beats. (From Bonke, 1968).*

et al. (1969) calculated that in the isolated right atrium the standard deviation of an arbitrary sample of 10 normal subsequent intervals was less than 1.1 ms, with a mean cycle length between 300 and 360 ms.

We compared those values with the values in recent literature (Fig. 3) and with the mean cycle length that was recorded in our own experiments on isolated rabbit atria (Fig. 4). From literature we extracted 44 publications (ref.) in which the rate of beating of the isolated rabbit atrium was stated explicitly or

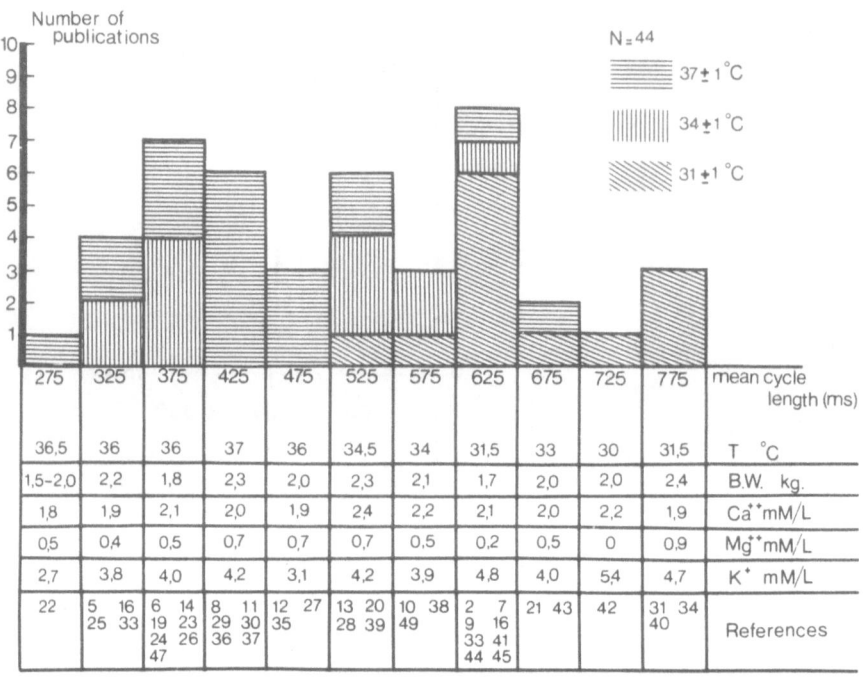

FIGURE 3 *Distribution of the mean cycle length of the isolated rabbit heart as it was found in 44 recent publications. The width of a class of cycle length is 50 ms. The values for T (temperature), B.W. (body weight) and Ca^{++}/Mg^{++}/K^{+} (perfusion fluid) are the mean values that were used in the studies that are grouped together in a certain class.*

could be estimated from graphs. The cycle length was divided into bins having a width of 50 ms, the shortest bin being from 250 to 299 and the largest 750-799 ms. Within these outer limits there is thus a wide variability. To find out possible clues to scale down this variability also the experimental temperature (T), the body weight of the animals (B.W.) and the concentration of ions that are known to have chronotropic effects were taken into account. The figures given in Fig. 3 are mean values of the ionic compositions from the experiments in a certain bin. From the parameters considered only the temperature of the perfusion fluid seems to correlate with the recorded cycle length. The correlation that has been established earlier (Altman, 1959) between body weight and intrinsic rate could not be confirmed, possibly because most investigators use young-adult rabbits having a body weight between 2 and 3 kg. The same holds true for the ionic concentrations used. $[Ca^{++}]$ seldomly exceeds the range between 1.8 and 2.2 mM; if magnesium is added at all, the $[Mg^{++}]$ concentration is generally 0.5 mM, $[K^+]$ varies between 2.7 and 5.6. Although it can be stated that the lowest K^+ concentration coincides with a high cardiac rate, and the highest concentration with a low rate, the correlation is weaker than with temperature.

In 35 experiments we localized the site of the pacemaker within the sinus node and we correlated the site of pacemaker dominance and the intrinsic rate. The localization was performed as described previously (Lu, 1970; Bleeker et al., 1980). After the recording of the rhythm of the intact preparation the sinus node and the attached atrial muscle was cutted into halves, separating the nodal area into a superior part and an inferior part. Mostly the preparation was cut 0.5 - 1 mm below the site of pacemaker dominance (Mackaay et al., 1980). After the separation of the two halves, the rate of beating of both parts was recorded simultaneously.

As can be seen in Fig. 4 (upper part), the intact preparation that was kept at a temperature of 38 °C has a mean cycle length that falls nicely into the relevant part of the histogram in Fig. 3. The B.W. of our rabbits was between 2.0 and 3.0 kg, the ionic composition of the perfusion fluid was: $[Ca^{++}]$ 2.2 mM/l, $[Mg^{++}]$ 0.6 mM/l, $[K^+]$ 5.6 mM/l. Even under constant experimental conditions like temperature and ionic composition of the superfusion fluid, there is a large variability in intrinsic cycle length. When the preparation is cutted into two parts, both parts show a regular beating rate, that in most cases differs from the other one. In the present group of experiments, the cycle length of the preparation prior to the separation was 384 ± 46.4 (SD) ms; after the separation and equilibration, the cycle length of the superior part was 377 ± 44 ms and of the inferior part 388 ± 38 ms. In most cases the superior part beat faster than the inferior with an average time difference of 11 ± 5.8 ms (p < 0.05). A correlation could be established between the beating rate of the total preparation and the difference in cycle length between the isolated superior and inferior part. The lower portion of Fig. 4 shows the regression line; this line crosses the abscissa at a cycle length of about 425 ms. This means that in preparations with cycle lenghtes shorter than 425 ms mostly the upper part beats faster than the lower part; when the cycle length of the total

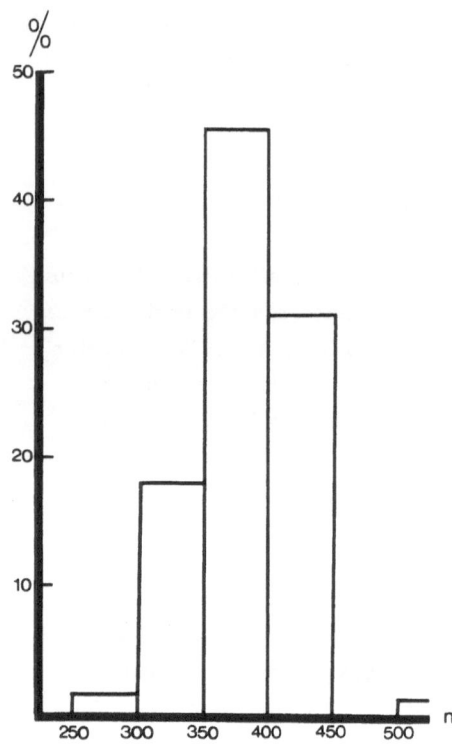

FIGURE 4 *Top: interval   histogram   of the   mean length of the cardiac cycle of 35 isolated rabbit atria.   For the   com-position   of   this   histogram   the cycle length was measured about 2 hours   after the isolation of the heart from the ani-mal.*

Bottom: Relation   between   the   cycle length of the total right atrium prepar-ation (same as in upper part of figure) and   the   difference   in   cycle   length between the upper and lower part of the sinus   node (for details see text).   y = 0.275 x - 116.48;   r = 0.372 (n = 35) (p < 0.025)

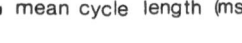

mean cycle length (ms)

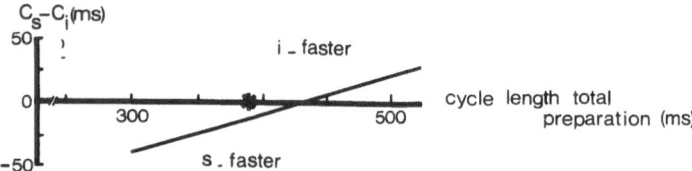

preparation   is   more   than 425 ms, probably the lower portion beats faster than the upper portion.

We think that this relation is caused by a variability of the site of   the dominant   pacemaker   within   the   sinus   node.   As the majority of the isolated hearts beat with a cycle length shorter than 425 ms, as a rule the dominant pacemaker is located in the upper portion of the sinus node, as was demonstrated earlier by mapping of the activation pattern of the sinus node (Bleeker et al., 1980). The intrinsic rate of the pacemaker fibers in the upper portion of the node seems to be faster than that of the lower portion of the node. When however, by a certain influence the spontaneous activity of the upper part is delayed, the lower part can take over pacemaker function. We conclude that in the isolated rabbit heart the variability in the intrinsic heart is accompanied by and perhaps even caused by a variability in the location of the primary pacemaker within the sinus node. There are many factors that can induce short-term shifts of the pacemaker within the sino-atrial node (see for example Mackaay et al., this volume); apparently there are also factors that can induce also long-term shifts in the cardiac pacemaker that are not identified as yet.

Comparing now the rate and rhythm of the isolated sinus node with that in the awake rabbit we must conclude that in the awake animal the cardiac rate is higher than from the isolated sinus node, while the rhythm is more irregular. The higher rate in the intact animal is not caused by an exclusive action of the accelerant nerves because if the vagal activity is reduced by sino-aortic deafferentiation the heart rate still increases; so we conclude that the relative short cycle length in the awake rabbit is the product of a synchronous action of the two divisions of the autonomic system; fluctuations in the activity of both divisions are held responsible for the irregularity that is a characteristic of the innervated heart.

The intrinsic rhythm of the rabbit sinus node is very regular, with only a small interbeat variance in cycle length. The mean cycle length of the heart beat of different animals shows a large variability that is correlated with the site of the dominant pacemakers inside the sinus node.

REFERENCES

1. Altman, P.L.: Handbook of Circulation, Dittmer, D.S. and Grebe, R.M., eds., W.B. Saunders, Philadelphia, pp. 81-83, 1959.

2. Angelakos, E.T., Maker, J.T. and Burlington, R.F.: Arrest of spontaneous atrial activity by cold at different potassium concentrations. Arch. Int. Physiol. Bioch., 79: 857-871, 1971.

3. Bleeker, W.K., Mackaay, A.J.C., Masson-Pevet, M., Bouman, L.N. and Becker, A.E.: Functional and morphological organization of the rabbit sinus node. Circ. Res., 46: 11-22, 1980.

4. Bonke, F.I.M.: De atrium extrasystole. Thesis, Amsterdam, 1968.

5. Bonke, F.I.M., Bouman, L.N. and van Rijn, H.E.: Change of cardiac rhythm in the rabbit after an atrial premature beat. Circ. Res., 24: 533-544, 1969.

6. Bonke, F.I.M., Bouman, L.N. and Schopman, F.J.G.: Effect of an early atrial premature beat on activity of the sinoatrial node and atrial rhythm in the rabbit. Circ. Res., 29: 704-715, 1971.

7. Bonke, F.I.M.: Electrotonic spread in the sinoatrial node of the rabbit heart. Pfluegers Arch., 339: 18-23, 1973.

8. Bouman, L.N., Gerlings, E.D., Biersteker, P.A. and Bonke, F.I.M.: Pacemaker shift in the sinoatrial node during vagal stimulation. Pfluegers Arch., 302: 225-267, 1968.

9. Carrier, G.O. and Bishop, V.S.: The interaction of acetylcholine and norepinephrine on heart rate. J. Pharmacol. Exp. Ther., 180: 31-37, 1972.

10. Courtney, K.R., Jensen, R.A. and Davis, E.E.: Sodium ions affect adrenergic control of sinoatrial rate. J. Mol. Cell. Cardiol., 11: 237-244, 1979.

11. Cramer, M., Siegel, M., Bigger jr., J.Th. and Hoffman, B.F.: Characteristics of extracellular potentials recorded from the sinoatrial pacemaker of the rabbit. Circ. Res., 41: 292-300, 1979.

12. Deck, K.A.: Dehnungseffekte am spontananschlagenden isolierten Sinusknoten. Pfluegers Arch., 280: 120-130, 1964.

13. Dorticos, F.R. and Garcia-Barreto, D.: Electrophysiological effects of droperidol on sinoatrial nodal fibers. Arch. Int. Pharmacodyn, 240:

137-142, 1979.

14. Freeman, S.E. and Turner, R.J.: Effects of temperature change and adrenaline on sinoatrial and atrioventricular nodal potentials. Cardiovasc. Res., 8: 443-450, 1974.

15. Jose, A.D. and Collison, D.: The normal range and determinants of the intrinsic heart rate in man. Cardiovasc. Res., 4: 160-167, 1970.

16. Kodama, J., Goto, J., Ando, S., Toyama, J. and Yamada, K.: Effects of rapid stimulation on the transmembrane action potentials of rabbit sinus node pacemaker cells. Circ. Res., 46: 90-99, 1980.

17. Lenfant, J.: Analyse des proprietes de la membrane myocardique sino-auriculaire: genese de l'activite spontanee. Theses, Poitiers, 1972.

18. Lu, H.H.: Shifts in pacemaker dominance within the sinoatrial region of cat and rabbit hearts resulting from increase of extracellular potassium. Circ. Res., 26: 339-346, 1970.

19. Mackaay, A.J.C., Op 't Hof, T., Bleeker, W.K., Jongsma, H.J. and Bouman, L.N.: Interaction of adrenaline and acetylcholine on cardiac pacemaker function. Functional Inhomogeneity of the rabbit sinus node. J. Pharmacol. Exp. Ther., 214: 417-422, 1980.

20. Masuda, M.O. and Paes de Carvalho, A.: Sinoatrial transmission and atrial invasion during normal rhythm in the rabbit heart. Circ. Res., 37: 414-421, 1975.

21. Nishi, K., Yoshikawa, Y., Sugahara, K. and Monoka, T.: Changes in electrical activity and ultrastructure of sinoatrial nodal cells of the rabbit's heart exposed to hypoxic solution. Circ. Res., 46: 201-213, 1980.

22. Noma, A.: Mechanisms underlying cessation of rabbit sinoatrial node pacemaker activity in high potassium solutions. Jap. J. Physiol., 26: 619-630, 1976.

23. Noma, A. and Irisawa, H.: The effect of sodium ion on the initial phase of the sinoatrial pacemaker action potentials in rabbits. Jap. J. Physiol., 24: 617-632, 1974.

24. Noma, A. and Irisawa, H.: Effects of Na^+ and K^+ on the resting membrane potential of the rabbit sinoatrial node cell. Jap. J. Physiol., 25: 287-302, 1975.

25. Noma, A. and Irisawa, H.: Membrane currents in the rabbit sinoatrial node cell as studied by the double microelectrode method. Pfluegers Arch., 364:

45-52, 1976.

26. Paes de Carvalho, A., De Mello, W.C. and Hoffman, B.F.: Electrophysiological evidence for specialized fibertypes in rabbit atrium. Am. J. Physiol., 196: 483-488, 1959.

27. Prystowsky, E.N., Grant, A.O., Wallace, A.G. and Strauss, H.C.: An analysis of the effects of acetylcholine on conduction and refractoriness in the rabbit sinus node. Circ. Res., 44: 112-120, 1979.

28. Roberts, L.A. and Hughs, M.J.: Chronotropic response of spontaneously beating rabbit atria to hyperosmotic media. Am. J. Physiol., 233: H228-H233, 1977.

29. Senges, J., Mizutani, T., Pelzer, D., Brachmann, J., Sonnhof, U. and Kuebler, W.: Effect of hypoxia on the sinoatrial node, atrium and atrioventricular node in the rabbit heart. Circ. Res., 44: 856-863, 1979.

30. Senges, J., Hennig, E., Brachmann, J., Pelzer, D., Mizutani, T. and Kuebler, W.: Effects of orciprenaline on the sinoatrial and atrioventricular nodes in presence of hypoxia. J. Mol. Cell. Cardiol., 12:135-147, 1980.

31. Seyama, I.: Characteristics of the rectifying properties of the sinoatrial node cell of the rabbit. J. Physiol. (London), 225: 379-397, 1976.

32. Seyama, I.: Effect of gryanotoxine I on SA node and right atrial myocardia of the rabbit. Am. J. Physiol., 235: C136-C142, 1978.

33. Seyama, I.: Characteristics of the anion channel in the sinoatrial node cell of the rabbit. J. Physiol. (London), 294: 447-460, 1979.

34. Shimamoto, K. and Toda, N.: Modifications by propranolol of the response of isolated rabbit atria to endogeneous and exogeneous noradrenaline. Br. J. Pharmacol. Chemo. Ther., 32: 539-545, 1968.

35. Spear, J.F., Kronhaus, K.D., Moore, E.N. and Kline, R.P.: The effect of brief vagal stimulation on the isolated rabbit sinus node. Circ. Res., 44: 75-88, 1979.

36. Steinbeck, G., Allessie, M.A., Bonke, F.I.M. and Lammers, W.J.E.P.: Sinus node reponse to premature atrial stimulation in the rabbit studied with multiple microelectrode impalements. Circ. Res., 43: 695-704, 1978.

37. Steinbeck, G., Allessie, M.A., Bonke, F.I.M. and Lammers, W.J.E.P.: The effect of ouabain on the isolated sinus node preparation of the rabbit studied with microelectrodes. Circ. Res., 46: 406-414, 1980.

38. Strauss, H.C. and Bigger jr., J.Th.: Electrophysiological properties of

the rabbit sinoatrial perinodal fibers. Circ. Res., 31: 490-506, 1972.

39. Taniguchi, T., Fujiwara, M., Ja Lee, J. and Hidaka, H.: Effect of acetyl-choline on the norepinephrine induced positive chronotropy and increase in cyclic nucleotides of isolated rabbit sinoatrial node. Circ. Res., 45: 493-504, 1979.

40. Taylor, J.J., d'Agrosa, L.S. and Burns, E.M.: The pacemaker cell of the sinoatrial node of the rabbit. Am. J. Physiol., 235: H407-H412, 1978.

41. Toda, N.: Influence of sodium ions on the membrane potential of the sino-atrial node in response to sympathetic nerve stimulation. J. Physiol. (London), 196: 677-691, 1968.

42. Toda, N.: Electrophysiological effects of potassium and calcium ions in the sinoatrial node in response to sympathetic nerve stimulation. Pfluegers Arch., 310: 45-63, 1969.

43. Toda, N. and West, Th.: Interactions of K, Na and vagal stimulation in the sinoatrial node of the rabbit. Am. J. Physiol., 212, 416-423, 1967.

44. Toda, N. and West, Th.: Interaction between Na, Ca, Mg and vagal stimula-tion in the sinoatrial node of the rabbit. Am. J. Physiol., 212: 424-430, 1967.

45. Turlapaty, P.D.M.V. and Carrier sr., O.: Influence of magnesium on calcium induced responses of atrial and vascular muscle. J. Pharmacol. Exp. Ther., 187: 86-98, 1973.

46. Wit, A.L. and Cranefield, P.F.: Effect of verapamil on the sinoatrial and atrioventricular nodes of the rabbit and the mechanism by which it arrests reentrant atrioventricular nodal tachycardia. Circ. Res., 35: 413-425, 1974.

47. Yamaguchi, I., Obayashi, K. and Mandel, W.J.: Electrophysiological effects of verapamil. Cardiovasc. Res., 12: 597-608, 1978.

48. Yamaguchi, I., Singh, B. and Mandel, W.J.: Electrophysiological actions of mexiletine on isolated rabbit atria and canine ventricular muscle and Purk-inje fibers. Cardiovasc. Res., 13: 288-296, 1979.

49. Yamasaki, J., Fujiwana, M. and Toda, N.: Effects of intracellularly ap-plied cyclic 3', 5''-adenosine monophosphate and dibutyryl cyclic 3', 5'-adenosine monophosphate on the electrical activity of the sinoatrial nodal cells of the rabbit. J. Pharmac. Exp. Ther., 190: 15-20, 1974.

MODE OF ACTION OF ACETYLCHOLINE ON THE RABBIT SA NODE CELL

Wolfgang Osterrieder, Qin-fei Yang[*], Wolfgang Trautwein

INTRODUCTION

Achetylcholine is known to shorten the action potential and to slow the heart rate. The effects are thought to be due to an increase of the K permeability of the cell membrane and to a decreased slow inward current. These effects will be called the muscarinic response because they can be prevented by atropine. Characteristic features of the muscarinic response are the slow time course and a pronounced latency between the stimulus and the beginning of the response (Castillo and Katz, 1955; Hutter and Trautwein, 1956; Toda and West, 1965). The increase in potassium permeability has directly been shown in flux measurements with ^{42}K (Harris and Hutter, 1956) as an increased efflux of potassium on application of ACh to the frog and turtle sinus venosus and auricles. Also, in constant current experiments on mammalian atrial muscle, a reversal potential for the effect of ACh was demonstrated which exhibited by its dependence on $[K]_o$ the feature of potassium electrode (Trautwein and Dudel, 1958). In recent voltage-clamp studies on different structures and species a strong reduction of the Ca^{++}-carried slow inward current by ACh was reported (Giles and Noble, 1976; TenEick et al., 1976; Ikemoto and Goto, 1977; Hino and Ochi, 1980).

In the present article results concerning the ACh-activated potassium cur-

[*] Dr. Yang is a recipient of the Alexander von Humboldt-Stiftung; permanent address: Department of Physiology, School of Chinese Traditional Medicine, Peking, China.

rent as well as the influence of ACh on the slow inward current in the rabbit SA node are described. Using the two-microelectrode voltage-clamp technique it became possible to study the kinetics of the ACh-activated K channel, to measure the conductance of the single channel from the ACh-induced current fluctuations and to give an estimate of the density of the muscarinic receptors in the sinus node preparation used.

We have further recorded muscarinic responses (current or hyperpolarization) on ionophoretic application of ACh and reconstructed such responses with a slow time course and an apparent delay. The computer calculation of a model included the kinetics of the receptor and the diffusion within the preparation.

METHODS

The dissection procedure of the rabbit sinus node, the applied voltage-clamp technique as well as the composition of the used Tyrode and test solutions are described elsewhere (Noma and Irisawa, 1976; Noma and Trautwein, 1978). The electronic apparatus, the principle of the measurement of ACh-induced current fluctuations including the analysis can be found at Noma **et al.**, 1978a. The ionophoretical method as well as the computer simulation of the muscarinic response has recently been published (Osterrieder **et al.**, 1980; Osterrieder et al., 1981).

RESULTS

EFFECT OF ACH ON THE MEMBRANE CURRENTS

The influence of ACh on the slow inward current in the SA node was studied in voltage-clamp experiments. Fig. 1 shows membrane currents accompanying 300 ms depolarizations from -40 mV (where the net current is around zero) to -10 mV before (A) and after 2.5×10^6 M ACh (B) in absence and presence of D 600 (super-

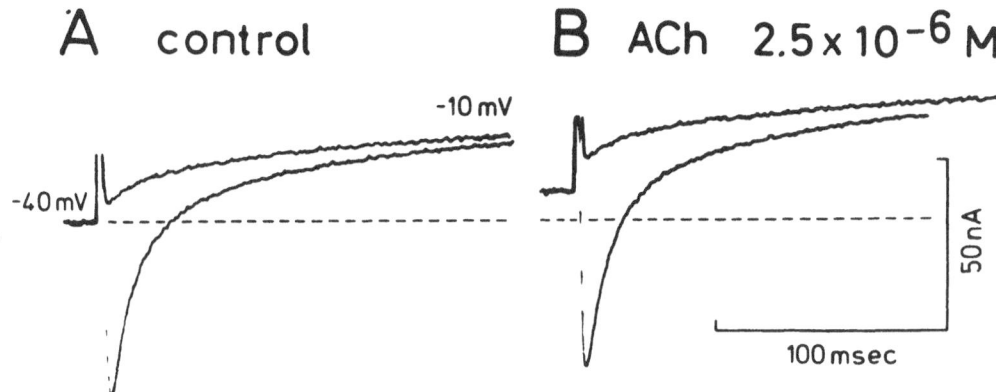

FIGURE 1 *Membrane currents in response to a voltage-jump from the holding potential of -40 mV to -10 mV, A) before, B) in presence of 2.5 x 10^{-6} M ACh. Two currents are superimposed in each panel, the upper trace is recorded after blocking the slow inward current by D 600 (10^{-7} g/ml), the lower trace is control. Horizontal broken lines indicate zero current. Note the shift in outward current by ACh. (From Noma and Trautwein, 1978, Fig. 1)*

imposed traces). Following the capacitive outward transient on depolarization the subsequent negative inward peak (in reference to the holding current) at about 10 ms is taken as the peak of the slow inward current (i_{si}). Thereafter, i_{si} decays in a mono-exponential fashion. i_{si} is superimposed on a voltage-dependent, instantaneous background outward current and a slowly rising time- and voltage-dependent potassium current (i_K). Therefore, after reaching a negative peak both mechanisms, the inactivating i_{si} and the slowly activating i_K lead to the typical current traces, shown in this figure. In the presence of ACh (2.5 x 10^{-6} M, Fig. 1B) the total current is shifted in positive direction before and during the potential step (outward direction). The clamp protocol is then repeated in the presence of D 600, a "calcium antagonist". It is a common observation that i_K generally is depressed by D 600 (Kass and Tsien, 1975; Nawrath et al., 1977). However, since the depression of i_K is not alwways a regular finding (see Fig. 3, Nawrath et al., 1977), also in the experiment the potassium outward current was not altered by the drug. The magnitude of the slow inward current was then calculated as the difference between the superim-

posed traces in A and B and remains unaffected by ACh. Even at   higher   concentrations   of   ACh   up to 10^{-4} M a clear reduction of the slow inward current, as
reported for mammalian and frog atrial strips (Giles and Noble,   1976;   TenEick
et al.,   1976;   Ikemoto and Goto, 1977) and guinea pig papillary muscle (Hino
and Ochi, 1980), is not seen. In our preparation a depression of i_{si} does   presumably not contribute to the muscarinic response.

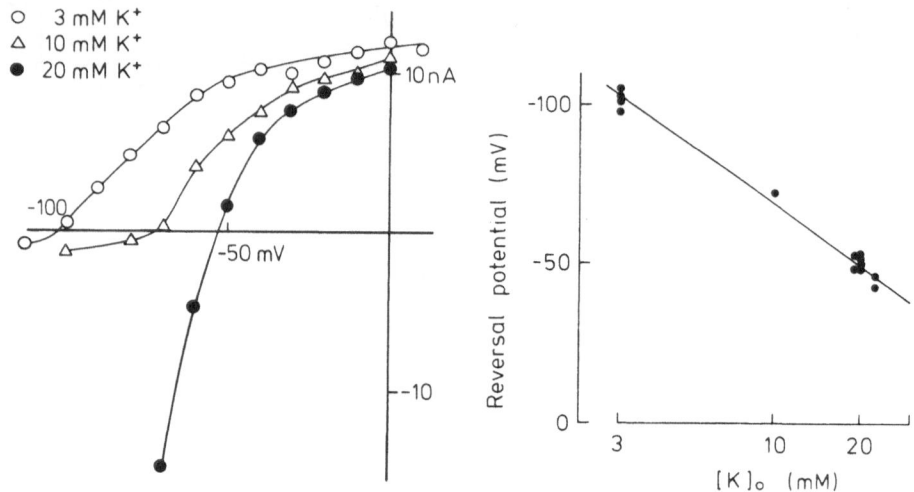

FIGURE 2 *A) Steady state IV-relations of the ACh induced K current at different*
$[K]_o$ *(open circles 3 mM, triangle 10 mM and filled circles 20 mM $[K]_o$).   ACh was*
applied ionophoretically during the test pulse. The bends of the curve towards
the   abscissa   at the low $[K]_o$ at potentials negative to the reversal potentials
are probably due to depletion of potassium at the outer vicinity of the   plasma
membrane.   B) Nernst plot of the reversal potentials of the ACh-induced current
determined by the intercept of the potassium current with the voltage axis like
in A. (From Noma and Trautwein, 1978, Figs. 9 and 10)

In order to demonstrate that the drug-activated outward current is due to a
potassium   current and to establish the IV-relation, $[K]_o$ was varied in the perfusate. The effect of 3 different external K concentrations on the   ACh-induced
outward   current   and   its   reversal   potential   is   shown   in Fig. 2 (Noma and
Trautwein, 1978). The drug was applied ionophoretically for 2.3 s   during   voltage-clamp   steps   to different potentials. The IV-relations (Fig. 2A) display

anomalous rectification like several other potassium currents in cardiac tissue; the intercepts with the voltage axis represent the reversal potentials. In B the reversal potentials (linear scale) measured in several experiments are plotted against $[K]_o$ on a logarithmic scale. The regression line has a slope of 60 mV for a tenfold change of $[K]_o$, as expected from the Nernst equation for a potassium electrode. This result suggests that the ACh-induced current is highly specific for potassium ions.

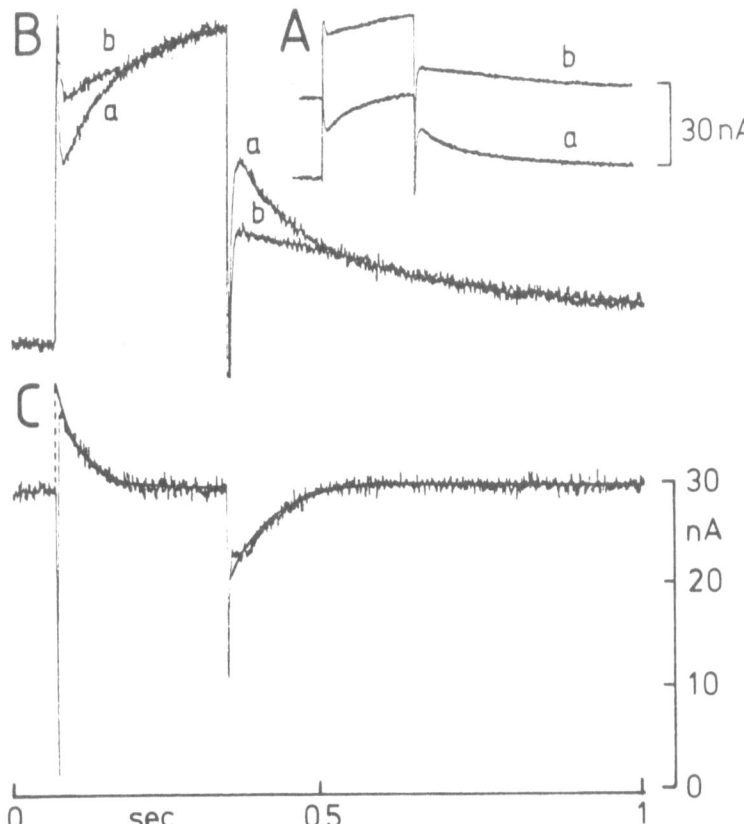

FIGURE 3 A) Currents in response to voltage jumps from -40 mV to -10 mV, before (a) and in the presence of 2.5 x 10^{-6} M ACh (b). The Tyrode solutions contained D 600 (5 x 10^{-7} g/ml). B) Both currents are superimposed with regard to the holding current at -40 mV. C) Computer subtraction of the control current a from current b. (From DiFrancesco et al., 1980, Fig. 2)

RELAXATION OF THE ACH-INDUCED POTASSIUM CURRENT

The question arises whether the ACh opens a new specific ion channel or increases i_K and/or the time-independent background current. This problem could be
solved in experiments (see Fig. 3), where the membrane was voltage-clamped from
-40 mV to -10 mV for 300 ms in control Tyrode and in the presence of 2×10^{-6} M
ACh, both solutions containing D 600. The result of such an experiment is demonstrated in Fig.   3A,   again   showing an ACh-induced extra K current which
shifts the net current in positive direction (trace b). When the currents (control a, and in presence of ACh, b) were superimposed with reference to the holding current at a higher magnification than in A (Fig. 3B), it   became obvious
that the pacemaker current i_K was not affected by ACh (during and after the test
pulse), but that there are considerable differences between the two traces early
on depolarization and repolarization. The difference, reflecting the time dependence of the ACh-induced current, is seen more clearly in a subtraction of
the current traces (Fig. 3C). After the depolarizing step the current is initially large and declines to a steady level and, vice versa, after repolarization the current is initially small, this time slowly rising to a steady state.
The time course of the ACh-induced current is adequately described by a single
exponential (solid lines Fig. 3C). This time dependence is called relaxation.
Relaxation was a regular observation both in the absence and the presence of
D 600 as well as in low (3 mM) and high (20 mM) $\left[K\right]_o$. In this context it is
worthwhile to note that relaxation is not due to accumulation of extracellular
potassium (DiFrancesco et al., 1980). This time-dependence of the additional
current excludes an effect of ACh on the potassium background current as proposed for the frog's atrium (Garnier et al., 1978).

Relaxation is a regular finding in many synapses. The interpretation of
relaxation in the SA node is based on two assumptions: 1) An individual ion
channel associated with an agonist-binding receptor site can exist in two
states, namely closed and open:

$$\text{(closed)} \; \underset{\alpha}{\overset{\beta\,'(A)}{\rightleftharpoons}} \; \text{(open)} \tag{1}$$

The fluctuations between the two states are described by the overall opening rate constant $\beta'(A)$ which includes all possible intermediate steps between the two states, and the rate constant α for the closing of the channel. It will be shown below that α does not depend on the agonist concentration. 2) If one rate constant, or both in a different way, is voltage dependent, relaxation with the time constant τ occurs after voltage steps:

$$\tau = 1/(\alpha + \beta'(A)) \tag{2}$$

The time constant of relaxation of the ACh-induced current depends on the membrane potential in a way similar to that of the nicotinic receptor, i.e. relaxation occurs faster the more positive the membrane potential. However, the absolute values of the time constants are much larger in the muscarinic than in the nicotinic receptor. In addition, the time constants are the same at 3 and 12 mM $[K]_o$, indicating that the kinetics of the ACh-induced K current, flowing through a drug-activated potassium channel, does not depend on the external potassium concentration (Noma et al., 1979b).

SINGLE CHANNEL CONDUCTANCE AND DENSITY OF THE ACH-ACTIVATED POTASSIUM CHANNELS

The individual potassium channel, activated by ACh, stays open for an average open time, then closes. On increasing the agonist concentration, the channel will open more often which results in a larger current. The transitions between the open and the closed state of ACh-activated channels give rise to current fluctuations as demonstrated in the experiment of Fig. 4. The membrane potential was clamped to -40 mV and ACh was applied at increasing concentrations in the perfusate (2×10^{-5}, 2×10^{-4} and 5×10^{-4} M from top to bottom). As shown in the low gain DC record (A) the activated outward current was larger the higher the agonist concentration. During the ACh application the current remained nearly constant, i.e. desensitization was negligible. In B the current is highly AC-magnified and digitized. The bandwidth of the control signal increases with increasing ACh concentrations in the perfusate, but seems to decrease again at the largest concentration. The current fluctuations originating from the transitions of the ACh-activated potassium channels were evaluated in two ways, by means of the spectral distribution of power density and the variance.

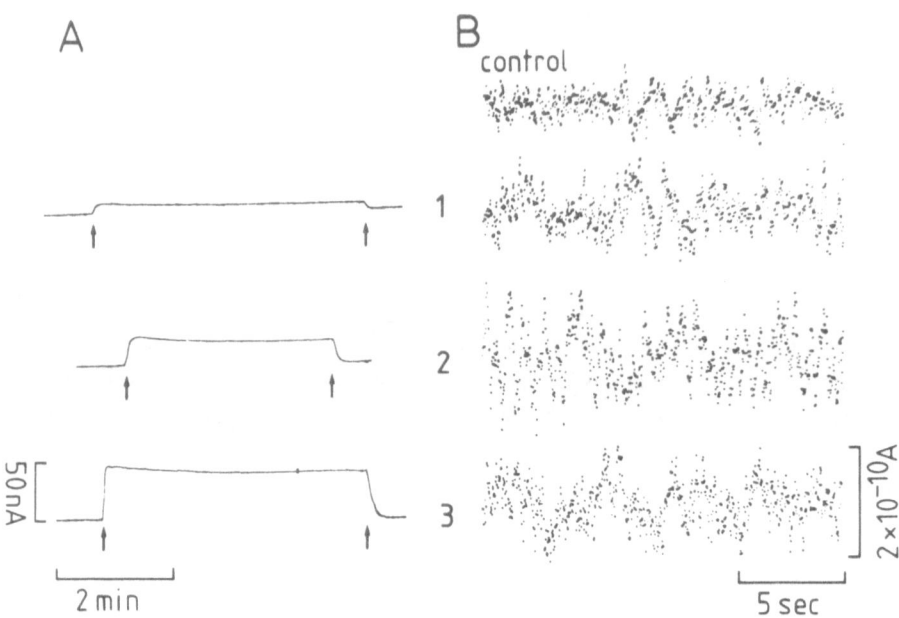

FIGURE 4 *Application of ACh in concentrations of 2 x 10^{-5} M (traces 1), 2 x 10^{-4} M (traces 2) and 5 x 10^{-4} M (traces 3), A) at low gain DC penrecording of the clamp current at -40 mV, B) high gain AC recording, digitalized. (From Noma et al., 1979a, Fig. 4)*

Fig. 5A is an example of the spectral distribution of the power density of the ACh-induced current fluctuations. The spectrum is the difference obtained by subtracting the spectrum under control conditions from that recorded during ACh application (10^{-4} M). This difference, plotted in a double-logarithmic scale, is the spectral power density produced by the activation of K channels by ACh. The power density distribution could be fitted by a Lorentzian curve (e-quation see legend), which is exptected if in a sequence of reactions one step is rate-limiting. The evaluation yields numerical values of the single channel conductance γ (Anderson and Stevens, 1973). The single channel conductance for this ACh-operated potassium channel has a value of about 3.8 pS (γ = 3.79 $\pm$ 1.25 pS, n = 21) at -40 mV, i.e. in 3 mM $\left[K\right]_o$ a unit current of about 0.22 pA flows through each individual open channel (Noma et al., 1979a; Noma et al., 1979b). From the total current and the unit current through the indi-

A

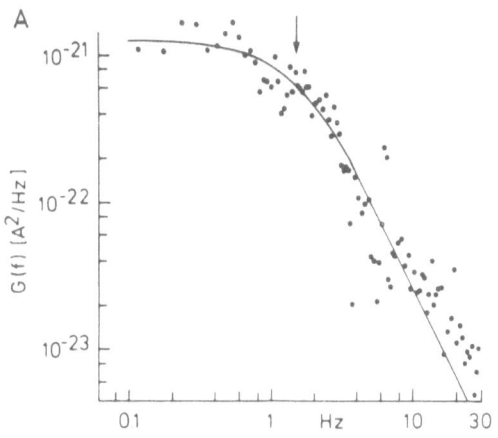

B

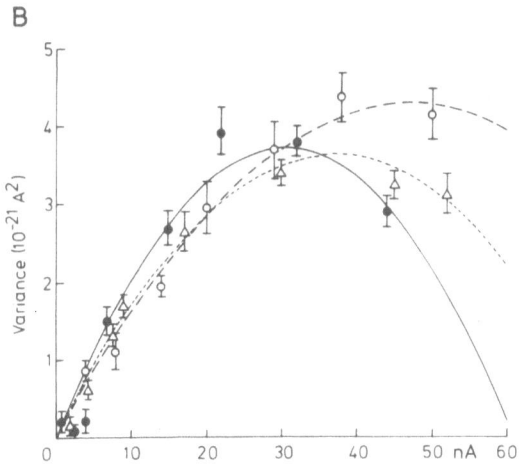

FIGURE 5 A) Power density spectrum of ACh-induced current fluctuations, obtained by a Fast Fourier Transform algorithm. Solid line: Least square fit using the Lorentzian curve $G(f)=G(0)/(1+(f/f_c)^2)$ with the parameters $G(0)=1.22 \times 10^{-21}$ A^2/Hz and $f_c = 1.47$ Hz (see arrow). B) Plot of the variance σ of the ACh-induced current fluctuations against the ACh-induced current I (3 different experiments). Vertical bars: Standard errors of the mean variance obtained by subtracting the mean variance of control frames (up to 20) from the variance of each of the frames (6 - 20) recorded in presence of ACh. Solid and broken curves obtained by a fitting procedure to the data using equation (3). (From Noma et al., 1979a, Figs. 5 and 6B)

vidual channel, the number of open channels can be determined. The spectrum does also contain by the corner frequency, f_c, information on the average open time of the channel. f_c is the frequency where the power density equals half that of the plateau level. Corner frequency (0.96 ± 0.25 Hz, n = 21) and time constant of relaxation are related by $\tau = 1/2 \pi f_c$ and lead to an average open time of the channel of about 100 ms.

The analysis of the variance of the ACh-induced current fluctuations vs. the ACh-activated current does not give information on the kinetics of the channel. The variance, σ^2, is related to the single channel conductance γ , the drug-induced current I, the maximum current I_{max} (the current if all available channels are open) and the driving force $E-E_K$ by means of the following equation (Begenisich and Stevens, 1975):

$$\sigma^2 = \gamma \cdot I \cdot (1 - I/I_{max}) \cdot (E - E_K) \tag{3}$$

The equation predicts a maximum of the variance at $I_{max}/2$ and a decline to zero when the current approximates I_{max}. The computer fit to the data of three experiments (Fig. 5B) yields the same value for the single channel conductance γ (3.71 $\pm$ 0.48 pS, n = 7), as determined above. I_{max} is given by the intercept with the abscissa. It is worth mentioning that the ACh-induced current hardly exceeds the maximum in the variance-current relation (Fig. 5B). This indicates that at high ACh concentrations the overall forward rate constant controlling the agonist binding and the subsequent channel transition from the closed to the open state and the backward rate constant are of similar magnitude (see below). I_{max} allows to estimate the total number of receptors in a preparation. Considering the total surface of the sinus node cells, as determined from measurements of the capacitive current, a low density of channels of 0.7 per μm^2 was calculated (Noma et al., 1979a).

DETERMINATION OF THE RATE CONSTANTS IN THE REACTION SCHEME FOR THE MUSCARINIC RECEPTOR

The reported data only describe that ACh opens one way or another a specific voltage-dependent K channel, but do not give information about the intermediate reaction sequence, how ACh operates its channel. In the endplate the Katz-Miledi model (Katz and Miledi, 1972) describes the reaction of acetylcholine with the nicotinic receptor. Therefore, we tested whether or not this model can also apply for the action of ACh on the muscarinic receptor. The Katz-Miledi model includes a fast binding step of the agonist (concentration A) to its receptor (R). The inactive agonist-receptor complex ((AR) = closed channel) then undergoes a relatively slower conformational change to the active, conductive form (AR* = open channel):

$$A + R \xrightarrow[k_2]{k_1} AR \xrightarrow[\alpha]{\beta} AR^* \qquad\qquad (4)$$

k_1, k_2, α and β are the rate constants as indicated in the reaction scheme. The assumption that only one molecule binds to its receptor is in line with the finding of a unity Hill coefficient, as found in atrial muscle (Glitsch and Pott, 1978) and in the SA node (Osterrieder et al., 1981). The mono-exponential time course of relaxation and the Lorentzian shape of the spectral power density of the ACh-induced current fluctuations suggest the existence of a rate-limiting step in the reaction scheme for the muscarinic receptor. In the Katz-Miledi model the overall rate constant $\beta'(A)$ (see equation (1)) can be expressed in terms of the apparent dissociation constant $K_D = k_2/k_1$, the ACh concentration (A) and the rate constant β for the opening of the channel by the following equation (Colquhoun and Hawkes, 1977; Osterrieder et al., 1980):

$$\beta'(A) = \beta/(1 + K_D/A) \qquad\qquad (5)$$

Information on the rate constants α and $\beta'(A)$ can be derived from the ACh-induced current recorded from the dose-response curve. This current, I(A), is proportional to the current I_{max}, which depends on the total number of ACh-operated ionic channels available in each preparation, and on the actual fraction of open channels described by $\beta'(A)/(\alpha + \beta'(A))$ at a given agonist concentration (also see equation (1)):

$$I(A) = \beta'(A)/(\alpha + \beta'(A)) \cdot I_{max} \qquad\qquad (6)$$

Another information is derived from the finding that the time constant of relaxation is strongly dependent on the agonist concentration (equation 2). Dividing the equation (6) through (2), an expression for $\beta'(A)$ in terms of three measurable data is derived:

$$I(A)/\tau(A) = \beta'(A) \cdot I_{max} \qquad\qquad (7)$$

In order to obtain, on the basis of this model, numerical values for $\beta'(A)$ and

α, the following three types of experiment were combined in the same preparation (Osterrieder et al., 1980): the measurement of the current in the dose-response curve (I(A)), the time constant of relaxation at different ACh concentrations (τ(A)), and the measurement of the current fluctuations to obtain I_{max}. With this information α was computed by subtracting β'(A) from the reciprocal time constant τ(A)$^{-1}$.

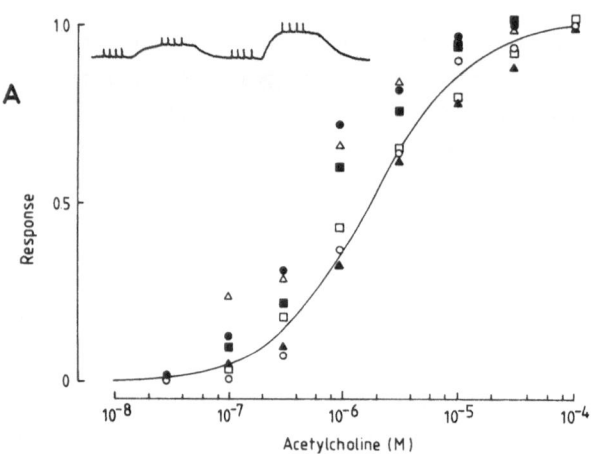

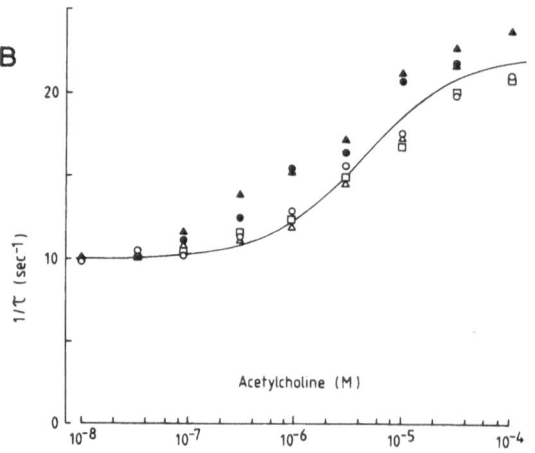

FIGURE 6 A) Dose-response curve of 6 experiments. The amplitude of the maximum response was taken to 1 and the current values were normalized. Inset: Clamp protocol. B) The relation between the reciprocal of the time constant of relaxation and the ACh concentration. In A and B the Tyrode's contained neostigmine (10 g/ml). The smooth curves are fits to the open circles using the values for α and β'(A) of Fig. 7 with equations (2) and (6). (From Osterrieder et al., 1980, Figs. 2 and 4)

The dose-response curve was obtained using the experimental procedure as outlined in the inset of Fig. 6. To a voltage-clamped preparation increasing concentrations of ACh were applied in the perfusate. The normalized currents from 6 experiments were plotted against the respective ACh concentration (Fig. 6A). The apparent dissociation constant K_D is at about 10^{-6} M. For the measurement of τ at different agonist concentrations (Fig. 6B) the membrane was depolarized for 300 ms four times from -40 mV to -10 mV before and during each perfusion (see also inset). The currents during each run were averaged and the average during ACh application was subtracted from the respective control average current; time constants of relaxation were fitted by the computer as shown in Fig. 3. The reciprocal time constant (Fig. 6B) strongly depended on the agonist concentration and ranged from 100 ms for very low to 45 ms for high ACh concentrations. Finally, the noise measurement performed in the same preparation yielded the value of I_{max} as described in Fig. 5B.

For each of these experiments $\beta'(A)$ was calculated following equation (7), and α was computed by the above mentioned procedure. A representative example for the agonist-concentration dependence of $\beta'(A)$ and α is shown in Fig.7. It shows that the rate constant α of about 10 s^{-1} is largely independent of the agonist concentration, whereas $\beta'(A)$ rises between 10^{-8} and 10^{-4} M ACh from zero to approximately 11.7 s^{-1}. The solid curve is a computer fit to the experimentally determined values of $\beta'(A)$ using equation (5) from the Katz-Miledi model considering a value of 12.3 s^{-1} for β; the K_D value is taken from the corresponding dose-response curve in Fig. 6 ($K_D = 4.2 \times 10^{-6}$ M). It is worthwhile to note that $\beta'(A)$ reaches a plateau as examplified in the inset (linear concentration scale). This result justifies the assumption that the channel transitions between the closed and open state are the rate-limiting steps. If the binding of the agonist would be rate-limiting, the overall rate constant would still rise with increasing agonist concentration (Colquhoun and Hawkes, 1977). The mean values for α and β, determined from 6 experiments, were 10.1 s^{-1} and 12.0 s^{-1}, K_D was 1.7×10^{-6} M.

THE TIME COURSE OF THE MUSCARINIC RESPONSE ON IONOPHORETIC APPLICATION OF ACH

The muscarinic response, as reported by potential measurements (hyperpolarizations) with its delay and slow rise time is mediated by the activation of an

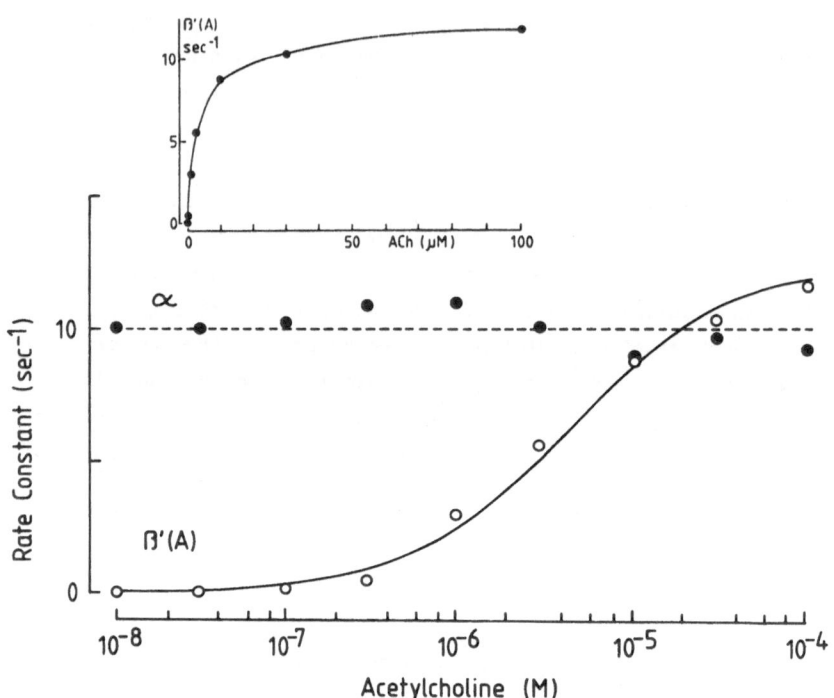

FIGURE 7   *The relation between the rate constants α and β'(A) and the ACh concentration.   Same experiments as presented by open circles in Fig. 6.   The smooth curve is the best fit using the equation (5) with β = 12.3 s^{-1}.   The theoretical line for α is the average of 9 values (from Osterrieder et al., 1980, Fig.
7).   Inset: β'(A) plotted on linear scale.*

ACh-generated potassium channel, as shown by the data presented so far. The attempt was made to reconstruct the time behaviour on the basis of the Katz-Miledi
model, since intermediate events between the binding of ACh and the opening of
the channel, e.g. elevation of the intracellular cGMP level, have been proposed. In the experiment shown in Fig. 8A the preparation was   voltage-clamped
at -40 mV. A third electrode filled with ACh was placed on the surface of the
preparation, and between the arrows ACh was released ionophoretically. The current response develops slowly and has its peak at about 700 ms. The flat onset
of the response, the apparent delay, has been reported to be in the order of 100
ms (Purves, 1976; Hill-Smith and Purves, 1978; Pott, 1979). Another factor,

however, which can influence the shape of the response is the diffusion from the agonist source to the receptors sparsely distributed in the preparation. This is suggested in the experiment shown in Fig. 8B.

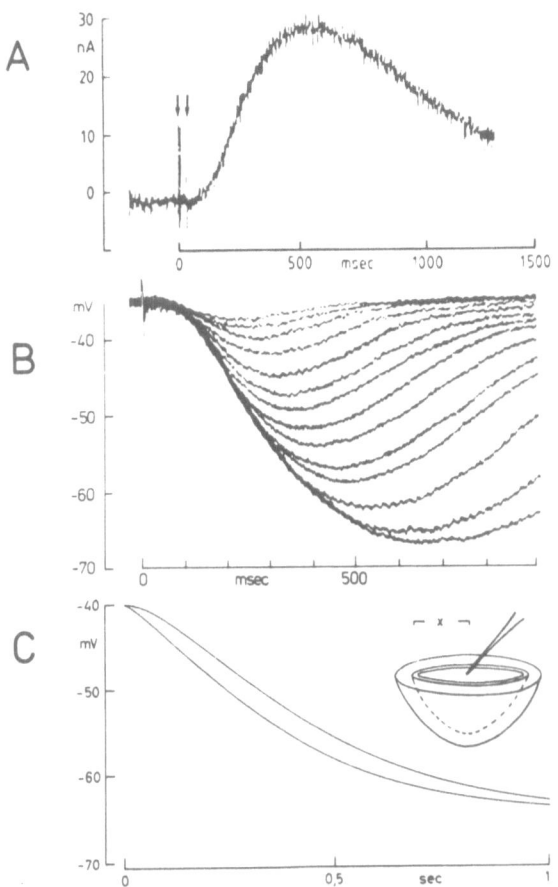

FIGURE 8 A) Experimental record of the membrane current in response to ionophoretic application of ACh. Duration of the releasing pulse (indicated by the arrows) is 33 ms and the strength is 50 nA. (From Osterrieder et al., 1980, Fig. 8A). B) Hyperpolarizations recorded after ionophoretic application of ACh. The releasing pulse varied from 1 ms (smallest response) to 330 ms duration (largest response). The beginning of the pulse is indicated by the electrical artefact. C) Model calculation of the muscarinic response. The upper trace was calculated including the rate constants for the opening and closing of the ion channel ($\beta = 12$ s^{-1} and $\alpha = 10$ s^{-1}). In the lower curve this rate–limiting step was not considered. Inset: Geometry of the model preparation. (From Osterrieder et al., 1981, Figs. 1A and 6A)

In this experiment the preparation was arrested by D 600 and the membrane potential was recorded. At time zero, as indicated by the electrical artefact, increasing amounts of ACh were released. Upon increasing ACh concentrations, the peak time gets longer. The explanation could be that, the more ACh is released, more receptors located more distant from the tip of the pipette can be reached. The recruitment of more ACh-activated K channels increases the response, the peak time rises because the drug has to diffuse along the distance.

We have reconstructed the hyperpolarizing response and the current response on ionophoretic application on the basis of the kinetics and low density of the receptors. The model for the stimulation of the muscarinic response was a half spheric preparation (radius 100 μm) with the tip of the ACh pipette located on the surface (for details of the computation see Osterrieder et al., 1980; Osterrieder et al., 1981). The preparation was divided into shells with increasing radii in increments of 5 μm. The receptors were assumed to be distributed homogeneously with a "volume density" estimated from the total number of receptors and the volume of the standard preparation. ACh diffuses radially into the preparation, its concentration expressed by the equation (Purves, 1977; Dreyer et al., 1978)

$$A(x,t) = \frac{M}{8 \cdot (\pi D t)^{1.5}} \cdot \exp(- \frac{x^2}{4Dt} - k_H t) \tag{8}$$

where an amount M of ACh is released instantaneously at time $t = 0$. D is the diffusion coefficient and k_H is the rate constant for the hydrolysis of ACh by the tissue cholinesterase. Inside the preparation the drug probably diffuses slower because of the binding to non-specific sites in the clefts and therefore less molecules reach the receptors. For this reason D was reduced to 8×10^{-6} $cm^2 s^{-1}$, half that for free diffusion. For each successive time step of computation (1 or 2 ms) the average concentration was calculated in each shell. At each time step $\beta'(A)$ was calculated, and time constant $\tau = 1/(\alpha + \beta'(A))$ and the fraction $\left[\beta'(A)/(\alpha + \beta'(A))\right]$ of open channels (cf. equ. (6)) were determined. On the basis of the fraction of open channels in each shell and the density of the receptors, the contribution of each shell to the total current was computed. For the calculation of the hyperpolarization the potential dependence of α (cf. Noma and Trautwein, 1978) and the input impedance of the preparation (1 MOhm) were included. The result of the reconstruction of the muscarinic response is illustrated in Fig. 8C. The computation of the response considering the rate-limiting step in the Katz-Miledi model has an apparent delay of about 30 ms as observed in our experiments. The delay seems to result from the small values of $\beta'(A)$ in the shells distant from the tip of the pipette where the ACh concentration is low. In the lower trace α and $\beta'(A)$ were not considered and there is no delay, nevertheless the rising phase to the peak is slow. Under the unrealistic assumption that agonist source and point-shaped preparation are 2 μm apart, the result of the calculation had a different shape: after a short releasing pulse the ACh concentration reached its maximum after 1 ms whereas the maximum response occurred about 30 ms later; a delay was not seen. The calculations suggest that the slow time course of the muscarinic response is mainly caused by diffusion in a preparation with a low receptor density, and that the apparent delay is due to the kinetics of the muscarinic receptor.

The model calculations were tested under a variety of external conditions (Osterrieder et al., 1981). One example is the activity of the tissue cholinesterase. It has strong influence on the shape of the muscarinic response after ionophoretic application of ACh. This is shown in Fig. 9 for the wash-out of neostigmine, a cholinesterase inhibitor. The hyperpolarizations were recorded in intervals of 5 min. Duration and peak time of the response are clearly shortened. In the simulation the inhibitory effect of neostigmine was taken into account by increasing the k_H value in equation (8) from 0 to 5 s^{-1}. The results of the experiments and calculations were in good agreement.

SUMMARY

The measurements suggest that ACh opens a specific potassium ion channel. The single channel conductance is at about 3.7 pS (in 3 mM $[K]_o$, and the muscarinic receptors are distributed with a low density (0.7 μm^2). The Katz-Miledi model is appropriate to describe the kinetics of the channel with a fast binding of the agonist to the receptor and slow channel transitions (opening, closing). The muscarinic response on ionophoretic application of the drug can be calculated on the basis of the rate constants β and α for the channel transitions and the diffusion in the preparation. A chemical mediator like cGMP or intermediate

A

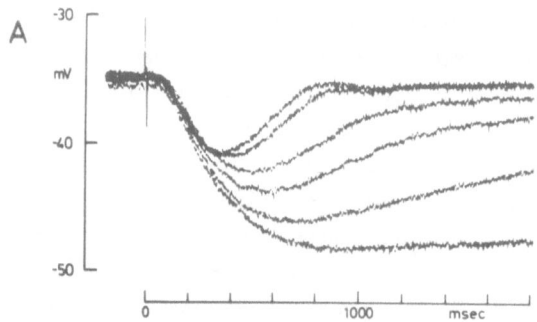

3

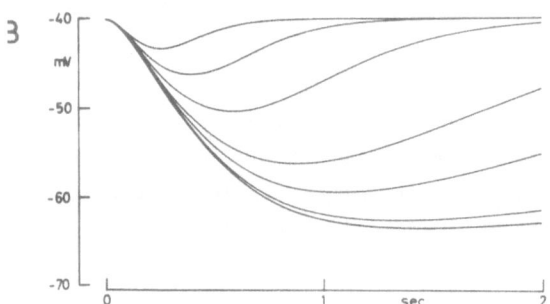

FIGURE 9 *Effect of cholinesterase: Comparison of experiment and calculation. A) Hyperpolarizations after ionophoretic application of ACh were recorded in intervals of 5 min during the wash-out of neostigmine (10^{-7} g/ml). The Tyrode's contained D 600 (5×10^{-9} g/ml) to arrest the preparation. Releasing pulse of 10 ms duration and 10 nA strength. B) The wash-out of neostigmine was simulated by increasing k_H from 0.1 s^{-1} (lowest trace) to 5 s^{-1} (uppermost trace). (From Osterrieder et al., 1981, Figs. 4B and 7B)*

reaction steps are not required to explain the apparent delay and the slow time course of the response. In the rabbit SA node a dual effect of ACh like in other structures, i.e. a reduction of the slow inward current in addition to an increase of the potassium conductance, has not been found.

ACKNOWLEDGEMENT

The authors wish to thank Dr. D. Pelzer for reading and discussing the manuscript. The financial support of the SFB 38 (Membranforschung), project G 1, is gratefully acknowledged.

REFERENCES

Anderson, C.R. and Stevens, C.F.: Voltage clamp analysis of acetylcholine produced endplate current fluctuations at frog neuromuscular junction. J. Physiol. (London), 235: 655-691, 1973.

Begenisich, T. and Stevens, C.F.: How many conductance states do potassium channels have? Biophys. J., 15: 843-846, 1975.

Castillo del, J. and Katz, B.: Production of membrane potential changes in the frog's heart by inhibitory nerve impulses. Nature, 175: 1035, 1955.

Colquhoun, D. and Hawkes, A.G.: Relaxation and fluctuations of membrane currents that flow through drug-operated channels. Proc. R. Soc. Lond. B., 199: 231-262, 1977.

DiFrancesco. D., Noma, A. and Trautwein, W.: Seperation of current induced by potassium accumulation from acetylcholine induced relaxation current in the rabbit SA node. Pfluegers Arch., 387: 83-90, 1980.

Dreyer, F., Peper, K. and Sterz, R.: Determination of dose-response curves by quantitative ionophoresis at the frog neuromuscular junction. J. Physiol. (London), 281: 395-419, 1978.

Garnier, D., Nargeot, J., Ojeda, C. and Rougier, O.: The action of acetylcholine on background conductance in frog atrial trabeculae. J. Physiol. (London), 274: 381-396, 1978.

Giles, W. and Noble, S.J.: Changes in membrane currents in bullfrog atrium produced by acetylcholine. J. Physiol. (London), 261: 103-123, 1976.

Glitsch, H.G. and Pott, L.: Effects of acetylcholine and parasympathetic nerve stimulation on membrane potential in quiescent guinea-pig atria. J. Physiol. (London), 279: 655-668, 1978.

Harris, E.J. and Hutter, O.F.: The action of acetylcholine and the movements of potassium ions in the sinus venosus of the heart. J. Physiol. (London), 133: 58P, 1956.

Hill-Smith, I. and Purves, R.D.: Synaptic delay in the heart: an ionophoretic study. J. Physiol. (London), 279: 31-54, 1978.

Hino, N. and Ochi, R.: Effect of acetylcholine on membrane currents in guinea-pig papillary muscle. J. Physiol. (London), 307: 183-197, 1980.

Hutter, O.F. and Trautwein, W.: Vagal and sympathetic effects on the pacemaker fibres in the sinus venosus of the heart. J. Gen. Physiol., 39: 715-733, 1956.

Ikemoto, Y. and Goto, M.: Effects of ACh on slow inward current and tension components of the bullfrog atrium. J. Mol. Cell. Cardiol., 9: 313-326, 1977.

Kass, R.S. and Tsien, R.W.: Multiple effects of calcium antagonists on plateau currents in cardiac Purkinje fibers. J. Gen. Physiol., 66: 169-192, 1975.

Katz, B. and Miledi, R.: The statistical nature of the acetylcholine potentials and its molecular components. J. Physiol. (London), 224: 665-699, 1972.

Nawrath, H., TenEick, R.E., McDonald, T.F. and Trautwein, W.: On the mechanism underlying the action of D 600 on slow inward current and tension in mammalian myocardium. Circ. Res., 40: 408-414, 1977.

Noma, A. and Irisawa, H.: Membrane currents in the rabbit sinoatrial node cell as studied by the double microelectrode method. Pfluegers Arch., 364: 45-52, 1976.

Noma, A, and Trautwein, W.: Relaxation of the ACh-induced potassium current in the rabbit sinoatrial node cell. Pfluegers Arch., 377: 193-200, 1978.

Noma, A., Peper, K. and Trautwein, W.: Acetylcholine-induced potassium current fluctuations in the rabbit sinoatrial node. Pfluegers Arch., 381: 255-262, 1979a.

Noma, A., Osterrieder, W. and Trautwein, W.: The effect of external potassium on the elementary conductance of the ACh-induced potassium channel in the sinoatrial node. Pfluegers Arch., 381: 263-269, 1979b.

Osterrieder, W., Noma, A. and Trautwein, W.: On the kinetics of the potassium channel activated by acetylcholine in the SA node of the rabbit heart.

Pfluegers Arch., 386: 101-109, 1980.

Osterrieder, W., Yang, Q.-f. and Trautwein, W.: The time course of the muscarinic response to ionophoretic acetylcholine application to the SA node of
the rabbit heart. Pfluegers Arch., 389: 283-291, 1981.

Pott, L.: On the time course of the acetylcholine-induced hyperpolarization in
quiescent guinea-pig atria. Pfluegers Arch., 380: 71-77, 1979.

Pott, L. and Pusch, H.: A kinetic model for the muscarinic action of acetylcholine. Pfluegers Arch., 383: 75-77, 1979.

Purves, R.D.: Function of muscarinic and nicotinic acetylcholine receptors.
Nature, 261: 149-151, 1976.

Purves, R.D.: The time course of cellular response to ionophoretically applied
drugs. J. Theor. Biol., 65: 327-344, 1977.

TenEick, R., Nawrath, H., McDonald, T.F. and Trautwein, W.: On the mechanism
of the negative inotropic response of acetylcholine. Pfluegers Arch., 361:
207-213, 1976.

Toda, N. and West, T.C.: Changes in sinoatrial transmembrane potentials on
vagal stimulation of the isolated rabbit atrium. Nature, 205: 808-809,
1965.

Trautwein, W. and Dudel, J.: Zum Mechanismus der Membranwirkung des Acetylcholin an der Herzmuskelfaser. Pfluegers Arch., 266: 324-334, 1958.

INTERACTION OF ADRENALINE AND ACETYLCHOLINE

ON SINUS NODE FUNCTION

Albert J.C. Mackaay, Tobias Op 't Hof, Wim K. Bleeker,
Habo J. Jongsma and Lennart N. Bouman

INTRODUCTION

Already 25 years ago T.C West (1955) described the first microelectrode study of the sinus node. Since then many investigators have been concerned with sinus node function (Brooks and Lu, 1972; Bonke, 1978). Although highly sophisticated techniques have been applied, it looks today that the definite words about the sinus node cannot yet be written. West's own observations gave already an indication of some of the problems involved. Describing the electrical activity recorded from single nodal cells, he defined "the true pacemaker" as the site which "depolarizes earlier than any other region during any one cardiac cycle". He established that this "true pacemaker activity" was not confined to a fixed site, he could easily induce shifts of pacemaker dominance by adding drugs like acetylcholine and adrenaline. Those observations indicated that the sinus node is functionally inhomogeneous, at least in its responses to autonomic mediators. Several pacemakers are capable to drive the sinus node and those pacemakers show different responses. Thus, one single pacemaker cell is not representative for the sinus node as a whole. Sinus nodal cells are coupled electrically (Bonke, 1973; Masson-Pevet et al., 1979; Bukauskas et al., 1981), so the configuration of the electrical activity recorded from single cells depends not only on their own activity, but also on changes of the activity of surrounding cells (Bonke, 1978; Mackaay et al., 1980a). West (1955) already emphasized this in stating that "analysis of drug effects in the pacemaker region is complicated by the apparent shifts in the pacemaker activity". Several papers concerning the autonomic control of the function of the mammalian sinus node published afterwards (West et al., 1956; Toda and West, 1965; Vincenzi and West, 1965; Toda and Shimamoto, 1968; Spear et al., 1979) are subject to the mentioned complication. Recently the effects of adrenaline and acetylcholine were also studied in small, electrically homogeneous specimen of rabbit sinus nodal tissue (Noma and Trautwein, 1978; Brown et al., 1979), but here the problem of pacemaker shifts is exchanged for the question of the applicability of the results to other pacemakers in the inhomogeneous node.

This chapter concerns the function of the rabbit sinus node under the influence of adrenaline and acetylcholine, considering the responses of both the total sinus node and of separated parts containing the different pacemakers involved.

METHODS

Rabbits were anesthetized with 10 mg of fluanison + 0.2 mg of fentanyl base (Hypnorm) per kg i.m. The spontaneously beating sinus node preparation (Bleeker et al., 1980) was fixed in a tissue bath (5 ml) which was perfused continuously at a rate of 20 ml per min with a solution of the following millimolar composition: NaCl 130.6; KCl 5.6; $NaHCO_3$ 24.2; $CaCl_2$ 2.2; $MgCl_2$ 0.6; glucose 11.1 and sucrose 13.2. The solution was equilibrated with 95 % O_2 and 5 % CO_2. The pH was 7.4. Temperature was kept constant within 0.1 $^{\circ}$C at 38 $^{\circ}$C. l-Adrenaline bitartrate (Adr) and acetylcholine bromide (Ach) were administered by adding small amounts of a concentrated solution to the bathing fluid through a mixing device.

A unipolar surface electrogram was derived from the inferior part of the crista terminalis and the tachogram was recorded continuously. Irregular beating preparations were discarded. Transmembrane potentials were recorded by means of the conventional glass microelectrode technique. Activation maps of the nodal area were made as previously described (Bleeker et al., 1980). The activation moment of the cells (the moment at which depolarization was halfway between maximal diastolic potential and the top of the action potential) was timed with respect to the steep deflection of the atrial surface electrogram by on-line and off-line computer analysis. The earliest discharging cell group under standard conditions was usually located in the superior part of the sinus node (Bleeker et al., 1980).

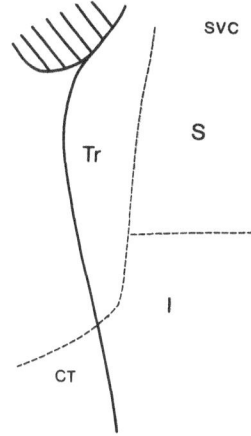

FIGURE 1 Separation of the sinus node preparation in a transitional zone (Tr) and a superior part of the compact zone (S) and an inferior part of the compact zone (I). The criteria for the separation are described in the Methods. CT = crista terminalis; SVC = superior vena cava.

In three preparations we separated the total preparation into three parts. One part containing the primary pacemaker (S) (the superior part of the compact sinus node), another containing the Adr-center (I) (the inferior part of the compact sinus node) and the third containing the Ach-center (Tr) (the transitional part of the sinus node) (fig. 1). To this end we first discriminated electrophysiologically the compact part of the sinus node. As a criterium we used an action potential upstroke velocity less than 5 V/s. At the crista terminalis border of this zone we marked the tissue iontophoretically by 1 % Alcian Blue (Bleeker et al., 1980). Next we cut the preparation along these marked sites by means of a razor blade. So we obtained a transitional zone and a compact zone. The primary pacemaker was within the compact zone. This zone was cut 0.5 mm caudal from the primary pacemaker in order to separate the primary pacemaker from the Adr-center (Mackaay et al., 1980b). The longitudinal cut parallel to the crista terminalis, i.e. the separation of the transitional from the compact zone induced often irregularities. Such preparations were discarded. It is emphasized that a cut perpendicular to the crista terminalis nearly always delivers two regularly beating (superior and inferior) parts of the sinus node (Mackaay et al., 1980b).

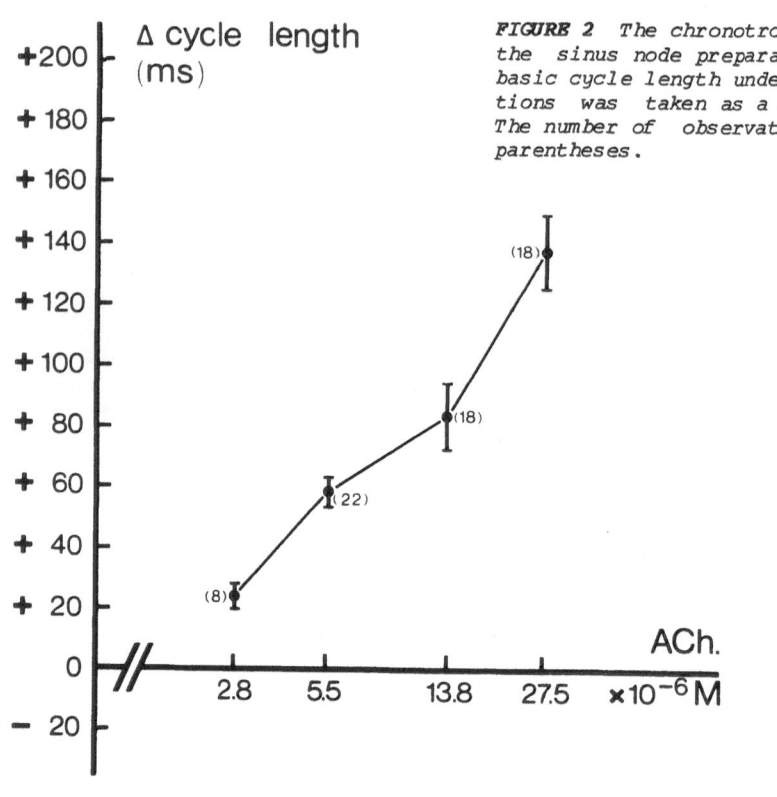

FIGURE 2 *The chronotropic response of the sinus node preparation to Ach. The basic cycle length under standard conditions was taken as a reference (0 ms). The number of observations is between parentheses.*

RESULTS

THE EFFECT OF ACETYLCHOLINE IN THE TOTAL SINUS NODE
Addition of Ach causes a dose-dependent deceleration of the preparation (fig. 2). A continuous impalement of the primary pacemaker (fig. 3A-C), made during the addition of Ach (11×10^{-6} M), confirmed the results of West et al. (1955, 1956). The most prominent change in the electrical activity of the node concerns the activation pattern. Under standard conditions the impaled cell meets the criteria of a dominant pacemaker cell (fig. 3A). It discharges earlier than any other site (32 ms before the atrial time reference) with a smooth transition between a prominent phase of diastolic depolarization and the action potential upstroke. Under Ach the activation order is reversed. The cell is activated late in the cardiac cycle, 9 ms after the atrial time reference (fig.

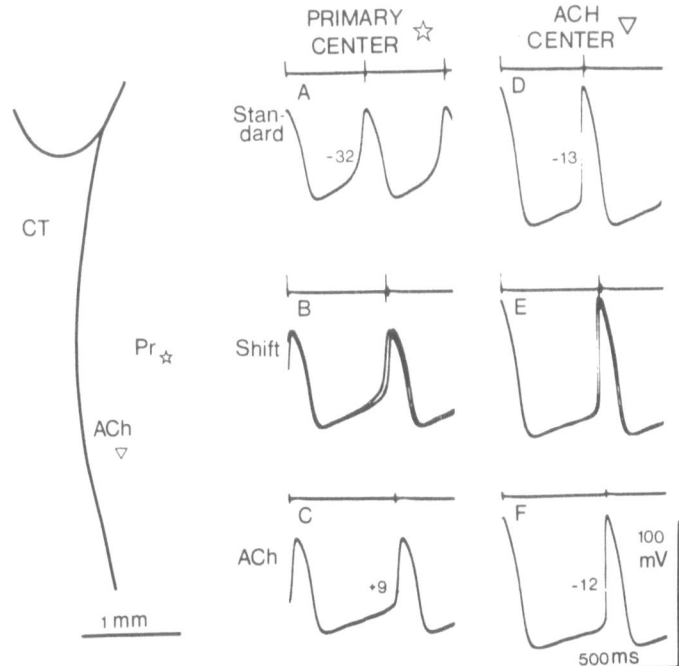

FIGURE 3 An Ach-induced pacemaker shift. CT = crista terminalis; Pr ☆ = primary dominant center under standard conditions; Ach (▽) = Ach-induced center. Continuous impalements. A: primary center, standard conditions. Cycle length 389 ms, amplitude 62 mV, upstroke velocity 1.4 V/s, discharge 32 ms before atrial reference; B: primary center, Ach concentration between 0 and 11 x 10^{-6} M. Cycle length 468 and 476 ms. Superimposed action potentials were taken 10 s after each other. Note the changed atrial electrogram; C: primary center, 11 x 10^{-6} M Ach. Cycle length 503 ms, amplitude 63 mV, upstroke velocity 2.2 V/s, discharge 9 ms after atrial reference; D: Ach-center, standard conditions.   Cycle length 394 ms, amplitude 92 mV, upstroke velocity 11.3 V/s, discharge 13 ms before atrial reference; E: Ach-center, Ach concentration between 0 and 11 x 10^{-6} M. Cycle lengths 497 and 502 ms. Superimposed action potentials were taken immediately after each other. Note the changed atrial electrogram; F: Ach-center, 11 x 10^{-6} M Ach. Cycle length 515 ms, amplitude 90 mV, upstroke velocity 7.8 V/s, discharge 12 ms before atrial reference.

In conclusion, Ach induced a shift of dominance away from the impaled site. The normal action potential of the primary center can be described as a slow response, with a small amplitude and without an overshoot. Under Ach the diastolic depolarization rate becomes smaller. The observed shift of pacemaker dominance

can explain the increased upstroke velocity. Fig. 3B shows two action potentials, superimposed when the shifting of the pacemaker just had started.

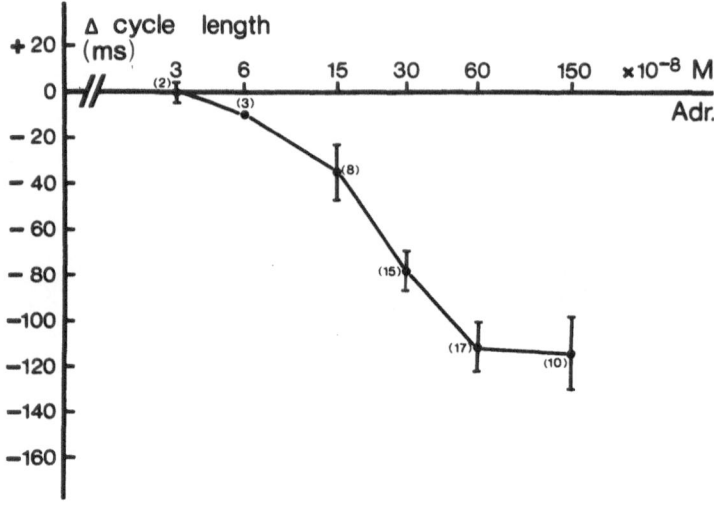

FIGURE 4 *The chronotropic response of the sinus node preparation to Adr. The
basic cycle length under standard conditions was taken as a reference (0 ms).
The number of observations is between parentheses.*

Next we mapped the site of the Ach-induced pacemaker. It was located 1 mm lower
in the node, nearer to the crista terminalis (fig. 3). Comparison of the
electrical activity recorded here (fig. 3D) under standard conditions with that
from the primary pacemaker (fig. 3A) shows a considerably higher upstroke velocity (11.3 instead of 1.4 V/s) and also a considerably larger action potential
amplitude (92 instead of 62 mV) in the subsidiary pacemaker.
Both the action potential parameters and the location in the node suggest that
it concerns a focus of transitional cells (Bleeker et al., 1980). In this
center addition of Ach gave a slightly reduced rate of diastolic depolarization
and a decreased action potential upstroke velocity (from 11.3 to 7.8 V/s, fig.
3F), but for both changes the altered activation pattern and the disappearance
of the influence of overdrive suppression, due to the action of Ach has to be
taken into account (fig. 3E). The action potential amplitude was not signifi-

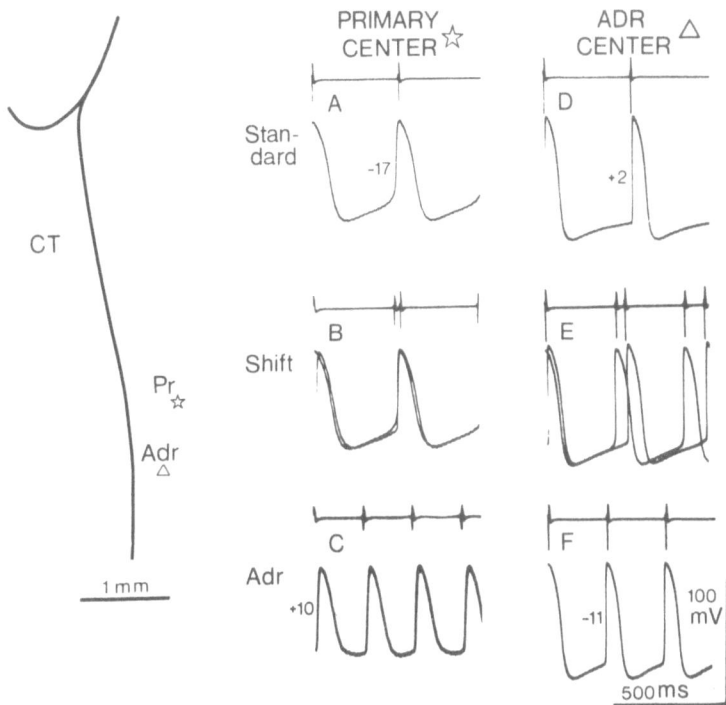

FIGURE 5 *An Adr-induced pacemaker shift. CT = crista terminalis; Pr ☆ = primary dominant center under standard conditions; Adr (△) = Adr-induced center. Continuous impalements. A: primary center, standard conditions. Cycle length 380 ms, amplitude 84 mV, upstroke velocity 5.5 V/s, discharge 17 ms before atrial reference; B: primary center, Adr concentration between 0 and 150 x 10⁻⁸ M. Cycle length 391 and 365 ms. Superimposed action potentials were taken 2 s after each other. Note the changed atrial electrogram; C: primary center, 150 x10⁻⁸ M Adr. Cycle length 216 ms, amplitude 74 mV, upstroke velocity 4.9 V/s, discharge 10 ms after atrial reference; D: Adr-center, standard conditions. Cycle length 379 ms, amplitude 104 mV, upstroke velocity 18.3 V/s, discharge 2 ms after atrial reference; E: Adr-center, Adr concentration between 0 and 60 x10⁻⁸ M. Cycle lengths 349 and 310 ms. Superimposed action potentials were taken 19.6 s after each other. Note the changed atrial electrogram; F: Adr-center, 60 x10⁻⁸ M Adr. Cycle length 257 ms, amplitude 97 mV, upstroke velocity 14.0 V/s, discharge 11 ms before atrial reference. The different atrial electrograms in C and F (150 and 60 x10⁻⁸ M Adr) suggest that the distance of the shift might be influenced by the Adr concentration.*

cantly altered in neither of the two pacemakers (n = 10, primary pacemaker; n = 15, Ach-induced pacemaker). All changes were reversible by returning to standard conditions.

THE EFFECT OF ADRENALINE IN THE TOTAL SINUS NODE

Addition of Adrenaline causes a dose-dependent acceleration of the preparation (fig. 4). Fig. 5 shows that also in this response more than one pacemaker is involved. Under standard conditions the impaled cell again meets the criteria of a dominant pacemaker (fig. 5A, compare with fig. 3A). It discharges 17 ms earlier than the atrial time reference. Under Adr (150×10^{-8} M) the primary pacemaker - located already relatively low in this node, which goes always hand in hand with a larger action potential amplitude, a higher upstroke velocity and a relatively small lead in time to the atrial time reference - lost its dominance. It now discharged 10 ms after the atrial time reference (fig. 5C). There is a marked decrease in diastolic depolarization rate. Next we mapped the site of the Adr-induced pacemaker. It was located 1 mm lower than the primary one. It preceded the atrial time reference by 11 ms (fig. 5F), while it had been following the atrial time reference by 2 ms under standard conditions (fig. 5D). This cell had a large action potential amplitude and also a high upstroke velocity. From these data it seems that we are dealing with a cell from the transitional zone. However, we have established by light microscopy that the Adr-center is located within the tail of the compact zone (unpublished data). As stated above, the changes in diastolic depolarization rate and upstroke velocity are influenced by the pacemaker shift. On average, Adr induced a small, but significant decrease in action potential amplitude in the primary center (n = 13) and no significant change in the subsidiary pacemaker (n = 10). All changes were reversible by returning to standard conditions.

THE COMBINED EFFECT OF ADRENALINE AND ACETYLCHOLINE
IN THE TOTAL SINUS NODE

We studied the effect of simultaneous addition of Ach and Adr, both on rate and on the activation pattern (Mackaay et al., 1980b). In 14 experiments (Table I) we first added Ach (concentration range $5.5 - 13.8 \times 10^{-6}$ M) to the bathing fluid. Cycle length increased from 394 to 462 ms (a and b in Table I). Then we added 60×10^{-8} M Adr, which gave rise to a decrease in cycle length of only 22

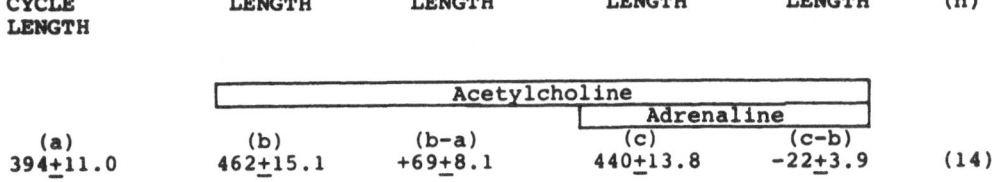

BASIC CYCLE LENGTH	CYCLE LENGTH	Δ CYCLE LENGTH	CYCLE LENGTH	Δ CYCLE LENGTH	(n)
	Acetylcholine				
			Adrenaline		
(a)	(b)	(b-a)	(c)	(c-b)	
394±11.0	462±15.1	+69±8.1	440±13.8	-22±3.9	(14)

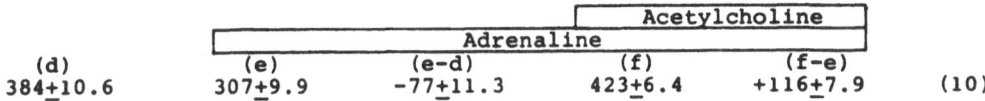

			Acetylcholine		
	Adrenaline				
(d)	(e)	(e-d)	(f)	(f-e)	
384±10.6	307±9.9	-77±11.3	423±6.4	+116±7.9	(10)

TABLE I   Chronotropic responses to Ach and to Adr and to both Ach and Adr of the total sinus node preparation. a: standard conditions; b: 5.5-13.8 x 10⁻⁶ M Ach; c: 5.5-13.8 x 10⁻⁸ M Ach + 60 x 10⁻⁸ M Adr; d: standard conditions; e: 30-60 x 10⁻⁸ M Adr; f: 30-60 x 10⁻⁸ M Adr + 5.5 x 10⁻⁶ M Ach.

ms (i.e. from 462 to 440 ms). This figure can be compared with data from fig. 4, where 60×10^{-8} M Adr alone gave a decrease in cycle length of 112 ± 10.4 ms. We conclude therefore that the Adr response is reduced in the presence of Ach.

In 10 experiments (Table I) we first added Adr (concentration range $30-60 \times 10^{-8}$ M) to the bathing fluid. Cycle length decreased from 384 ms to 307 ms (d and e in Table I). Then we added 5.5×10^{-6} M Ach, which prolonged the cycle length by 116 ms. This figure may be compared with data from fig. 2, where 5.5×10^{-6} M Ach alone gave an increase in cycle length of 59 ± 5.2 ms. So the Ach response is enhanced in the presence of Adr.

Fig. 6 shows the effects of the addition of Adr, of Ach and of Adr and Ach together on the electrical activity recorded from the primary pacemaker (fig. 6A-C) and from the Ach-induced pacemaker (fig. 6D-G). Fig. 6A shows that the primary pacemaker precedes the atrial time reference by 54 ms. The addition of Ach brings the pacemaker to a more inferior location (fig. 6, compare with fig. 3). The action potentials from these both centers, the primary one and the Ach-induced one however, follow the atrial time reference by a large arrear when only Adr is present (fig. 6C and 6F). We have no good impalements from the

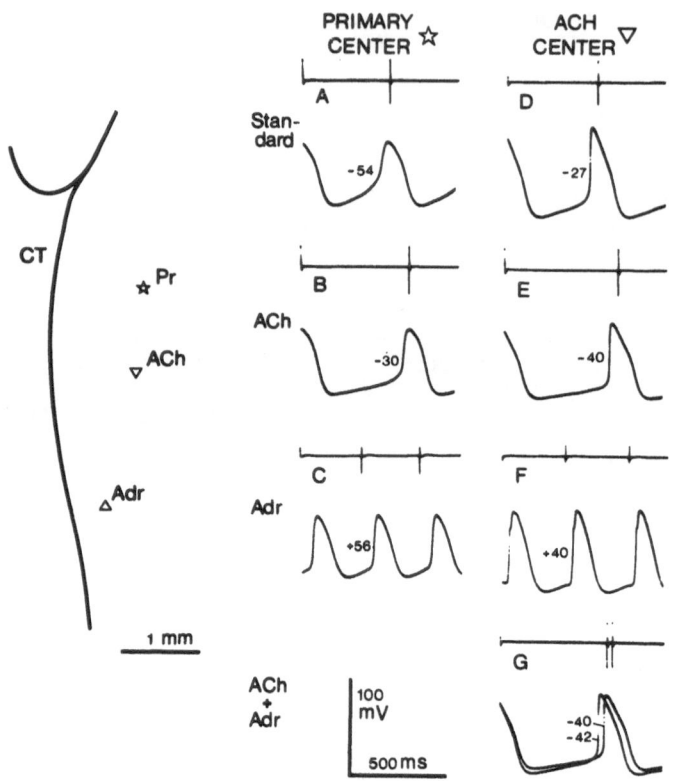

FIGURE 6 *Shifts induced by Ach, Adr and the combined presence of Ach and Adr. CT = crista terminalis; Pr* ⭐ *= primary dominant center under standard conditions; Ach (∇) = Ach-induced center; Adr (△) =Adr-induced center. Continuous impalements. A: primary center, standard conditions. Cycle length 438 ms, amplitude 65 mV, upstroke velocity 1.4 V/s, discharge 54 ms before the atrial reference; B: primary center, 11 x 10[-6] M Ach. Cycle length 545 ms, amplitude 67 mV, upstroke velocity 2.3 V/s, discharge 30 ms before atrial reference; C: primary center, 60 x 10[-8] M Adr. Cycle length 302 ms, amplitude 62 mV, upstroke velocity 3.2 V/s, discharge 56 ms after the atrial reference; D: Ach-center, standard conditions. Cycle length 440 ms, amplitude 92 mV, upstroke velocity 10.4 V/s, discharge 27 ms before atrial reference; E: Ach-center, 11 x 10[-6] M Ach. Cycle length 552 ms, amplitude 76 mV, upstroke velocity 10.4 V/s, discharge 40 ms before the atrial reference; F: Ach-center, 60 x 10[-8] M Adr. Cycle length 292 ms, amplitude 81 mV, upstroke velocity 6.3 V/s, discharge 40 ms after the atrial reference; G: Ach center, 60 x 10[-8] M Adr + 11 x 10[-6] M Ach. Cycle length 526 ms, amplitude 81 mV, upstroke velocity 10.1 V/s, discharge 42 ms before atrial reference.*

Adr-center, which was located still more inferiorly. It is important to stress
that the Ach-center which followed the atrial time reference under Adr by 40 ms
(fig. 6F), maintains its dominance under Ach (fig. 6E), when both Ach and Adr
are present (fig. 6G). In fig. 6G we superimposed the action potentials from
the Ach-center under Ach alone (same action potential as in fig. 6E) and under
the combined presence of Ach and Adr. Summarized, under the simultaneous addition of Adr+Ach the Ach-induced pacemaker dominates. The small chronotropic
response to Adr in the presence of Ach thus reflects the small response of the
Ach-center. So the Ach-center is neither very responsive to Ach nor to Adr. In
this pacemaker Ach gave a decrease in action potential amplitude, partly reversed by the simultaneous addition of Adr.

THE EFFECTS OF Ach AND Adr ON ISOLATED PACEMAKERS

In the foregoing sections we described pacemaker shifts during the addition of
Ach and Adr. Ach brings pacemaker dominance toward cells which are less responsive to its deceleratory action than the primary pacemaker, while under Adr the
most accelerated cells will take the lead. According to West (1955) pacemaker
shifts complicate the analysis of drug effects. The chronotropic response of
the total sinus node reflects the response of a pacemaker only if and as long as
this pacemaker dominates. We cannot measure the responses of the individual pacemakers involved as long as they are coupled to each other. In a previous
study (Mackaay et al., 1980b) we separated the primary pacemaker in the superior part of the node from the caudally located subsidiary ones. But those isolated inferior parts appeared to be still inhomogeneous, the reaction of the
Ach-induced pacemaker still predominated. So we were still not able to measure
the Ach response of the Adr-center. We tried to overcome this incomplete isolation by separating the compact center from the transitional zone of the node and
within the compact center the superior part from the inferior part (see Methods). The results are presented with reservation as the number of observations
is limited (see Methods). From three preparations the results are summarized in
fig. 7. The results indicate that the Ach-pacemaker is only little responsive
to Ach as well as to Adr and that the Adr-pacemaker is very sensitive to both
Adr and Ach. The large response to Ach of the primary center and the very large
response to Ach of the Adr-induced center can only be observed when these
centers have been isolated. Otherwise these responses are obscured by the fact

that under Ach the Ach-center takes the lead, even when also Adr is present. It can be concluded that the compact part of the sinus node is more responsive to the chronotropic action of Adr and Ach than the transitional nodal fibers. Within the compact node the caudal portion has the largest responsiveness.

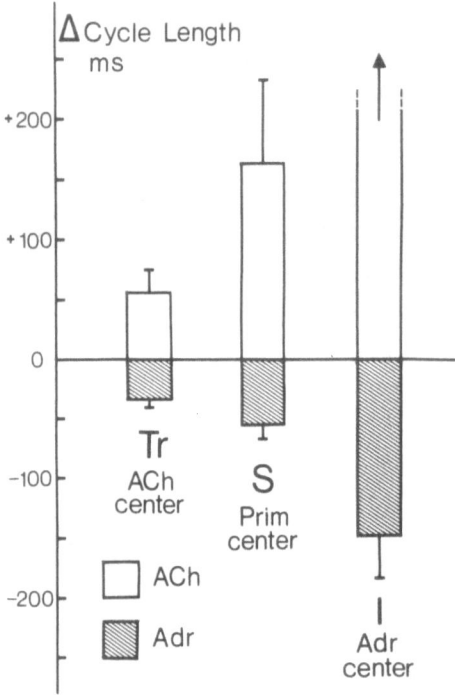

FIGURE 7 *The chronotropic responses of the three described centers (see Methods) to Ach and Adr. The number of observations was three. The arrow above the Ach-response of the Adr-center means that 1 out of 3 preparations became quiescent. The end of the solid lines depicts the averaged value of the other two preparations.*

DISCUSSION

This study concerns sinus node function, illustrated by its responses to adrenaline and acetylcholine. We documented three centers with respect to Adr and Ach (fig. 7).

-an Ach-induced center, little responsive to both drugs.

-an Adr-induced center, very responsive to both drugs.

-a primary center with intermediate responsiveness.

This demonstrates that the sinus node cannot be considered as one homogeneous generator of the cardiac impulse. Within the node several pacemakers are capa-

ble of originating the impulse and are actually doing so during several interventions.   Lu (1970) demonstrated a gradual pacemaker shift due to elevation of
the external potassium concentration toward the inferior part of the sinus node.
We have described similar shifts after lowering the temperature and reduction of
the 'extracellular calcium concentration (Mackaay et al., 1980a).   This study
documents a pacemaker shift toward the tail of the node under Adr. So within
the compact center pacemakers in the superior part differ from those in the inferior part. In addition, the compact center differs from the transitional zone
along the crista terminalis. Steinbeck et al. (1980) described dominance of
cells in the transitional zone during the addition of toxic doses of ouabain,
the same cells dominate after reduction of the sodium concentration to 50 % (unpublished data). We presume that the Ach-induced center is located within this
zone. So the Ach-induced pacemaker probably consists of transitional cells.
All taken together there is overwhelming evidence that sinus node function concerns the activity of several pacemakers which differ functionally.   And this
functional inhomogeneity should be taken into account in a review of sinus node
studies (see Brooks and Lu, 1972). Within the sinus node there are differences
in basic rhythmicity (Lu, 1970; Mackaay et al., 1980b). The actual relations
between the pacemakers may vary from preparation to preparation, reflected in
the site of pacemaker dominance and in the basic cycle length of the node (Opt
Hof et al., 1981a, submitted; Bouman et al., 1981, this volume). In our
preparations we found a conspicious variation in the site of the dominant pacee-
maker (Bleeker et al., 1980; Mackaay et al., 1980a,b). Most of the preparations were driven by a pacemaker within the superior part of the compact node
("the true pacemaker", characterized by a low maximal diastolic potential, 55-60
mV, low upstroke velocity, 1-3 V/s, no action potential overshoot, see West,
1955; Paes de Carvalho et al., 1959; Sano and Yamagishi, 1965; Bouman
et al., 1968).   Sometimes the dominant pacemaker was located in the inferior
part (see for instance fig. 5) or in the transitional zone and those pacemakers
differed in their action potential parameters and in their responses to interventions. In this chapter we showed that Ach can fix the pacemaker in the transitional zone, thus reducing the Adr response of the sinus node. Interventions
which selectively accelerate the "true pacemaker" or depress the
other,subsidiary pacemakers, will fix pacemaker dominance in the superior part
of the compact node and they will increase the arrear in basic cycle length of

the other, subsidiary pacemakers. So interventions that influence the differences in intrinsic cycle length between primary and subsidiary pacemakers are
expected to influence the responsiveness of the total sinus node to Ach and Adr.
As such an intervention we propose the elevation of the Mg-concentration (Opt
Hof et al., 1981b). Although high Mg (6.0 mM) decelerates the primary dominant pacemaker, it stabilizes its leading position. This is explained by the
fact that the other, subsidiary pacemakers decelerate still more. Thus high Mg
enlarges the lead of the primary dominant pacemaker to the subsidiary ones.
Elevation of the Mg-concentration is thus expected to reduce the acceleration
under isoproterenol (see Hashimoto et al., 1974) or enhance the deceleration
under Ach (see Somjen and Baskerville, 1968) by preventing a pacemaker shift.
The total preparation will then respond conform part S in our fig. 7. At low
temperature, the responses to Adr and Ach are more pronounced than at 38 $^{\circ}$C
(Ach: Toda et al., 1976; Vincenzi and West, 1965; Adr: Toda and Shimamoto,
1968) because of the lower position of the dominant pacemaker (Mackaay et al.,
1980a). We presume that at low temperature cells are leading with a larger responsiveness to both Adr and Ach. This large responsiveness to Ach might be un-
covered because of the large arrear in intrinsic cycle length of the Ach-induced
center at low temperature.

The functional inhomogeneity of the sinus node is also pertinent to the results obtained in small sinus node preparations. The description of the isolation procedure (Noma and Irisawa, 1976; Irisawa, 1978) suggests that the preparations are derived from the lateral border of the node. This fits with the
characteristics of the recorded action potentials (amplitude 93 mV, overshoot 25
mV, $\dot{V}_{max}$ 16 V/s, inferred from recordings of Brown et al., 1979), which differ
considerably from the "true pacemaker" activity (West, 1955) and more resemble
transitional cell activity (Strauss and Bigger, 1972; Bleeker et al., 1980).
In fact the magnitude of the chronotropic response to 5×10^{-7} g/ml (Brown et
al., 1979, fig. 15) nicely fits with our results in transitional cells.
Because differences in membrane potential level and the related electrical activity are also observed in the small preparations (membrane resting potential
level ranging from -34 to -45 mV and related action potential amplitudes from 61
to 73 mV, Noma and Irisawa, 1975), we suggest that the functional inhomogeneity
of the total sinus node is related to differences in local membrane currents
responsible for spontaneous activity rather than based on the hyperpolarizing

influence of the adjacent atrium.

ACKNOWLEDGEMENTS

The authors wish to thank mr. Arnold Meijer and mr. Wim Schreurs for valuable technical advice. Ir. Anton van Gent is thanked for writing computer programs.

REFERENCES

Bleeker, W.K., Mackaay, A.J.C., Masson-Pevet, M., Bouman, L.N. and Becker, A.E.: Functional and morphological organization of the rabbit sinus node. Circ. Res., 46: 11-22, 1980.

Bonke, F.I.M.: Electrotonic spread in the sinoatrial node of the rabbit heart. Pfluegers Arch., 339: 17-23, 1973.

Bonke, F.I.M.: A general introduction about the current status of the electrophysiology of the sinus node. In: The Sinus Node. Structure, Function and Clinical Relevance, Bonke, F.I.M., ed., Martinus Nijhoff, The Hague, pp. 225-232, 1978.

Bouman, L.N., Gerlings, E.D., Biersteker, P.A. and Bonke, F.I.M.: Pacemaker shift in the sinoatrial node during vagal stimulation. Pfluegers Arch., 302: 255-267, 1968.

Bouman, L.N., Op 't Hof, T., Mackaay, A.J.C., Bleeker, W.K. and Jongsma, H.J.: On the intrinsic cardiac rhythm, this volume, 1981.

Brooks, C.McC and Lu, H.H.: The sinoatrial pacemaker of the heart. Charles C. Thomas, Springfield, Illinois, 1972.

Brown, H.F., DiFrancesco, D. and Noble, S.J.: Cardiac pacemaker oscillation and its modulation by autonomic transmitters. J. Exp. Biol., 81: 175-204, 1979.

Bukauskas, F.F., Gutman, A.M., Kisunas, K.J. and Veteikis, R.P.: Electrical

cell coupling in rabbit sinoatrial node and atrium: experimental and theoretical evaluation, this volume, 1981.

Hashimoto, K., Suzuki, Y. and Chiba, S.: Influence of calcium and magnesium
ions on the sinoatrial pacemaker of the canine heart. Tohuku J. Exp.
Med., 113: 187-196, 1974.

Irisawa, H.: Ionic currents underlying spontaneous rhythm of the cardiac primary pacemaker cells. In: The Sinus Node. Structure, Function and Clinical
Relevance, Bonke, F.I.M., ed., Martinus Nijhoff, The Hague, pp. 368-375,
1978.

Lu, H.H.: Shifts in pacemaker dominance within the sinoatrial region of cat and
rabbit hearts resulting from increase of extracellular potassium. Circ.
Res., 26: 339-345, 1970.

Mackaay, A.J.C., Bleeker, W.K., Op 't Hof, T. and Bouman, L.N.: Temperature
dependence of the chronotropic action of Ca. J. Mol. Cell. Cardiol.,
12: 433-443, 1980a.

Mackaay, A.J.C., Op 't Hof, T., Bleeker, W.K., Jongsma, H.J. and Bouman, L.N.:
Interaction of adrenaline and acetylcholine on cardiac pacemaker function.
J. Pharmacol. Exp. Ther., 214: 417-422, 1980b.

Masson-Pevet, M., Bleeker, W.K. and Gros, D.: The plasma membrane of leading
pacemaker cells in the rabbit sinus node. Circ. Res., 45: 621-629, 1979.

Noma, A. and Irisawa, H.: Effects of Na^+ and K^+ on the resting membrane potential of the rabbit sinoatrial node cell. Jap. J. Physiol., 25: 287-302,
1975.

Noma, A. and Irisawa, H.: Membrane currents in the rabbit sinoatrial node cell
as studies by the double microelectrode method. Pfluegers Arch., 364:
45-52, 1976.

Noma, A. and Trautwein, W.: Relaxation of the Ach-induced potassium current in
the rabbit sinoatrial node cell. Pfluegers Arch., 377: 193-200, 1978.

Op 't Hof, T., Mackaay, A.J.C., Bleeker, W.K., Jongsma, H.J. and Bouman, L.N.:
Dependence of the chronotropic effects of adrenaline and acetylcholine and
of the site of the dominant pacemaker on cycle length in the rabbit sinus
node. J. Pharmacol. Exp. Ther., submitted, 1981a.

Op 't Hof, T., Mackaay, A.J.C., Bleeker, W.K., Jongsma, H.J. and Bouman, L.N.:
Magnesium and sinus node function. Magnesium Bulletin, accepted, 1981b.

Paes de Carvalho, A., DeMello, W.C. and Hoffman, B.F.: Electrophysiological

evidence   for   specialized   fiber   types   in   rabbit   atrium.   Amer.   J.
Physiol., 196: 483-488, 1959.

Sano, T. and Yamagishi, S.: Spread of excitation from the sinus   node.   Circ.
Res., 16: 423-430, 1965.

Somjen, G.G. and Baskerville, E.N.: Effect of excess magnesium on vagal   inhibition and acetylcholine sensitivity of the mammalian heart in situ and
in vitro. Nature, 217: 679-680, 1968.

Spear, J.F., Kronhaus, K.D., Moore, E.N. and Kline, R.P.: The effect of   brief
vagal   stimulation   on   the   isolated   rabbit sinus node. Circ. Res., 44:
75-88, 1979.

Steinbeck, G., Bonke, F.I.M., Allessie, M.A. and Lammers, W.J.E.P.: The effect
of ouabain on the isolated sinus node preparation of the rabbit studied
with microelectrodes. Circ. Res., 46: 404-414, 1980.

Strauss, H. and Bigger, J.T.: Electrophysiological properties of the rabbit
sinoatrial perinodal fibers. Circ. Res., 31: 490-505, 1972.

Toda, N. and West, T.C.: Changes in sinoatrial node transmembrane potentials
on vagal stimulation of the isolated rabbit atrium. Nature, 205: 808-809,
1965

Toda, N., Fu, W.L.H. and Osumi, Y.: Age-dependence of the chronotropic response to noradrenaline, acetylcholine and transmural stimulation in isolated rabbit atria. Jap. J. Pharmacol., 26: 359-366, 1976.

Toda, N. and Shimamoto, K.: The influence of sympathetic stimulation on
transmembrane potentials in the s-a node. J. Pharmacol. Exp. Ther.,
159: 298-305, 1968.

Vincenzi, F.F. and West, T.C.: Modification by calcium of the release of autonomic mediators in the isolated sinoatrial node. J. Pharmacol. Exp.
Ther., 150: 349-360, 1965.

West, T.C: Ultramicroelectrode recording from the cardiac pacemaker.   J.
Pharmacol. Exp. Ther., 115: 283-290, 1955.

West, T.C., Falk, G. and Cervoni, P.: Drug alteration of transmembrane potentials in atrial pacemaker cells. J. Pharmacol. Exp. Ther., 117:
245-252, 1956.

CONDUCTION IN THE SINUS NODE AND

ITS MODIFICATION BY AUTONOMIC DRUGS

Felix I.M. Bonke, Maurits A. Allessie, Victor A.J. Slenter
and Roland Kengen

INTRODUCTION

Studying the electrophysiology of the sinus node of the rabbit, it is important
to realize that the node is not a homogeneous structure (Bleeker et al.,
1980); the consequence is that it is necessary to define carefully which part
of the node is under study and under which conditions. One of the possible experimental procedures is to make an activation map of the whole sinus node area,
as is shown in the contribution of Masson-Pevet et al. in this book.
Figure 1 gives an example of such an activation map. In the left diagram the
spread of an impulse through the sinus node is indicated. With one microelectrode more than 50 impalements were made subsequently and all recordings were
made together with a record of a surface electrogram of the crista terminalis.
Then all recordings were time aligned taking the earliest moment of spontaneous
discharge as zero reference (for a more detailed description, see Steinbeck
et al., 1978). This map shows that the impulse arising in the dominant pacemaker fibers does not take the shortest route toward the atrium. Conduction
from the pacemaker center directly toward the atrium is very slow or perhaps
even blocked; there seems to be a preferential conduction from the pacemaker
center toward the cranial end of the crista terminalis. In this case the crista
terminalis was reached 24 ms after the spontaneous discharge of the dominant pacemaker. This figure also demonstrates that the propagation toward the caval
area is very slow and might even be blocked (see Masson-Pevet et al., this volume). The right map of figure 1 shows the propagation of an ectopic impulse
from the atrium into the sinus node following a premature atrial beat (given

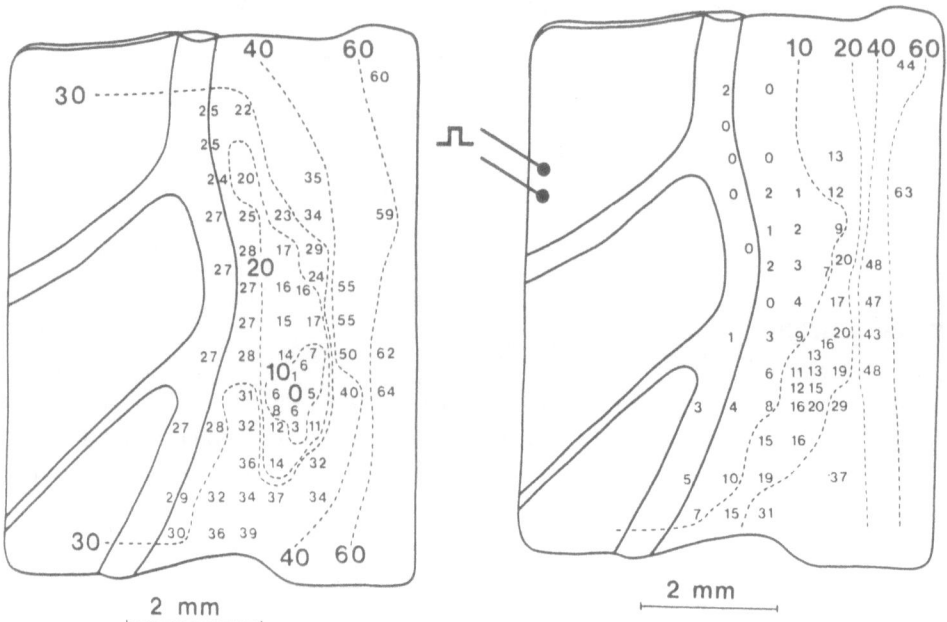

FIGURE 1 *Maps of antegrade and retrograde sinoatrial conduction as constructed from time measurements of more than 50 impalements of sinus node fibers. During spontaneous rhythm (basic cycle length 440 ms) the earliest moment of spontaneous discharge is taken as zero reference (left map). Following a single premature atrial beat with a coupling interval of 370 ms, the activation of the crista terminalis is taken as zero reference (right map).*
    The activation times of the fibers are given in milliseconds and the stippled lines are isochronic lines. (From: Steinbeck et al., 1978. With permission of the American Heart Association).

about 50 ms before the next spontaneous beat was expected). The premature impulse invades from the atrium the sinus node over a broad front (activation of the crista terminalis is taken as zero reference) and a preferential pathway through the node cannot be distinguished. The conduction of the impulse toward or through the caval area is slower than in the other parts of the sinus node. In this case retrograde conduction (from crista terminalis toward dominant pacemaker area) is faster than antegrade sinoatrial conduction, 15 ms versus 24 ms.

However, such conclusions about the conduction velocity or conduction time, might be less realistic, since a certain time difference between two neighbouring points does not allow us to calculate the conduction velocity. It is possible - and perhaps even likely - that the impulse is not using the shortest way between the two points. Therefore it is better to try to force the impulse via a predetermined route through the sinus node and then perhaps the conduction properties of sinus node fibers can be studied. We made a preparation that enables us to study this by cutting the atrial part of the preparation in such a way that an impulse could travel from one atrial part toward the other only via a bridge of sinus node fibers.

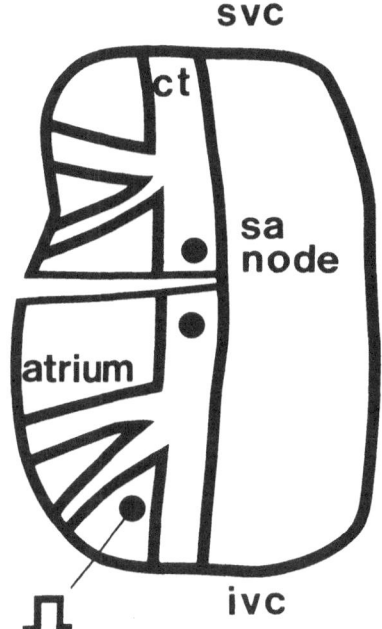

FIGURE 2 *Diagram of the preparation. The atrium is cut perpendicularly on the crista terminalis and the incision is extended through the crista terminalis (= CT). The two black dots on the crista terminalis indicate the position of the two surface electrodes. SVC = superior vena cava. IVC = inferior vena cava.*

METHODS

Young New Zealand rabbits (1.5 - 2.5 kg) were killed by a blow in the neck. The heart was removed as quickly as possible and put into cold Tyrode solution. Then a preparation including the superior vena cava and the inferior vena cava, and the right atrial appendage was made. This preparation did not contain the

AV nodal region and the interatrial septum also was cut away. The preparation was mounted in a tissue bath with the endocardial surface uppermost. The perfusion fluid contained in mM: NaCl 130, KCl 5.6, $CaCl_2$ 2.2, $MgCl_2$ 1.7, $NaHCO_3$ 24, NaH_2PO_4 1.2, glucose 11, and saccharose 13. The temperature was kept constant at 37 $^{\circ}C$ $\pm$ 0.1 $^{\circ}C$ and the pH was 7.35 $\pm$ 0.05. The fluid was oxygenated with a gas mixture of 95 % O_2 and 5 % CO_2 and entered the tissue bath at the bottom, whereas it was sucked off from the surface at a rate of 50 ml/min.

We made an incision in the atrium as indicated in Fig. 2. The preparation was paced via a stimulating electrode at one of the atrial parts of the preparation - in fig. 2 this is at the caudal part. Two surface electrodes - bipolar, chlorided teflon-coated silver wire - were placed on the crista terminalis near the incision and these electrodes were considered as the entrance to and the exit of a bridge of sinus node tissue. In the preliminary experiments which we will describe in this paper, we supposed that the impulse is conducted through the fibers at the sino-atrial border just beside the incision and that these fibers form the bridge of sinus node tissue; it is reasonable to assume that the impulse will also invade the center of the node, but conduction in this area will be much slower or might even be blocked. Therefore, the shortest route between the "entrance electrode" and the "exit electrode" is supposed to be formed by sino-atrial border (or transitional zone) fibers. In the future, this assumption has to be proven by careful microelectrode studies in which the activation pattern in the sinus node area will be mapped.

The protocol of the experiments was as follows: after the incision was made and the recording electrodes were placed at the crista terminalis, we positioned a stimulating electrode at one side of the atrium. Then the preparation was paced with stimuli having an intensity of twofold threshold and a duration of 1 ms. Not only the effect of pacing but also the effect of premature stimuli after a series of 10 basic atrial stimuli, was studied. Then a stimulating electrode was positioned at the other atrial part and the whole procedure was repeated. In almost all preparations - we have studied so far - the effects of pacing as well as of premature stimuli were the same for both positions of the stimulating electrode. For the rest of the experiment we then used one position of the stimulating electrode.

In most experiments, we lengthened the incision into the sinus node. For the first incision - thus through the crista terminalis just till the sinoatrial border - the condition can be made that the spontaneous discharge rate of the sinus node is not altered by the procedure. When the incision is lengthened into the nodal area, the spontaneous rate of the sinus node will change as soon as the dominant pacemaker in the center of the node is damaged or is influenced by changes in the tension of the preparation.

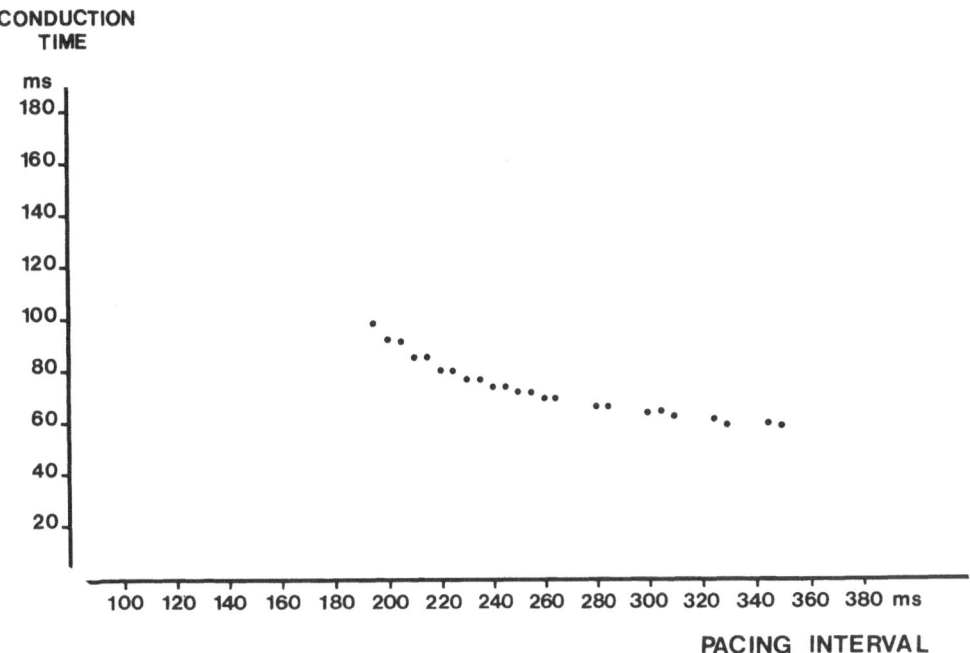

FIGURE 3 *The relation between the pacing interval and the conduction time (i.e. the time delay between the activation of the two surface electrodes on the crista terminalis).*

RESULTS

CONDUCTION THROUGH THE SINUS NODE

Figure 3 shows the effect of pacing the lower (caudal) part and it is obvious that the faster the rate the slower the conduction (the conduction time is longer). The shortest interval that was followed was 195 ms in this experiment. The conduction time was 99 ms, indicating the time the impulse needed to travel from the "entrance electrode" toward the "exit electrode". If we paced with a shorter interval (190 ms or shorter) not all impulses were followed within the sinus node and we could record a typical Wenckebach-phenomenon. The longest conduction time is 170 % of the conduction time during pacing with 3 Hz.

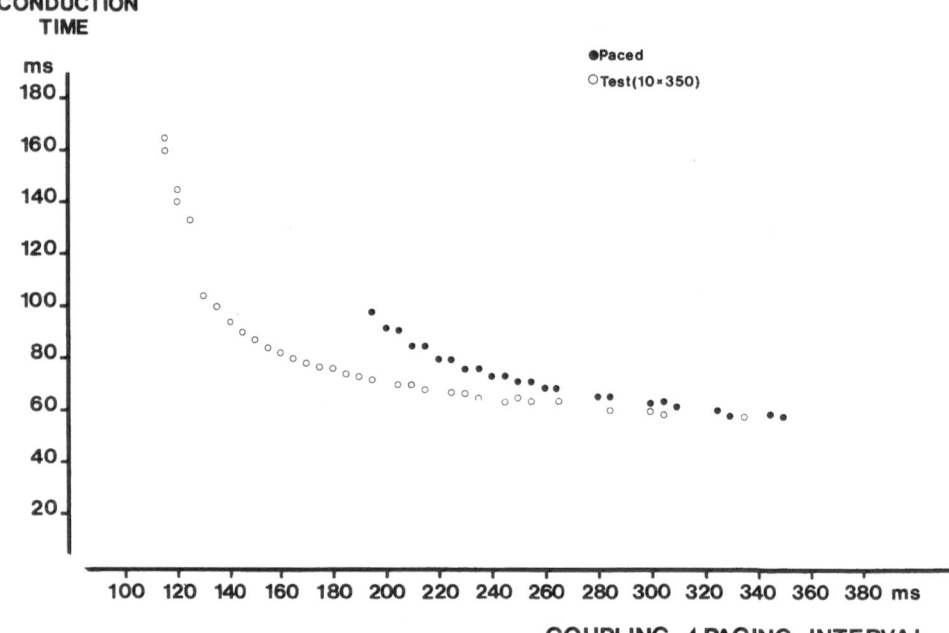

FIGURE 4 *The relation between the pacing interval and the conduction time (as figure 3) in combination with the relation between the coupling interval (i.e. the interval between the last stimulus of a series of ten and the premature stimulus) and the conduction time. Note that one single premature impulse can be conducted through the SA node with a much more pronounced prematurity and with a much longer conduction delay than impulses of a series of rapid pacing.*

Figure 4 shows the effect of pacing (as in figure 3), but also the relation between the coupling interval (i.e. the interval between the last basic beat of a series of ten and the premature beat) and the conduction time (i.e. the latency between the entrance electrode and the exit electrode).

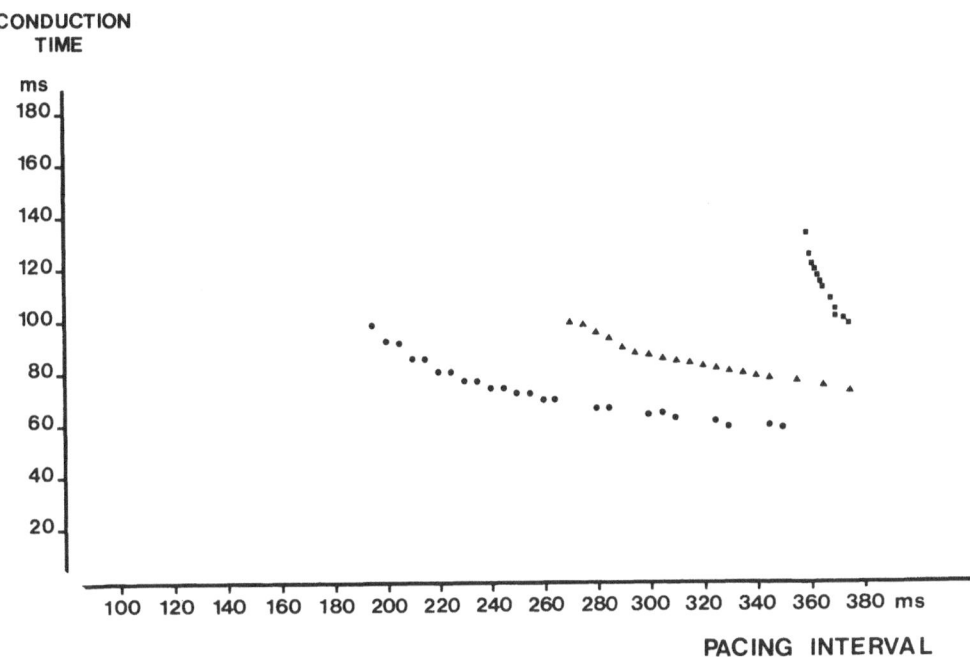

FIGURE 5 *The relation between the pacing interval and the conduction time. The dots have to do with the situation in which the incision was just through the crista terminalis (thus the same as in figure 3). The triangles refer to the situation in which the incision was extended into the sinus node about 1 mm, whereas the squares point to the situation in which the incision has extended again about 1 mm.*

One single premature impulse will be conducted with a much more outspoken prematurity than the impulses during pacing. So, in this example, a premature beat with a coupling interval of 115 ms was conducted through the sinus node. The conduction time in case of such an early premature impulse was 270 % of the time necessary for the conduction of the basic-drive impulses (we stimulated the atrium ten times with an interval of 350 ms and then gave a premature impulse).

If we lengthened the incision into the sinus node and thus forced the impulse to travel deeper in to the node, we could not pace with a shorter interval than 270 ms. Faster pacing was not accompanied with a 1:1 conduction. Further lengthening of the incision caused a further slowing of the maximal driving rate (shortest interval was 359 ms). This is showed in Figure 5. Thus, the more the impulse is forced to travel through the central nodal area, the more the conduction through the sinus node is slowed down as well as the more the conduction is depressed (i.e. the maximal rate that can be followed is decreased). This is not only the case if the preparation is paced, but also if a premature beat has to be conducted through the sinus node.

TABLE I

CONDUCTION THROUGH SINO-ATRIAL BORDER

Exp. no.	Minimal pacing interval (MPI) (ms)	Minimal coupling interval (MCI) (ms)	Conduction time at MPI (ms)	Conduction time at MCI (ms)	Conduction time at 3 Hz * (ms)
1	190	-	55	-	25
2	180	136	44	80	24
3	195	139	61	68	43
4	195	115	99	165	58
5	185	117	52	56	34
6	210	-	64	-	36
7	190	144	72	92	36
8	205	145	80	104	47
9	180	134	103	138	50
10	175	122	50	52	20
Mean	190.5	131.5	68.0	94.4	37.4

*In some experiments, the basic drive interval was 350 ms in stead of 333 ms.

In figures 3, 4 and 5, we showed results of a single experiment (no. 4 in tables I and II). In table I, the results of ten experiments are listed. In these experiments, the incision was made just through the crista terminalis allowing conduction through the sino-atrial border. We found that the minimal pacing interval - i.e. the fastest pacing rate - was about 190 ms. If the preparation was driven with a regular rate of 3Hz and premature stimuli were given after ten basic stimuli, the shortest possible coupling interval was 131.5 ms (mean of eight experiments, since in experiments no. 1 and 6, we did not test the effect of premature stimuli). The minimal coupling interval can be considered the effective refractory period of the fibers of the sinoatrial border.

Table I also gives the conduction time (= time necessary for the conduction of the impulse from the entrance electrode to the exit electrode) in the different situations, viz. during fast pacing, in case of the earliest premature stimulus and at regular drive at a rate of 3 Hz. These conduction times differed from experiment to experiment because the position of the recording electrodes varied and - of course - the damage of the preparation made by the incision was not always the same. Despite of these variations, we calculated the mean values of these conduction times and it turned out that the conduction of the impulse during fast pacing is almost twice as slow as during pacing with a rate of 3 Hz and an early premature impulse is conducted even about 2.5 times as slow as a basic impulse. In these ten experiments, the spontaneous beat-to-beat interval of the sinus node was between 350 and 400 ms and pacing with 3 Hz was therefore always possible.

TABLE II

CONDUCTION THROUGH CENTER OF SINUS NODE

Exp. no.	Minimal pacing interval (MPI) (ms)	Minimal coupling interval (MCI) (ms)	Conduction time at MPI (ms)	Conduction time at MCI (ms)	Conduction time at 3 Hz * (ms)
2	264	204	98	116	63
3	230	–	75	–	51
4	270	160	99	132	76
5	230	145	55	62	42
11	235	214	90	100	51
12	255	175	72	80	48
Mean	247.3	179.6	81.5	98.0	55.2

*In some experiments, the basic drive interval was 350 ms instead of 333 ms.

In some of the experiments listed in Table I, we lengthened the incision through the sino-atrial border and repeated the stimulation procedure. In two other experiments, the incision was made too deep into the sinus node area at the beginning of the experiment and we could not study the conduction properties of the sino-atrial border. These two experiments are included in Table II as experiments no 11 and 12. The fibers in the center of the sinus node could follow pacing with a rate of about 4 Hz (mean minimal pacing interval 247.3 ms) and the minimal coupling interval was about 180 ms. Comparison of the conduction times under different conditions reveals that in the center of the sinus node the slowing of the conduction never exceeds a factor of two.

THE EFFECT OF AUTONOMIC TRANSMITTERS

We added cholinergic drugs (acetylcholine or carbamylcholine) to the superfusing fluid in such a concentration that the spontaneous beat-to-beat interval of the sinus node increased with 100-150 ms. This caused a depression of the conduction through the sinus node. As is showed in figure 6, the shortest pacing interval is 250 ms in stead of 195 ms under control conditions. The conduction time at a pacing interval of 350 ms was longer than under control conditions, viz. 63 ms versus 58 ms.

Addition of catecholamines in a moderate concentration (we have chosen concentrations causing a shortening of the beat-to-beat interval of about 100 ms) had a positive dromotropic effect: the preparation could be paced faster than under control conditions (shortest pacing interval 170 ms instead of 195 ms) and at a pacing interval of 265 ms the conduction time is 12 ms shorter than under control conditions (see figure 6).

Therefore the conduction through the transitional zone of the sinus node is enhanced by catecholamines and depressed by cholinergic agents.

IS THERE DECREMENTAL CONDUCTION WITHIN THE SINUS NODE?

To investigate whether the impulse during fast pacing is conducted through a pathway in the transitional zone toward a site where conduction block occurs causing only some electrotonic potential changes in the fibers behind the site of block or that the conduction of the impulse was decremental causing failure of stimulation of the fibers at the end of the pathway in the sino-atrial border, we impaled with one single micro-electrode in the "sinus node bridge" subsequently at several sites and during each impalement, we applied several pacing rates. At a pacing interval of 220 ms, there is a Wenckebach conduction pat-

CONDUCTION
TIME

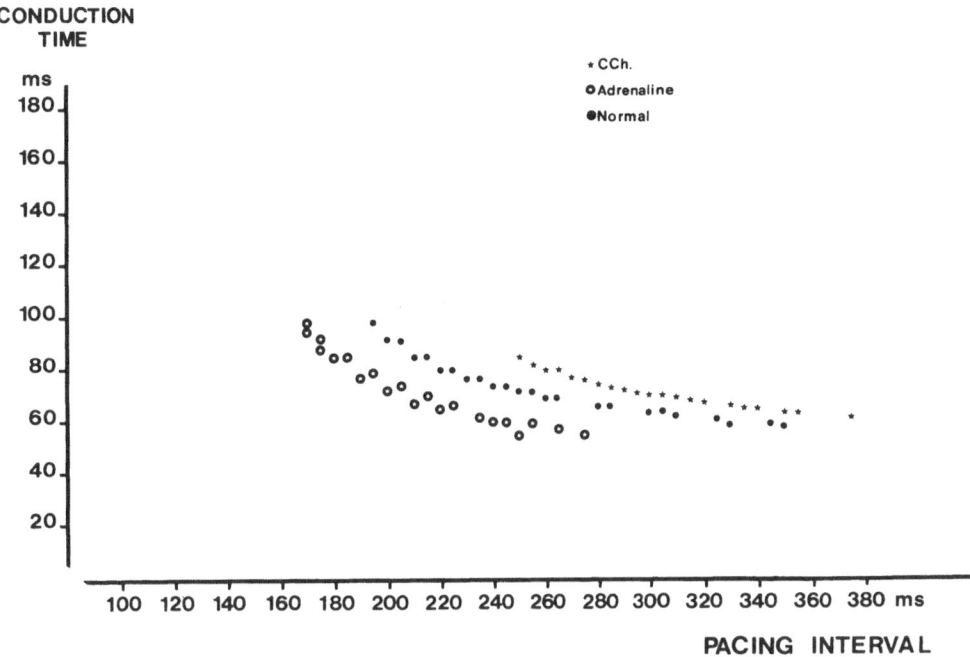

FIGURE 6 *The relation between the pacing interval and the conduction time under control conditions (the same as figure 3) and under influence of adrenaline or carbamylcholine. The conduction through the sinoatrial border (transitional zone) is enhanced by adrenaline, but depressed by carbamylcholine.*

tern. This is illustrated in figure 7.

In this figure - and the following one - the records of three different impalements are shown.   In each panel, the upper trace is the recording of the entrance electrode (the more caudal electrode on the crista terminalis), the   middle trace shows the action potential and the lower trace gives the surface electrogram of the exit electrode (more cranially positioned on the   crista termi-nalis).   In the panels at the right side, the traces are superimposed (the oscilloscope was triggered on the stimulus). In these fibers, the activation pat-

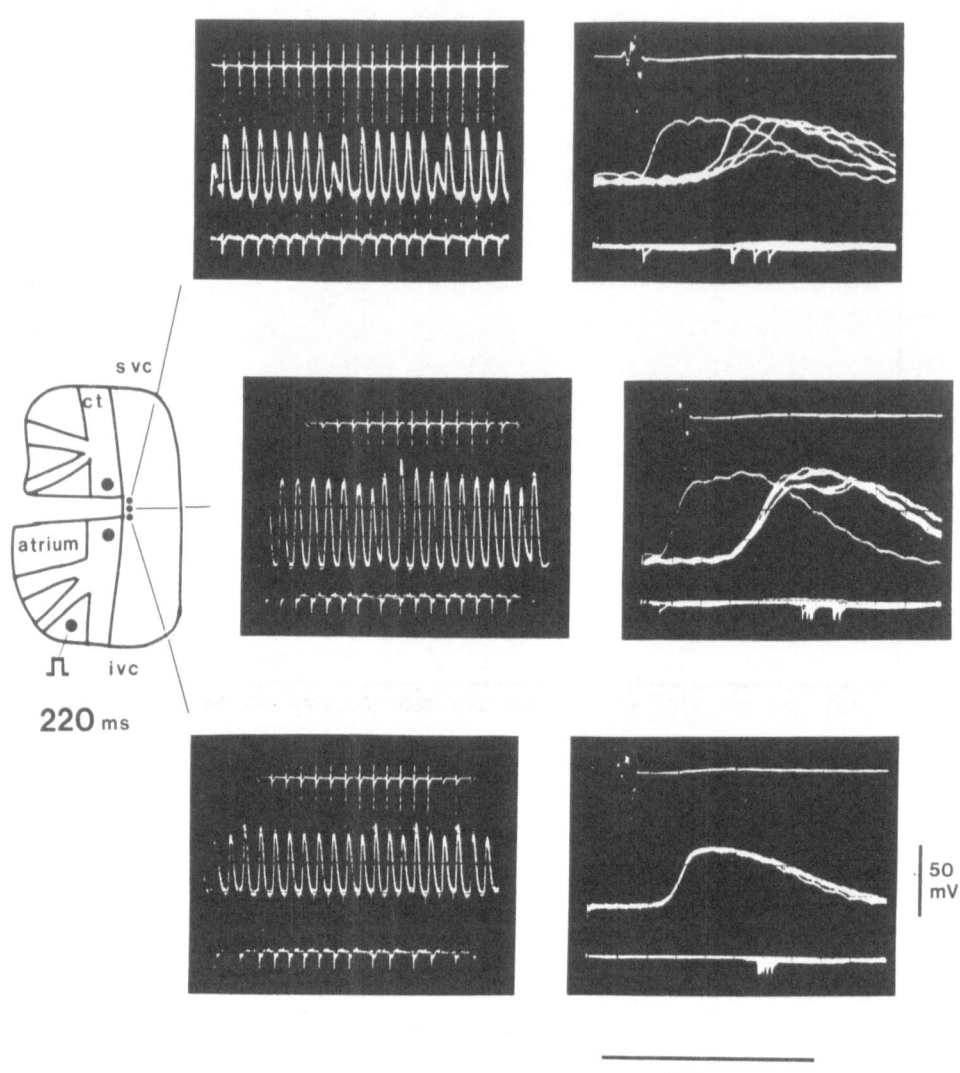

FIGURE 7 *Impulse conduction through the sinoatrial border during pacing with an interval of 220 ms. Three impalements were made subsequently. See text for further description. Note that in the lower panel at the left side the pacing interval was changed from 220 ms to 200 ms and as a consequence a 3:2 block occurred instead of the 8:7 block, present in the first half of this picture.*

tern is a bit complicated. Most stimuli are followed and the impulses are conducted through the entire bridge but one in eight (lower panel), one in nine
(middle panel) and one in six (upper panel) is not conducted. If conduction failed the pacemaker in the center of the node could come to a spontaneous discharge and the sinus node including the sino-atrial border is brought to discharge by this (normal) pacemaker. Because of the low speed of the oscilloscope
in the left-hand panels, this is difficult to perceive. However, in the middle
and upper panel at the right side, it is obvious that one action potential shows
a complete different relationship to the entrance as well as to the exit electrode as the other action potentials. In case of spontaneous discharge of the
sinus node, the exit electrode is reached earlier thhe entrance electrode
(complex on the lower trace preceeds the complex on the upper trace) and also
earlier than the impaled fiber. Since the electrogram of the entrance electrode
shows the same latency to the stimulus (nice superposition) it can be concluded
that the entrance electrode is activated via the stimulating electrode whereas
the sino-atrial border is under the control of the pacemaker in the center of
the sinus node for this single beat. The lower panel at the right does not show
this phenomenon, because only five sweeps were superimposed and it just happened
that all these impulses were conducted through the "sinus node bridge". This
phenomenon is rare and occurred only because the pacemaker in the center of the
node had a rather fast rate, viz. a beat-to-beat interval of 320 ms. If the
spontaneous rate of the pacemaker should have been lower, for instance 2.5 Hz or
less, than pacing with 4.5 - 5 Hz will easily overdrive the pacemaker completely
and no spontaneous dischrage will occur if a stimulus does not invade the sinus
node deep enough.

The upper right panel of this figure shows that the subsequent action potentials have a lower amplitude and a much slower rate or rise of the upstroke.

Figure 8 shows the effect of pacing with 5 Hz (interval 200 ms). Under
this condition, one stimulated impulse is conducted through the "sinus node
bridge", the following one is blocked and then the sinus node is discharged by
the pacemaker in the center of the node. This is nicely demonstrated in the
middle right panel where three sweeps are superimposed. The largest - and earliest - action potential is caused by the spontaneous discharge of the pacemaker. The second action potential is recorded in the case the driven impulse is
conducted through the sinus node toward the exit electrode, whereas the small

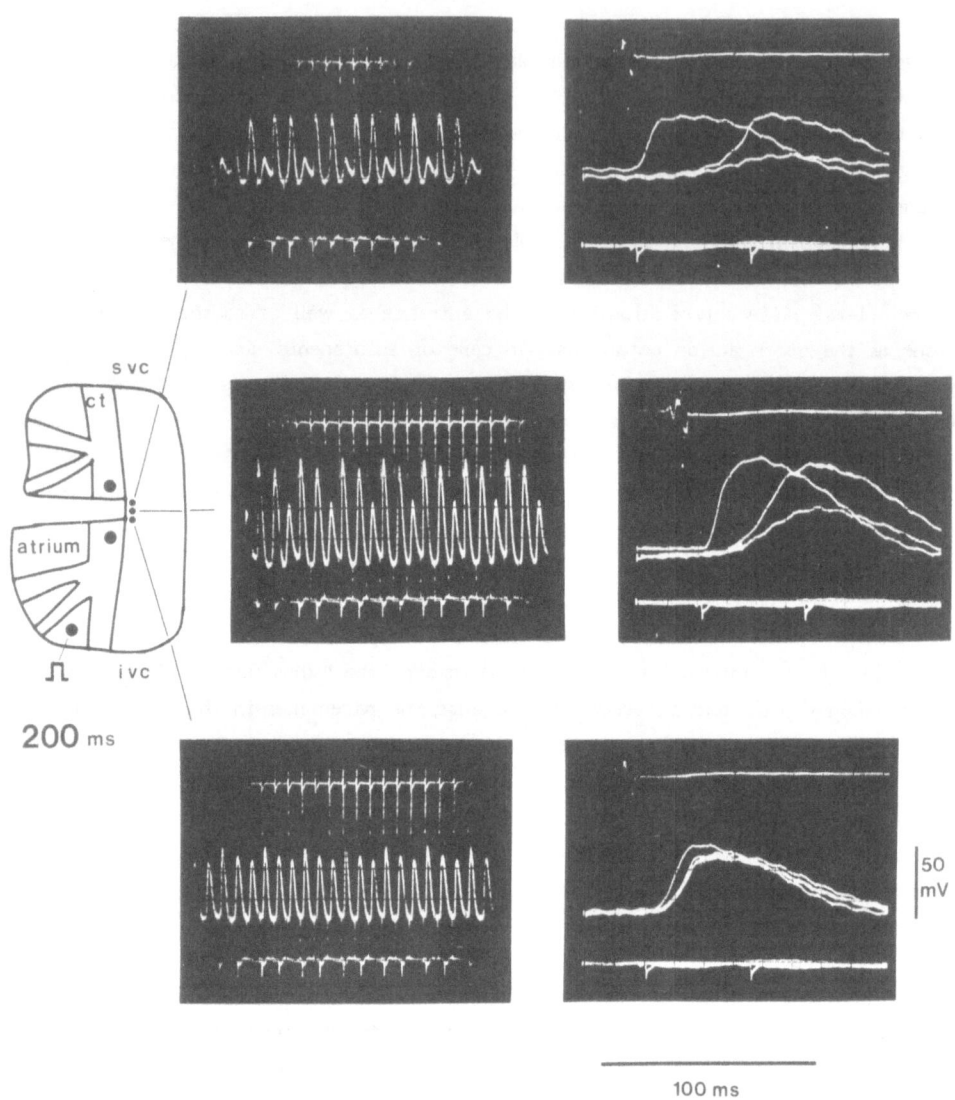

FIGURE 8 *Impulse conduction through the sinoatrial border during atrial pacing with 5 Hz (200 ms interval). Three impalements were made subsequently. See text for further description.*

action potential is recorded during the conduction block. The lower right panel shows one action potential being larger than the other two and this one is caused by the spontaneous pacemaker discharge; the other two are equal and it can be concluded that at this site of the "sinus node bridge" there is no conduction block. The middle panel shows that the impulse that failed to be conducted is accompanied by a small action potential (amplitude less than 50 mV) and this is more outspoken in the upper panel. If we consider the small action potential in the upper panel as an electrotonic hump - although we do not have good criteria for this - we might conclude that the conduction of the impulse is blocked somewhere between the cranial and the middle sites of impalement (the distances between the sites of impalement were 0.5 mm). Although more careful study with microelectrodes is desired these two figures (7 and 8) strongly suggest that during fast pacing some impulses are conducted through the sino-atrial border with decrement and as a consequence, cannot be conducted through the whole "sinus node bridge".

DISCUSSION

With this preparation it is possible to study the conduction properties of the sinus node. Although further evaluation of this method has to be done, some conclusions can be drawn from this - preliminary - study:

   * The sinus node of the rabbit is not able to follow a pacing rate of more than 5 - 6 Hz (for the fibers in the center of the node 4 Hz is the maximum); one premature impulse however, can be conducted with a more pronounced prematurity than a series of impulses.

If the maximal pacing rate for the sino-atrial border is about 6 Hz, it can be concluded that these sinus node fibers never can be part of a circular pathway in which an impulse travels causing a supraventricular tachycardia with a rate of more than 6 Hz. For the fibers in the center of the node, it can be stated that they cannot play a role in circus-movement tachycardia with frequencies above 4 Hz. Thus, supraventricular circus-movement tachycardias with a fast rate have to be purely atrial tachycardias. We (Allessie et al., 1973) demon-

strated   that   in the left atrium of the rabbit - and also in the right although
we did not publish data about that - tachycardias with a rate between 6   and   10
Hz (or even higher under special conditions) can be induced by a single premature stimulus and that these tachycardias are based on a circus movement of   the
impulse   in   a   circuit   of   which   the   diameter   was less than 10 mm (Allessie
et al., 1977).

The data in Table I show that the mean conduction time of an   early   premature impulse is about 90 ms. This means that an atrial impulse being blocked on
its way into the sinus node except for one single entrance, can   travel   through
the sino-atrial   border during such a long time that reexcitation of the atrium
is possible. The refractory period of atrial fibers is between   60   and   80   ms
(these   values   we   have   found in all our experiments with right or left atrial
preparations of the rabbit;   see also Allessie et al., 1976) and   the   excitability of the atrial fibers adjacent to the sinus node, will be restored after
the foregoing premature activation at the moment, the impulse in the sinus   node
will find an exit to the atrium. Thus, a single "sinus echo" has to be possible
and we already demonstrated this in an isolated right atrium of the rabbit (Allessie and Bonke, 1979).

[*] The conduction through the border of the sinus node (transitional   zone)   is
    enhanched by catecholamines and depressed by cholinergic drugs.
The conduction velocity is directly related to the rate of rise of the depolarization   of   the   fibers   during   the   action   potential.   In   the fibers of the
sino-atrial border two currents are important for   the   depolarization (Lipsius
and Vassalle, 1978a, b), viz. the fast inward current - carried by sodium ions
- and the slow inward current - carried by   calcium   and   probably   sodium   ions
(Kohlhardt et al., 1976; Noma and Irisawa, 1976). The slow inward current is
stimulated by catecholamines (Reuter, 1975; Vassort et al., 1969) and is diminished   by   acetylcholine (Giles   and   Tsien,   1975;   TenEick et al., 1976;
Lipsius and Vassalle, 1978a). We might therefore expect that decrease   of   the
slow inward current will cause a lowering of the rate of rise of the depolarization of fibers in the sino-atrial border whereas increase of   the   slow   inward
current   will be accompanied by an increase of the depolarization rate. In this
way,   the   observed   changes   in   conduction   velocity   in   the   fibers   of   the
sino-atrial   border   under the influence of autonomic transmitters can be explained.

REFERENCES

Allessie, M.A., Bonke, F.I.M. and Schopman, F.J.G.: Circus movement in rabbit atrial muscle as a mechanism of tachycardia. Circ. Res., 33: 54-62, 1973.

Allessie, M.A., Bonke, F.I.M. and Schopman, F.J.G.: Circus movement in rabbit atrial muscle as a mechanism of tachycardia. II. The role of non-uniform recovery of excitability in the occurrence of unidirectional block, as studied with multiple microelectrodes. Circ. Res., 39: 168-177, 1976.

Allessie, M.A., Bonke, F.I.M. and Schopman, F.J.G.: Circus movement in rabbit atrial muscle as a mechanism of tachycardia. III. The "leading circle" concept: a new model of circus movement in cardiac tissue without the involvement of an anatomical obstacle. Circ. Res., 41: 9-18, 1977.

Allessie, M.A. and Bonke, F.I.M.: Direct demonstration of sinus node reeentry in the rabbit heart. Circ. Res., 44: 557-568, 1979.

Bleeker, W.K., Mackaay, A.J.C., Masson-Pevet, M., Bouman, L.N. and Becker, A.E.: Functional and morphological organization of the rabbit sinus node. Circ. Res., 46: 11-22, 1980.

Giles, W. and Tsien, R.W.: Effects of acetylcholine on membrane currents in frog atrial muscle. J. Physiol. (London), 246: 64P-66P, 1975.

Kohlhardt, M., Figulla, H.R. and Tripathi, O.: The slow membrane channel as the predominant mediator of the excitation process of the sinoatrial pacemaker cell. Basic Res. Cardiol., 71: 17-26, 1976.

Lipsius, S.L. and Vassalle, M.: Dual excitatory channels in the sinus node. J. Mol. Cell. Cardiol., 10: 753-767, 1978a.

Lipsius, S.L. and Vassalle, M.: Characterization of a two-component upstroke in the Sinus Node subsidiary pacemakers. In: The sinus node. Structure, Function and Clinical Relevance, Bonke, F.I.M., ed., Martinus Nijhoff, The Hague, pp. 233-244, 1978b.

Masson-Pevet, M.: this volume, 1981.

Noma, A. and Irisawa, H.: Effects of calcium ion on rising phase of the action potential in rabbit sinoatrial node cells. Jap. J. Physiol., 26: 93-99, 1976.

Reuter, H.: Ueber die Wirkung von Adrenalin auf den cellulaeren Ca-Umsatz des Meerschweinchen-vorhofs. Naunyn-Schmiedebergs Arch. Pharmakol., 251:

401, 1965.

Steinbeck, G., Allessie, M.A., Bonke, F.I.M. and Lammers, W.J.E.P.: Sinus-node response to premature atrial stimulation in the rabbit studied with multiple microelectrode impalements. Circ. Res., 43: 695-704, 1978.

TenEick, R., Nawrath, H., McDonald, T.F. and Trautwein, W.: On the mechanism of the negative inotropic effect of acetylcholine. Pfluegers Arch., 361: 207-213, 1976.

Vassort, G., Rougier, O., Garnier, D., Sauviat, M.P., Coraboeuf, E., Gargouil, Y.-M.: Effects of adrenaline on membrane inward currents during the cardiac action potential. Pfluegers Arch., 309: 70, 1969.

THE EFFECTS OF BRIEF VAGAL AND SYMPATHETIC STIMULATION

ON RATE AND RHYTHM CHANGES IN THE SINUS NODE

E. Neil Moore, Joseph F. Spear and Kenneth D. Kronhaus

INTRODUCTION

How the parasympathetic and sympathetic nervous system influence the rate of pacemaker generation and conduction within the sinus node is a subject that has fascinated electrophysiologists for many years. Our early studies in the dog using brief vagal and brief sympathetic nerve stimulation demonstrated that there was a considerable difference in the time course between the effects of the parasympathetic and sympathetic nervous system (Spear and Moore, 1973). The acceleration of sinus node rate caused by brief stellate stimulation was observed to be a gradual acceleration followed by a gradual slowing. The effects of vagal stimulation on sinus rhythm were more brief and more complex. Brief vagal stimulation resulted in an initial slowing of sinus rhythm followed by a transient period of acceleration in which the spontaneous rate sometimes actually exceeded the control sinus rate followed by a second period of sinus slowing. This phenomena of anomalous acceleration following brief vagal stimulation was shown first by Brown and Eccles in 1934 in studies on the cat sinus node. Since Brown and Eccles' early studies it has been shown that this acceleratory component is not due to a simultaneous stimulation of sympathetic fibers since beta adrenergic blockade does not eliminate the anomalous acceleratory component observed following brief vagal stimulation (Levy et al., 1970; Spear and Moore, 1973). Also, acceleration of the sinus node resulting from sympathetic stimula-

These studies were supported in part by grants from the National Heart, Lung and Blood Institute.

tion occurs at a much later time and has a longer duration than the anomalous acceleration observed following brief vagal stimulation. Iano et al. (1973) prevented the initial sinus slowing produced by vagal stimulation by overdrive pacing of the sinus node to maintain the control sinus rate and observed that anomalous acceleration was still present. Even when the sinus node was not allowed to initially slow the period of acceleration was not shifted in time nor duration. The injection of acetylcholine directly into the sinus node artery also resulted in the same bimodal slowing interceded by a period of acceleration as observed with vagal stimulation (Chiba et al., 1975). Thus, variations in presynaptic release of acetylcholine patterns are not causing anomalous acceleration. However, atropine does eliminate both the inhibitory and acceleratory responses to vagal stimulation. Since atropine does not prevent the release of acetylcholine, the mechanism(s) for this complex time course of vagal effects appeared to be due to: 1) the intrinsic response of the sinus node to acetylcholine, 2) acetylcholine-induced release of some secondary mediator, such as K^+, 3) due to a shift of the pacemaker site following vagal stimulation or 4) changes in sinoatrial conduction. Since vagal stimulation is known to increase the potassium efflux from the atrium due to an increased membrane conductance to potassium, we utilized the potassium sensitive microelectrode technique to follow extracellular potassium changes associated with vagally produced slowing and acceleration of the sinus node. We also mapped sinus pacemaker site and sinoatrial conduction during brief vagal stimulation.

METHODS

Experiments were carried out on rabbits weighing 1-3 kg anesthetized with intravenous sodium pentobarbital (30 mg/kg). The chest was opened and the heart rapidly excised and the atrium opened in the manner described by Paes de Carvalho et al. (1959). The heart was superfused with Tyrode's soluttion and gassed with 95% oxygen and 5% carbon dioxide. Temperature was maintained at 37 ^{o}C. In most experiments propranolol was added (1 mg/liter) to eliminate sympathetic activity. Vagal stimulation was carried out by previously described modification of the technique of Vincenzi and West (1963). Close bipolar silver stimulating electrodes were placed on the endocardial surface of the superior vena cava in the region where vagal fibers innervating the sinus node are located. A 100 ms duration burst of 4 ms constant current rectangular pulses occurring at a frequency of 100 Hz was used for vagal stimulation. The intensity of vagal stimulation was submaximal and ranged between 0.1 and 1.0 mA. Maximal vagal stimulation using this duration and frequency in the various preparations produced increases in the interval between sinus beats ranging between a 60 to 220 percent change above the control sinus rate. The magnitude of response to vagal stimulation remained stable throughout the course of the experiments. Standard glass microelectrodes were used to record transmembrane potentials and double barreled potassium sensitive microelectrodes used to record extracellular potassium activity from the sinus node region. The double barreled potassium microelectrodes were made using techniques previously described (Spear et al., 1979). The tip resistance of the potassium sensitive microelectrodes was about 1,000 MOhm and the tip diameters were 3-4 m. The time constant response to rectangular test pulses was 15-20 ms. The reference barrel had a response time constant of 0.2 ms. Electrodes had sodium to potassium selectivities of 1/60 and slopes of 50 to 60 mV for a 10-fold change in potassium activity.

RESULTS

A schematic illustration of the isolated rabbit sinus node preparation used in most of the studies is presented in Figure 1A. SVC refers to the superior vena cava, AO to the aorta, IVC inferior vena cava, CS coronary sinus, TV tricuspid valve, AM atrial muscle, and CT crista terminalis. It can be noted that extracellular bipolar stimulating electrodes labeled VS are located on the endocardial surface of the SVC at the upper part of this drawing. These extracellular bipolar electrodes were used for vagal stimulation. SN1 and SN2 note the location of two microelectrodes within the sinus node region (stippled area). A bipolar electrode labeled CT recorded electrograms from the crista terminalis and the AM bipolar electrodes recorded from atrial muscle. Analog records recorded

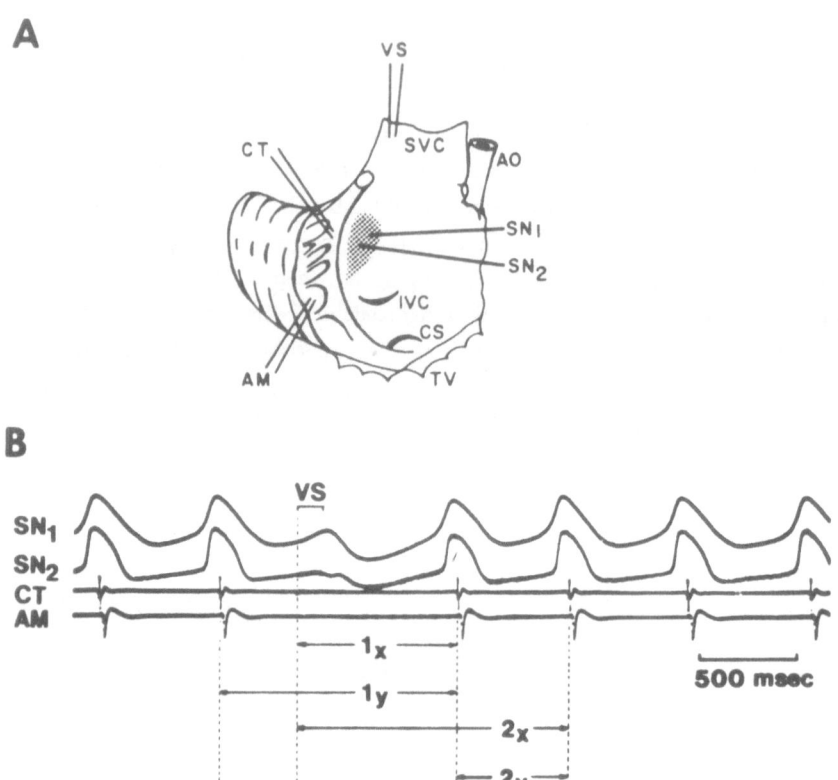

FIGURE 1 A schematic of the isolated rabbit atrial preparation (A) and selected analog records demonstrating the effect of brief vagal stimulation (B). In A, SVC indicates the superior vena cava, AO indicates the aorta, IVC indicates the osteum of the inferior vena cava, and CS indicates the osteum of the coronary sinus node. VS indicates the approximate location of the bipolar vagal stimulating electrodes. CT indicates the crista terminalis recording bipolar electrode, and AM indicates the location of the atrial muscle, bipolar recording electrode. SN1 and SN2 are the relative positions of the sinus node transmembrane potential recordings. In B, SN1 is a transmembrane potential recording from the primary pacemaker site within the sinus node. SN2 is a recording from a more peripheral subsidiary pacemaker; CT is the crista terminalis bipolar electrogram; and AM is the atrial muscle bipolar electrogram. 1x and 1y indicate the time interval from vagal stimulation to the CT activation and the interval between CT activations measured to generate the data point indicated by 1 in Figure 2A; 2x and 2y indicate similar intervals measured to generate the date point indicated by 2 in Fig. 2A. (Spear et al., 1979, by permission of the American Heart Association, Inc.)

from this isolated rabbit sinus node preparation during a short 100 ms burst of vagal stimuli are presented in Fig. 1B. SN1 was the sinus node pacemaker cell (upper trace) and SN2 a latent pacemaker cell. CT and AM are bipolar electrograms recorded from the crista terminalis and atrial muscle. At the time labeled VS vagal stimulation was applied and resulted in low amplitude non-propagated action potentials in both the SN1 and SN2 cells. Conduction to the crista terminalis and atrial muscle failed. The vertical lines indicate intervals used to plot points 1 and 2 in the graph in Fig. 2A.

Figure 2A graphically presents the effects of brief vagal stimulation upon sinus node pacemaker function. The method for constructing the graph was suggested originally by Brown and Eccles (1934) and consists of plotting the interval between the beginning of vagal stimulation and the subsequent sinus node response (1x) on the X axis against the interval between the two sinus node responses closing that interval on the Y axis (1Y). In Fig. 2A, point 1 from Fig. 1B represented the maximal observed sinus slowing and point 2 exhibited anomalous acceleration and was plotted from intervals 2X and 2Y in Fig. 1B. Thus, the interval between the onset of vagal stimulation and the first sinus node response was plotted against the interval between the two sinus responses closing that interval; this system of plotting was continued for subsequent sinus node intervals until no effect of vagal stimulation on sinus rate was observed. In this way, a graph showing the effects of vagal stimulation on sinus rate (CT-CT interval) could be plotted as in Fig. 2A. The onset of vagal stimulation occurred at time 0.0 (far left) and each division on the X axis represents two seconds. The effects of sympathetic stimulation were eliminated by the presence of 1 mg/L of propranolol.

In other isolated rabbit sinus preparations, the effects of brief sympathetic stimulation upon sinus rate was evaluated. In Fig. 2B, atropine (1 mg/L) was added to the Tyrode's solution and then the vagosympathetic fibers coursing along the endocardial surface of the SVC were stimulated using the same method mentioned previously. Note that following sympathetic stimulation an acceleration of sinus rate occurred and that the duration of this sinus acceleration was much longer than were the effects of brief vagal stimulation. Each time division on the X axis in Fig. 2B denotes a time period of 2 seconds. Also, note that sympathetic stimulation resulted in a smooth acceleration and deceleration of sinus rate rather than the brief bimodal response observed following vagal

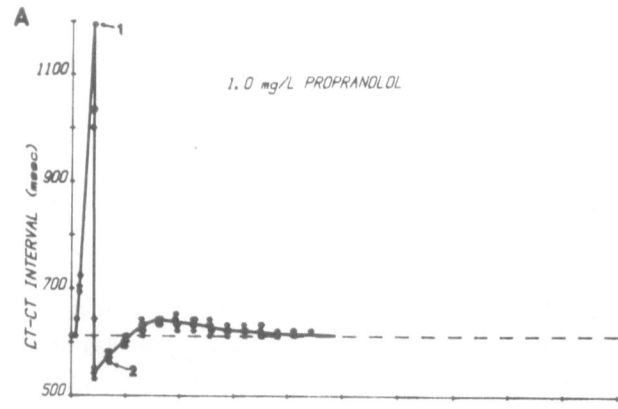

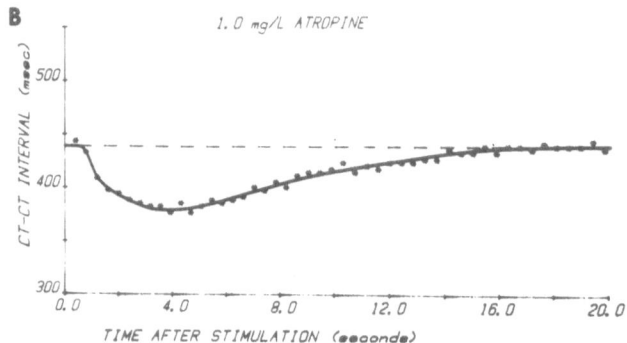

FIGURE 2 *A comparison of the time courses of changes in atrial rate following vagal or sympathetic stimulation. The common abscissa is the time after stimu-lation. The ordinates are the coupling intervals between activations of the crista terminalis following either vagal (A) or sympathetic stimulation (B). The data presented in A are from the same preparation as that in Fic g. 1. Propranolol (1 mg/liter) was added to the superfusate to eliminate the B-adrenergic influences; 1 and 2 indicate data points generated from the analog record of Fig. 1B. In a different preparation (B), atropine (1 mg/liter) was added to the superfusate to eliminate vagal influences. (Spear et al., 1979, by permission of the American Heart Association, Inc.)*

stimulation. In electrophysiological studies done in intact dogs similar ef-fects of sympathetic and vagal stimulation upon sinus node pacemaker function were observed following brief vagal and sympathetic nerve stimulation (Spear and

Moore, 1973). Thus, this isolated rabbit sinus node-vagus preparation exhibits similar time courses for sinus acceleration and slowing following sympathetic and parasympathetic stimulation. There was no direct effect on the sinus node using this method of stimulating the autonomic nerve fibers since when both propranolol and atropine were added to the perfusate the brief electrical stimuli had no effect whatsoever upon the sinus rate. Thus, the great difference in the time course of sinus acceleration produced by sympathetic stimulation points out that sympathetic effects do not account for the anomalous acceleration observed with vagal stimulation.

Another possibility for the anomalous acceleration that occurs following brief vagal stimulation is that a shift of the sinus pacemaker site occurs. Fig. 3 presents data from an experiment concerning whether anomalous acceleration can occur in the absence of a shift in the primary pacemaker site. In this study, detailed mapping of the onset of activation at 46 different sites in the sinus node-right atrial preparation were made during vagal stimulation. Representative transmembrane potentials recorded from a primary sinus node pacemaker cell (SN) simultaneously with bipolar electrograms recorded from the crista terminalis (CT) are presented in Fig. 3A. A single microelectrode was used to impale the different sites noted by solid circles in Fig. 3B. Transmembrane potentials were recorded from the area of the primary pacemaker region (darkly stippled area) as well as from regions outside of the area of pacemaker activity. The sequence of activation map for a spontaneous sinus beat is shown in the upper right hand graph labeled "Beat 1." Zero (0) indicates the primary pacemaker site and isochronic time lines are drawn at 5 ms intervals. Conduction time between the sinus node and the crista terminalis during spontaneous sinus rhythm was 38 ms as shown in the analog records in this figure and the spontaneous sinus cycle length was 470 ms. The brief vagal stimulation applied just after beat 1 (labeled VS below the second CT response) resulted in considerable slowing of sinus rate but was of too low an intensity to cause sinus block. The crista terminalis response following beat 1 occurred 646 ms after the sinus response labeled 1 and represents a 38% slowing of atrial rate. Part of the vagally induced slowing of atrial rate was a result of slowing of sinoatrial conduction time. This can be noted by the fact that the interval between the two sinus node transmembrane potentials was 635 ms while the interval between the two corresponding crista terminalis responses was 647 ms. Therefore, conduction

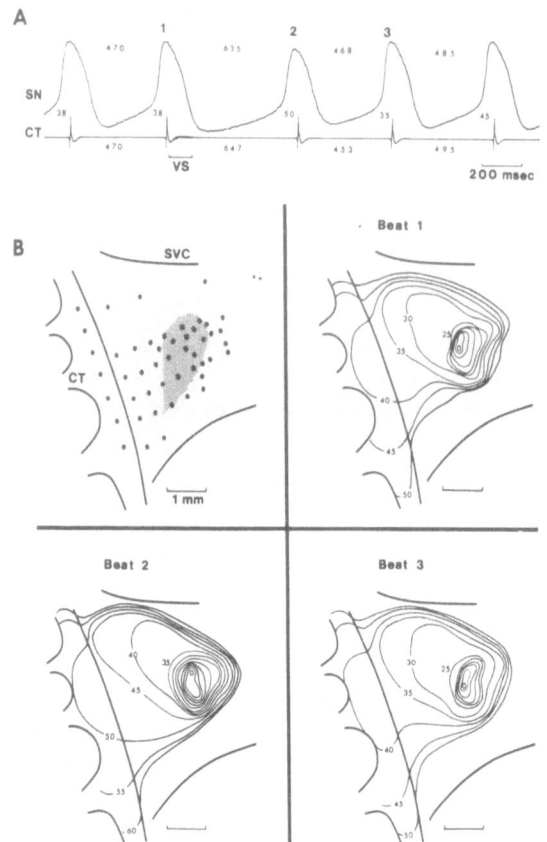

FIGURE 3 *The effect of vagal stimulation on the sequence of activation of the sinus node in the isolated rabbit atrium. Selected analog records obtained from the primary pacemaker site of the sinus node (SN) and the crista terminalis (CT) are presented in A. The coupling intervals in ms for the sinus node action potentials and crista terminalis are indicated. VS indicates the time of vagal stimulation. Vagal stimulation was applied earlier in the cardiac cycle in this figure as compared to that in Fig. 1B and 4B. This accounts for the difference in the appearance of the effect of vagal stimulation on the sinus node action potential configurations between this figure and Fig. 1B and 4A. In B in the upper left quadrant, the recording sites used in the activation map are indicated by the filled circles. The stippled area indicates the region from which sinus node action potentials were recorded. The 1, 2 and 3 in A indicate the beats for which the conduction sequence maps in B were determined. The isochronous lines of the conduction sequence maps define 5 ms intervals. (Spear et al., 1979, by permission of the American Heart Association, Inc.)*

from the sinus node to crista terminalis response for the beat labeled "2" required 50 ms rather than 38 ms as observed prior to vagal stimulation. Most of the vagally produced slowing of sinoatrial conduction resulted from slow conduction within the primary pacemaker region. This can be noted in Fig. 3 by comparing the sequence of activation maps for beats 1 (upper right schematic) recorded during normal sinus rhythm and beat 2 (lower left schematic) recorded following vagal stimulation. In beat 1 note that it required about 25 ms before activity propagated out from the region of primary pacemaker activity (0) to the rest of the sinus node and atrium. Once leaving the area of primary pacemaker activity conduction occurred much more rapidly and activation of the rest of the atrium and crista terminalis resulted. The crista terminalis was completely activated by 50 ms. In the beat 2 sequence of activation map note that it required about 35 ms before activity propagated from the site of earliest pacemaker activity (0) to the rest of the sinus node and atrium. Slowing of sinoatrial conduction as a result of vagal stimulation is also demonstrated by the fact that it required 60 ms for the crista terminalis to be activated vs. 50 ms for beat 1 which preceded vagal stimulation. Thus, part of the initial slowing of atrial rate produced by vagal stimulation is due to slowing of propagation out from the site of primary pacemaker activity. Another major point of this illustration is that with this low level of vagal stimulation only a very minimal change in the site of pacemaker initiation occurs.

In the analog records (upper traces) presented in Fig. 3A, it can be noted that beat 3 represented a beat exhibiting anomalous acceleration. Note that the interval between crista terminalis responses for beat 3 was 453 ms vs. 470 ms for the spontaneous sinus node crista terminalis interval. The interval between the corresponding maximum rates of depolarization (phase 0) of the sinus node transmembrane action potentials labeled 2 and 3 was 468 ms while during spontaneous sinus rhythm (beat 1) the interval between responses was 470 ms. Another reason for the anomalous acceleration observed between beats 2 and 3 is accelerated conduction between the sinus node transmembrane potential and the crista terminalis region (35 ms vs. 38 ms). In analyzing the sequence of activation map of beat 3 (lower right schematic), it can be noted that the time required for exit from the primary pacemaker region for beat 3 was 25 ms which is similar to that for the control sinus response. Again, it can be noted that site of primary pacemaker activity did not shift in this preparation during beat

3, and corresponds closely to beat 1 and beat 2. Thus, the slowing and acceleration that occur following brief vagal stimulation do not necessarily result from pacemaker shifts when one uses submaximal vagal stimulation as done in these investigations. However, it is known that sinus node pacemaker shifts can occur as a result of vagal stimulation. We have observed vagally induced sinus node reentry and during reentry both acceleration and slowing resulted from shifting sinus node pacemaker activity (Spear and Moore, 1978).

Data illustrating how acceleration can occur between sinus node transmembrane potentials as a result of brief vagal stimulation is presented in Fig. 4. In A, transmembrane potentials were recorded from a primary pacemaker cell (SN1), a latent pacemaker cell (SN2) simultaneously with a crista terminalis (CT) electrogram. Vagal stimulation occurred at the time noted as VS in the crista terminalis electrogram. The actual sites of the transmembrane potential recordings for SN1 and SN2 are noted on a schematic diagram of the sinus node below (B). The interval between the third and fourth sinus and crista terminalis responses following vagal stimulation exhibit a slowing of sinus rate, while corresponding intervals between the fourth and fifth beats indicated by an asterisk exhibit an acceleration of sinus rate. In the SN1 transmembrane potential recorded from the primary pacemaker site during the acceleratory phase (asterisk) the maximum attained resting potential exhibit a depolarization while during sinus slowing the maximum resting potential was associated with a hyperpolarization. The straight lines below the SN1 and SN2 traces are drawn for emphasis of the maximum attained diastolic membrane potentials. In these studies, it could not be determined whether or not the threshold potential for an all-or-none response was altered as well. However, only in the primary pacemaker region was a depolarization of the maximum diastolic membrane potential observed. In regions of latent pacemaker activity, a membrane hyperpolarization was routinely observed. This hyperpolarization is evident in the latent pacemaker cell (SN2) during both sinus slowing and acceleration. A detailed mapping of individual sites within the sinus node-atrial preparation was made to determine those areas where depolarization was associated with the anomalous acceleration, as well as those areas associated with a hyperpolarization during the same anomalous acceleration. The results of this mapping are presented in Fig. 4B with pluses denoting those regions where depolarization was observed and minuses denoting regions where hyperpolarizations occurred. Open circles denote

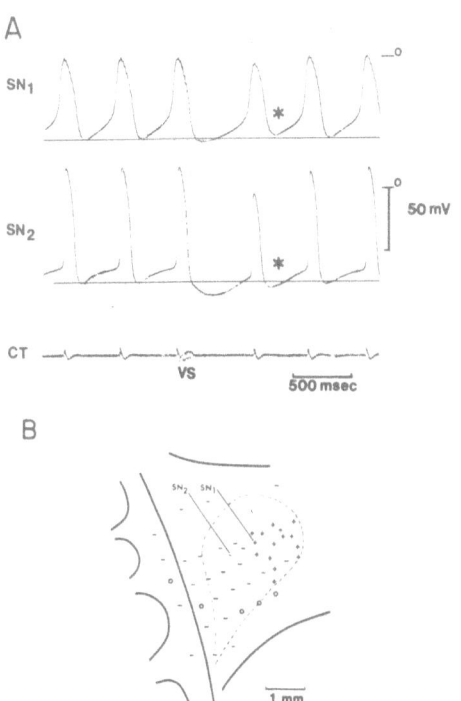

FIGURE 4 *The effect of vagal stimulation on the maximum diastolic potential of cells of the rabbit sinus node. SN1 is a record obtained from the primary pacemaker region of the sinus node. SN2 is a record obtained from a subsidiary pacemaker fiber, and CT is an electrogram recorded from the crista terminalis in an area excited earliest in the normal sequence of atrial activation. In the analog records, horizontal lines indicate the control maximum diastolic potential. Vagal stimulation was performed at the time indicated by VS. The changes in maximum diastolic potential were determined for the coupling interval indicated by the asterisk for the two cells shown in A as well as 44 additional recording sites. The timing and intensity of vagal stimulation was held constant for each of these sequential recordings. In B, a schematic of the sinus node is presented. The area bounded by the dashed lines indicates the region from which sinus node action potentials were recorded. SN1 and SN2 indicate the recording sites for the corresponding analog records presented in A. The plus signs in the schematic indicate those sites in which the maximum diastolic potential was depolarized at the time indicated by the asterisk in A. The minus signs indicate those sites in which the maximum diastolic potential was hyperpolarized at the time indicated by the asterisk in A. The zero indicate sites which showed no deviation from control maximum diastolic potential at this time. These data are from the same experiment as presented in Fig. 3. (Spear et al., 1979, by permission of the American Heart Association, Inc.)*

cells which had no change in the maximum attained resting potential during the
acceleratory phase that followed a brief vagal stimulation. It is evident that
in the primary pacemaker region depolarizations in the maximum attained resting
potential were observed while latent pacemaker cells always exhibited no change
or a hyperpolarization. Thus, since in the primary pacemaker region the maximum
attained resting potential was more towards the zero potential than in latent
pacemaker cells, it required less time to attain threshold for an all-or-none
response to be evoked. This depolarization of maximally attained resting potential in the primary pacemaker region we believe is one way that acceleration of
sinus rate occurs following brief vagal stimulation.

The difference between latent pacemaker (upper graph A) and primary pacemaker cells (lower graph B) in the maximal diastolic potential attained following brief vagal stimulation is presented in Fig. 5. The time after vagal stimulation is shown on the horizontal axis with time 0.0 being the instance when
vagal stimulation was initiated. It can be noted in "A", which represents the
hyperpolarization observed in a latent pacemaker cell, that immediately following vagal stimulation a maximal hyperpolarization is observed which over a time
course of less than two seconds returns to the baseline maximal diastolic potential. The horizontal dotted line represents the control maximum diastolic potential. The different effects of vagal stimulation upon primary pacemaker
cells is shown in the lower graph of Fig. 5. In the primary pacemaker cell,
the initial hyperpolarization is followed by a transient depolarization; the
transient depolarization has a similar time course for return to control maximum
diastolic potential as for the latent pacemaker hyperpolarizations. Note that a
more marked hyperpolarization occurred in the latent pacemaker fibers (14 mV)
than in primary pacemaker fiber (-8 mV).

One possible reason for the depolarization of the maximum attained diastolic potential in the primary pacemaker regions associated with anomalous acceleration occurring following vagal stimulation is an increase in potassium in the
extracellular fluids surrounding the primary pacemaker region. Acetylcholine is
known to increase potassium conductance. Thus, we did a series of experiments
using the potassium sensitive microelectrode technique to measure extracellular
potassium accumulation in the sinus node. Fig. 6 presents analog records recorded in an isolated rabbit sinus node preparation where simultaneous recordings were made from the crista terminalis (CT), primary sinus node pacemaker re-

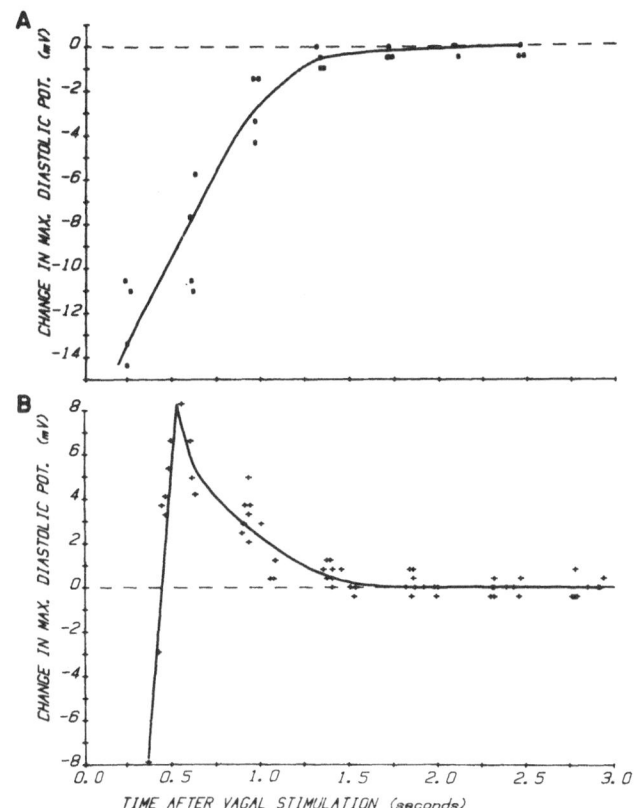

FIGURE 5 *The time course of changes in maximum diastolic potential following vagal stimulation. The graphs are plotted on a common time axis with seconds following vagal stimulation being indicated. The ordinates are the change in the maximum diastolic potential from control in mV. In A are records obtained from a single impalement of a sinus node subsidiary pacemaker cell. In B are records obtained from a single impalement in a cell in the primary pacemaker area in a different preparation. The data were generated by multiple stimulations with a fixed intensity and duration delivered at varying times relative to the spontaneous sinus interval. Negative values indicate hyperpolarization; positive values indicate depolarization. (Spear et al., 1979, by permission of the American Heart Association, Inc.)*

gion (SN), and extracellular potassium activity (V_K). Vagal stimulation was applied at the time of VS (lower trace). In this study a higher intensity of vagal stimulation was used than in the previous experiments. Strong vagal stim-

ulation in this instance resulted in a shift of the primary pacemaker site within the sinus node. This shift in sinus node pacemaker occurred after the second
SN action potential. Note that the third crista terminalis response occurred
when only a local non-propagated response was recorded in the sinus node fiber.

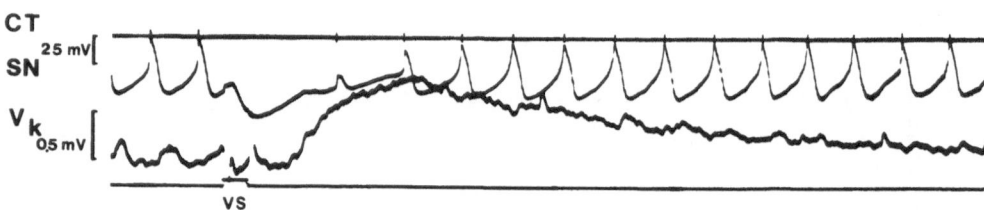

FIGURE 6 *Analog records obtained using a potassium-sensitive microelectrode positioned in the extracellular space of the sinus node. CT is a crista terminalis bipolar electrogram. SN is the transmembrane potential recording from the
dominant pacemaker area of the sinus node. V_K is a recording using a
potassium-sensitive microelectrode placed in the extracellular space adjacent to
the SN recording site. VS indicates the timing of vagal stimulation consisting
of 4 ms pulses at 100 Hz delivered at 2 mA intensity for 300 ms. The records in
A were obtained in the presence of propranolol (1 mg/liter) added to the superfusate.*

Note also that immediately following vagal stimulation there was a hyperpolarization in the impaled sinus node fiber and that the third SN action potential
was prevented. The accumulation of potassium in the extracellular space surrounding this region did not occur immediately. The maximum amount of potassium
accumulated in this instance in the extracellular space was 0.17 mmol, with a
peak occurring two seconds following vagal stimulation. Therefore, the hyperpolarization in the pacemaker cell and potassium accumulation within the extracellular space did not have the same time course. The clearing of the accumulated
potassium in the extracellular space required 14-16 seconds while the presence
of hyperpolarizing in the transmembrane potentials of the sinus node was over
within less than three seconds. The addition of atropine (1 mg/kg) to the Tyrode's superfusing the sinus node atrial preparation resulted in elimination of
the sinus slowing effects of vagal stimulation as well as elimination of the accumulation in extracellular potassium. The absence of any change in the potassium activity recorded following vagal stimulation in the presence of atropine

confirmed that the potassium-sensitive electrode was not measuring released acetylcholine nor influenced by the electrical stimulus train.

It is apparent that the bimodal slowing and anomalous acceleration of sinus
rate associated with brief vagal stimulation does not appear to have a simple
mechanism. Actually an interplay of a number of different factors must be associated with the vagal effects on sinus node rate. The data in Fig. 3 pointed
out that it is not necessary to have a shift in the primary pacemaker site in
order to have the anomalous acceleration and bimodal slowing of the sinus rate
following brief vagal stimulation. Also, we have already mentioned that the bimodal slowing and anomalous acceleration do not result from the initial slowing
of sinus rate, presynaptic effects or sympathetic activity. Our current working
hypothesis for the anomalous acceleration of the sinus rate following vagal
stimulation is shown in the graphs in Fig. 7.

We have used the same time axis following vagal stimulation with 0.0 denoting
the beginning of vagal stimulation. In the four graphs we have plotted the relationship between the interval between spontaneous atrial responses, (upper
graph), the change in maximum diastolic potential in the primary pacemaker fiber
(second graph), the accumulation of potassium in the extracellular space, (third
graph) and a hypothetical time course for the action of acetylcholine (lower
graph). The dotted vertical line coursing through all four graphs indicates the
time of maximum potassium accumulation in the extracellular space. This figure
emphasizes the fact that the early initial slowing of sinus rate is associated
with hyperpolarization in the primary pacemaker fibers as well as within latent
pacemaker fibers. The extracellular potassium accumulation occurs much later
and is far too slow to account for the initial sinus slowing. This early slowing of sinus rate must be associated with the release of acetylcholine which increases potassium conductance and produces an initial membrane hyperpolarization. The anomalous acceleration of sinus rate following the initial slowing
appears to be due both to decreasing coupling intervals between responses in the
primary pacemaker region as well as due to vagally induced changes in sinoatrial
conduction time. The decreased maximum diastolic potential (transient depolarization) in the primary pacemaker area may result from an increase in the membrane's sodium and/or calcium conductance as well as an increased potassium accumulation immediately outside of the primary pacemaker membrane. The time
course of recovery of depolarization (second graph) in the primary pacemaker

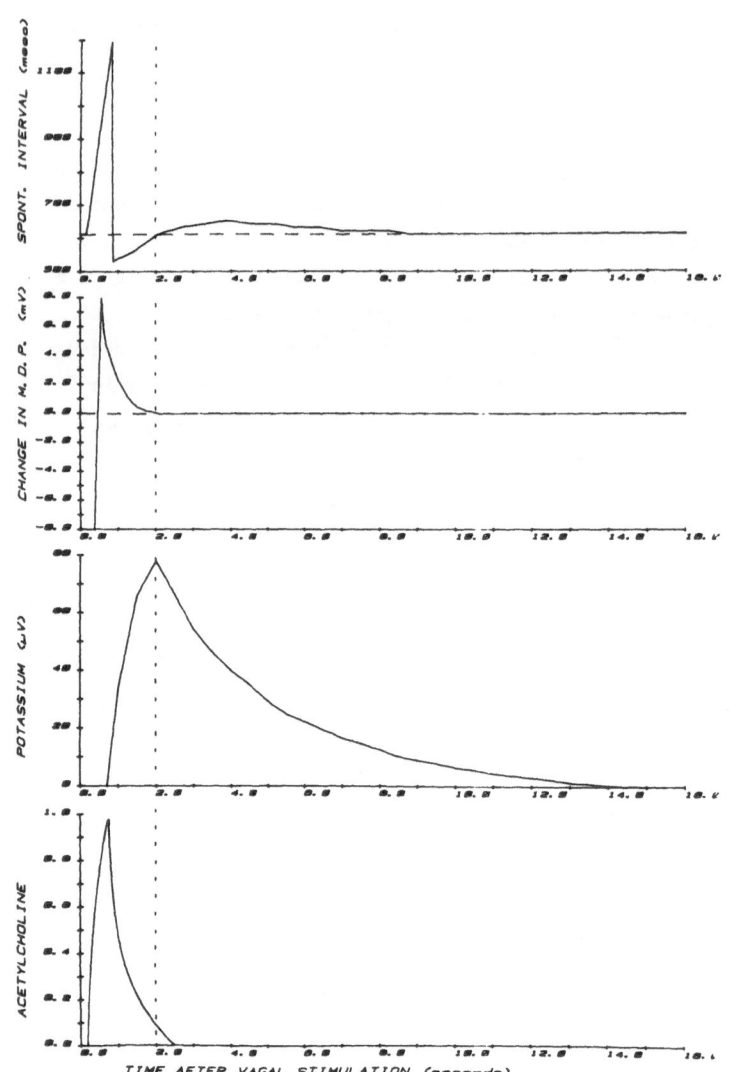

FIGURE 7 *The time course of effects following brief vagal stimulation upon the spontaneous sinus interval, the change in the maximum diastolic potential, extracellular potassium and the presumed changes in released acetylcholine are shown in this illustration. The dotted line indicates the peak of extracellular potassium recorded by the potassium-sensitive microelectrode. See text for discussion.*

site corresponds with the time course of acceleratory component in the sinus node intervals (upper graph). We did not observe any transient depolarization in maximum diastolic potential in pacemaker fiber in those experiments where a bimodal slowing separated by a period of anomalous acceleration was not observed following brief vagal stimulation. Also, preliminary results with a slow channel blocking agent (verapamil) eliminated the observed depolarization in the primary pacemaker site as well as the period of sinus node acceleration. Thus, our current data suggest that this anomalous acceleration may be associated with an increased sodium and/or calcium current within the primary pacemaker region which results in the observed depolarization in the maximum diastolic potential recorded in primary pacemaker fibers.

We believe that the secondary slowing following vagal stimulation is most likely associated with the extracellular accumulation of potassium and its slow elimination from the extracellular space. This slow accumulation and slow elimination of potassium we think is not associated with the presence of acetylcholine, as we believe acetylcholine has a brief action as schematically diagrammed in the lower graph. The fact that low intensities of brief vagal stimulation result in only slowing of the sinus node which lasts 2 seconds or less suggests that the action of acetylcholine is quite brief. The brief duration of action of acetylcholine is also supported by the brief period of hyperpolarization observed in the latent and primary pacemaker fibers; maximum membrane hyperpolarization effects were over within 2 seconds. Therefore, we believé that the secondary slowing of sinus rate observed following brief vagal stimulation is not associated with acetylcholine effects but rather may be due to the increased extracellular potassium concentration outside of the sinus node pacemaker membranes. As can be noted in Fig. 7, peak potassium accumulation was associated with the secondary slowing. The return of extracellular potassium to control levels is associated with a return of the sinus rate to control frequencies.

Thus, although there have been numerous experiments carried out to analyze

the effects of vagal stimulation upon sinus node pacemaker function, we still do
not fully understand either the secondary sinus slowing nor anomalous acceleration. It is encouraging to find that the response of the sinus node to vagal
and sympathetic stimulation in the isolated tissue bath is very similar to the
responses recorded in situ. Similarly, the finding that the rabbit sinus node
behaves similar to the canine sinus node presents the possibility of correlating
in situ canine experiments with isolated rabbit sinus node studies.

REFERENCES

Brown, G.L. and Eccles, J.C.: The action of a single vagal volley on the
    rhythm of the heart beat. J. Physiol. (London), 82: 211-240, 1934.

Chiba, S., Levy, M.N. and Zieske, H.: Chronotropic response to acetylcholine
    injected into the sinus node artery of the isolated atrium of the dog.
    Cardiovasc. Res., 9: 127-133, 1975.

Iano, T.L., Levy, M.N. and Lee, M.H.: An acceleratory component of the para-
    sympathetic control of heart rate. Am. J. Physiol., 224: 997-1005,
    1973.

Levy, M.N., Martin, P., Iano, T. and Zieske, H.: Effects of single vagal stim-
    uli on heart rate and atrioventricular conduction. Am. J. Physiol., 218:
    1256-1262, 1970.

Paes de Carvalho, A., De Mello, W.C. and Hoffman, B.F.: Electrophysiological
    evidence for specialized fiber types in rabbit atrium. Am. J. Physiol.,
    196: 483-488, 1959.

Spear, J.F. and Moore, E.N.: Influence of brief vagal and stellate nerve stim-
    ulation on pacemaker activity and conduction within the atrioventricular
    conduction system of the dog. Circ. Res., 32: 27-41, 1973.

Spear, J.F., Kronhaus, K.D., Moore, E.N. and Kline, R.P.: The effect of brief
    vagal stimulation on the isolated rabbit sinus node. Circ. Res., 44:
    75-88, 1979.

Vincenzi, F.F. and West, T.C.: Release of autonomic mediators in cardiac tis-
    sue by direct subthreshold electrical stimulation. J. Pharmacol. Exp.

Ther., 141: 185-194, 1963.

THE PHASE-DEPENDENT EFFECTS OF REPETITIVE BURSTS

OF VAGAL ACTIVITY ON HEART RATE[*]

Matthew N. Levy

About five decades ago, Brown and Eccles (1934) demonstrated that the negative chronotropic response of the heart to a brief vagal stimulus depended on its timing within the cardiac cycle. About four decades passed, however, before it was appreciated that the chronotropic response to sustained vagal activity also was influenced by the timing of the individual clusters of action potentials in the efferent nerve fibers.

In Japan, Suga and Oshima (1968,1969) noted that under appropriate conditions, a continuous, rhythmic oscillation of the heart rate was observed in response to tonic vagal stimulation at a constant frequency. When the vagal stimulation frequency (F_v) and heart rate (F_h) were almost the same, the rhythmic oscillation of the heart rate occurred at the "beat frequency"; that is, the oscillation frequency was equal to the absolute value of $F_v - F_h$. The rhythmic oscillations disappeared when $F_v = F_h$. Within a year, similar observations were also made by Reid (1969) in South Africa and by Levy et al. (1969) in the United States.

The pronounced oscillations in heart rate that can occur with constant frequencies of vagal stimulation (Levy et al., 1969) are shown in Figure 1. Note that at vagal stimulation frequencies of 1.7, 1.3, 1.2, and 1.1 Hz, the cardiac cycle length (P-P interval) varied rhythmically. Note also that the frequency of the rhythmic variation in cycle length changed as soon as the stimulation frequency was altered. The timing of each vagal stimulus (St) within the cardi-

[*]Supported by U.S.Public Health Service Grant HL 10951

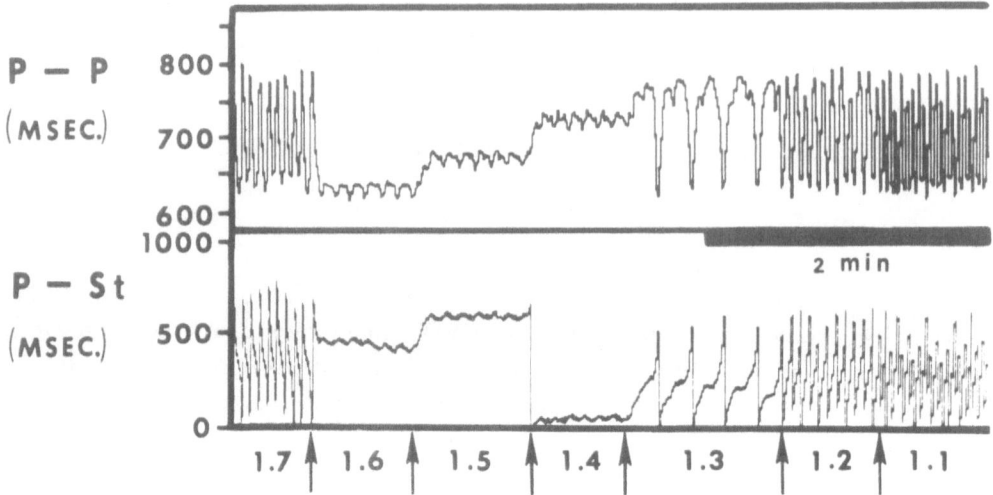

FIGURE 1 *The changes in cardiac cycle length (P-P interval, ms) and in the phase-lag between the beginnings of the P wave and the vagal stimulus (P-St interval, ms) during step changes in the frequency of efferent vagal stimulation in an anesthetized dog. The vagal stimulus frequency (Hz) is denoted by the number between arrows. (Modified from Levy et al., 1969, with permission of the American Heart Association, Inc.)*

ac cycle was measured with respect to the beginning of atrial depolarization (P wave). It is evident from the figure that the oscillations in cardiac cycle length were accompanied by fluctuations in the P-St interval, which denotes the phase-lag of the stimulus within the cardiac cycle.

At stimulation frequencies of 1.6, 1.5, and 1.4 Hz, the fluctuations in the P-P and P-St intervals almost disappeared. Note that as the stimulation frequency was decreased from 1.6 to 1.5 and then to 1.4 Hz, the cardiac cycle length progressively increased. This is a "paradoxical" response; it would ordinarily be predicted that a reduction in the frequency of stimulation of an inhibitory nerve would lead to a reduction in cycle length. It will become evident that the observed paradoxical response occurs because the SA nodal pacemaker cells become entrained by the repetitive neural activity in the efferent vagal nerve fibers. Consequently, as the vagal discharge frequency is decreased, the heart rate follows this change in frequency.

The signals shown in Figure 1 were stored on analog tape. When the signals recorded during vagal stimulation at frequencies of 1.3 to 1.6 Hz were input to an X-Y plotter, the graph shown in Figure 2 was obtained (Levy et al., 1969). The clusters of points recorded at frequencies of 1.4, 1.5 and 1.6 Hz are encircled. The other points on the graph were recorded at a stimulation frequency of 1.3 Hz. The curve of the cardiac cycle length as a function of the P-St interval expresses the variation in the negative chronotropic response to vagal stimulation that is evoked by a change in the timing of the stimuli. That a true causal relationship existed between P-P and P-St was verified by giving just one vagal stimulus per cardiac cycle, but by timing those stimuli so that they would be delivered at different times in successive cardiac cycles (Levy et al., 1969). The results were similar to those shown in Figure 2.

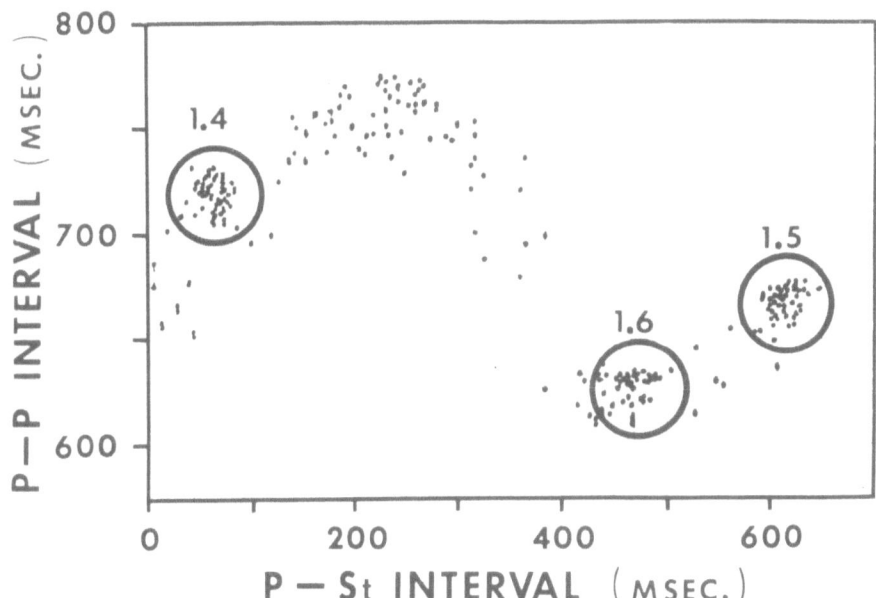

FIGURE 2 *Cardiac cycle length (P-P interval, ms) as a function of the P-St interval (ms) of efferent vagal stimuli. The data were taken from the identical experiment shown in Figure 1, at stimulation frequencies of 1.3 to 1.6 Hz. The data points recorded at stimulation frequencies of 1.4, 1.5 and 1.6 Hz are encircled; the remaining points were recorded at a stimulation frequency of 1.3 Hz. (From Levy et al., 1969, with permission of the American Heart Association, Inc.)*

In the experiment shown in Figure 2, the vagal stimuli had their maximum negative chronotropic effect when each stimulus was delivered about 230 ms after the P wave (i.e., at P-St = 230 ms). The minimum effect prevailed at a P-St interval of about 470 ms. Vagal stimulation at 1.6 Hz (Fig. 2) resulted in a minimal negative chronotropic response in this experiment, because the pacemaker cells became adapted to the vagal stimuli in a manner such that the P-St interval was about 470 ms. At this P-St interval, the P-P interval was 625 ms, which was precisely equal to the period between successive vagal stimuli; i.e., 0.625 s is the reciprocal of 1.6 Hz, the stimulation frequency. Hence, the ratio of heart beats to vagal stimuli was precisely 1:1.

When the vagal stimulation frequency was decreased to 1.4 Hz (Fig. 2), there was a readjustment of the pacemaker cells such that the stimuli fell at a P-St interval of about 60 ms. At this phase of the cardiac cycle, the pacemaker cells were much more responsive to the vagal stimuli than they were when the P-St interval was 470 ms (for a stimulus frequency of 1.6 Hz). At the P-St interval of 60 ms, the P-P interval was 715 ms, which was the reciprocal of the applied stimulation frequency (1.4 Hz). Again, the ratio of heart beats to vagal stimuli was 1:1.

The range of P-P intervals from the maximum to the minimum value in the phase response curve, such as that shown in Figure 2, defines the range over which 1:1 synchronization obtains. Within this range, an increase in stimulation frequency evokes an increase, rather than a decrease, in heart rate. As the stimulation frequency is increased, a shift in phase occurs such that the stimuli fall on a portion of the curve where each stimulus is less effective in prolonging the cardiac cycle.

Figure 3 shows that 1:1 synchronization is favored when the stimuli are delivered at P-St intervals which fall on the positive-slope regions of the phase-response curve. Negative feedback exists under such conditions. In Figure 3, S_s represents the P-St interval for a repetitive vagal stimulus that evokes stable synchronization, such as the stimulus at 1.4 Hz in Figure 2. Let P_1 to P_{14} represent a series of successive atrial depolarizations, and let S_1 to S_{14} represent a series of successive vagal stimuli. Let the period between successive stimulus pulses remain constant. If stable synchronization prevailed, any small changes in the P-P interval would be self-correcting, by virtue of the resultant change in the time-lag between P and S.

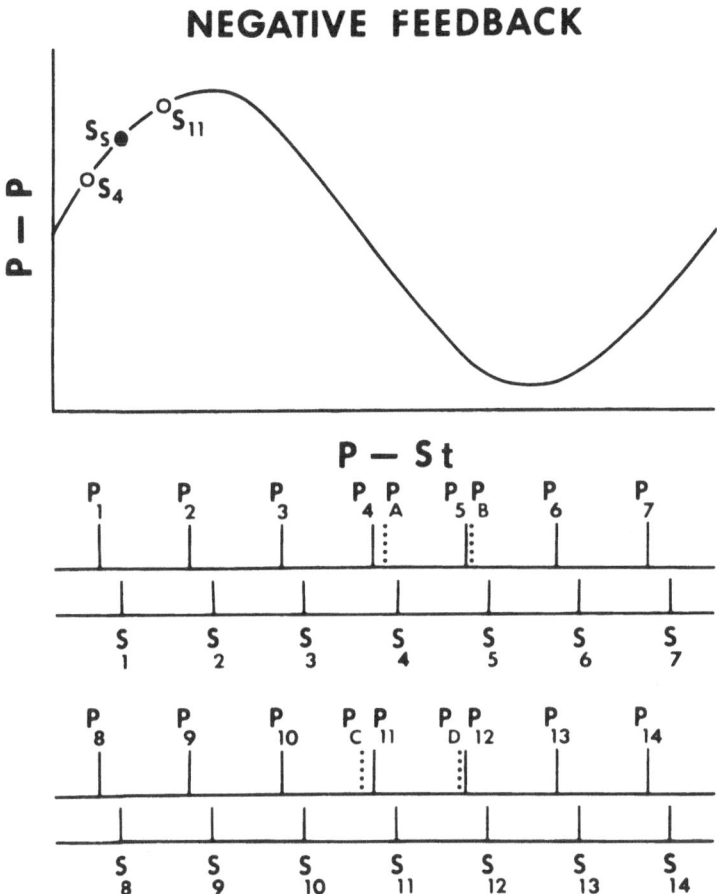

FIGURE 3 *Schema to illustrate the negative feedback that prevails when the vagal stimuli fall during the positive-slope region of the phase-response curve. S_s represents a stable equilibrium point. P_A and P_C represent transient changes in an otherwise constant cardiac cycle length. S_i represents the vagal stimuli, occurring at a constant frequency. (Modified from Levy et al., 1969, with permission of the American Heart Association, Inc.)*

Suppose, for example, that P_4 was delayed slightly (to P_A in Figure 3). The P_A - S_4 interval would be less than the preceding P-S intervals. The phase-response curve in Figure 3 indicates that the negative chronotropic effect of S_4 would be less than that of S_s; i.e., S_4 has a smaller ordinate value than does S_s. Hence, the resultant P_A - P_B interval would be less than the P_4 - P_5 interval. Within two or three beats, therefore, the time lags between P and S would stabilize again at a value virtually identical to the P_1 - S_1 interval.

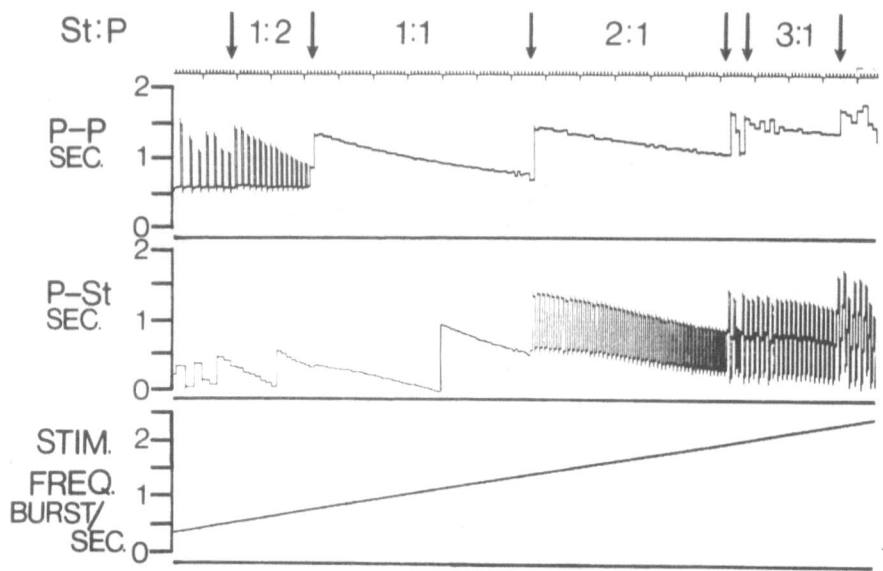

FIGURE 4 *The effect of a ramp-like increase in the burst frequency of efferent vagal stimulation on the P-P and P-St intervals in an anesthetized dog. Each vagal stimulus burst contained 10 pulses; the interval from one pulse to the next was 3 ms. The ratios between arrows denote the ratios of vagal stimulus bursts to heart beats. Downward deflections of the time marker indicate 10 s intervals. (From Levy et al., 1972, with permission of the American Heart Association, Inc.)*

Similarly, if a P wave were slightly premature (e.g., P_C in Figure 3), the P_C - S_{11} time-lag would be greater than the P_{11} - S_{11} time lag. S_{11} would come at a time on the phase-response curve at which the negative chronotropic effect was enhanced. Hence, the P_C - P_D interval would exceed the P_{11} - P_{12} interval, and within a few beats, the P-P interval would approach the constant interval between vagal stimulus pulses. In other words, over the positive-slope region, the phase-response relationship is such that any transient deviation in cardiac cycle length tends to be self-correcting. A short cycle tends to lengthen the next cycle, whereas a long cycle tends to abridge the next one.

When the vagal stimuli consist of repetitive bursts of pulses instead of evenly-spaced single pulses, the tendency for synchronization is exaggerated (Dong and Reitz, 1970; Levy et al., 1972). The spontaneous efferent vagal activity characteristically consists of a cluster of action potentials within each cardiac cycle (Jewett, 1964; Katona et al., 1970; Kunze, 1972).

The effect of stimulating the vagus nerves with periodic bursts of pulses is shown in Figure 4. In this experiment, the frequency of such stimulus bursts was progressively increased (bottom trace) as a linear function of time. It is evident that the cardiac cycle length (P-P interval, top trace) changed in an irregular fashion. In general, the P-P interval tended to increase as the stimulation frequency was raised. This reflects the negative chronotropic effect of the vagal stimulation. However, the course of the chronotropic response was characterized by a number of discontinuities. The numbers between the arrows along the top of the figure indicate the ratios of vagal stimulus bursts to heart beats. The heart was synchronized by the repetitive bursts of vagal stimuli in the ratios indicated. Within each entrainment zone, the response was paradoxical, in the sense that the heart rate tended to increase even as the frequency of stimulation of this strongly inhibitory nerve was being raised. For example, within the zone of 1:1 synchronization, the heart rate rose from 45 to 80 beats/min as the vagal stimulation frequency was being augmented from 45 to 80 bursts/min (i.e., from 0.75 to 1.33 Hz).

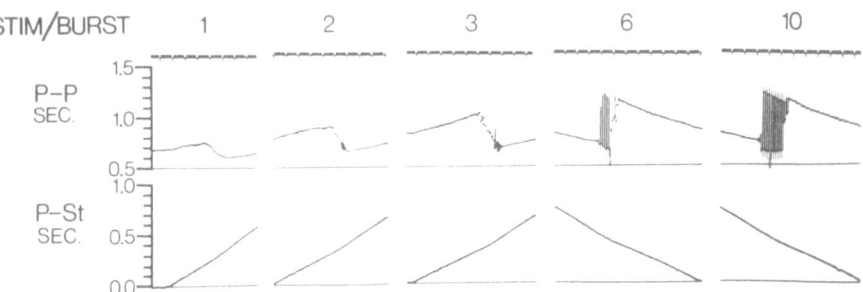

FIGURE 5 *The changes in P-P interval evoked by one burst of vagal stimuli each heart beat in an anesthetized dog. The phase-lag (P-St interval) of the burst was varied as a ramp-function of time. The numbers along the top of the figure denote the numbers of pulses per burst of vagal stimuli. Downward deflections of the time marker, 10 s. (From Levy et al., 1972, with permission of the American Heart Association, Inc.)*

When the vagal stimulator was programmed to deliver one   burst   of   pulses
each   cardiac   cycle,   but   the P-St interval was changed progressively so as to
gradually sweep the entire cycle, chronotropic   responses   were   obtained   which
were similar   to   those shown in Figure 5 (Levy et al., 1972). It is evident
that the P-P interval depended on the phase-relationship between atrial depolarization and the beginning of the stimulus burst (i.e., the P-St interval).

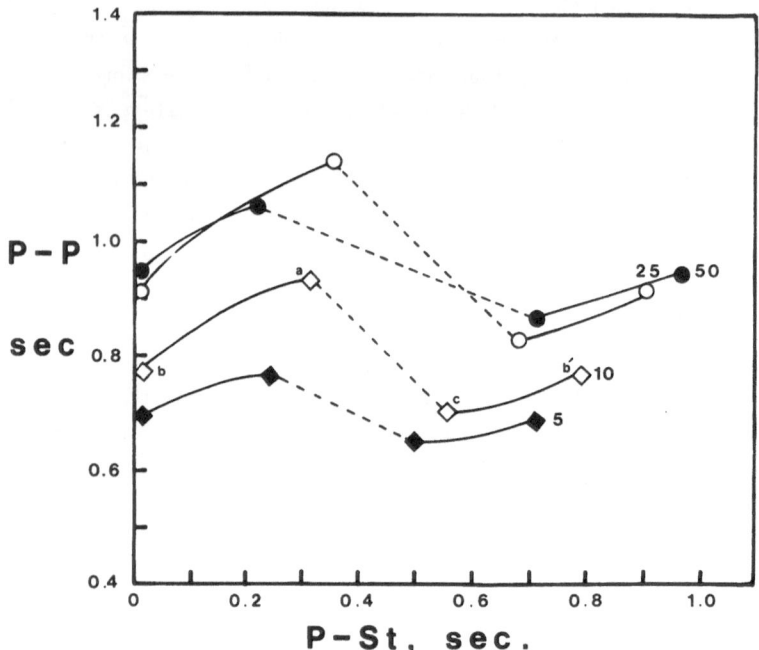

FIGURE 6 *The effect of changes in the interval between individual   pulses   (interpulse   interval)   in a vagal stimulus burst on the phase-response curve, in a
representative experiment on an anesthetized dog.   Stimulus bursts comprised 10
pulses, and one burst was given each heart beat.   The numbers along the right of
each curve denote the interpulse interval, in ms.   (From Levy et al., 1979, with
permission of the American Heart Association, Inc.)*

The number of stimulus pulses in each burst is indicated along the   top   of   the
figure.   It is apparent that the more pulses per burst, the greater the amplitude of the chronotropic response. The amplitude of   the   phase-response   curve

denotes the range of cardiac cycle lengths over which 1:1 synchronization will prevail. It is also evident from the figure that a pronounced arrhythmia appears when there are several pulses per burst (6 and 10 in the figure). Such instability occurs only on the negative-slope region of the phase-response curve, over which positive-feedback prevails (Levy et al., 1969, 1972).

The amplitude of the phase-response curve depends not only on the number of pulses within each burst of vagal stimuli, but also on the interval between the individual pulses (Levy et al., 1978). In the experiment shown in Figure 6, one burst of 10 pulses was delivered to the right vagus nerve each heart beat, and the P-St interval was systematically changed each beat in order to scan the entire cardiac cycle. The numbers to the right of each curve in the figure denote the time, in ms, between the individual pulses in a burst (i.e., the interpulse interval). The figure reveals that as the interpulse interval was increased from 5 to 10 and then to 25 ms, the mean P-P interval was lengthened concomitantly. The number of pulses per burst was not changed, and the number of bursts per minute actually decreased as the increased interpulse interval led to a reduction in heart rate. The results of this experiment therefore signify that the negative chronotropic effect of each stimulus burst became considerably more powerful as the interpulse interval was augmented over the range of 5 to 25 ms. Concomitant with the increase in the mean P-P interval as the interpulse interval was incremented within the range of 5 to 25 ms, there was also a greater amplitude of the phase-response curve. Hence, an increase in interpulse interval within that range exerts a greater synchronizing effect on the SA nodal pacemaker cells. It is likely that as the spacing between individual action potentials in the efferent vagal fibers is increased over the range of interpulse intervals from 5 to 25 ms, more acetylcholine is released from the nerve endings per pulse.

Intramural parasympathetic fibers were stimulated in isolated right atria preparations from rats, in order to activate neural fibers very close to the SA node (Stuesse et al., 1978). When one stimulus burst was delivered each cardiac cycle and the P-St interval was varied progressively, the chronotropic response varied with the P-St interval (Figure 7), just as in the intact, anesthetized dog preparations. There was only a brief phase-lag between the maximum response (point B, Fig. 7) and the minimum response (point A). This is illustrated graphically in Figure 8, where c represents the beginning of atrial depo-

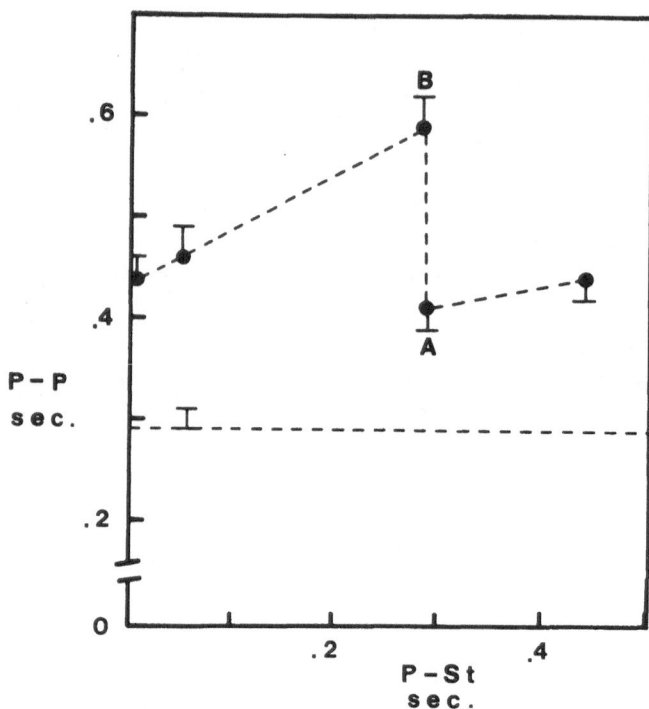

FIGURE 7 *Mean phase-response curve derived from isolated right atrial prepara-tions from 13 rats. One burst of stimuli was given to the intramural vagal fibers each heart beat. The bars indicate the standard errors of the mean. The dotted horizontal line indicates the mean P-P interval in the absence of vagal stimulation. (From Stuesse et al., 1978, with permission of the American Heart Association, Inc.)*

larization, b the beginning of the upstroke of the pacemaker action potential, and a the time of vagal stimulation. In the top panel, time a represents the time of minimal efficacy of the stimulus (i.e., point A in Fig. 7).

When the stimulus was applied only 5 to 10 ms earlier (time a in Fig. 8, bottom panel), the negative chronotropic effect of the vagal stimulus was maximal (point B in Fig. 7). Time a in the top panel of Figure 8 probably corresponds to the beginning of the period, in the experiments of Jalife and Moe (1979), during which acetylcholine failed to hyperpolarize the pacemaker cell membrane. These investigators postulated that this critical time marks the beginning of

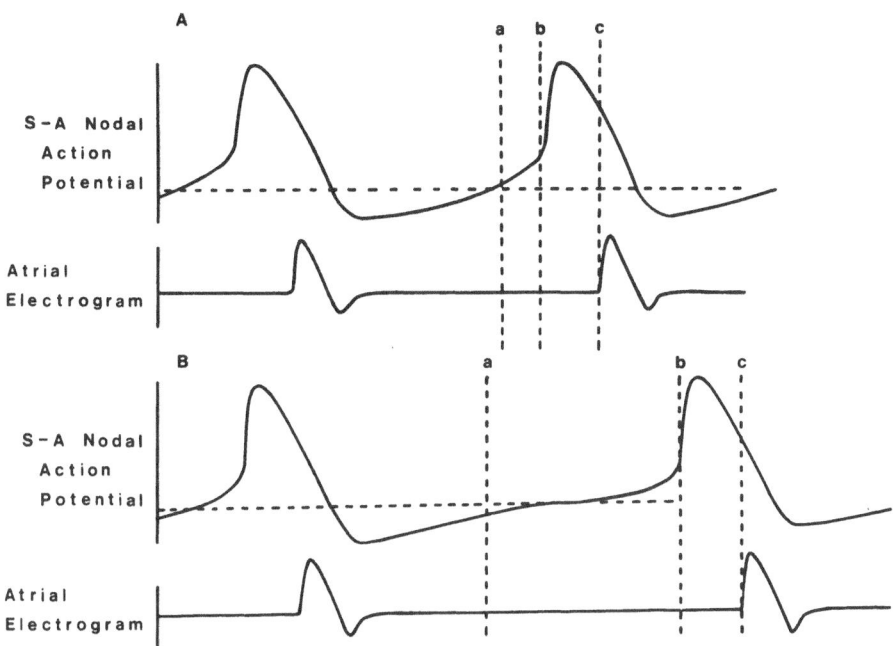

FIGURE 8 *Schema to illustrate the relationship between the timing of vagal stimuli (lines a), pacemaker cell depolarization (lines b), and atrial depolarization (lines c), in the isolated rat atrium in which the intramural vagal fibers are stimulated with one burst of pulses each cardiac cycle. The stimuli are given at the time of minimal efficacy in panel A, and at the time of maximal efficacy in panel B. (From Stuesse et al., 1978, with permission of the American Heart Association, Inc.)*

the activation of inward current responsible for the upstroke of the pacemaker cell action potential.

The profound influence of timing on the chronotropic effect of efferent vagal activity applies not only to cells in the SA node, but also to cells in the AV junction (Wallick et al., 1979). Phase-response curves were obtained from anesthetized dogs first while they were in an SA nodal rhythm (SANR), and then after an AV junctional rhythm (AVJR) had been instituted. It is evident from Figure 9 that the phase-response curves from the two regions have very similar characteristics, the principal disparities being that (1) the phase relationships differ, as reflected by the R-St intervals at which the maximum and

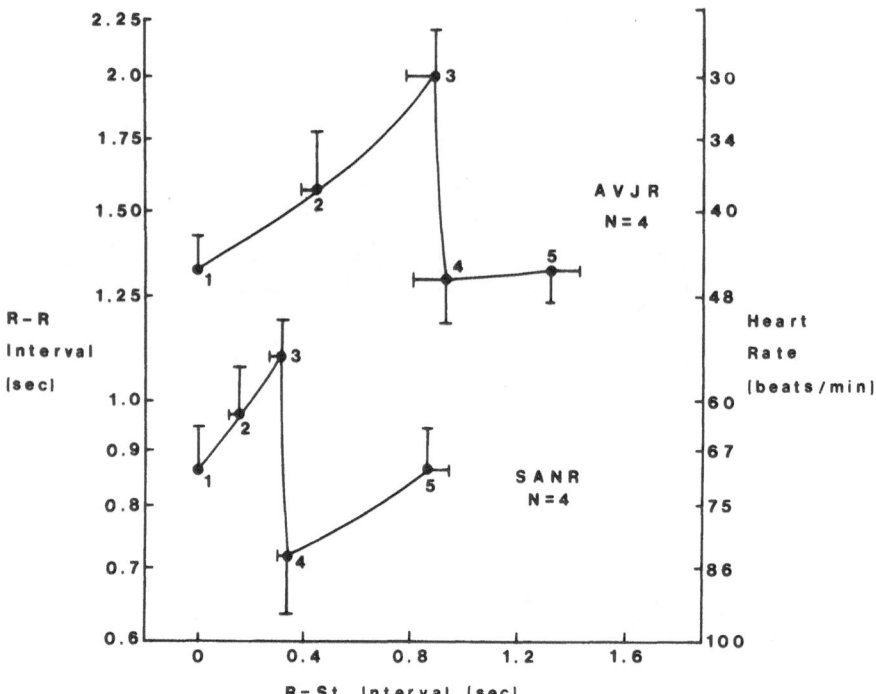

FIGURE 9 *The mean phase-response curves from 4 anesthetized dogs when they were in an SA nodal rhythm (SANR) and then in an AV junctional rhythm (AVJR). (From Wallick et al., 1979)*

minimum values occur, and (2) the R-R intervals for the AVJR are substantially greater than are those for the SANR, as expected.

The phase-dependent effects are evident even when the changes in efferent vagal activity are reflexly induced (Levy and Zieske, 1972). In Figure 10, the carotid sinus nerves were stimulated once each heart beat with a burst of electrical pulses, and the P-St interval was altered as a ramp-function of time. The resultant P-P interval varied reflexly with the P-St interval of the afferent neural stimulus. The amplitude of the phase-reponse curve was much less when the chronotropic response was evoked reflexly than when it was induced by direct stimulation of efferent vagal fibers. Hence, the phase-dependent effects are attenuated as the neural impulses are processed in the brain. However,

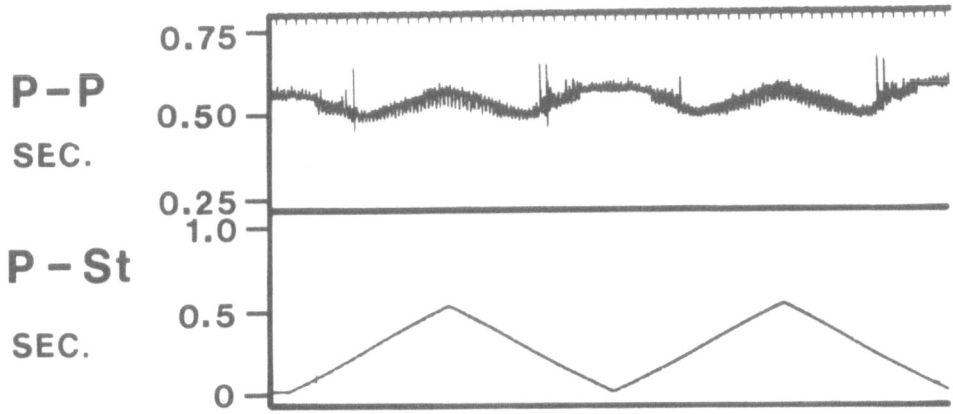

P-P

SEC.

P-St

SEC.

FIGURE 10 *The reflex changes in P-P interval with one burst of stimuli to the carotid sinus nerve each heart beat, in an aesthetized dog. The P-St interval was changed as a ramp-function of time. Downward deflections of the time marker, 10 s. (From Levy and Zieske, 1972, with permission of the Americal Heart Association, Inc.)*

pulse-synchronous bursts are prominent in the spontaneous activity recorded from efferent vagal nerve fibers as mentioned above. Therefore the phase-dependency must play some role in the neural regulation of the heart beat under natural conditions. The precise role of this factor under various physiological and pathological conditions remains to be established, however.

REFERENCES

Brown, G.L. and Eccles, J.C.: The action of a single vagal volley on the rhythm of the heart beat. J. Physiol. (London), 82: 211-240, 1934.

Brown, G.L. and Eccles, J.C.: Further experiments on vagal inhibition of the heart beat. J. Physiol. (London), 82: 242-257, 1934.

Dong, E., Jr., and Reitz, B.A.: Effect of timing of vagal stimulation on heart rate in the dog. Circ. Res., 27: 635-646, 1970.

Jalife, J. and Moe, G.K.: Phasic effects of vagal stimulation on pacemaker activity of the isolated sinus node of the young cat. Circ. Res., 45: 595-607, 1979.

Jewett, J.D.: Activity of single efferent fibers in the cervical vagus nerve of the dog, with reference to possible cardioinhibitory fibers. J. Physiol. (London), 175: 321-357, 1964.

Katona, P.G., Poitras, J.W., Barnett, G.O. and Terry, B.S.: Cardiac vagal efferent activity and heart period in the carotid sinus reflex. Am. J. Physiol., 218: 1030-1037, 1970.

Kunze, D.L.: Reflex discharge patterns of cardiac vagal efferent fibres. J. Physiol. (London), 222: 1-15, 1972.

Levy, M.N., Iano, T. and Zieske, H.: Effects of repetitive bursts of vagal activity on heart rate. Circ. Res., 30: 186-195, 1972.

Levy, M.N., Martin, P.J., Iano, T. and Zieske, H.: Paradoxical effect of vagus nerve stimulation on heart rate in dogs. Circ. Res., 25: 303-314, 1969.

Levy, M.N., Wexberg, S., Eckel, C. and Zieske, H.: The effect of changing interpulse intervals on the negative chronotropic response to repetitive bursts of vagal stimuli in the dog. Circ. Res., 43: 570-576, 1978.

Levy, M.N. and Zieske, H.: Synchronization of the cardiac pacemaker with repetitive stimulation of the carotid sinus nerve in the dog. Circ. Res., 30: 634-641, 1972.

Reid, J.V.O.: The cardiac pacemaker: effects of regularly spaced nervous input. Am. Heart J., 78: 58-64, 1969.

Stuesse, S.L., Levy, M.N. and Zieske, H.: Phase-related sensitivity of the sinoatrial node to vagal stimuli in the isolated rat atrium. Circ. Res., 43: 217-224, 1978.

Suga, H. and Oshima, M.: Modulation-characteristics of heart rate by vagal stimulation. Japan J. Med. Electron. Biol. Eng., 6: 465-471, 1968.

Suga, H. and Oshima, M.: Periodic variation of heart rate caused by repetitive electric stimulation of cardiac vagus nerve. J. Physiol. Soc. Japan, 31: 33-34, 1969.

Wallick, D.W., Levy, M.N., Felder, D.S. and Zieske, H.: Effects of repetitive bursts of vagal activity on atrioventricular junctional rate in dogs. Am. J. Physiol., 237: H275-H281, 1979.

ENTRAINMENT OF THE SA NODAL PACEMAKER BY

BRIEF VAGAL BURSTS IN RELATION TO AV CONDUCTION[*]

Jose Jalife, Philip Fraccola[**] and Gordon K. Moe

INTRODUCTION

Efferent vagal discharges do not occur at random but they tend to group in discrete bursts and to occur at periods that may hold harmonic relations to the cardiac cycle (Jewett, 1964; Katona et al., 1970). When the systolic pressure wave reaches the baroreceptor regions of the aorta and of the carotid sinuses it elicits a brief train of impulses in efferent cardiac vagal fibers (Iriuchijima and Kumada, 1963; Levy and Zieske, 1972). Brief bursts of discharges in efferent vagal fibers may result in phasic changes and entrainment of the sinoatrial pacemaker and in complex, frequency-dependent, interactions between the cardiac pacemaker and the vagal activity. Recently, it has been suggested that there might also be time-locked phasic changes of vagal effects on the atrioventricular (AV) conducting system (de la Fuente et al., 1969; Levy et al., 1969; Martin, 1977). Changes in conduction time or intermittent block, as in Wenckebach periodicity, could be induced by phasic efferent vagal discharges through a similar baroreceptive mechanism. However, the possibility of vagal

[*] Supported in part by grant HL19487 from NIH; by grant 79003 from the American Heart Association; and by a grant from the Research Foundation, S.U.N.Y.

[**] Philip Fraccola was a Summer Research Scholar at the Masonic Medical Research Laboratory.

involvement in AV conduction disturbanches is often dismissed because   there   is not a corresponding change in the sinoatrial pacemaker cycle.

In 1969 de la Fuente et al. reported that the time course of   vagal   effects   upon   the   sinus   node and upon the AV node are distinctly and discretely separate.   These effects on both systems are shifted in phase with   one   another depending   upon the heart rate.   This was also reported by Levy et al. (1969), who demonstrated a hysteresis loop in the relationship between sinoatrial   pacemaker   activity   and   AV   conduction   during periodic application of brief vagal stimuli scanning the pacemaker cycle. If vagal activity produces alterations in sinus nodal discharges which are out of phase with effects on AV conduction then it should be expected that at some frequencies of   vagal   discharge   effects   on heart   rate   would   be   predominant;   whereas at other frequencies AV conduction might be affected without apparent alterations in heart rate.

We undertook this study to extend de la Fuente's and Levy's observations in the   anesthetized   dog   and   to gain some insight about the dynamic interactions between the vagal discharge, the sinoatrial pacemaker and   the   atrioventricular conducting   system.   On the basis of these and other results from our laboratory (Jalife and Moe, 1979;   Jalife et al., 1980a) we have developed   a   theory   to explain the cellular mechanisms involved in these interactions.

METHODS

Dogs were anesthetized with sodium pentobarbital (35   mg/Kg I.V.).   Through   a midline   incision   the chest and neck were opened, the heart exposed and atrial, ventricular and His bundle electrograms, as well as lead II of the ECG were recorded.   The cervical portions of both vagi were dissected free from surrounding tissues and ligated.

To avoid interference of sympathetic responses to vagal   stimulation,   propranolol (1   mg/Kg I.V.) was administered 15-20 minutes prior to stimulation. Adrenergic blockade was maintained by complementary doses of   propranolol   every 2-3 hours.

The experimental protocol in these preparations consisted of three consecutive stages. In the first, we assessed the chronotropic effects of brief stimu-li applied every 30-60 sec to both vagal nerves scanning the spontaneous (free-running) sinoatrial pacemaker period. The spike of the atrial recording was used to trigger, after variable delay, a stimulator which delivered brief vagal trains consisting of 1-5 pulses, 5 or 10 ms in duration, 10-20 V in ampli-tude and 50 or 100 Hz in frequency. The stimuli were applied through bipolar shielded elecrodes attached to the caudal portions of the ligated vagi.

In the second stage we studied the effects of similar vagal bursts on atri-oventricular conduction. To avoid heart rate-dependent changes in AV conduc-tion, the heart was driven by rhythmic stimuli applied through bipolar stainless steel electrodes attached to the tip of the right atrial appendage. The driving cycle length was just slightly briefer (20 ms or less) than the free-running pa-cemaker cycle length. Brief vagal trains were also applied every 20-30 seconds scanning the driven cycle.

The results obtained in these initial stages were used to construct phase response curves (PRC's) for the effects of brief vagal bursts on SA nodal pace-maker activity and on atrioventricular conduction. The PRC's of both systems were compared in terms of latent periods, maximum inhibitory effects, and phasic relationships.

In the final stage, brief vagal stimuli were applied at constant periods of 200 to 1500 ms in 20-50 ms steps. To measure the steady state interactions between the periodic vagal stimuli and the SA and AV nodes the control free-running pacemaker period and AV conduction time were determined during at least 2 minutes. Vagal stimuli were then applied at a constant driven period for about 20 to 50 cycles, until a stable pattern of interaction between the vagal discharge and the nodal systems was established. This was followed by 2 minutes of recovery in the absence of vagal stimulation.

RESULTS

DIFFERENT TIME COURSES OF VAGAL EFFECTS
Brief bursts of vagal activity produced clearly separate changes of sinoatrial

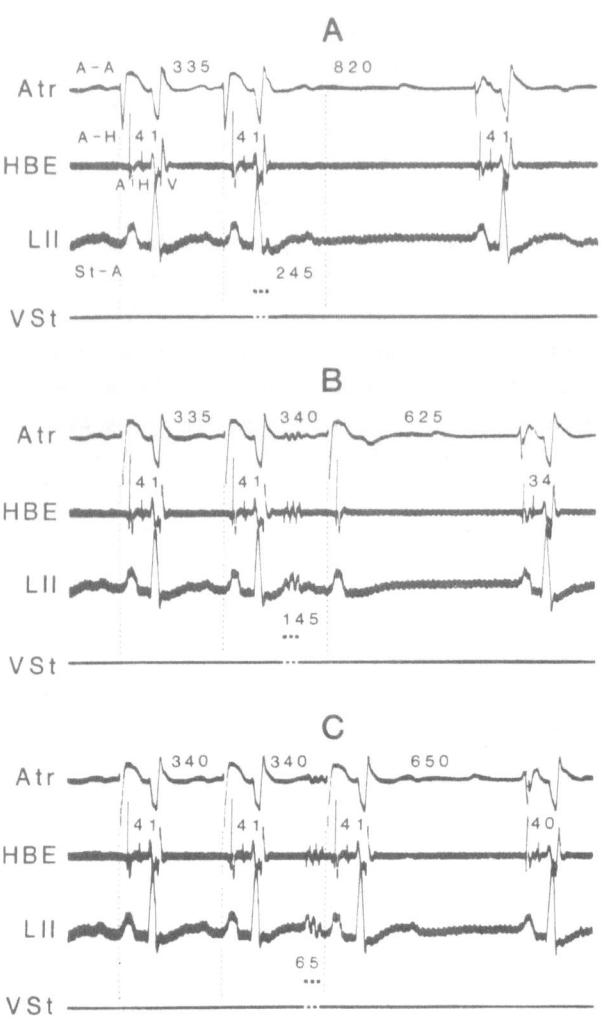

FIGURE 1 *Temporal differences of inhibitory effects on heart rate and atrioven-tricular conduction: In all panels Atr is the atrial electrogram recorded very near to the sinoatrial pacemaker zone; HBE is a His bundle electrogram. LII is Lead II of the ECG and VST indicates vagal stimulus timing. In this and subse-quent figures, A-A indicates sinoatrial pacemaker cycle length; A-H is the in-terval between the atrial septal activation in HBE and the His bundle spikes. ST-A is the interval between the beginning of the vagal stimulus and the sinoa-trial discharge. All intervals in ms. The dotted line indicates the free-running A-A interval Exp. 7-6-79.*

pacemaker activity and of atrioventricular conduction. These effects were out of phase with one another and they depended on the precise timing of the vagal input within the pacemaker cycle (de la Fuente et al., 1969). This is illustrated in figure 1, obtained from an experiment in the anesthetized open-chest dog.

In this experiment 50 ms trains of 3 stimuli 10 ms in duration and of supramaximal strength were applied every 60 seconds to both vagi at different phases of the free-running cardiac cycle. In all panels the top trace is an atrial (Atr) electrogram recorded through a pair of bipolar electrodes, attached to the epicardial surface of the right atrium, very close to the sinoatrial nodal region. The second trace is the His bundle electrogram (HBE) recorded by means of a bipolar catheter electrode inserted through the left carotid artery. The third trace is lead II of the ECG and the fourth trace is a record of the vagal stimulus (VSt). In panel A the spontaneous pacemaker cycle length (A-A interval) was 335 ms. AV conduction time, measured from the HBE as the difference between the atrial septal (A) and His bundle (H) spikes, was 41 ms under control conditions. The vagus nerves were stimulated during the second spontaneous cycle, 245 ms in advance of the third expected pacemaker discharge (dotted line), and the duration of this cycle was prolonged to 820 ms. Atrioventricular conduction, however, was not affected by this stimulus; the A-H interval in the delayed HB complexes of panel A was identical to the control (41 ms). When the position of the vagal stimulus was shifted to a later phase (panel B), the next A-A interval was prolonged very little and the cardiac pacemaker fired on schedule. The vagal effects on pacemaker activity were postponed to the following cycle which was prolonged to 625 ms. In contrast, the HBE trace in panel B shows that the vagal effects on atrioventricular conduction were maximal when the stimulus was applied late in the cycle, 145 ms in advance of the next expected pacemaker discharge. Indeed, after this stimulus the ensuing sinoatrial impulse was blocked somewhere in the AV node, as it is clearly apparent by the complete absence of His bundle and ventricular complexes following the first atrial spike after the stimulus (Figure 1, Panel B).

In panel C the vagal train was further delayed. In spite of the fact that this stimulus was delivered 65 ms in advance of the next expected sinoatrial discharge, and about 130 ms prior to the expected activation time of the His bundle, neither of the systems was altered during the stimulated cycle. Again, the vagal effects on the pacemaker were manifest during the following cycle, prolonged to 650 ms, whereas atrioventricular condition was, if anything, accelerated during this last event, perhaps as a result of prolongation of the preceding cycle. (See also the last HBE complex in Panel B).

Figure 2 shows phase response curves of sinoatrial pacemaker activity and atrioventricular conduction obtained from a similar preparation. The figure shows the results of two separate scans using 50 ms trains of vagal stimuli 10 ms in duration and 15 V in amplitude. The changes in the A-A interval (ΔA-A; black dots) plotted on the right ordinate were measured during the initial experimental stage (see methods). The cardiac pacemaker was allowed to beat spontaneously (free-running cycle = 520 ms) while the full cycle was scanned with vagal stimuli applied every 60 seconds. In the left ordinate are plotted the changes produced by the vagal input on the A-H interval (ΔA-H open triangles) during the second stage of the experiment, i.e. while the right atrium was driven at a constant cycle of 500 ms. This was done to avoid heart rate-dependent changes of AV conduction, and to obtain a more realistic picture of the time course of vagal effects on the A-H interval. Comparison of the two curves on the same axis is validated by the fact that both scans were performed at nearly identical heart rates and that both changes are plotted as functions of the same S-A interval, i.e. the time difference between the vagal stimulus and the next expected septal atrial activation. Figure 2 demonstrates striking differences in the time course of vagal inhibitory effect on the two systems. Effects on sinoatrial pacemaker activity are manifest at S-A intervals as long as 1000 ms; the PRC increases monotonically as S-A decreases up to a maximum A-A of 220 ms at an interval of 400 ms. Beyond this point the inhibitory effect decreased abruptly and disappeared completely when the stimuli were applied 200 ms or less in advance of the next discharge, i.e. during the latent period of the inhibitory effect (Brown and Eccles, 1934; Jalife and Moe, 1979). On the other hand, as shown by the open triangles, vagal stimuli applied at long S-A intervals did not affect AV conduction. In this experiment significant effects on the A-H interval were apparent only when the vagal train was applied 600 ms or less in advance of the next expected atrial septal activation. The PRC for the A-H interval increased more or less abruptly after this point and complete A-V block was the rule whenever the stimulus was presented at S-A intervals between 520 and 140 ms. Stimuli applied 100 ms before the scheduled

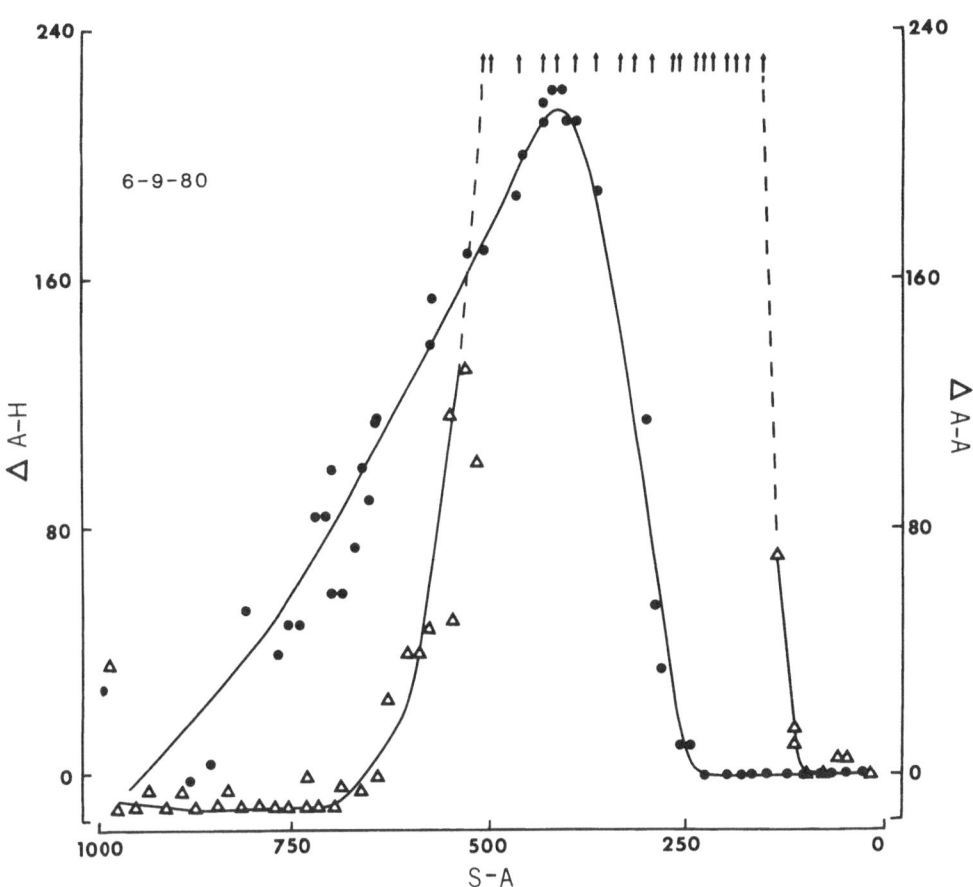

FIGURE 2 *Response curves showing phasic changes induced by brief vagal stimuli on pacemaker cycle length (ΔA-A; left ordinate) and AV conduction (ΔA-H; right ordinate), expressed in ms as functions of the vagal stimulus to atrial septal activation interval (S-A, abscissa). The black dots show the changes in A-A as the vagal train was applied at various phases of the spontaneous pacemaker period (520 ms). The open triangles illustrate ΔA-H with vagal stimuli scanning the driven A-A cycle of 500 ms. Atrioventricular block is indicated by the arrows pointing upward.*

atrial cycle were no longer affective in prolonging the ensuing A-H interval. The results of figure 2 confirm de la Fuente's experiments and clearly show a conspicuous separation in the PRC's of pacemaker activity and AV conduction.

Application of the vagal stimuli at very long S-A intervals inhibited pacemaker activity without altering A-H interval. Yet, the latent period of the vagal in-hibitory effect on AV conduction was briefer (100 ms) than was the latent period of the effects on pacemaker activity, with both curves overlapping at intermediate S-A intervals. Although there was some variability in the shape of the PRC's that depended on whether the right or the left or both nerves were stimulated, on the duration and amplitude of the stimulus and on the relationship between the spontaneous cycle length and the duration of the vagal effect (Jalife and Moe, 1979), a constant separation of the phase response curves of both systems was always observed in our experiments.

THE ENTRAINMENT PARADIGM

After prolongation by a brief vagal train, the pacemaker period does not immediately return to its free-running period. The primary phase of prolongation of the first and sometimes the second pacemaker cycle is followed by a phase of relative or actual abbreviation occurring 0.8 to 1 second after the stimulus and by a final phase of lesser prolongation lasting several seconds (Brown and Eccles, 1934; Iano et al., 1973; Jalife and Moe, 1979). The primary inhibitory and acceleratory components are critically dependent upon the position of the vagal stimulus within the pacemaker cycle, whereas the secondary inhibitory component does not show such a dependency. Triphasic curves have also been described for the vagal effects on AV conduction. However, only the primary change in the A-H interval appears to be a direct result of vagal activity (Spear and Moore, 1973; Martin, 1975).

The existence of a phasic response of cardiac pacemaker activity to the vagal effect, plus the fact that the changes in pacemaker cycle length are out of phase with the changes in the A-H interval (Figure 1 and 2), suggest that during the application of repetitive vagal stimuli complex patterns of interaction should develop between the vagal activity and the two nodal systems, depending upon the frequencies of vagal discharge. The presence of the primary phases of inhibition and acceleration indicates that periodic application of vagal stimuli should entrain the pacemaker to beat at frequencies both above and below its own intrinsic rate. However, the secondary inhibitory effect should build up with repetition, should force the pacemaker cycle toward a new steady state and should contribute to a lack of actual acceleration once the new steady

state is reached. At the same time, as suggested by the PRC of the A-H interval
(Figure 2), phasic changes in atrioventricular conduction time should also be
produced by the repetitive vagal bursts. These changes should depend upon the
frequency of stimulus application, upon the heart rate and upon the position of
the stimulus within the affected cycle. This is precisely what happens.
In the experiment illustrated in figure 3 the free-running A-A interval varied
between 360 and 370 ms and sinoatrial impulses propagated across the A-V node
with an average A-H interval of 50 ms. Each column of graphs represents the effects during 15 consecutive beats on A-A and A-H intervals (black dots and triangles on top and middle panels, respectively), produced by brief vagal trains
(50 ms) applied at three different interstimulus intervals and occurring at
phases indicated by the VS-A interval (black squares in bottom panel). The column at the left shows tha vagal effects during the last 15 of a series of 30
beats when both vagi were stimulated at an interstimulus interval (S-S) of 900
ms, i.e. at a cycle that was almost 3 times longer than the free-running pacemaker period of 360 ms. At this rate, the vagal effects were much more predominant on the pacemaker, which was forced to oscillate at periods that varied
between 420 and 600 ms (mean = 536 ms) from one cycle to another. The duration
of these periods was clearly dependent upon the interval between the vagal stimulus and the atrioventricular discharge (VS-A). Note that even though at this
frequency the individual vagal stimuli induced great variations in the duration
of the pacemaker period as they wandered through the cycle, only those occurring
at intermediate VS-A intervals (< 390; > 210 ms) induced slight prolongations
of the A-H interval. When the S-S interval was prolonged to 950 ms (middle column), the pacemaker was forced to decelerate from its stable free-running period of 370 ms to cycle lengths that varied between 440 and 590 ms, with an average A-A interval of 531 ms. Although, as with S-S = 900 ms (left column), at
this frequency the vagal stimuli did not occur at stable VS-A intervals during
each consecutive pacemaker cycle, the variations in the cycle length were somewhat smaller and more homogeneous. This is clearly apparent between the 6th and
17th beats during which the vagal stimuli occurred every other sinus beat with
increasing VS-A intervals (middle column, black squares). In contrast, at this
frequency, vagal effects on the A-H interval became clearly apparent. Indeed,
the 4th stimulus in this run, which occurred at VS-A of 230 ms, induced only a
moderate change in the 8th pacemaker discharge (A-A = 480 ms black dots in mid-

J. Jalife **et al.**

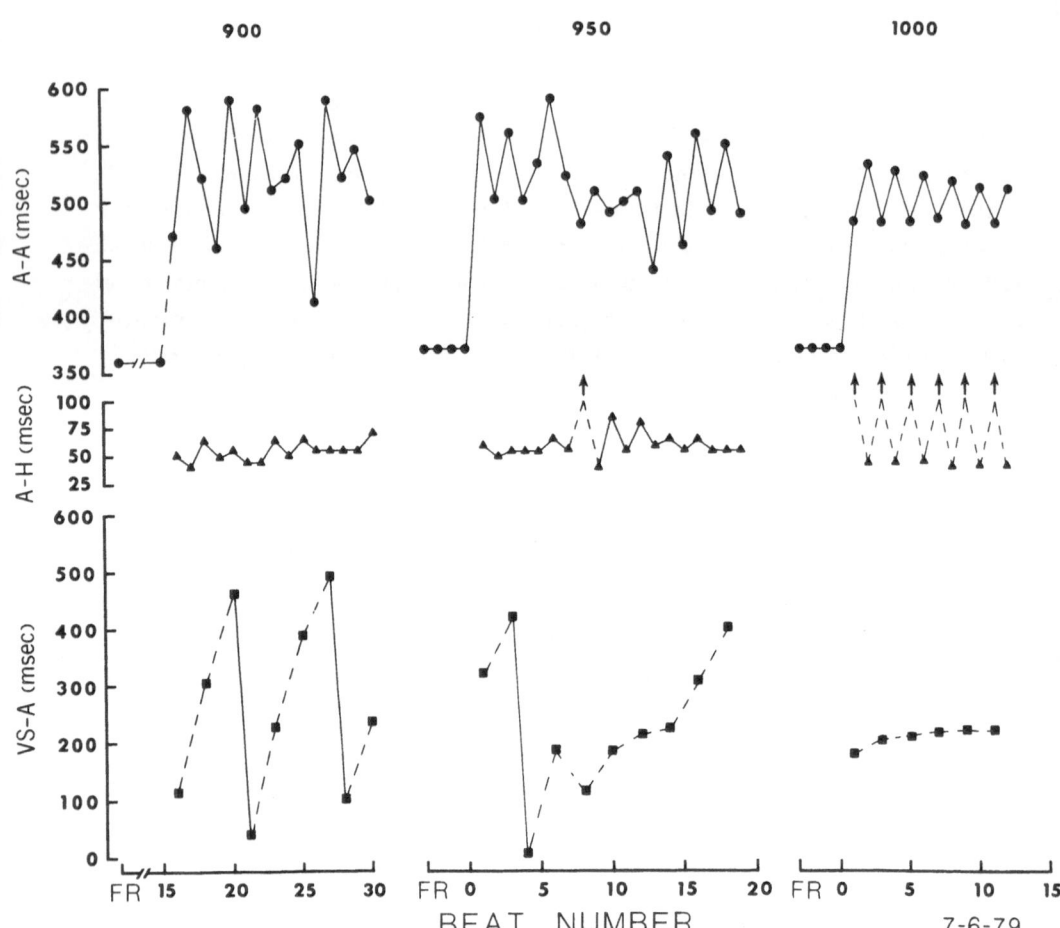

FIGURE 3 *Sequential changes in the A-A, A-H and VS-A intervals in an open chest dog preparation during application of repetitive vagal bursts at three different S-S periods (900, 950 and 1000 ms). FR = free-running pacemaker period. The control A-H interval was 50 ms for all runs. Upward arrows indicate complete atrioventricular block. See text for further description.*

dle column), but, as indicated by the arrow pointing upward (black triangles), it effectively blocked atrioventricular propagation of this impulse.

The middle column of figure 3 also shows that even though AV conduction rapidly recovered after the 8th beat (the A-H interval was only 40 ms during the

9th beat), the following vagal inputs occurred at intermediate but increasing VS-A intervals, and induced decreasing delays in AV conduction, giving the appearance of damped oscillations in the A-H curve. Also, at this frequency (S-S = 950), the largest variations in A-H interval occurred during cycles in which the oscillations in A-A interval were minimal. Stable entrainment of the pacemaker is apparent in the right column of figure 3, in which we plotted the results obtained at S-S intervals of 1000 ms. As shown by the black squares in the bottom panel, stable entrainment at 1:2 was almost immediately reached at this frequency. The stimuli occurred every other pacemaker discharge at VS-A intervals that were almost constant and the pacemaker was "locked in" to fire at cycles that were between 480 and 530 ms with an average of about 500 ms. On the other hand, since at this frequency all vagal stimuli occurred at VS-A between 180 and 240 ms and in spite of the fact that the A-A interval was relatively unchanged, every other sinoatrial discharge was blocked in the AV node, and a constant pattern of 2:1 AV block was manifest.

Analog recordings from a similar experiment are shown in figure 4. This illustration, obtained from the same dog preparation as figure 1, demonstrates the strong dependence of the A-A and A-H intervals on the timing of the vagal input during repetitive stimulation of both nerves. As in figure 1, the top trace in all panels is the atrial electrogram, the second trace is a His bundle electrogram, the third trace is lead II of the ECG and the fourth trace is a record of the stimulus artifact, to indicate its timing. The method used in this experiment were essentially the same as those of figure 3, but the records presented in figure 4 illustrate only the steady state conditions at each S-S interval. All traces in this figure were obtained 10-15 beats after repetitive stimulation had started.

In panel A the vagal nerves were stimulated repetitively at a constant S-S interval of 850 ms. At this frequency the entrainment ratio $(\frac{A - A}{S - S})$ was 0.65 and the individual stimuli occurred at different phases of the pacemaker cycle (VSt in panel A). In the steady state, pacemaker discharges were forced to occur at A-A intervals between 275 and 590 ms, with brief and long cycles alternating in a one to one manner. At the same time, and probably as a result of the heart rate-dependence of atrioventricular conduction, long A-A cycles were followed by brief A-H intervals and vice versa. It was only after the last stimulus in panel A that a somewhat longer A-H interval (62 ms) was apparent

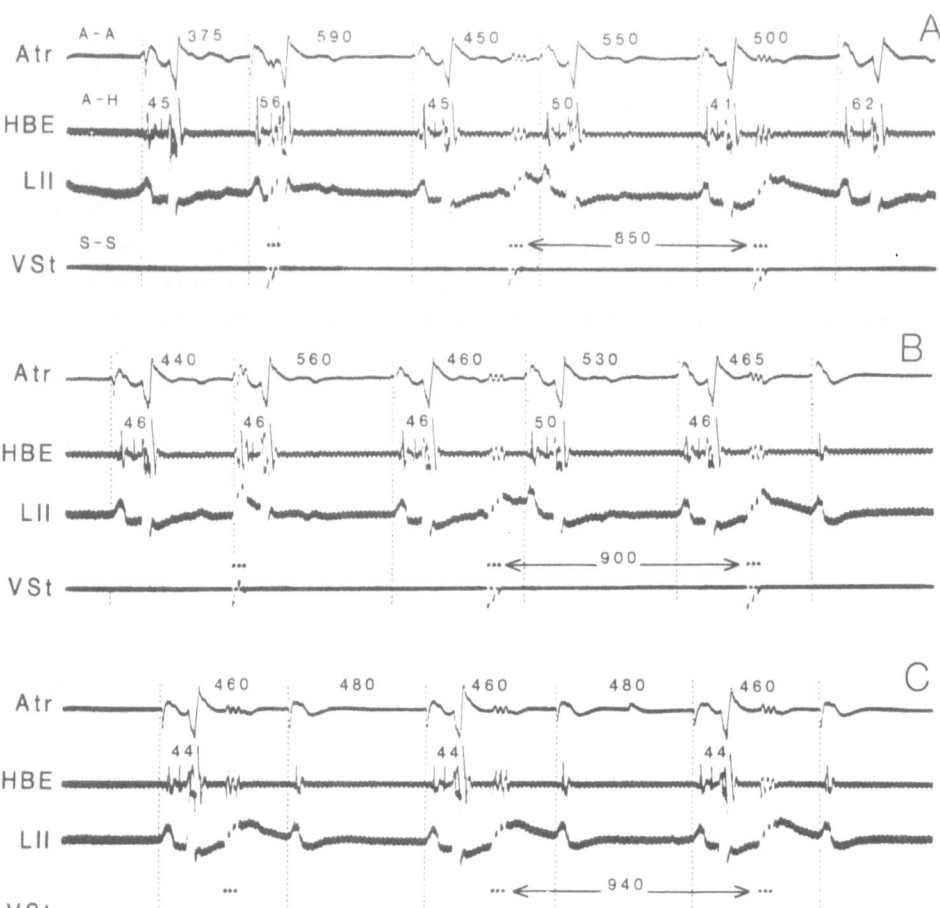

FIGURE 4 *Entrainment of the sinoatrial pacemaker and changes in atrioventricular conduction induced by repetitive vagal stimuli in the same experiment as in figure 1. Dotted lines indicate entrained pacemaker cycle and show the phase relations between the vagal stimulus and the sinoatrial discharge. All intervals are in ms.*

even though it was preceded by a relatively long cycle. This was probably due to the timing of the vagal stimulus which, in this example, occurred 290 ms in advance of an already delayed sinoatrial discharge producing only a moderate increase in AV conduction time. On the other hand, the other two stimuli in this

panel occurred at phases that were either too early or too late to alter the A-H
interval. This is also apparent for the first two vagal stimuli in panel B in
which the pacemaker was entrained to beat at an average $\frac{A - A}{S - S}$ of 0.59 and to
discharge at alternating cycles of 440 and 560 ms. Note that in this panel the
A-H interval during the initial five cycles was practically unchanged. However,
during this run the phase relations changed in such a way for the consecutive
beats, that the last stimulus in panel B occurred 230 ms in advance of the last
sinoatrial discharge and blocked propagation to the ventricles. In the clinic
this pattern would have been labeled as "alternating heart rate with 5:6 intermittent AV block of the Mobitz type II".

In panel C, the S-S was increased to 940 ms, and stable 1:2 entrainment resulted $(\frac{A - A}{S - S} = 0.5)$ with pacemaker cycles varying only by 20 ms but with an
accompanying pattern of 2:1 atrioventricular block as the vagal bursts occurred
at constant intervals, 225 ms in advance of every other sinoatrial discharge.

ONE-TO-ONE ENTRAINMENT AND WENCKEBACH

Patterns of entrainment of the sinoatrial pacemaker with periodic vagal inputs
within the range of 1:1 are illustrated in figure 5, obtained from a similar experiment in which the free running pacemaker period was 550 ms and the control
A-H interval was 90 ms. Again, all panels represent steady state modulation
patterns of A-A and A-H intervals by repetitive 90 ms vagal bursts (5 pulses 10
ms duration; 15 V amplitude), at S-S intervals indicated by the number on the
bottom trace of each panel. In panel A, the vagal nerves were driven with repetitive trains at an S-S interval of 590 ms. At this frequency, the pacemaker
was entrained to beat at an average cycle of about 910 ms $(\frac{A - A}{S - S} = 1.54)$ with
small variations in pacemaker cycle length, but with alternating first degree AV
block. Long and brief A-H intervals alternated from beat to beat as the vagal
trains occurred at apparently random phases in the pacemaker cycle. In B, S-S
was increased to 790 ms. At this stimulus frequency the entrainment ratio was
about 1.05 and there were also relatively small variations in pacemaker cycle
length (average A-A = 845 ms). However, as the stimuli occurred progressively
earlier in the entrained cycle, they induced progressively greater delays in the
A-H intervals, yielding the typical pattern of first degree AV block with Wenckebach periodicity, (Mobitz type I).

In panel C, the stimulus period was further increased to 800 ms.

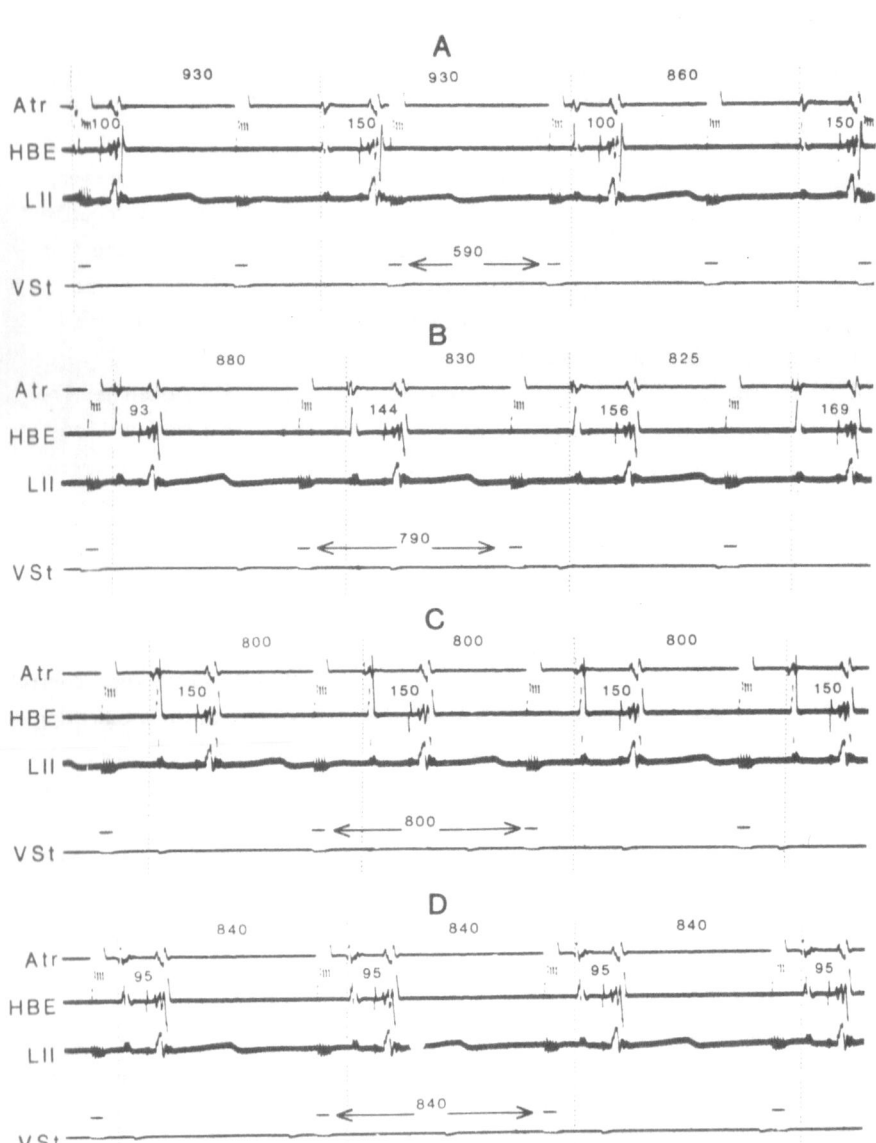

FIGURE 5 *Stable entrainment of the sinoatrial pacemaker and patterns of AV conduction delay during vagal stimulation at four relatively long stimulus periods. The numbers on the first, second and fourth traces of all panels indicate A-A, A-H and S-S intervals respectively.*

Entrainment occurred at the ratio of 1.0 and the pacemaker was forced to beat at a constant period of 800 ms. Each vagal stimulus occurred at a constant phase within the pacemaker period and preceded the subsequent atrial activation by 190 ms. Note that at this entrainment ratio the effects on the AV node persisted and first degree AV block was apparent but with a constant A-H interval of 150 ms. In panel D, the S-S interval was prolonged still further. At this frequency (840 ms), 1:1 entrainment persisted and was stable, but the AV nodal block disappeared (A-H = 95 ms); most propably because the stimuli occurred now at a constant VS-A interval of 100 ms and they were too late to have an effect on the immediately following A-H interval (see also figure 2).

TWO-TO-ONE AND HIGHER

Entrainment of the pacemaker can also occur at 1.5, 2.0, 3.0 and higher $(\frac{A \ -}{S \ -}$ $\frac{A}{S})$ ratios. When the vagal nerves are stimulated at relatively high frequencies, two or more stimuli may occur within one pacemaker cycle and their inhibitory effects may fuse to induce greater changes in the A-A and A-H intervals. However, even at high frequencies, the vagal effects on the two systems will depend on phase relationships and apparent changes will predominate on the AV node or on the sinus node depending on the rate of the vagal stimulus. A striking example is illustrated in figure 6 taken from an experiment in which the interaction patterns induced by repetitive 50 ms vagal trains (3 pulses) were studied at S-S intervals that were incremented from 200 to 1000 ms in 20 ms steps. Only three complete runs at the fastest stimulus rates are shown. As in figure 3, the top panels show the free-running and entrained A-A intervals at each one of three S-S periods. The middle graphs illustrate the A-H interval under control conditions and during vagal stimulation. The bottom graphs indicate the coupling interval (VS-A) between the vagal stimulus and the entrained sinoatrial discharge. In the left column of figure 6 the free-running period was 380 ms and the control A-H was 65 ms. At the S-S of 200 ms, two or three vagal trains occurred within a single cycle. When stimulation started the pacemaker cycle length (A-A) changed rapidly from the control value to a maximum of 585 ms during the second, third and fourth cycles. This was also coincident with development of complete atrioventricular block during these initial cycles. Perhaps due to the development of receptor desensitization at this high stimulus frequency (Jalife et al., 1980b), the inhibitory effects were not maintained des-

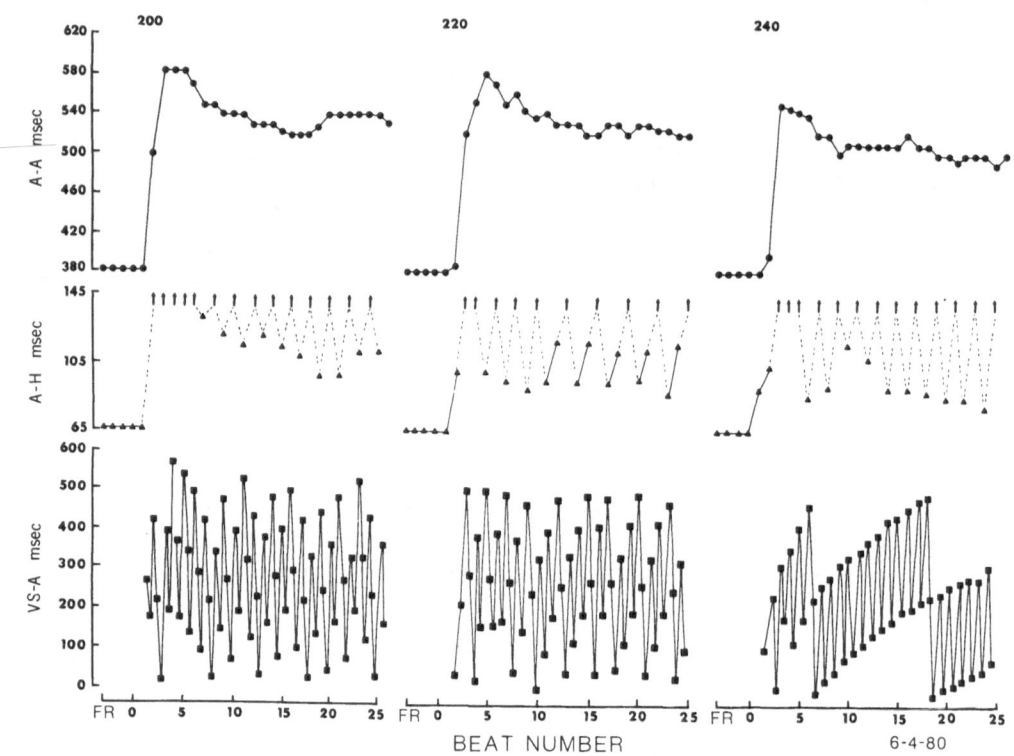

FIGURE 6   Entrainment and atrioventricular conduction changes induced by brief vagal trains at relatively fast frequencies and occurring at coupling intervals indicated by VS-A (bottom graphs). The S-S intervals were 200, 220 and 240 ms on left middle and right columns, respectively. Exp. June 9, 1980.

pite periodic vagal stimulation, and the pacemaker cycle length gradually decreased to be entrained at a new steady state period that ranged between 520 and 540 ms. This was accompanied by a gradual recovery of the A-H interval toward a final steady state pattern of 2:1 AV block. As shown in the second column, during stimulation at a slightly longer S-S interval (220 ms), entrainment of the pacemaker persisted at an average period of 525 ms when the new steady state was reached, but the AV nodal pattern now stabilized at the level of 3:2 block with Wenckebach periodicity. In the left column, when the S-S was further prolonged to 240 ms, steady state entrainment of the pacemaker was maintained at a period of 515 ms. Yet, contrary to expected, the decrease in the stimulation frequency was not accompanied this time by a further relief of the vagal effects on the A-H interval. In fact, there was a paradoxical increase of these effects and the pattern returned to that of 2:1 atrioventricular block. Even though in this experiment the pacemaker was forced to beat at similar entrained periods at all three frequencies, the patterns of interaction between the vagal stimulus and the pacemaker period varied significantly from one rate to the other. As shown by the VS-A graphs at S-S of 200 ms, 2 and 3 consecutive stimuli occurred alternately with each pacemaker cycle with patterns that repeated periodically every 4-8 sinus beats. At 220 these patterns became somewhat disorganized and did not show any apparent periodicity. Finally, at S-S of 240 ms there was a clearly defined pattern with 2 stimuli moving in about 10 ms steps and occurring at progressively later phases in the pacemaker cycle. In the steady state this pattern would have repeated itself every 13th sinus beats at which time 3 stimuli would have occurred within one pacemaker cycle and would have reset the intial conditions.

DISCUSSION

Brief trains of stimuli applied to the vagus nerves scanning the cardiac pacemaker cycle induce inhibitory effects on sinoatrial pacemaker activity and atrioventricular conduction with time courses that are distinctly separate from each other. The vagal effects on the two systems can be described by phase response curves (figure 2), that permit a quantitative description of these temporal differences and can be used to predict higher order interactions between the vagus nerves, the sinoatrial pacemaker and the atrioventricular conducting system during the application of repetitive vagal bursts. One of these predictions

relates to the ability of the vagal burst to correct the   spontaneous   pacemaker
period   by   an amount that depends on the timing of the stimulus, and to entrain
the pacemaker to beat at periods that may hold fixed and harmonic relations   to
the stimulus period (figures 3-6).   Cardiac pacemakers behave like other biological oscillators (Pittendrigh, 1965;   Winfree, 1970;   Winfree,   1977;   Pinsker,
1976;   Jalife et al., 1980a);   they show a periodically varying sensitivity to
brief perturbations and thus can be entrained by repetitive applications of such
perturbing stimuli as depolarizing or hyperpolarizing current pulses (Jalife and
Moe, 1976;   Jalife et al., 1980a), electrotonic depolarizations across an area
of   depressed excitability (Jalife and Moe, 1979a) and brief vagal stimuli (Levy
et al., 1969;   Levy et al., 1970;   Reid, 1969;   Jalife and Moe, 1979b).   In
every   case,   the   sensitivity of the pacemaker to the stimulus is a function of
the time of stimulus application within the pacemaker cycle.

    Other predictions are related to the ability of the vagal burst to induce
phasic   changes   in   AV conduction that also depend upon the stimulus timing but
that are out of phase with the changes in the sinoatrial pacemaker cycle. As a
result of these temporal differences, overt alterations of AV conduction predominate at some entrainment frequencies at which the cardiac pacemaker may fire at
relatively constant rates (figure 6);   whereas, at other frequencies, arrhythmic
patterns of sinoatrial discharge may be manifest with no apparent changes in AV
conduction time (Fig.   3).   At each level of entrainment, the manifest heart
rate and conduction patterns are functions of the intensity and duration of the
vagal stimulus train, of its position within the entrained cycle, and of the op-
erative ratio of the entrained pacemaker period and the entraining stimulus period $(\frac{A - A}{S - S})$.

    Our experiments confirm and expand previous studies by de la Fuente et al.
(1969) and by Levy et al. (1969) in anesthetized open chest dog preparations.
These two groups studied the time course of the effects of brief vagal bursts on
SA node and AV node using two different approaches. De la Fuente et al.
(1969) applied single vagal stimuli to the right or left vagus at various intervals after atrial driving stimuli or after the spontaneous pacemaker discharge.
In their experiments, they used a protocol very similar to that employed by us
in the   construction of the curves illustrated in figure 2, and they found that
the delay of the SA nodal discharge during the   primary   inhibitory effect occurred only when the vagal train preceeded the expected atrial response by at

least 300 ms. Maximum effect occurred at about 400 ms and decreased to almost zero at one second. In contrast, effects on AV transmission were present even when the vagal stimulus preceeded the atrial discharge (recorded close to the sinoatrial region) by less than 50 ms. Maximal AV nodal effects occurred at 150 ms and were nearly over at 500 ms. Levy et al. (1969) studied similar interactions during repetitive application of the vagal burst at preset timings during the pacemaker period. These authors demonstrated that the time course of effects on AV conduction and on pacemaker cycle follow similar response curves, but they are approximately 180° out of phase with each other. Maximal delays of sinoatrial pacemaker activity occurring at earlier intervals (VS-A 430 ms), and the maximal inhibition on AV conduction occurring at the later times (VS-A 230 ms).

In confirmation of those studies, our experiments also revealed temporal differences in the PRC's of both systems. In five anesthetized dog preparations in which PRC's were constructed for the inhibitory effects during stimulation of both vagal nerves, we found that the peak effects on sinoatrial pacemaker activity occurred at VS-A intervals that ranged between 350 and 420 ms with latent periods between 180 and 250 ms. The maximal effect on the A-H interval occurred at intervals as brief as 120 ms in advance of the next expected discharge and in some experiments (c.f. figure 2) it extended to about 500 ms. The latent period for the AV nodal effects ranged between 60 and 100 ms in advance of the next expected discharge and it was invariably briefer than the latent period for the changes in pacemaker activity.

Spear and Moore (1973), studied vagal effects on the sinus escape interval after a period of rhythmic atrial stimulation, and on the A-H interval scanning the driven atrial cycle with brief vagal trains. These authors measured threshold requirements for inhibitory effects and demonstrated that AV nodal conduction was less sensitive to the vagal effects than sinoatrial pacemaker activity, but they were unable to show temporal differences in the response of the two systems to the phasic vagal input. In the analysis of their results, Spear and Moore (1973) used the interval between the vagal stimulus and the atrial escape beat (V-Ax) as a time base to plot the effects on sinoatrial pacemaker activity, and they showed that these effects had a latency (about 200 ms) and time course that were similar to the latency and time course of the changes in A-H interval. However, these changes were plotted as a function of the vagal stimulation to the His bundle activation time (V-h; see Spear and Moore, 1973; their figure 9).

We recognize that the plotting method used by Spear and Moore may in fact get closer to showing the "true" latency (see Jalife and Moe, 1979b) for the vagal inhibitory effects on each independent nodal system. However, in our opinion, this method does not permit a direct comparison in "real time" of the dynamic interactions of the vagal input with the two nodes. Although in our study we always applied supramaximal stimuli and we did not observe different sensitivities, our results clearly show that there is a definite separation in both the latent period and the time course when the phase response curves are compared to each other on the same horizontal axis (c.f. figure 2). Plotted in this manner, the phase response curves can be used to predict, at least qualitatively, differential frequency-dependent effects of the vagal burst on the SA node and on the AV node during repetitive stimulation.

The cellular mechanisms of the complex interactions demonstrated in this study are not entirely understood. Yet, several pieces of information are available in the literature that may provide some insight into these mechanisms. First, ever since the studies of Brown and Eccles (1934), it is known that the effects of brief vagal bursts on pacemaker activity follow an inhibitory curve consisting of several components: a latent period of about 200 ms, a phase of major prolongation of the first and sometimes the second pacemaker cycle, a brief phase of relative or actual acceleration at about one second after the stimulus, and a final phase of lesser prolongation that may last up to 10 seconds. The existence of this triphasic curve has been confirmed in several laboratories (Levy et al., 1970; Dong and Reitz, 1970; Iano et al., 1973; Spear and Moore, 1973; Spear et al., 1979; Jalife and Moe, 1979b). Second, it is also well established that vagal stimulation or application of exogenous acetylcholine can produce membrane hyperpolarization and can decrease the slope of phase-4 depolarization in sinoatrial pacemaker cells (del Castillo and Katz, 1955; Hutter and Trautwein, 1956; Brooks and Lu, 1972). Hyperpolarization of AV nodal cells in the N zone also attends vagal stimulation (West and Toda, 1967). Secondary inhibitory effects have also been described for this system, but they have been attributed to heart rate and interval dependence rather than to direct vagal effects on the AV node (Spear and Moore, 1973; Martin, 1975; Martin, 1977).

Third, recent experiments by Jalife and Moe (1979b) have established that
the phase of primary inhibition in the triphasic curve is directly due to hyperpolarization (figure 7) of the sinoatrial pacemaker cell.

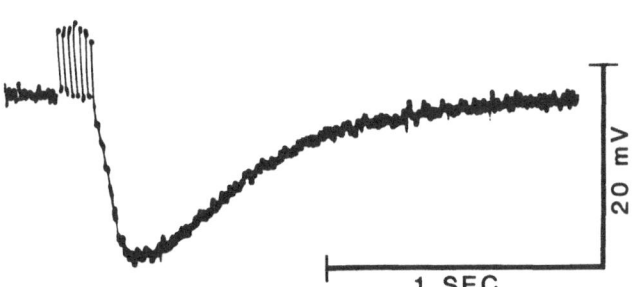

FIGURE 7 *Hyperpolarization of a quiescent sinoatrial pacemaker cell induced by
a relatively brief (110 ms) vagal train in an isolated vagus-SA node preparation
of the young cat. Spontaneous activity was abolished by continuous superfusion
with 2.2 x 10^-6 M verapamil (Jalife and Moe, 1979b) during 30 minutes. Top
trace = stimulus monitor; bottom trace = highly amplified transmembrane potential recording. Resting membrane potential = -56 mV. Hyperpolarization began
after a latency of 100 ms, reached a maximum of 16.8 mV and recovered exponentially with a half time of about 700 ms. (Jalife and Moe, unpublished).*

This hyperpolarization lasts approximately one second depending on the train duration. In spontaneously beating preparations the primary phase of hyperpolarization may be followed by a postinhibitory rebound that may, in fact, accelerate
the next expected pacemaker discharge, depending on the timing of the stimulus
within the pacemaker cycle (Jalife and Moe, 1979b). After these events, there
is no further change in maximum diastolic potential unless a new stimulus is applied. In contrast, the secondary inhibitory effect is associated with a progressive decrease in the slope of phase-4 depolarization during subsequent
beats. The shape and amplitude of the primary inhibitory and acceleratory components are functions of the intensity and duration of the vagal stimulus train,
of its temporal position within the pacemaker cycle and of the spontaneous frequency of the pacemaker. On the other hand, the secondary inhibitory effects is

less sensitive to changes in the spontaneous frequency or to the timing of the vagal stimulus. Finally, recent experiments from our laboratory (Jalife and Moe, unpublished observations) indicate that the "true" latencies and time courses of hyperpolarizations induced by brief vagal stimuli in quiescent sinoatrial and AV nodal cells are not very different from each other.

All these bits of information suggest to us that the differential behavior of the two nodal systems in response to brief vagal stimuli results from voltage-and-time dependent changes in the sensitivity of the nodal cells to the hyperpolarizing action during the primary inhibitory effect.

Consider for a moment a hypothetical experiments in the "armchair" model of vagus nerve-SA node-AV node interactions depicted in figure 8. Let the top tracings in both panels be the His bundle electrograms in which atrial, His and ventricular spikes are drawn for each beat. Let the other tracings be idealized transmembrane potential recordings from a sinoatrial pacemaker cell (SAN), an AV nodal cell (AVN) in the N zone of the node, an a fiber in the main trunk of the His bundle. Suppose that these tracings belong to an anesthetized dog as in, for example, figure 1, and that its sinoatrial pacemaker is beating spontaneously at a cycle length of, let's say, 540 ms, with activation reaching the AV nodal cell with a delay of 85 ms.

Now, let's apply a 50 ms train of 3 stimuli to both vagi at a phase that is 210 ms in advance of the third expected sinoatrial discharge (figure 8, panel A). After a latency of about 100 ms, the vagal train would hyperpolarize the sinoatrial pacemaker cell (Jalife and Moe, 1979b), and would delay its approach to threshold by about 450 ms. If we also suppose - and we have reason to do so (Jalife and Moe, unpublished) - that the latency and the time course of hyperpolarization are within a similar range in the two types of nodal cell, then the vagal train in panel A of figure 8 would also hyperpolarize the AVN cell after a certain latency (between 100 and 200 ms in our unpublished experiments). Because hyperpolarization of AVN would follow a similar time course as that of SAN, and because the AV nodal cell would be recovered at the time in which the pacemaker would fire, the inhibitory effect on AV conduction would not be manifest on the His bundle electrogram at this time. AV conduction of the delayed discharge could be, in fact, abbreviated, perhaps as a result of a long preceeding cycle (Spear and Moore, 1973; Martin, 1975), perhaps as a result of a postinhibitory rebound in the membrane potential of the AV nodal cell (Jalife and

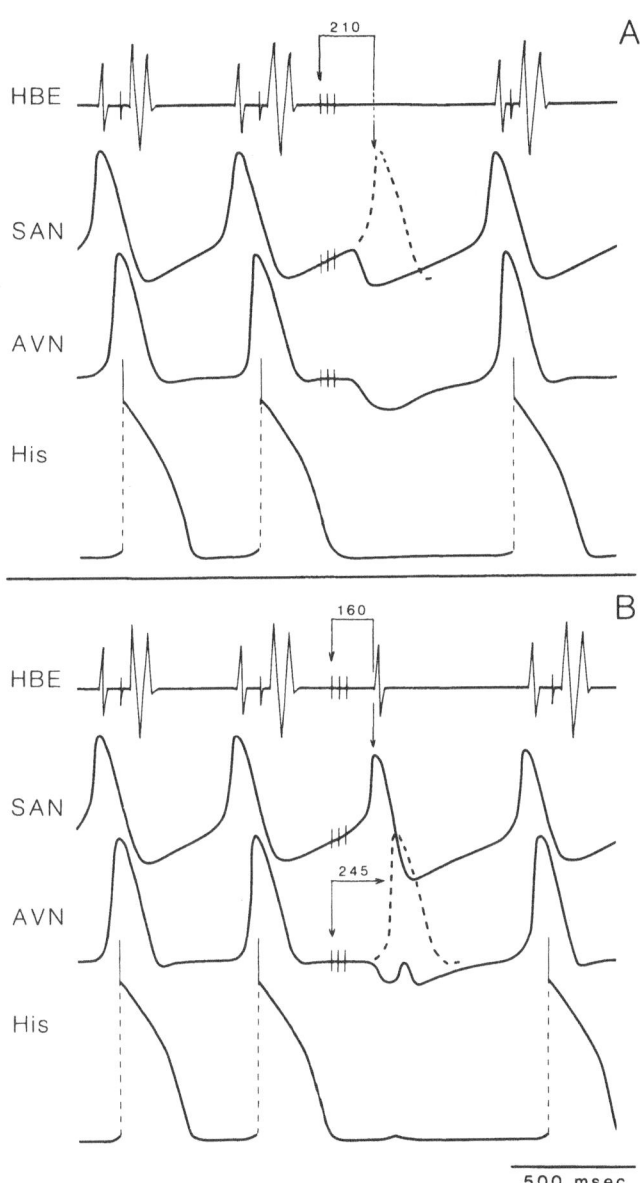

FIGURE 8 *"Armchair" model of vagus-SA node-AV node interactions. See text for description.*

Moe, 1979b) or, perhaps as a result of a combination of these two mechanisms.

In panel B of figure 8 we have moved the position of the stimulus to a later phase and applied it 160 ms in advance of the next expected sinoatrial discharge, or 245 ms in advance of the next AV nodal activation time. As the PRC for sinoatrial pacemaker activity in figure 2 indicates, this stimulus would have been too late to delay the pacemaker discharge because, by the time of termination of the 100 ms latency for hyperpolarization, the sinoatrial pacemaker would have been very close to, or would have already reached threshold and fired an action potential. Indeed, the inhibitory effects would have been manifest during the following cycle as a hyperpolarization of SAN and as a delay of its approach to threshold. In contrast, since the PRC for the AV nodal effects in figure 2 assures us that the latent period for these effects occurs when the vagal stimulus is applied only 100 ms or less in advance of the next sinoatrial pacemaker discharge, sufficient time (245 ms) would be available for hyperpolarization to start in the AV nodal cell before it is activated by the sinus beat (figure 8, panel B). As a result of this hyperpolarization, the discharge of sinus origin would not reach threshold in the AVN cell and complete AV block would be apparent in HBE as a lack of His bundle and ventricular spikes following atrial activation; a pattern very similar to that recorded in the in vivo experiment of figure 1. Again, since the hyperpolarizing response of both systems is short lived, after one second or so, the primary inhibitory effect would disappear and would give way to the secondary components of the inhibitory curves.

Of course, this is just a hypothesis, but in our opinion, this model would be directly applicable to the situation in which repetitive vagal stimuli are used. Under these circumstances, the buildup of the secondary inhibitory component after several consecutive beats would force the pacemaker to beat at slower steady state frequencies but, as demonstrated in figure 3 to 6 it would not interfere with the phasic changes induced by the primary inhibitory effects of the individual vagal trains.

These experiments have clear implications in terms of mechanisms, diagnosis and treatment of rhythm disturbances, and they suggest that in the analysis of complex arrhythmias associated with AV conduction disturbances, it is important to consider the time intervals between the possible phasic discharge of the vagus and the next event in the cardiac cycle. At some intervals and heart

rates, changes in conduction time or intermittent AV block of the Mobitz types I
or II, could be reflexly induced through baroreceptor stimulation by the systolic pulse wave, even with a complete absence of manifest rhythm disturbances
(c.f. figure 6). At other intervals and heart rates, loss of stable entrainment of the sinoatrial pacemaker by the reflexly mediated vagal burst could lead
to the development of complex disrhythmias, in the presence of apparently normal
and undisturbed atrioventricular conduction.

ACKNOWLEDGEMENT

The authors thank Mr. Henry Talarico for his technical assistance in some of
the experiments.

REFERENCES

Brooks, C.McC. and Lu, H-H.: The sinoatrial pacemaker of the heart. Thomas,
    Springfield, IL, 1972.

Brown, G.L. and Eccles, J.C.: The action of a single vagal volley on the
    rhythm of the heart beat. J. Physiol. (London), 82: 211-241, 1934.

Del Castillo, J. and Katz, B.: The membrane potential changes in frog's heart
    produced by inhibitory nerve impulses. Nature (London), 175: 1035, 1955.

De la Fuente, D., Jedlicka, J. and Moe, G.K.: Time course of vagal effects on
    SA and AV nodes. Fed. Proc., 28: 269, 1969.

Dong, E. and Reitz, B.A.: Effects of timing of vagal stimulation on heart rate
    in the dog. Circ. Res., 27: 635-646, 1970.

Hutter, O.F. and Trautwein, W.: Vagal and sympathetic effects on the pacemaker
    fibers in the sinus venosus of the heart. J. Gen. Physiol., 39:
    715-733, 1956.

Iriuchijima, J. and Kumada, M.: Efferent cardiac vagal discharge in response to electrical stimulation of sensory nerves. Jap. J. Physiol., 13: 599-605, 1963.

Jalife, J. and Moe, G.K.: Effect of electrotonic potentials on pacemaker activity of canine Purkinje fibers in relation to parasystole. Circ. Res., 39: 801-808, 1976.

Jalife, J. and Moe, G.K.: A biological model of parasystole. Am. J. Cardiol., 43: 761-772, 1979a.

Jalife, J. and Moe, G.K.: Phasic effects of vagal stimulation on pacemaker activity of the isolated sinus node of the young cat. Circ. Res., 45: 595-608, 1979b.

Jalife, J., Hamilton, A.J., Lamanna, V.R. and Moe, G.K.: Effects of current flow on pacemaker activity of the isolated kitten SA node. Am. J. Physiol., 238 (Heart Circ. Physiol. 7): H307-H316, 1980a.

Jalife, J., Hamilton, A.J. and Moe, G.K.: Desensitization of the cholinergic receptor at the sinoatrial cell of the kitten. Am. J. Physiol., 238 (Heart Circ. Physiol. 7): H439-H448, 1980b.

Jewett, J.D.: Activity of single efferent fibers in the cervical vagus nerve of the dog, with special reference to cardioinhibitory fibers. J. Physiol. (London), 175: 321-357, 1964.

Katona, P.A., Poitras, J.W., Barnett, G.D. and Terry, B.S.: Cardiac vagal efferent activity and heart period in the carotid sinus reflex. Am. J. Physiol., 218: 1030-1037, 1970.

Levy, M.N., Martin, P.J., Iano, T. and Zieske, H.: Paradoxical effects of vagus nerve stimulation on heart rate in dogs. Circ. Res., 25: 303-314, 1969.

Levy, M.N., Martin, P.J., Iano, T. and Zieske, H.: Effects of single vagal stimulus on heart rate and atrioventricular conduction. Am. J. Physiol., 218: 1256-1262, 1970.

Levy, M.N. and Zieske, H.: Synchronization of cardiac pacemaker with repetitive stimulation of the carotid sinus nerve in the dog. Circ. Res., 30: 634-641, 1972.

Martin, P.J.: Dynamic vagal control of atrial-ventricular conduction: theoretical and experimental studies. Ann. Biomed. Eng., 3: 275-295, 1975.

Martin, P.J.: Paradoxical dynamic interaction of heart period and vagal activity on atrioventricular conduction in the dog. Circ. Res., 40: 81-89, 1977.

Pinsker, H.M.: Aplysia bursting neurons as endogenous oscillators. II. Synchronization and entrainment by pulsed inhibitory synaptic input. J. Neurophysiol., 40: 544-556, 1976.

Pittendrigh, C.A.: On the mechanism of entrainment of a circadian rhythm by light cycles. In: Circadian Clocks, Aschoff, J., ed., Amsterdam, North Holland, pp. 277-297, 1965.

Reid, J.V.O.: The cardiac pacemaker: Effects of regularly spaced nervous input. Am. Heart J., 78: 58-64, 1969.

Spear, J.F. and Moore, E.N.: Influence of brief vagal and stellate nerve stimulation on pacemaker activity and conduction within the atrioventricular conducting system of the dog. Circ. Res., 32: 27-41, 1973.

Spear, J.F., Kronhaus, K.D., Moore, E.N. and Kline, R.P.: The effect of brief vagal stimulation on the isolated rabbit sinus node. Circ. Res., 44: 75-88, 1979.

West, T.C. and Toda, N.: Response of the AV node of the rabbit to stimulation of the intracardiac cholinergic nerves. Circ. Res., 20: 18-31, 1967.

Winfree, A.T.: Integrated view of resetting a circadian clock. J. Theor. Biol., 28: 327-374, 1970.

Winfree, A.T.: Oscillatory glycolysis in yeast: the pattern of phase resetting by oxygen. Arch. Biochem. Biophys., 149: 388-401, 1972.

Winfree, A.T.: Phase control of neural pacemakers. Science, 197: 761-763, 1977.

PROPERTIES OF THE FAST SODIUM CHANNEL AND OF THE MUSCARINIC RECEPTOR DURING DEVELOPMENT OF EMBRYONIC HEART CELLS IN OVO AND IN VITRO

Michel Lazdunksi, Jean-Francois Renaud, Georges Romey,
Michel Fosset, Jacques Barhanin and Alain Lombet

INTRODUCTION

During ontogenesis of the chick embryonic heart (and also of the mammalian heart) two important properties of the excitable membrane which play a role in the regulation of the rate of the pacemaker system appear to follow a drastic differentiation. These two properties are the physiological expression of the fast Na^+ channel inhibitable by tetrodotoxin and the negative inotrope effect due to the interaction of acetylcholine with its muscarinic receptor.

This paper describes an analysis using both biochemical and physiological techniques of the mechanism of the differentiation of the fast Na^+ channel and of the muscarinic response, throughout the heart ontogenesis both in ovo using hearts themselves and in vitro using cell cultures.

DIFFERENTIATION OF THE FAST Na^+ CHANNEL IN EMBRYONIC HEART CELLS

Two inward currents underlie the action potential in adult cardiac muscle (Rougier et al., 1968) a fast Na^+ current specifically blocked by tetrodotoxin (TTX) (Rougier et al., 1968; Reuter, 1973; Trautwein, 1973) and (ii) a slow current which is carried by Ca^{2+} and Na^+ ions, insensitive to TTX and blocked by verapamil and D_{600} (Trautwein, 1973; Kohlhardt et al., 1972). For the first few days after the beat begins in chick embryonic heart (2-4 days in ovo), the inward current responsible for the rising phase of the action potential is similar to the slow inward current in the adult heart; it is sensitive to D_{600} but not to TTX (Shigenobu and Sperelakis, 1972; McDonald et al., 1972; Sperelakis and Shigenobu, 1972; Shigenobu et al., 1974). A TTX-sensitive fast Na^+ channel appears only after the 4th day of incubation (Shigenobu and Sperelakis, 1971; McDonald et al., 1972; Sperelakis and Shigenobu, 1972). Other molecules are also specific for the fast Na^+ channel. Polypeptide neurotoxins such as sea anemone toxins (ATX_{II}) slow down the inactivation process (Romey and Lazdunski, 1975; Rathmayer and Beress, 1976; Romey et al., 1976; Bergman et al., 1976) and compounds like veratridine or batrachotoxin permanently open the fast Na^+ channel essentially be removing the inactivation process (Ulbricht, 1969; Ohta et al., 1973; Sperelakis and Pappano, 1969). These latter toxins have been applied to chick embryonic heart cells cultured in aggregates at different stages of differentiation.

ATX_{II}, the major polypeptide toxin from Anemonia sulcata (Wunderer et al., 1976) has several effects on the action potential of aggregates from 3-, 7- and 16-day-old embryonic hearts. At all stages of development the application of ATX_{II} provokes the appearance of a marked plateau phase (the lowest concentration of ATX_{II} giving a detectable effect is 0.1 µM; maximum effects appear at 1 µM) (Fig. 1).

These effects are reversible by washing. When looking at the maximum upstroke velocity of cardiac action potentials, $\dot{V}_{max}$, one observes that the value of $\dot{V}_{max}$ for 16-day aggregates is not significantly affected by 1 µM ATX_{II} (120 + 20 V/s and 125 + 15 V/s, ATX_{II}-treated and control, respectively; mean + S.E., N = 25 aggregates). In contrast, in 3-day-old aggregates, 1 µM ATX_{II} provokes an increase in $\dot{V}_{max}$ from 12.5 + 3 V/s (control) to 25 + 4 V/s (mean + S.E., N = 20). This observation suggests that ATX_{II} unmasks non functional Na^+ channels (Romey et al., 1980). This is supported by the fact that although the control action potential of 3-day aggregates is TTX-insensitive, the plateau phase induced by ATX_{II} is reversed by 0.1 µM TTX (Fig. 1A) and with TTX treatment the $\dot{V}_{max}$ returns to its control value. If TTX (0.1 µM) is added before ATX_{II} (1 µM), the effects of the polypeptide toxin are prevented. The action of TTX on 16-day aggregates treated with ATX_{II} is presented for comparison in Fig. 1C. Table I

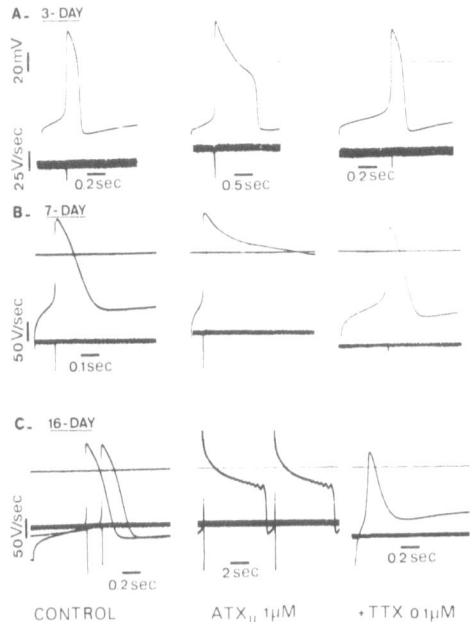

FIGURE 1 *Electrical activities of cardiac cells cultured in aggregates for 2 days from A: 3-day; B: 7-day: C: 16-day-old embryonic hearts. These aggregates retain the electrical properties of the embryonic hearts from which they were prepared. Left: control. Midle: effect of 1 μM ATX$_{II}$. Right: effect of 0.1 μM TTX on ATX$_{II}$-treated aggregates. In A: left and right, evoked action potentials; middle, spontaneous action potential. In C: left, spontaneous and evoked action potentials; middle, spontaneous action potential; right, evoked action potential at the end of a strong hyperpolarizing pulse of current; this action potential is identical to that obtained after treatment with 0.1 μM TTX alone. In each record, the higher trace is the zero voltage line and the lower trace gives dV/dt. Electrical activities were only recorded from aggregates having a diameter between 50 and 100 μm. In order to remove the resting sodium inactivation, the maximum upstroke velocity (V_{max}) was systematically measured on stimulated action potentials produced at the end of an hyperpolarizing pulse of current of 5 to 10 s duration.*

Cardiomyoblasts from 3-day to 16-day-old chick embryos were cultured using a previously described technique (Renaud, 1980). After 24 hours of culture, the majority of the cells formed spherical aggregates measuring between 40 and 150 μm in diameter. Glass capillary microelectrodes were used for intracellular recording and stimulation. They were filled with an equal mixture of 3 M KCl and 4 M potassium acetate and had resistance ranging between 20 and 60 MOhm. The microelectrode was connected to a negative capacitance electrometer (WPI-M707) containing an active bridge nettwork which permits recording and stimulation through the same microelectrode. ATX$_{II}$ was prepared according to Beress et al., 1975.

gives $\dot{V}_{max}$ values recorded at different stages of development in ovo after 2 days in culture, in the absence and presence of neurotoxins.

TABLE I

Embryonic age (days)	3	4	7	11	14	16
			$\dot{V}_{max}$(V/s)			
Control	12±3	52±5	80±9	95±10	118±15	125±20
ATX_{II}(1 µM)	25±4	75±5	85±9	100±10	120±15	120±15
ATX_{II}(1 µM) + TTX (0.1 µM)	12±3	8±2	10±3	5±1	5±1	5±1

All values are mean ± SE of 20 to 30 measurements.

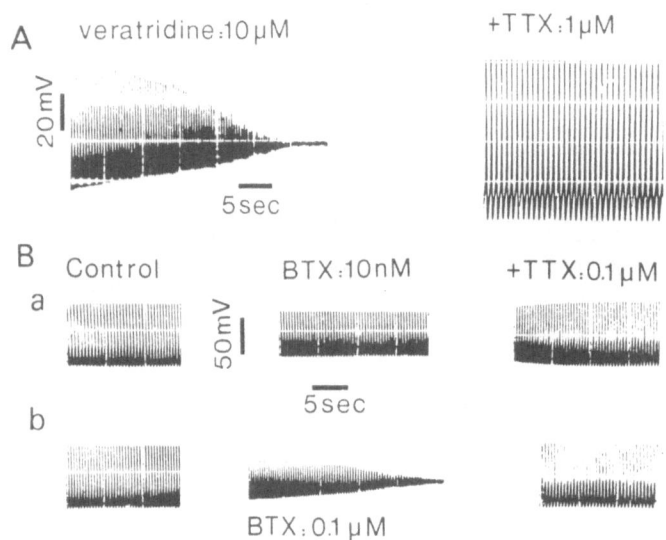

FIGURE 2 Effects of veratridine and batrachotoxin (BTX) on 3-day aggregates kept 2 days in culture. A: effect of veratridine (10 µM). Left: after 2 min, the electrical activity was blocked by excessive depolarization. Right: 10 min after the addition of 1 µM TTX to the medium containing 10 µM veratridine, the electrical activity was recovered but with a lower beating frequency. B: effect of batrachotoxin 10 nM (a) and 0.1 µM (b). Left: control. Middle: (a) 40 min after the addition of the toxin; (b) 2 min after the addition of the toxin, the electrical activity was blocked by excessive depolarization. Right: the initial electrical activity was recovered in a and b after the addition of 0.1 µM TTX to the medium containing 10 nM and 0.1 µM batrachotoxin.

Veratridine and batrachotoxin also have receptors in 3-day aggregates (Fig. 2). Both toxins block electrical activity by excessive depolarisation; addition of TTX after veratridine or batrachotoxin can restore the initial electrical activity.

The development of Na^+ channels in embryonic cardiac cells can also be followed in vitro (Nathan and DeHaan, 1978). The evolution of the $\dot{V}_{max}$ during in vitro differentiation of the fast Na^+ channel with both ATX_{II} and TTX is shown in Fig. 3 and Table II. Results are similar to those previously described for the in vivo differentiation of the fast Na^+ channel. Values for $\dot{V}_{max}$ recorded at different stages of development both in ovo and in vivo, in the absence and presence of neurotoxins, are indicated in Table I. These latter results indicates that an adult-like behavior corresponds to $\dot{V}_{max} > 90$ V/s, a value which can be reduced by TTX to less than 15 V/s. Using this criterion, the data indicate that the in ovo development of fast Na^+ channels is essentially achieved in embryonic heart cells after 7 days of incubation. In the in vitro experiments, aggregates formed from 3-day-old cells reach an adult-like behavior after 5 days in culture. ATX_{II} increases $\dot{V}_{max}$ by a factor of two at the early stage of development, when $\dot{V}_{max}$ in the control is TTX-insensitive. This ATX_{II}-induced increase of $\dot{V}_{max}$ gradually disappears with the culture duration and is absent when the control $\dot{V}_{max}$ reaches an adult-like value of 80-90 V/s.

The in vitro differentiation of the fast Na^+ channel is completely prevented by cycloheximide at 20 μg/ml, a concentration which blocks protein synthesis in these cells (Table II). Cycloheximide arrests development in cardiac aggregates at the early stage of development, since values of $\dot{V}_{max}$ in the control and in neurotoxin-treated cells are essentially the same for 3-day aggregates after 2 days in culture and for those maintained 4 days in culture in the presence of cycloheximide.

These results indicate that the membrane of 3-day-old embryonic heart cells contains Na^+ channels in a "silent" form. These "silent" channels are not electrically excitable, but are chemically excitable by a variety of neurotoxins (ATX_{II}, veratridine, batrachotoxin) which are known to slow down or to remove the Na^+ inactivation process. This type of Na^+ channel has already been described for non impulsive cells (Lowe et al., 1978; Romey et al., 1979).

The presence of silent Na^+ channels that cannot be activated electrically

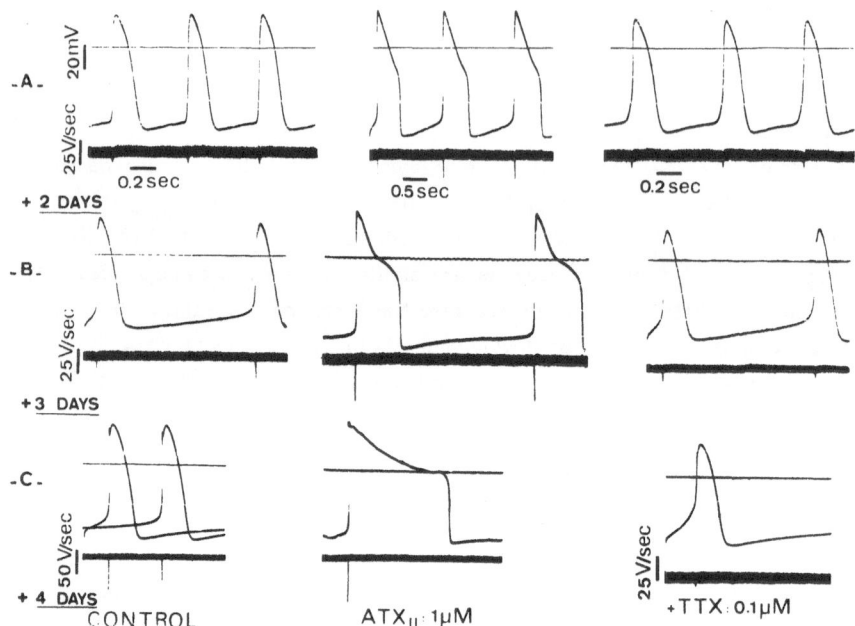

FIGURE 3. *Electrical activity of cardiac cells from 3-day-old chick embryos cultured for (A) 2 days, (B) 3 days and (C) 4 days. Left: control. Middle: effect of 1 μM ATX$_{II}$-treated aggregates. Right: effect of 0,1 μM TTX on ATX$_{II}$-treated aggregates. In A: left and right, spontaneous activity; middle, evoked activity. In B: left and right evoked activity; middle, spontaneous activity. In C: left, spontaneous and evoked action potentials; middle, spontaneous action potential; right, evoked action potential. In each record, the higher trace is the zero voltage line and the lower trace gives dV/dt.*

TABLE II

Days in culture	2	3 $\dot{V}_{max}(V/s)$	4	5
Control	12±3	26±5	60±5 *12±3	90±6
ATX$_{II}$(1 μM)	25±4	42±5	82±6 *23±4	95±7
ATX$_{II}$ + TTX (1 μM) (0.1 μM)	12±3	11±2	9±2 *10±1	6±1

*After 2 days of incubation in presence of cyclohexi-mide (20 μg/ml). All values are mean ± SE of 20 to 30 measurements.

but that can be "unmasked" by ATX_{II} is confirmed by voltage-clamp analysis carried out with aggregates from 3- and 11-day-old embryonic hearts, (Fig. 4).
ATX_{II} (1 µM) provokes a significant increase of the peak inward current that is
sensitive to TTX in aggregates from 3-day-old embryonic hearts after 3 days in
culture (we have been unable to test the same aggregates after only 2 days in
culture). This increase is of the order of 50% as compared to 15% only for
11-day-old aggregates after 3 days in culture.

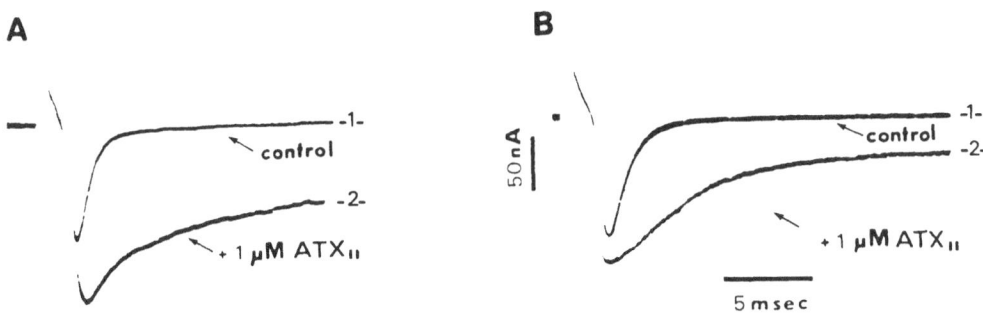

FIGURE 4 *Voltage clamp analysis of ATX_{II} action on the transient inward current
of cardiac cells cultured in aggregate form. A. Aggregate from 3-day-old embryonic heart cultured for 3 days. The aggregates were preincubated with 1 µM
D600 to block the slow Ca^{2+}/Na^+ channel. The membrane potential was clamped at
-30 mV after a step change from a holding potential of -70 mV. (1) Control;
(2) After 5 min exposure to 1 µM ATX_{II}, note the substantial increase of the
peak inward current (50%) and the decreased rate of inactivation. B. Aggregate
from 11-day-old embryonic heart cultured for 2 days. (1) Control, same procedure as in A; (2) 5 min after exposure to 1 µM ATX_{II}. The effect of ATX_{II} was
an increase of the peak inward current (15%) and a decrease of the inactivation
rate of the inward current. The increase of the peak inward current is less
pronounced for the 11-day-old stage than for the 3-day-old stage.*

Tritiated etylenediamine-tetrodotoxin ([³H]en-TTX) is a highly radiolabelled derivative of TTX which associates to the tetrodotoxin itself (Chicheportiche et al., 1980). The binding properties of [³H]en-TTX on cardiac homogenates have been previously characterized (Lombet et al., 1980). Inset Fig. 5
shows the binding properties of [³H]en-TTX to the TTX receptor of cardiac cells
from 11-day-old chick embryos. Specific binding to these cells is a saturable

process and the half maximal saturation of the receptor is observed around 1.6 nM. Fig. 5A shows Scatchard plots for the specific association of $[^3H]$ en-TTX to intact heart homogenates, to monolayers and aggregates in culture. The linearity of Scatchard plots demonstrates that $[^3H]$ en-TTX binds to a single class of sites. Under these conditions maximal binding capacities (BM) and dissociation constants (K_D) are similar for monolayers, aggregated heart cells and fresh non-cultured hearts from 11-day-old chick embryos (Fig. 5A).

TABLE III

Age in ovo (days)	3	6	11	14	16	21
B_M (fmol/mg protein)	16	28±3	60±6	80±5	62±4	100±10
K_D (nM)		1.3	1.6	1.8	1.6	3.8
n_H		0.9	1.1	1.1	1.2	

	Days after plating in vitro					
Aggregates	1	2	3	4	6	4 monolayers
B_M (fmol/mg protein)	42±4	43±4		41±4	42±3	60±9
K_D (nM)	1.9	1.5	–	0.8	0.9	1.5
n_H	0.9	1.1	–	1.0	1.2	0.9

Fig. 5B and Table III show that the maximal number of binding sites for $[^3H]$ en-TTX increase during the course of development in ovo. Moreover, the TTX receptor is already present very early, at the third day of development, thereby confirming that the Na^+ channel exists in the young embryonic heart prior to detectable TTX sensitivity.

All the previous data taken together indicate (i) that Na^+ channels seen as receptors for TTX are present very early (at 3 days in ovo) during the embryonic development (ii) that the number of TTX receptors increases about 6 times between day 3 and day 21 in ovo (iii) that the properties of the TTX receptor (number of sites and affinity) are essentially the same in aggregate cultures from 11-day-old ventricles which are totally sensitive to TTX with regard to beating properties, and in monolayer cultures, from the same 11-day-old ventricles, which are largely insensitive to TTX. (iv) that the small number of TTX binding sites which are present in embryonic hearts at the earliest stages of

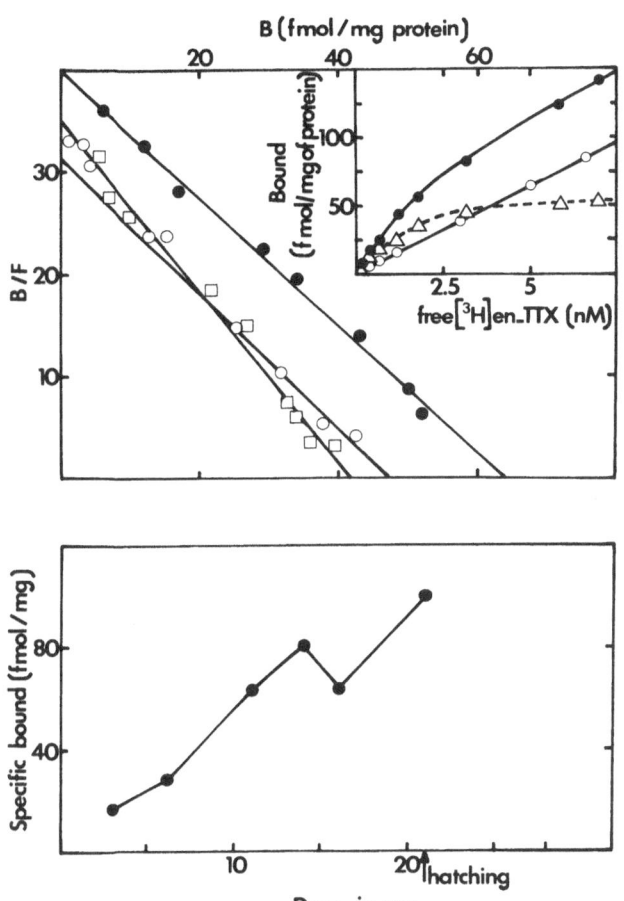

FIGURE 5 Binding of $[^3H]$en-TTX to embryonic heart cells. A. Scatchard plots computed from specific $[^3H]$en-TTX binding to 11-day-old ventricle homogenates (●) and to homogenates of monolayers (○) and aggregates (□) obtained from 11-day-old embryonic heart cells cultured during 4 days. B/F is the ratio of bound over free ligand and B is bound ligand. Inset: Binding of $[^3H]$en-TTX to 11-day-old ventricle homogenates. Total $[^3H]$en-TTX binding (●) and non-specific binding (○) were made in parallel in the absence and presence of 5 μM TTX. Specific binding (△) is represented in dotted line, calculated by subtracting non-specific from total binding. In this typical example, constant of dissociation (K_D) and maximum binding capacity (B_M) values of 1.6 nM and 62 fmol/mg protein were obtained respectively. B. Evolution of the number of $[^3H]$en-TTX binding sites are given for hearts from 3 to 21 days of development (●).

development belong to the Na$^+$ channels which are in a silent form i.e. to channels that cannot be activated electrically but that can be revealed by toxins like veratridine, batrachotoxine or ATX$_{II}$ which affect the gating system of the Na$^+$ channel (v) that the physiological development of a fast Na$^+$ channel during heart ontogenesis is due both to the transformation of the silent form into a functional form of the Na$^+$ channel and to an increase of the total number of Na$^+$ channels.

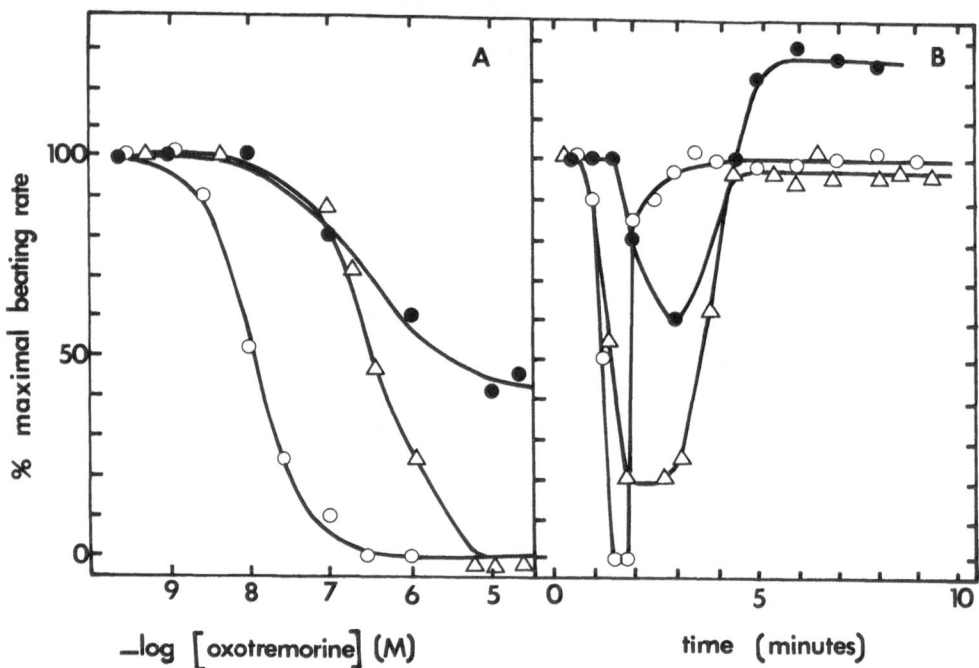

FIGURE 6 *Action of oxotremorine on the rate of beating of developing chick embryonic heart. Beatings were recorded with an electro-optical device, previously described by Fayet et al., 1974, and calculated every 15-30 s. A. Dose-response curves for oxotremorine on 3 (●), 6 (△) and 11-day-old (○) chick embryonic hearts. B. Desensitization of the response to 1 μM oxotremorine on 3 (●), 6(△) and 11-day-old (○) chick embryonic hearts. Beating rate was plotted as percentage of control rate at a given concentration of oxotremorine. All these effects were blocked by 1 μM atropine. Each point represents the average of values obtained with 4 hearts.*

COMPARATIVE PROPERTIES OF THE IN OVO AND IN VITRO
DIFFERENTIATION OF THE MUSCARINIC CHOLINERGIC RECEPTOR
IN EMBRYONIC HEART CELLS

In the chick embryo, the heart starts contracting spontaneously at the 9th somite stage (33–38 hr after fertilization (Romanoff, 1960)).

At this early stage of development the chick heart is susceptible to chemical and electrical stimuli. Vagal innervation of the myocardium does not occur until after 5 days of development and onset of functional cholinergic neurotransmission does not take place until the 11th day in ovo (Pappano and Loeffelholz, 1974). It has been shown that the cardioinhibitory effects of acetylcholine both in early and late embryonic stages may be blocked by atropine a muscarinic cholinergic antagonist (Coraboeuf et al., 1970; Loeffelholz and Pappano, 1974; Pappano and Loeffelholz, 1974). This suggests the presence of muscarinic cholinergic receptors in the developing chick even prior to detectable cardiac innervation. The sensitivity of embryonic heart to oxotremorine increases with age (Fig. 6A). Changes in sensitivity to oxotremorine are accompanied by changes in rates of activation and desensitization of the muscarinic receptor (Fig. 6B). The onset of oxotremorine action as well as the desensitization process are more rapid in older than younger embryonic hearts and desensitization is accompanied by a significant positive chronotropic effect of oxotremorine in 3-day-old heart (Fig. 6B). All these effects are blocked by 1 μM atropine. The previously reported insensitivity of cardiac cells cultured in form of monolayer to acetylcholine (Sperelakis and Lehmkuhl, 1965) is also found with oxotremorine (Fig. 7A).

In contrast, aggregated cardiac cells from 3- and 11-day-old chick embryos respond by a negative chronotropic effect to oxotremorine application. This effect is completely suppressed by application of 1 μM atropine. However, a difference in sensitivity to oxotremorine persists between the 3- and 11-day-old aggregates cultured 3 days. Half maximal inhibition (ID_{50}) being 0.3 μM and 0.004 μM respectively (Fig. 7A). The desensitization process is faster for 11-day-old than for 3-day-old aggregates ((Fig. 7B).

When 11-day-old embryonic hearts are cultured in form of aggregates their sensitivity to acetylcholine after only 2 days in culture is very similar to that of the 3-day-old heart (Fig. 8A). A reversion of the acetylcholine sensi-

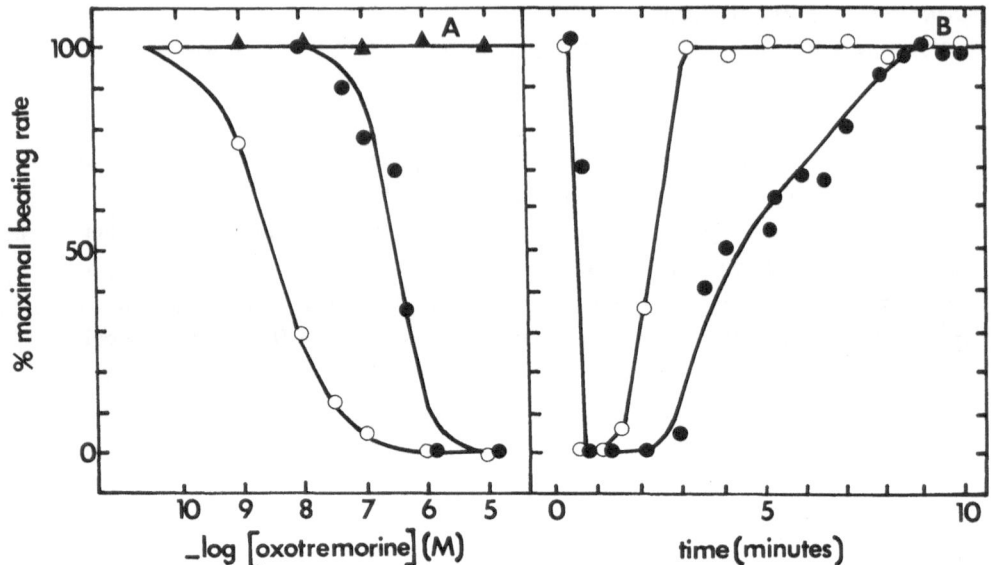

FIGURE 7   *Action of oxotremorine on the rate of beating of cultured cardiac cells. Cardiac cells in culture were obtained according to Renaud, 1980. A. Dose-response curves for oxotremorine on heart cells cultures as aggregates from 3 (●) and 11-day-old (O) chick embryos and monolayers (▲) from 11-day-old chick embryos. All cells were kept 3 days in culture before experiments. Oxotremorine triggers a negative chronotropic effect and stops the beat at 1 μM with 3-day-old aggregates and 0.3 μM with 11-day-old aggregates respectively. Conversely, monolayers were insensitive to oxotremorine. B. Desensitization of the response to 1 μM oxotremorine on 3-day-old (●) and 11-day-old (O) heart cells cultured in the form of aggregates during 3 days. The beating rate at a given concentration of oxotremorine was plotted as percentage of the control rate. All these effects were blocked by 1 μM atropine. Each point represents an average of values obtained with 5-7 hearts. Negative chronotropic effects were only recorded from aggregates having a diameter of 80 to 120 μM with spontaneous rate of beating ranging between 100 and 120 beats/min at 37 °C.*

tivity from the late to the early embryonic stage of development has clearly occured. Then, when the same aggregates are kept in culture over long enough periods of time, they gradually develop an increased sensitivity to acetylcholine showing that a differentiation of the acetylcholine response occurs in culture. The ID_{50} value for the action of the acetylcholine decreases by a factor of 200 between day 3 and day 10 in culture (Fig. 8A). The gradual increase of the sensitivity of aggregates to acetylcholine during differentiation in culture is

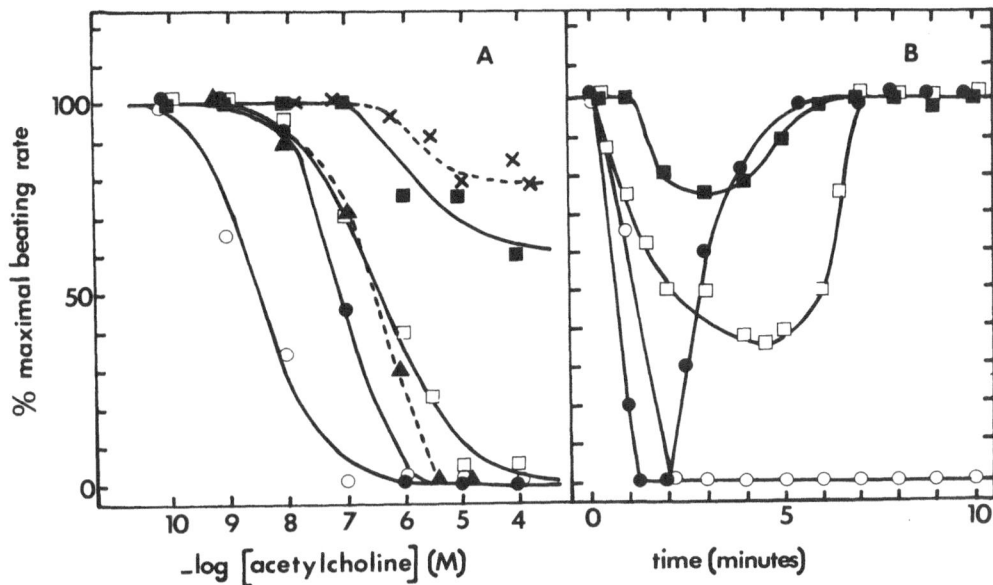

FIGURE 8 *Action of acetylcholine on 11-day-old chick embryonic hearts aggregates and intact hearts. A. Dose-response curve of intact hearts (dotted lines) from 3 (✖) and 11-day-old (▲) chick embryos and from aggregates after 2 (■), 3 (□), 4(●) and 10 days (○) in culture.*
B. Desensitization of the response to 1 μM acetylcholine on aggregates after 2 (■), 3 (□), 4 (◗) and 10 days (○) in culture. Experiments were carried out in the presence of 10 M eserine. Each point represents the average of values obtained with 5-7 aggregates and 4 hearts.

accompanied by changes in the desensitization properties (Fig. 8B). The negative chronotropic effect of muscarinic agents has been associated with changes in K^+ permeability (Mallart and Trautmann, 1973; Pappano, 1972). Then it may be that the maturation of functional muscarinic system is linked to the development of an adequate permeability for K^+. Young hearts have a very low K^+ permability and this increases markedly so that, at about day 12, the final adult value is attained (Carmeliet et al., 1975; Sperelakis et al., 1975).

It has been proposed that the chronotropic effect of muscarinic agents could be associated with an elevation of cyclic GMP levels (George et al., 1970; Lee et al., 1972). The intracellular level of cyclic GMP is not changed by high concentrations of muscarinic agonists in embryonic hearts taken

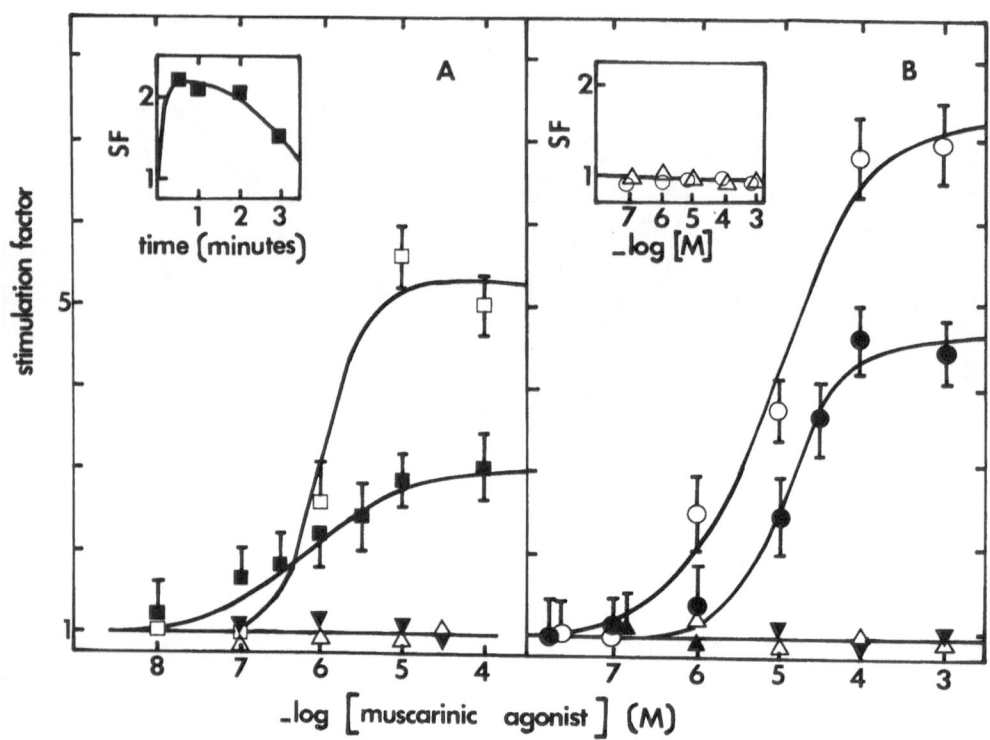

FIGURE 9 *Effect of muscarinic agonists on cyclic GMP content of intact chick embryonic hearts and heart cells in culture. A. Dose-response curves for oxotremorine on 3 (△), 6 (▼), 11 (●) and 16-day-old (□) chick embryonic hearts. Inset: Time course of cyclic GMP accumulation when 11-day-old chick embryonic hearts are treated with 1 µM oxotremorine. B. Dose-response curves for carbamylcholine on 3 (△), 6 (▼), 11 (●) and 16-day-old (○) intact chick embryonic hearts. Inset: Effects of oxotremorine and carbamylcholine on monolayers (○) and aggregated heart cells (△) obtained from 11-day-old chick embryonic hearts and kept 3 days in culture. SF means stimulation factor. Each point represent the average of 5 experiments. Vertical bars indicate the standard error (+ S.E.). Cyclic GMP contents were determined according to Delaage et al., 1975, by a radio immunoassay method. Proteins were determined by the method of Hartree, 1972, using bovine serum albumine as a standard.*

before 6 days of incubation. For hearts taken at 11 and 16 days of incubation both oxotremorine and carbamylcholine give an substantial increase (3 to 7.5 times) in the cyclic GMP content of the intact hearts (Fig. 9A and 9B). However, the negative chronotropic effect of carbamylcholine or oxotremorine in aggregates from 11-day-old hearts is not accompanied by a stimulation of the intracellular amount of cyclic GMP (inset Fig. 9B). This latter observation is of particular importance since it shows that the increase of cyclic GMP level triggered by the action of muscarinic agonists on cardiac cells is not essential for the production of the negative chronotropic effect and it is very unlikely that the transition from the physiologically unresponsive to the physiologically responsive state of the cardiac cell is due to the coupling between the muscarinic receptor which merely binds acetylcholine or its agonists and the enzyme system which regulates cyclic GMP levels. If such a coupling were essential for the maturation of the muscarinic response, it should also be observed during the in vitro differentiation of cardiac aggregates.

The most widely used radiolabelled ligand for biochemical studies of the muscarinic receptor is a very potent muscarinic antagonist, quinuclidinyl benzylate ($[^3H]$QNB).

The specific binding of $[^3H]$QNB to monolayers and aggregates is a saturable process (Fig. 10A); half maximum saturation ($K_{0.5}$) of the muscarinic receptor is observed at 0.4 nM $[^3H]$QNB and 0.9 nM $[^3H]$QNB at 37 °C for monolayers and aggregates respectively. Scatchard plots for the specific association of $[^3H]$QNB to aggregates and monolayers give maximum binding capacity of 170 and 500 fmol $[^3H]$QNB specifically bound per mg of cell protein (Fig. 10B). The Hill coefficient is 1.0 and 1.1 respectively indicating no cooperativity. The relative potency of cholinergic agents in displacing $[^3H]$QNB binding from monolayers and aggregates are quite similar (Fig. 11). Muscarinic agonists are less potent to displace than muscarinic antagonists. Binding of antagonists is characterized by Hill coefficient near 1., whereas values for agonists binding are significantly less than 1.0 as previously observed in other biological systems (Birdsall et al., 1978; Young, 1974) and in heart (Cavey et al., 1977; Field et al., 1978). The biochemical properties of the muscarinic receptor in terms of Hill coefficient and affinity of binding to muscarinic agonists and antagonists are nearly the same for aggregates and monolayers. However, the maximal binding capacity for monolayers and aggregates are different (Fig. 10). The

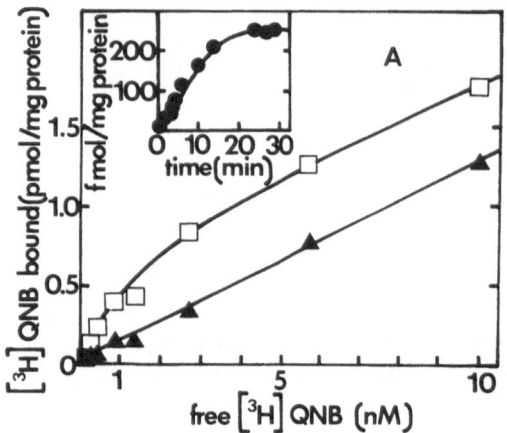

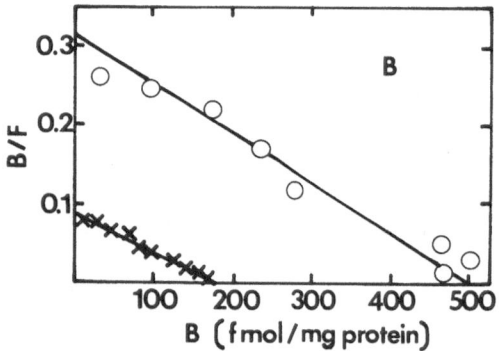

FIGURE 10 Binding of $[^3H]QNB$ to heart cells in culture. A. Increasing amount of $[^3H]QNB$ were incubated 40 min at 37° C with monolayers obtained from 11-day-old heart cells. The experiment was first carried out in the absence of atropine to measure the total binding capacity (□). Then in the presence of 10 M atropine to measure the nonspecific binding (▲), the specific binding being measured by the difference between the two curves. Inset: time course of the specific association of 0.9 nM $[^3H]QNB$ binding to monolayers. B. Scatchard plots computed from specific $[^3H]QNB$ binding to monolayers (O) and to homogenates of aggregates (✕) obtained from 11-day-old heart cells cultured during 3 days. B/F is the ratio specific of bound over free ligand and B is bound ligang. The nonspecific binding of $[^3H]QNB$ to homogenates of aggregates never exceeded 5% of the total binding capacity.

maximal number of binding sites for $[^3H]QNB$ and the dissociation constant of the QNB muscarinic receptor complex do not vary significantly in the course of the maturation in culture of aggregates (Fig. 12). Also, the maximal number of binding sites for $[^3H]QNB$ is not significantly different for embryonic hearts taken between 3 and 16 days of development (Fig. 12). This latter finding confirms the observations reported by Galper et al., 1977 and disagrees with those reported by Sastre et al., 1977.

It is not yet possible to describe in detail the molecular differences between a functional and a non-functional muscarinic receptor. However, the rate of degradation of the muscarinic receptor in embryonic cardiac cells in mo-

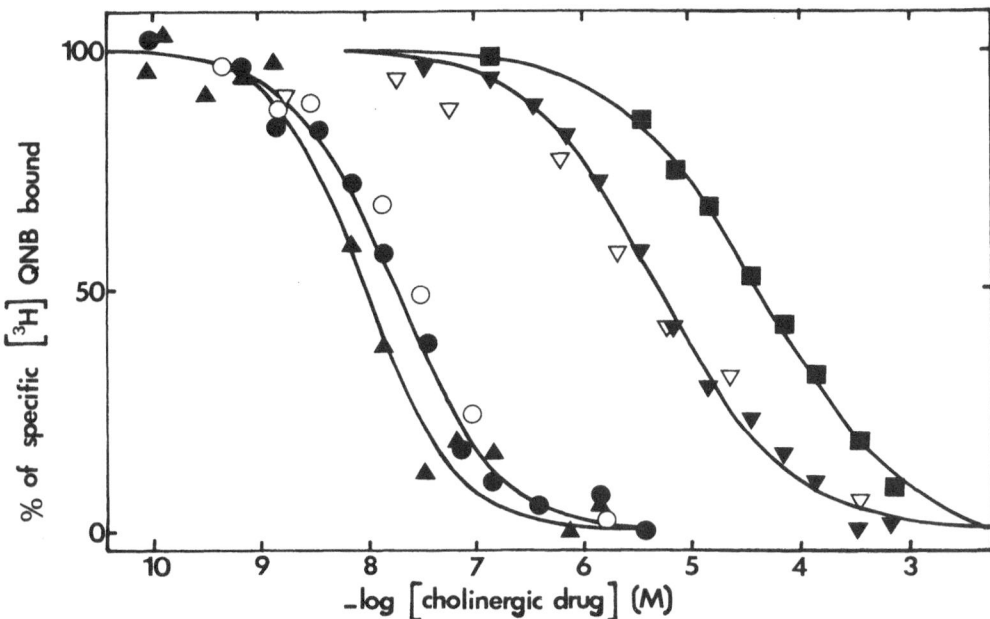

FIGURE 11 *Displacement of $[^3H]$QNB by various concentrations of muscarinic agonists and antagonists on 11-day-old embryonic heart cells cultured 3 days. 0.4 and 0.9 nM $[^3H]$QNB were respectively incubated 35 min at 37 °C with homogenate of aggregates (open symbols) and monolayers (black symbols) in the presence of the indicated concentration of muscarinic agents. Scopolamine (▲), atropine (●,○), oxotremorine (▼,▽) and pilocarpine (■). Specific $[^3H]$QNB binding compared to total binding was 65-70% with monolayers and 95% with homogenates of aggregates. Each point is the average of duplicate experiments.*

nolayer and aggregate culture suggests that the two forms of receptors exhibit different properties of degradation.

The non-functional muscarinic receptor in monolayers of cardiac cells is not very stable in culture once protein synthesis has been blocked; it is degraded with half-time of 14 hr. Under identical conditions, the functional muscarinic receptor in cardiac aggregates remains perfectly stable over a period of 20 hr (Fig. 13). A parallel may be made between the properties of degradation of the muscarinic receptor in cardiac cells and those of the nicotinic receptor of skeletal muscle. Junctional and extrajunctional nicotinic receptors appear

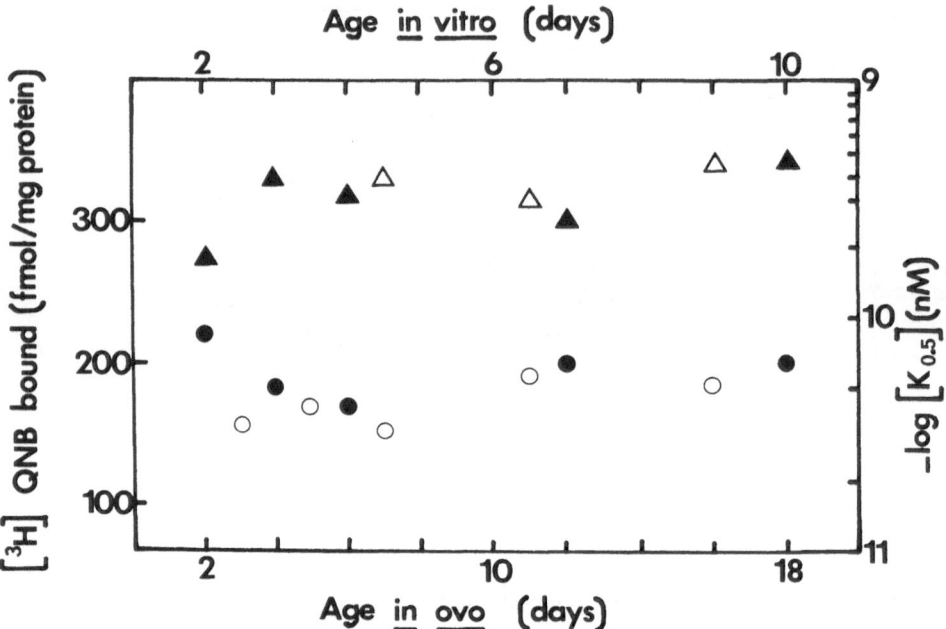

FIGURE 12 Evolution of the properties of muscarinic receptors in the intact embryonic chick hearts and aggregated cells in culture. Values of number of sites
are given for hearts from 3 to 16 days of development (O) and for aggregated
cells from 11-day-old embryonic hearts (●) at 2, 3, 4 and 10 days of culture and
$K_{0.5}$ values for hearts: (△), and for aggregates: (▲). Maximal number of sites
for $[^3H]QNB$ were computed from Scatchard plots. When the Hill number is 1.0,
$K_{0.5}$ is calculated from the ED_{50} value by the formula:

$$ED_{50} = K_{0.5} \ (1 + [QNB]/K_{QNB})$$

where $[QNB]$ is the concentration of free $[^3H]QNB$ at half dissociation and K_{QNB} is
the dissociation constant of the QNB-heart membrane complex (Cavey et al.,
1977).

to be similar but distinct molecules, they have differences in their isoelectric
points and differences of affinities for nicotinic agents like d-tubocurarine
(Brockes and Hall, 1975), the half-time of degradation of extra-junctional nicotinic receptor is 8-10 hr and of junctional receptor is approximatively 6 days.
The stability of an extra-junctional receptor is clearly comparable to the stability of a non-functional muscarinic receptor. The stability of a junctional
receptor is comparable to that of a physiologically active muscarinic receptor.
It is conceivable that the existence of a physiologically inactive (or nearly

inactive) muscarinic receptor in cardiac cell monolayers and younger embryonic hearts is simply due to inadequate kinetics of the activation desensitization system of the muscarinic receptor. If desensitization is much faster than activation no physiological response will be observed.

Differentiation of a physiological response to muscarinic agents seems to be clearly linked to molecular events which occur after ligand binding to the muscarinic receptor. It does not seem that a coupling between agonist binding and guanylate cyclase stimulation is necessarily involved.

CONCLUSION

In chick embryonic heart cells the degree of functionality of the sodium channel follows that observed for the muscarinic receptor (i) in monolayers of cardiac cells when there is no sensitivity to acetylcholine or to its agonists, there is no sensitivity to tetrodotoxin (Sperelakis and Lehmkuhl, 1965) (ii) cardiac cells cultivated as aggregates retain the properties of sensitivity to tetrodotoxin found in the embryonic hearts from which they were isolated (McLean and Sperelakis, 1976; Romey et al., 1980) (iii) an in vitro development of the sodium channel has been obtained. It has been seen (Renaud et al., 1980) that the absence of muscarinic response did not mean an absence of a muscarinic receptor. Similarly, the absence of a functionally active fast sodium channel does not mean that the machinery of the channel is absent in the membrane. It has been shown in fact that the receptors of toxins specific for the fast sodium channel (tetrodotoxin, veratridine, sea anemone toxin) are present even when the channel is not physiologically expressed (Romey et al., 1979; Romey et al., 1980). It is suggested that the absence of functionality of the fast sodium channel at the early stage of embryonic development or in culture (in form of monolayer) is due to kinetics of inactivation (closing process) of the channel which are faster than kinetics of activation (opening process). Then, the immature or "silent" sodium channel would in a way resemble a desensitized state for a muscarinic receptor. Maturation in the case of the fast sodium channel would make inactivation kinetics slower than activation kinetics. This maturation

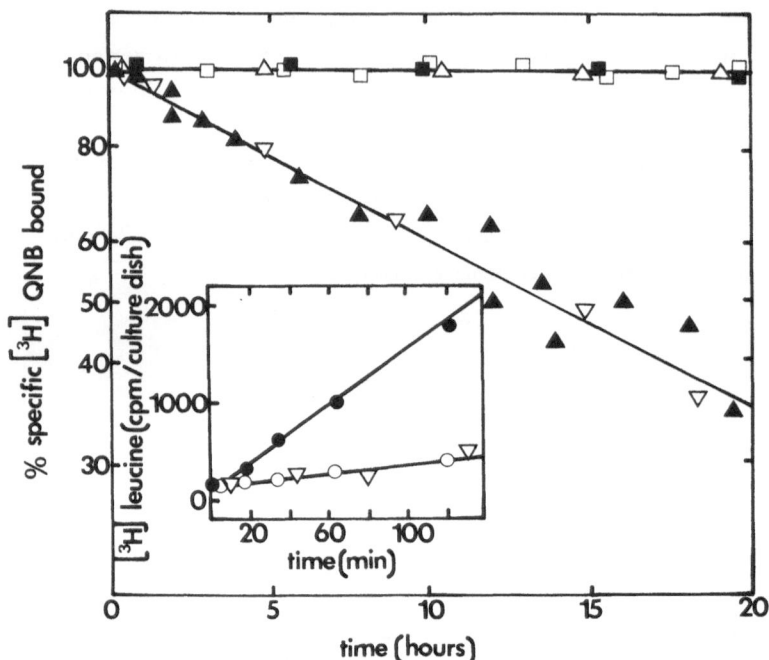

FIGURE 13 *Rate of degradation of the muscarinic receptor in 11-day-old chick em-bryonic heart cells cultured 4 days in form of monolayer and aggregate. Monolayers (▲,△,▽) and aggregates (■,□) were incubated in complete growth medium with (▲,■) or without (△,▽) cycloheximide (20 µg/ml) at 37 °C or with puromycin (▽) at 20 µg/ml. 0.9 nM [³H]QNB was used for binding. Specifically bound [³H]QNB was determined as usual. Inset: Incorporation of [³H]leucine (0.25 µCi) in the absence (●) or in the presence of cycloheximide (20 µg/ml) (O) or of puromycin (20 µg/ml) (▽) in monolayers of cardiac cells. The effects of puromycin and cycloheximide on protein synthesis were measured using techniques developed by Devreotis and Fambrough, 1975, in their studies of the cholinergic nicotinic receptor.*

would occur in parallel with the biosythesis of new Na$^+$ channels in ovo.

Finally, the fact that one can obtain an in vitro differentiation of the muscarinic response to acetylcholine and of a sensitivity to tetrodotoxin of the fast sodium channel are direct indication that innervation is not necessary for the development and the maintenance of acetylcholine and tetrodotoxin sensitivity in the embryonic heart. One last conclusion is that the biochemical detection of binding sites for [³H]QNB or [³H]en-TTX does not provide any information

about the presence or absence of a physiological cholinergic response and   of   a
fast sodium channel functionality.

ACKNOWLEDGMENTS

This work was supported by the Centre National de la Recherche Scientifique,   by
the   Institut National de la Santé et de la Recherche Médicale (Grants 78.1.0665
and 80.30.10) and by the Fondation pour la Recherche Médicale. The authors   are
grateful to M.T.   Ravier and M.C.   Lenoir for their expert technical assistance.

REFERENCES

Beress, L., Beress, R.   and Wunderer, G.:   Purification   of   three   polypeptides
    with   neuro and cardiotoxic activity from the sea anemone Anemonia sulcata.
    Toxicon, 13:   359-367, 1975.

Bergman, G., Dubois, J.M., Rojas, E.   and Rathmayer, W.:   Decreased rate of   so-
    dium   conductance inactivation in the node of Ranvier induced by a polypep-
    tide toxin from sea anemone.   Biochem.   Biophy.   Acta., 455:   173-184,
    1976.

Birdsall, N.J.M., Burgen, A.S.V.   and Hulme, E.C.:   The binding of   agonists   to
    brain muscarinic receptors.   Mol.   Pharmacol., 14:   723-736, 1978.

Brockes, J.P.   and Hall, Z.W.:   Acetylcholine receptors in normal and denervated
    rat   diaphragm muscle II: comparison of junctional and extrajunctional re-
    ceptors.   Biochemistry, 14:   2100-2106, 1975.

Carmeliet, E., Horres, C.R., Lieberman, M.   and Vereecke, J.S.:   Potassium   per-
    meability in the chick heart: change with age external K, and valinomycin.
    In: Developmental   and   Physiological   Correlates   of   Cardiac   Muscle.
    Lieberman, M.   and   Sano,   T., eds., Raven Press, New York, pp.   103-116,
    1975.

Cavey, D., Vincent, J.P. and Lazdunski, M.: The muscarinic receptor of heart cell membranes: Association with agonists, antagonists and antiarrhythmic agents. FEBS Lett., 84: 110-114, 1977.

Chicheportiche, R., Balerna, M. Lombet, A., Romey, G. and Lazdunksi, M.: Synthesis of new highly radioactive tetrodotoxin derivatives and their binding properties to the sodium channel. Eur. J. Biochem., 104: 617-625, 1980.

Coraboeuf, E., Obrecht-Coutris, G. and Le Douarin, G.: Acetylcholine and the embryonic heart. Amer. J. Cardiol., 25: 285-291, 1970.

Delaage, M., Roux, D. and Cailla, H.L.: Recent advances in cyclic nocleotide radioimmunoassay. In: Nato Advanced Study Institute on Cyclic Nocleotides, Paoletti, R., ed., Elsevier-North-Holland Biomedical Press, Amsterdam, 1977.

Devreotis, P.N., and Fambrough, D.M.: Acetylcholine receptor turnover in membranes of developing muscle fibers. J. Cell Biol., 65: 335-358, 1975.

Fayet, G., Couraud, F., Miranda, F. and Lissitzky, S.: Electro-optical system for monitoring activity of heart cells in culture: Application to the study of several drugs and scorpion toxin. Eur. J. Pharmac., 27: 165-174, 1974.

Fields, J.Z., Roeske, W.R., Morkin, E. and Yamamura, H.I.: Cardiac muscarinic cholinergic receptors: Biochemical identification and characterization. J. Biol. Chem., 253: 3251-3258, 1978.

Galper, J.B., Klein, W. and Catterall, W.A.: Muscarinic acetylcholine receptors in developing chick heart. J. Biol. Chem., 23: 8692-8699, 1977.

George, W.J., Polson, J.B., O'Toole, A.G. and Goldberg, N.D.: Elevation of guanosine 3', 5'-cyclic phosphate in rate heart after perfusion with acetylcholine. Proc. Natl. Acad. Sci. USA, 66: 398-403, 1970.

Hartree, E.F.: Determination of protein: a modification of the lowry method that gives a linear photometric response. Anal. Biochem., 48: 422-427, 1972.

Higgings, C.B., Vatner, S.F. and Braunwald, E.: Parasympathetic control of the heart. Pharmacol. Rev., 25: 119-155, 1973.

Kohlhardt, M., Bauer, B., Krause, H. and Fleckenstein, A.: Differentiation of the transmembrane Na and Ca channels in mammalian cardiac fibers by use of specific inhibitors. Pfluegers Arch., 335: 309-322, 1972.

Lee, J.P., Kuo, J.F. and Greengard, P.: Role of muscarinic cholinergic receptors in regulation of guanosine 3', 5'. Monophosphate content in mammalian brain, heart muscle and intestinal smooth muscle. Proc. Natl. Acad. Sci. USA, 69: 3287-3291, 1972.

Loeffelholz, K. and Pappano, A.J.: Ontogenetic changes in pacemaker activity in chick. J. Pharmacol. Exp. Ther., 191: 479-486, 1974.

Lombet, A., Renaud, J.F., Chicheportiche, R. and Lazdunski, M.: A cardiac tetrodotoxin-binding component: biochemical identification, characterization and properties. Biochemistry 20: 1279-1285, 1981.

Lowe, D.A., Bush, B.M.H. and Ripley, S.H.: Pharmacological evidence for "fast" sodium channels in nonspiking neurones. Nature, 274: 289-290, 1978.

Mallart, A. and Trautmann, A.: Ionic properties of the neuromuscular junction of the frog; effects of denervation and pH. J. Physiol. (London), 234: 553-567, 1973.

McDonald, T.F., Sachs, H.G. and De Haan, R.L.: Development of sensitivity to tetrodotoxin in beating chick embryo hearts, single cells and aggregates. Science, 176: 1248-1250, 1972.

McLean, M.J. and Sperelakis, N.: Retention of fully differentiated electrophysiological properties of chick embryonic heart cells in culture. Devel. Biol., 50: 134-141, 1976.

Nathan, R.D. and De Haan, R.L.: In vitro differentiation of fast Na^+ conductance in embryonic heart cell aggregates. Proc. Natl. Acad. Sci. USA, 75: 2776-2780, 1978.

Ohta, M., Naharashi, T. and Keeler, R.F.: Effects of veratrum alkaloids on membrane potential and conductance of squid and crayfish giant axons. J. Pharmacol. Exp. Ther., 184: 143-154, 1973.

Pappano, A.J.: Sodium-dependent depolarization of non-innervated embryonic chick heart by acetylcholine. J. Pharmacol. Exp. Ther., 180: 340-350, 1972.

Pappano, A.J. and Loeffelholz, K.: Ontogenesis of adrenergic and cholinergic neuroeffector transmission in chick embryo heart. J. Pharmacol. Exp. Ther., 191: 468-478, 1974.

Rathamayer, W. and Beress, L.: The effect of toxins from Anemonia sulcata (coelenterata) on neuromuscular transmission and nerve action potentials in the crayfish (Astacus Leptodactylus). J. Comp. Physiol., 109: 373-382,

628 M. Lazdunski **et al.**

1976.

Renaud, J.F.: Use of cell cultures as tool to elucidate physiological, pharmacological and biochemical membrane properties of the embryonic heart. Biol. Cellulaire, 37: 97-104, 1980.

Renaud, J.F., Barhanin, J., Cavey, D., Fosset, M. and Lazdunski, M.: Comparative properties of in ovo and in vitro differentiation of the muscarinic cholinergic receptor in embryonic heart cells. Devel. Biol., 78: 184-200, 1980.

Reuter, H.: Divalent cations as charge carriers in excitable membranes. Prog. Biophys. Mol. Biol., 26: 1-43, 1973.

Romanoff, A.L.: In: The Avian Embryo: Structure and Functional Development, McMillan Company, New York, 1960.

Romey, G. and Lazdunski, M.: Scorpion and sea anemone neurotoxins actions on axonal membrane. 5th International Biophysics Congress, Copenhagen, 503, 1975.

Romey, G., Abita, J.P., Schweitz, H., Wunderer, G. and Lazdunski, M.: Sea anemone toxin: a tool to study molecular mechanisms of nerve conduction and excitation-secretion coupling. Proc. Natl. Acad. Sci. USA, 73: 4055-4059, 1976.

Romey, G., Jacques, Y., Schweitz, H., Fosset, M. and Lazdunksi, M.: The sodium channel in non-impulsive cells. Interaction with specific neurotoxins. Biochim. Biophys. Acta, 556: 344-353, 1979.

Romey, G., Renaud, J.F., Fosset, M. and Lazdunksi, M.: Pharmacological properties of the interaction of a sea anemone polypeptide toxin with cardiac cells in culture. J. Pharmacol. Exp. Ther., 213: 607-615, 1980.

Rougier, O., Vassort, G. and Stampfi, R.: Voltage-clamp experiments frog atrial heart muscle fibers wwith the sucrose-gap technique. Pfluegers Arch., 301: 91-108, 1968.

Sastre, A., Gray, D.B. and Lane, M.A.: Muscarinic cholinergic binding sites in the developing avian heart. Devel. Biol., 55: 201-205, 1977.

Shigenobu, K. and Sperelakis, N.: Development of sensitivity to tetrodotoxin of chick embryonic hearts with age. J. Mol. Cell. Cardiol., 3: 271-286, 1971.

Shigenobu, K., Schneider, J.A. and Sperelakis, N.: Blockade of slow Na^+ and Ca^{++} currents in myocardial cells by verapamil. J. Pharmacol. Exp.

Ther., 190: 280-288, 1974.

Sperelakis, N. and Lehmkuhl, D.: Insensitivity of cultured chick heart cells to autonomic agents and tetrodotoxin. Am. J. Physiol., 209: 693-698, 1965.

Sperelakis, N. and Pappano, A.J.: Depolarization of cultured heart cells by a lipid soluble acetylcholine analoque. Am. J. Physiol., 217: 625-629, 1969.

Sperelakis, N. and Shigenobu, K.: Changes in membrane properties of chick embryonic heart during development. J. Gen. Physiol. 60: 430-453, 1972.

Sperelakis, N., Shigenobu, K. and McLean, M.J.: Membrane cation channels: changes in developing hearts, in cell culture and in organ culture. In: Developmental and Physiological Correlates of Cardiac Muscle. Lieberman, M. and Sano, T., eds., Raven Press, New York, pp. 209-234, 1975.

Trautwein, W.: Membrane currents in cardiac muscle fibers. Physiol. Rev., 53: 793-835, 1973.

Ulbricht, W.: The effect of veratridine on excitable membranes of nerve and muscle. Ergeb. Physiol. Biol. Chem. Exp. Pharm., 61: 18-71, 1969.

Wunderer, G., Fritz, H., Wachter, E. and Machleidt, W.: Amoni-acid sequence of a coelenterate toxin: Toxin II from anemonia sulcata. Eur. J. Biochem., 68: 193-198, 1976.

Young, J.M.: Desensitization and agonist binding to cholinergic receptors in intestinal smooth muscle. FEBS Lett., 46: 354-356, 1974.

INITIATION OF TRANSMITTER SECRETION BY ADRENERGIC NEURONS

AND ITS RELATION TO MORPHOLOGICAL AND FUNCTIONAL

INNERVATION OF THE EMBRYONIC CHICK HEART [*]

Achilles J. Pappano and Dennis Higgins [**]

INTRODUCTION

Innervation by a terminal adrenergic axon in the right ventricle of a 7 day chick is shown in Fig. 1. The varicose region contains small granular vesicles, a characteristic inclusion of adrenergic axons. These vesicles are storage sites for norepinephrine (NE), the sympathetic adrenergic transmitter. At this stage of development, the axon can take up exogenous NE, synthesize NE from precursors, store NE in vesicles and release NE by exocytosis.

There are divergent views about the time that such sympathetic adrenergic fibers enter the avian heart and begin to function. Some have assumed that sympathetic innervation occurs at the 5th incubation day, that is, five days after fertilization (McCarty et al., 1960; Ignarro and Shideman, 1968; Culver and Fischman, 1977; Alexander et al., 1979). Previous work in our laboratory has supported a different conclusion, namely that, sympathetic innervation was not evident until the end of the second week of life in ovo and that sympathetic transmission occurred toward the end of the third week in ovo (reviewed in Pappano, 1977).

[*] The research was supported by grants from USPHS (HL-13339) and the American Heart association of Greater Hartford, Inc.
[**] Recipient of a fellowship from the Pharmaceutical Manufacturers Association Foundation.

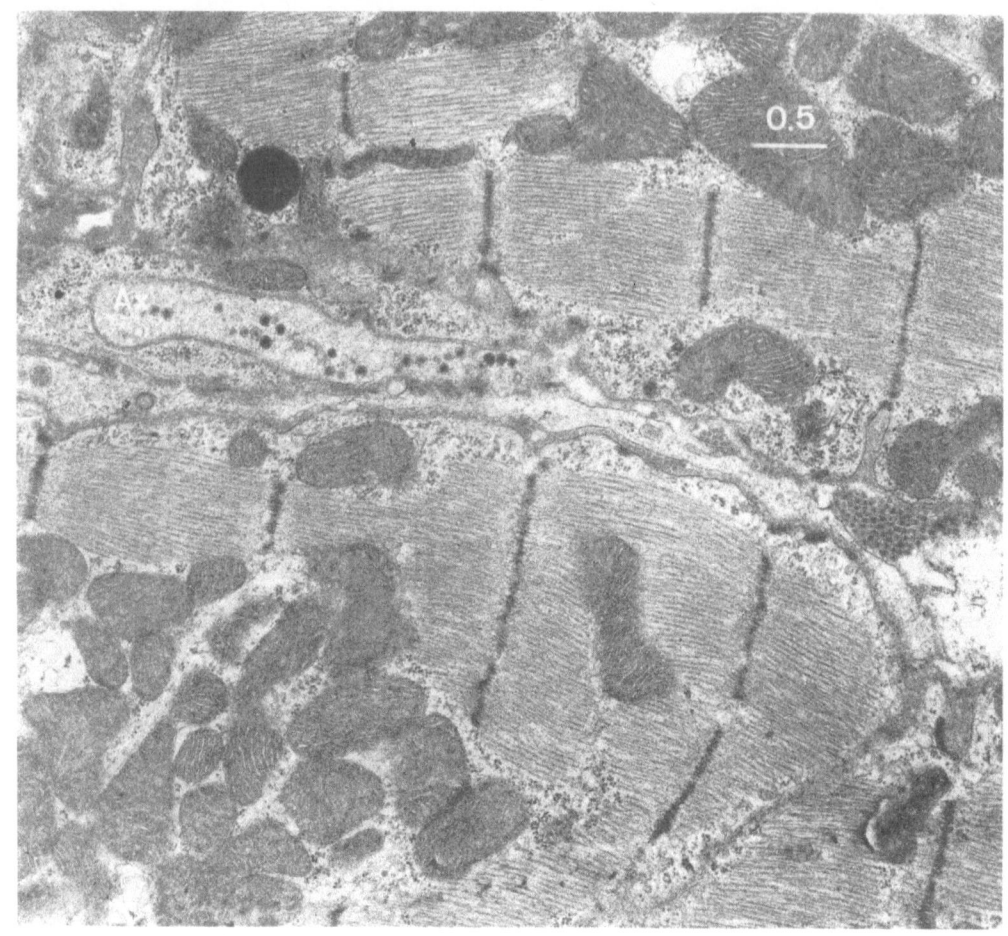

FIGURE 1 *Electron micrograph of ventricular muscle in the heart of a chick 7 days after hatching. An adrenergic axon (Ax) lies between cardiac muscle cells. The axon displays characteristics small granular vesicles. Calibration, 0.5 μm.*

Since it has been proposed that the sympathetic innervation has a trophic influence on cardiac muscle, namely, on DNA synthesis (Claycomb, 1976) and on the synthesis of TTX-sensitive Na channels (Shigenobu and Sperelakis, 1972), a more accurate picture of the development of sympathetic innervation could provide a better understanding of the possible trophic effects on cardiac muscle.

A delay or lag of several days occurs between the first appearance of axons displaying an adrenergic phenotype and the detection of transmitter release by neuroeffector transmission (Higgins and Pappano, 1981b; Pappano and Loeffelholz, 1974). The delay is evident in the mammalian heart (Lau and Slotkin, 1979; Seidler and Slotkin, 1979; Standen, 1978; MacKenzie and Standen, 1980) and in the avian heart (Pappano, 1977). In order to study the mechanism(s) involved in the delay between morphological and functional innervation, it is essential to ascertain the disposition of norepinephrine (NE) in developing adrenergic axons. Therefore, experiments were done to determine when adrenergic axons: 1.) could first be detected by histochemical methods, 2.) could first stimulate beta-adrenergic receptors on postsynaptic cells, and 3.) could first secrete NE. For this purpose, the ability of adrenergic axons to accumulate, retain and release tritiated NE (^{3}H-NE) was studied systematically.

With this experimental format, we addressed the following questions. When can the adrenergic axon first secrete transmitter? What stages are involved in the development of secretory function and how are these expressions of the adrenergic phenotype "programmed" during development? Finally, how does secretion in newly formed axons compare to that in axons from mature animals and how is it related to the proposed trophic effects on cardiac muscle?

METHODS

The histochemical procedures for the glyoxylic acid determination of tissue catecholamines in the embryonic chick heart have been given previously (Higgins and Pappano, 1979). Determination of neurally-evoked release of norepinephrine by field stimulation and by tyramine in the sinoatrial pacemaker (Pappano and Loeffelholz, 1974; Pappano, 1976) and in the right ventricle (Higgins and Pappano, 1981a) was done with isolated tissues superfused with Tyrode's solution and prepared for recording by methods standard for this laboratory. The disposition of L- 7-^{3}H -norepinephrine (^{3}H-NE) was used to study the accumulation, retention and release of exogenous transmitter by the avian heart at different times during development. A detailed description of the procedures used in the experiments with ^{3}H-NE can be found elsewhere (Higgins, 1980; Higgins and Pappano, 1981b).

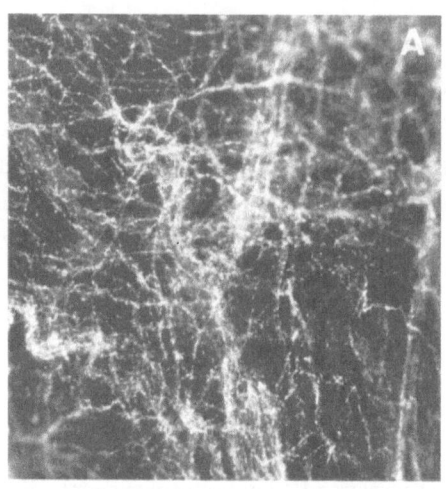

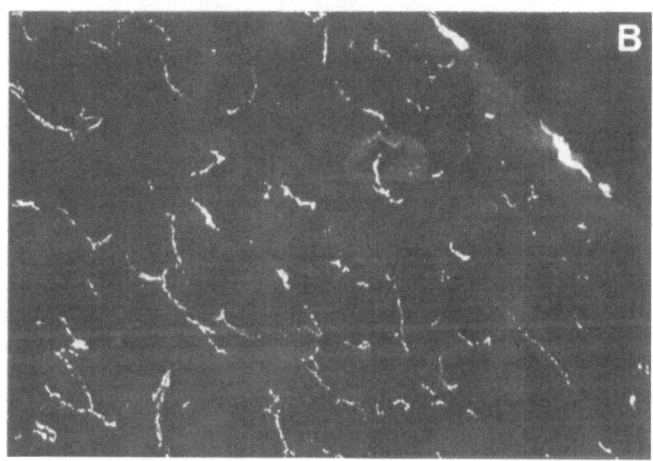

FIGURE 2 *Adrenergic innervation in chick heart 7 days after hatching. Glyoxylic acid was used for the fluorescent histochemical demonstration of catecholamine-containing axons in the sinoatrial region (A) and in the right ventricle free wall (B). (Adapted from Higgens and Pappano, 1979).*

RESULTS

HISTOCHEMICAL EXPERIMENTS - GROWTH AND DEVELOPMENT OF ADRENERGIC AXONS

Axons that displayed a green fluorescence characteristic of catecholamine containing structures were first observed in epicardial nerve trunks in the sinoatrial region and in the right ventricular free wall on the 11th incubation day. The fluorescence intensity could be increased by pre-incubation in alpha-methylnorepinephrine, an amine that can be accumulated and stored within adrenergic axons of the embryonic heart (Higgins and Pappano, 1979). Axons appeared in sinoatrial region and in the base of the right ventricle by the 14th incubation day; they displayed a smooth appearance. Varicose adrenergic fibers were detected in the sinoatrial region and right ventricle by the 16th incubation day. However, the density was very low and the density did not attain that of the adult until one week after hatching (cf. Bennett and Malmfors, 1970). As in the mammalian heart, the density of innervation was greater in the sinoatrial pacemaker (Figure 2A) than in the right ventricle (Figure 2B).

FIELD STIMULATION EXPERIMENTS - ONSET OF NEUROEFFECTOR TRANSMISSION

The occurrence of adrenergic transmission to sinoatrial pacemaker cells was indicated by propranolol-sensitive acceleration of the pacemaker caused by field stimulation (Figure 3). Adrenergic transmission to the sinoatrial pacemaker was first detected on the 19th incubation day (Pappano and Loeffelholz, 1974).

By contrast, the onset of adrenergic transmission to ventricular muscle cells was first observed on the 16th incubation day. The procedure used to detect the positive inotropic effect of endogenously released catecholamines is shown in Figure 4. Clearly, the ability of endogenously released catecholamine to increase ventricular contractions (ΔA) eventually attains the same force as that produced by exogenously applied isoproterenol (ISO,ΔB). This is shown in Figure 5 where the first significant positive inotropic effect to field stimulation is registered on the 16th incubation day. This action of endogenously released norepinephrine is antagonized by propranolol, which blocks postsynaptic beta-adrenergic receptors, and by guanethidine (Figure 5), which prevents the release and storage of norepinephrine.

Whereas the beta-adrenergic mechanism had been incorporated into cardiac

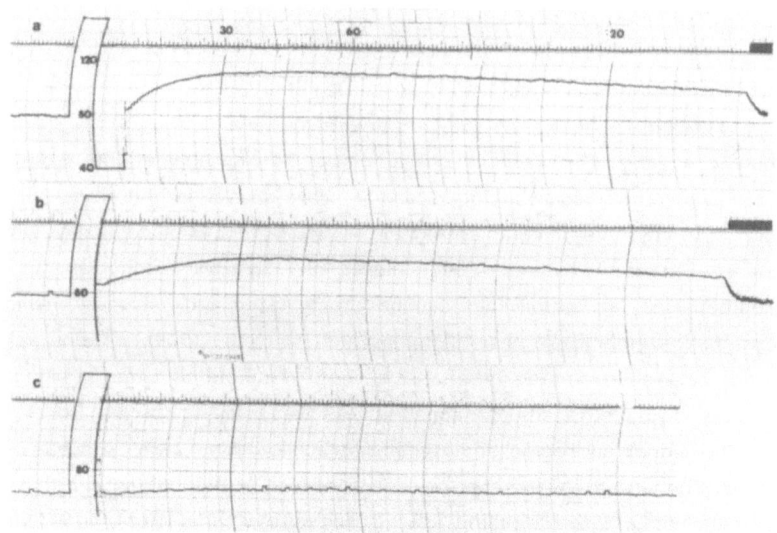

FIGURE 3 *Autonomic transmission to sinoatrial pacemaker from hatched chick. Ordinate: impulse frequency (action potentials min⁻¹); abscissa: time (s). Field stimulation (50 V, 0.5 ms, 30 Hz for 5 s) applied during the time indicated by the upward deflection of the pen writer recording at the beginning of each trace. a, control (inhibition followed by acceleration). b, in atropine (3 x 10⁻⁷ M). c, in propranolol (3 x 10⁻⁷ M) plus atropine.*

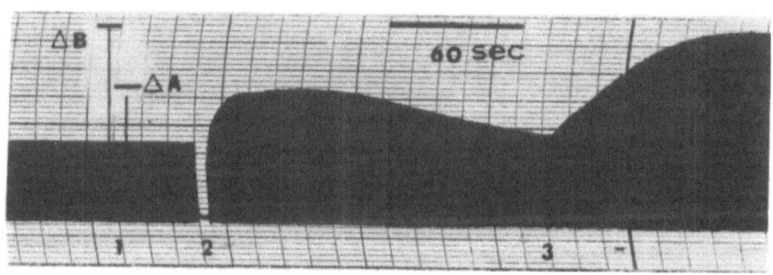

FIGURE 4 *Adrenergic transmission to the right ventricle (18th incubation day). 1. control contraction (3 Hz) in the presence of atropine (3 x 10⁻⁷ M). 2. field stimulation (30 Hz for 5s). 3. superfusion with isoproterenol (10⁻⁶ M) begins. Maximum change in contraction by field stimulation is ΔA; maximum change in contraction caused by isoproterenol is ΔB. (From Higgins and Pappano, 1981, with permission of the publishers of Developmental Biology).*

cells within a day or so after spontaneous contractions had begun (reviewed in Pappano, 1977), the sensitivity of the beta-receptors to ISO diminished at the time that sufficient endogenous NE was released to allow neuroeffector transmission (Higgins and Pappano, 1981a; Loeffelholz and Pappano, 1974). In order to examine the relationship between functional innervation and subsensitivity of the beta-receptor, functional innervation was delayed by administration of reserpine into the yolk sac. Injection of reserpine (10 µg in 50 µl/egg) on the 11th incubation day delayed the onset of neuroeffector transmission until some time after hatching (Higgins and Pappano, 1981a).

For example, on the 18th incubation day $\Delta A/\Delta B$ averaged 44% in untreated animals and only 3% in reserpine-treated animals. Measurements of the sensitivity to ISO (expressed as ED_{50}, the concentration needed to produce half the maximum effect) in these experiments are given in Table I. There was no difference in the time of occurrence or in the magnitude of the subsensitivity when the onset of transmission had been delayed by reserpine. Moreover, reserpine did not interfere with the normal increase in heart weight when it delayed the onset of adrenergic transmission.

The discrepancy between the onset of adrenergic transmission to the sinoatrial pacemaker and to the right ventricle was due to the difference in the experimental temperature. The original experiments with the sinoatrial pacemaker were done at 30 °C and transmission was detected on the 19th day. When the temperature was raised to 37 °C, the same temperature used in the experiments with the right ventricle, adrenergic transmission was detected on the 16th incubation day. Because postsynaptic sensitivity to ISO was similar at 30 ° and 37 °C, the effect of temperature on transmission is probably due to an action on the release of transmitter.

Attempts to increase endogenous stores of adrenergic transmitter were not successful in promoting adrenergic transmission. Incubation of the sinoatrial region and of the right ventricle in norepinephrine (1 µM) for up to one hour did not allow an earlier detection of adrenergic transmission to the pacemaker or to ventricular muscle (Pappano and Loeffelholz, 1974; Higgins and Pappano, 1981b). Therefore, experiments were done with ^{3}H-NE in order to ascertain the disposition and release of transmitter.

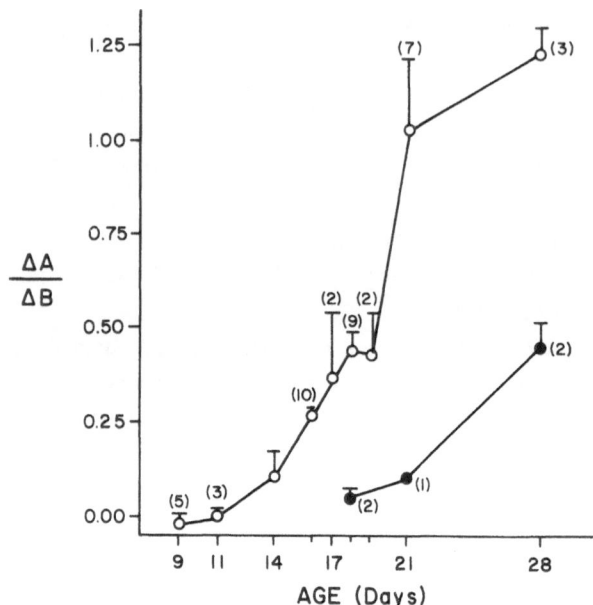

FIGURE 5 *Development of adrenergic transmission to the right ventricle. Abscissa: A/ B (see Figure 4 for definition); abscissa: age in days (21 days = hatching). 0, control (means +SEM); ●, 30 minutes after 20 µM guanethidine. Number of experiments in parenthesis. (From Higgins and Pappano, 1981, with permission of the publishers of Developmental Biology).*

TABLE I

EFFECT OF RESERPINE ON SENSITIVITY TO ISOPROTERENOL

Age	Control	Reserpine
14 i.o.[a]	5.3 ± 1.1 (7)[b]	6.4 ± 1.0 (3)
18	35.2 ± 4.9 (12)	27.8 ± 4.4 (4)
19	30.2 ± 4.7 (4)	26.3 ± 3.7 (4)
21 (hatching)	7.9 ± 1.8 (7)	8.7 ± 3.2 (4)

[a] in ovo (i.o.)
[b] Values are ED_{50} $(x10^{-9}$ M; means $\pm$ SEM (N). Drug treatment had no significant effect (analysis of variance, $P > 0.05$).

RADIOACTIVE TRACER EXPERIMENTS - ACCUMULATION, RETENTION AND RELEASE OF ^{3}H-NE

The size of the right ventricle made it more suitable for a comparison of the results of histochemical, physiological and radiochemical experiments. Therefore, this tissue was used for tracer studies; the similarities in the innervation of and transmission to the sinoatrial pacemaker and right ventricle indicate that the results obtained with ^{3}H-NE in the right ventricle apply also to the sinoatrial pacemaker.

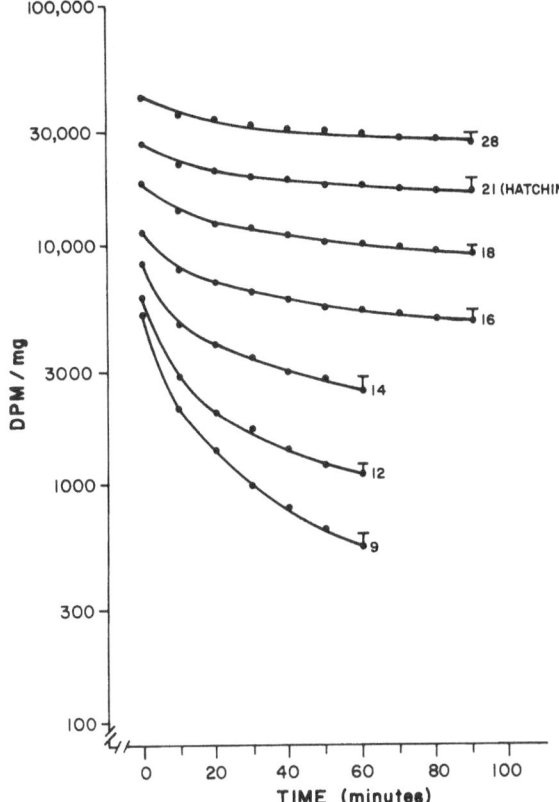

FIGURE 6 *Ontogenetic changes in accumulation and retention of [3]H. Ordinate: Disintegration per minute (DPM) in 1 mg of ventricular tissue; abscissa: time (min) after removal from incubation medium containing ^{3}H-NE. Age in days (after fertilization) given next to each line (28 = 7 days after hatching; 9 = 9 day embryo). Points are means and standard error bars are given at end of each trace. (From Higgins and Pappano, 1981, with permission of the publishers of Developmental Biolog).*

The results presented in Figure 6 illustrate that the accumulation and re-tention of ^{3}H-NE are a function of the age of the chick from which the heart was isolated. After a 1 hour incubation in ^{3}H-NE, the accumulation of label is gre-atest at the 28th day (i.e., 7 days after hatching) and least on the 9th day. (The age of the animal is given with reference to the day of fertilization de-signated as zero.) In addition to the 8-fold increase of ^{3}H-NE accumulation at t = 0 between the 9th incubation day and 7 days after hatching, there was a decrease of the rate of ^{3}H-NE washout from the tissue. For example, after a 1 hour washout in nonradioactive Tyrode's solution, the right ventricle of a 7 day chick contained 68% of the ^{3}H present at t = 0 whereas the ventricles of a 9 day embryo contained only 11%. There are two other features of these experiments that should be mentioned. First, there was no increase of ^{3}H retention between 1 and 3 weeks after hatching. Second, chromatographic analysis revealed that over 90% of the ^{3}H content of the right ventricle of hatched chicks was ^{3}H-NE (Andrenyak et al., 1980). These measurements were made at 90 minutes after having begun washout in nonradioactive Tyrode's solution.

TABLE II

EFFECTS OF COCAINE AND RESERPINE ON TISSUE ^{3}H CONTENT[a]

Age (days)[b]	Control	Cocaine[c]	Reserpine[d]
21 a.h.	25,533 ±4,620(3)	–	–
7 a.h.	29,100 ±2,310(18)	7,790 ±884(3)	5,730 ±536(2)
21 (hatching)	17,900 ±2,130(7)	–	4,900 –
18 i.o.	10,100 ±904(18)	2,270 ±834(3)	3,710 ±424(6)
14 i.o.	2,480 ±267(14)	692 ±22(2)	1,060 ±51(2)
12 i.o.	1,140 ±78(14)	631 ±110(2)	955 ±284(2)
9 i.o.	560 ±61(4)	552 ±138(4)	–

[a] Mean ± SE (N) of tissue ^{3}H content (DPM/mg) after 60 minutes of passive efflux.
[b] After hatching (a.h.); in ovo (i.o.).
[c] Cocaine (9 µM) was present throughout the experiment.
[d] Dose for 7-day-old chicks is 5 mg/kg, intraperitoneally at 24 and 48 hours before experiment. Embryos received 1 dose of 10 µg/egg. Embryos tested on days 18 and 21 were injected on day 11; other embryos were injected on day 7.

Cocaine (9 µM) blocks the neuronal uptake of NE (Iversen, 1967). By incubating in the presence of ^{3}H-NE and cocaine, it was possible to discern a cocaine-sensitive compartment of ^{3}H-NE no earlier than the 12th incubation day

(Table II). The size of this compartment, which is an indicator of the neuronal compartment, increased 42-fold between the 12th incubation day and 7 days after hatching.

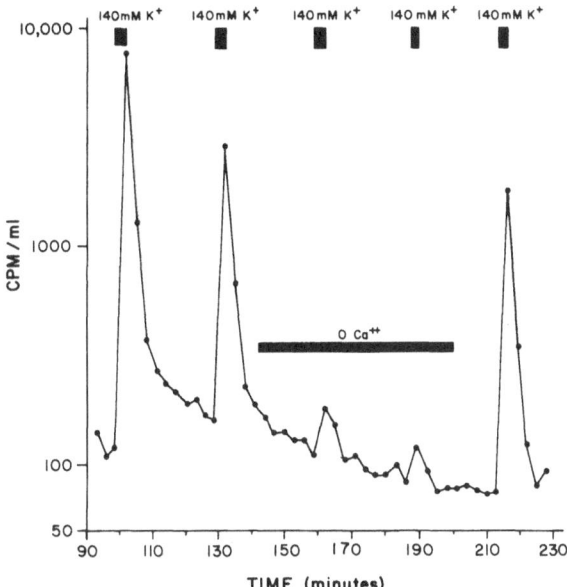

FIGURE 7 *Release of ^3H by elevated K and its dependence upon Ca^{2+} in right ventricle of a chick, 7 days after hatching. Ordinate: counts per minute (CPM) in 1 ml of medium during a 3 min. collection period; abscissa: time (min) after removal from incubation medium containing ^3H-NE. Bars indicate 3 min. exposure to solution with 140 mM KCl. Calcium was withdrawn from the medium from the 142nd min. to the 201st min. (From Higgins and Pappano, 1981, with permission of the publishers of Developmental Biology).*

Reserpine blocks the storage of NE by vesicles in adrenergic neurons (Kirshner, 1962). Pretreatment of embryonic chicks (10 μg reserpine/egg administered into the yolk sac) and of hatched chicks (5 mg/kg, intraperitoneally at 24 and 48 hours before experiment) permitted the detection of a reserpine-sensitive compartment of ^3H-NE no earlier than the 14th incubation day. The size of this compartment increased 16-fold between the 14th incubation day and 7 days after hatching.

The release of ^3H was produced by different stimuli: elevated (140 mM) K^+, electrical stimulation and tyramine. Release of ^3H by elevated K^+ (Na^+ was reduced to maintain tonicity) in a right ventricle from a chick 7 days after hatching is shown in Figure 7. Elevation of external K to 140 mM (the usual concentration was 5.4 mM) produced a prompt increase in the rate at which ^{3}H left the tissue. Most of the release (85%) occurred in the three minute period of exposure to elevated K$^+$. A second exposure to elevated K$^+$ (minutes 127-130 in Fig. 7) produced a similar increase in the overflow of ^{3}H. Removal of Ca^{2+} largely eliminated the stimulatory effect of elevated K$^+$ (3rd and 4th exposures in Figure 7). The effect of Ca^{2+} deprivation was promptly reversed as shown by the results of the 5th exposure to elevated K$^+$. It is noteworthy that 78 $\pm$ 2% (N = 3) of the ^{3}H released was identified as ^{3}H-NE. Only 9.7 $\pm$ 4.0% of the ^{3}H released passively was ^{3}H-NE.

The release of ^{3}H by elevated K$^+$ was diminished by pretreatment with reserpine or 6-hydroxydopamine as well as by removal of Ca^{2+}. However, tetrodotoxin (TTX, 3 x 10^{-7} M) had no effect on the release of ^{3}H by elevated K$^+$. The release by elevated K$^+$ was not the result of reduced Na$^+$ content.

The earliest detection of a release of ^{3}H by elevated K$^+$ was on the 12th incubation day. Release of ^{3}H was probably from a neuronal store since it was inhibited by pretreatment either with reserpine (to prevent storage) or by cocaine (to prevent ^{3}H-NE from entering the neuronal compartment). Release of ^{3}H from adrenergic nerves by elevated K$^+$ increased by 225-fold between the 12th incubation day and 7 days after hatching.

Electrical field stimulation (50 mA, 5 ms, 30 Hz for 60 s) also produced a prompt increase of the rate of ^{3}H overflow from the tissue (90% of the increase occurred in the first 3 minutes). The results in Figure 8 illustrate the reproducible increments in ^{3}H overflow caused by field stimulation in a right ventricle from a chick 6 days after hatching. Tetrodotoxin reversibly blocked the increased overflow of ^{3}H caused by electrical stimulation of intracardiac nerves (3rd field stimulation period in Figure 8). Like elevated K$^+$, the stimulatory effect of electrical stimulation was antagonized by Ca^{2+} deficiency or by pretreatment with reserpine or 6-hydroxydopamine. Significant release of ^{3}H by electrical stimulation was first detected on the 14th incubation day. The size of this release had increased 33-fold by 7 days after hatching.

Tyramine (3 x 10^{-5} M) also increased the release of ^{3}H from the right ventricle. The results in Figure 9 show the stimulatory effect of tyramine in the ventricle of a chick 7 days after hatching. It is noteworthy that tyramine released ^{3}H in the absence of Ca^{2+} in the bathing medium (Figure 9). However, the stimulatory effect of tyramine was diminished by pretreatment with reserpine or

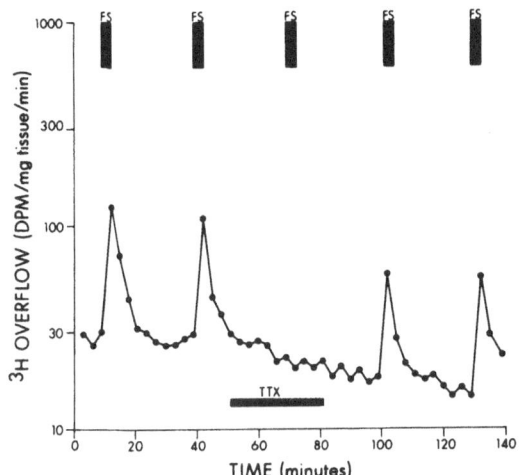

FIGURE 8 *Release of* ³*H by electrical stimulation from the right ventricle of a chick (6 days after hatching). Ordinate: ³H overflow (DPM/mg/min); abscissa: time (min). Zero time is 90 min. after removal from ³H-NE incubation medium. Bars indicate field stimulation (FS: 50 V, 5 ms, 3 Hz for 3 min). The horizontal bar marks a 30 min. exposure to 0.3 μM TTX.*

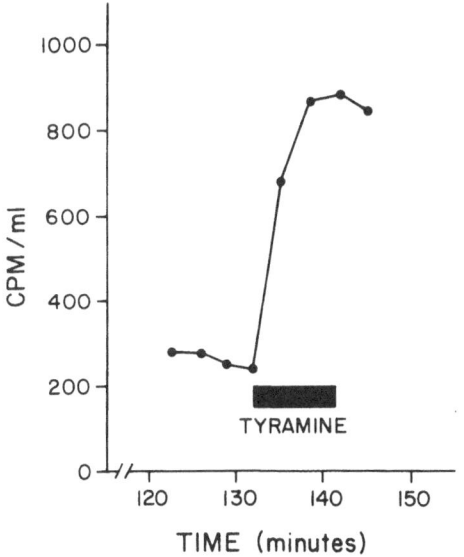

FIGURE 9 *Release of* ³*H by tyramine (3 x 10⁻⁵ M) from the right ventricle of a chick (7 days after hatching). Ordinate: ³H overflow (CPM/ml of medium); abscissa: time (min) after removal from incubation medium containing ³H-NE. The tissue was bathed in nominaly Ca²⁺-free solution from minute 111 to the end of the experiment. Tyramine was added at minute 132.*

6-hydroxydopamine. The stimulatory effect of tyramine was clearly present by the 16th incubation day.

TABLE III

DEVELOPMENTAL CHANGE IN THE FRACTION OF ^3H RELEASED
FROM NEURONAL COMPARTMENT

Age	K^+-Induced Fraction of ^3H in Neuronal Compartment[a]	Electrically-Induced Fraction of ^3H in Neuronal Compartment[a]
21 a.h.	.267+.012(3)	–
7 a.h.	.232+.013(8)	.147+.034(3)
21 i.o.	.155+.016(5)	
18 i.o.[b]	.147+.017(8)	.169+.018(3)
16 i.o.[c]	.123+.019(5)	
16 i.o.	.130+.019(3)	–
14 i.o.	.087+.018(6)	.062+.004(5)
12 i.o.	.097+.020(4)	

K^+-induced stimulation was a 3 minutes exposure to 140 mM KCl. Electrical stimulation consisted of 1 min of 30 Hz stimulation (50 mA, 5 ms). Data have been taken only from the first evoked release. Mean $\pm$ S.E. (N)

[a] Amount of ^3H released divided by the amount of ^3H which was in the neuronal compartment before stimulation. The neuronal compartment was defined as total tissue ^3H minus 560 DPM/mg (the amount in a 9 day embryo RV after 60 minutes of wash).
[b] 90 minute efflux period before stimulation.
[c] 60 minutes efflux period before stimulation.

The increments of released ^3H amounted to 225-fold and 33-fold for K^+- induced and electrical stimulation-induced overflow, respectively, during the course of development. However, when the fraction of tissue ^3H which is released from the neuronal compartment by either K^+ or electrical stimulation is considered, only a modest (about 3-fold in the case of elevated K^+) increase is observed during development.(Table III)

DISCUSSION

The chick embryo heart begins to contract spontaneously at about 33-38 hours after fertilization, soon after myofibrillogenesis was detected in ventricular myocytes (Manasek, 1968). Adrenergic receptors that mediate the positive chronotropic and positive inotropic effects of exogenously applied catecholamines are present as early as the 2nd incubation day in the sinoatrial pacemaker (Markowitz, 1931) and the 4th incubation day in ventricular muscle (McCarty et al., 1960). The receptors are blocked by propranolol and are classified as beta-adrenergic receptors (reviewed in Pappano, 1977).

The beta-adrenergic mechanism is incorporated into avian heart cells well in advance of sympathetic adrenergic innervation. Histochemical studies showed that axons containing catecholamines are present by the 11th incubation day (Higgins and Pappano, 1979). Sympathetic innervation of the embryonic avian heart has often been considered to occur by the 5th incubation day (reviewed in Romanoff, 1960). Recent observations with silver stains and histochemical fluorescence methods suggest a later ontogenetic appearance of adrenergic axons (Kirby et al., 1980), a conclusion in accordance with that reached in our laboratory (Higgins and Pappano, 1979). Sympathetic fibers do not reach the heart before the 10th incubation day; at this time the fibers are found in the bulbar region and in the atrium (Kirby et al., 1980). Fluorescent cells can be detected in the atrium at the 10th day provided that the preparations have been incubated in NE. Varicose fibers appear by the 14th incubation day according to Kirby et al., 1980; this is two days earlier than reported by us (Higgins and Pappano, 1979). The results of these two studies are in general agreement about the principal features of adrenergic axon development into the heart. It has been noted that the terminal adrenergic innervation of other organs in the chick can first be detected at the end of the second week of life in ovo. Thus, adrenergic axons are first detected on the 13th incubation day in the pupillary dilator muscle (Kirby et al., 1978) and in the intestinal tract (Epstein and Gershon, 1978). Taken altogether, these results indicate that axons, identified histochemically by their content of catecholamine, are not present in the embryonic avian heart until the 11th incubation day, almost one week after it had been assumed by others that adrenergic innervation had occurred (McCarty et al., 1960; Culver and Fischman, 1977). Moreover, the ability of exogenously applied NE (Kirby et al., 1980) and its alpha-methyl derivative (Higgins and Pappano, 1979) to permit a fluorescence signal from axons at a time when endogenous stores are minimal or absent, depends upon the rapid development of a neuronal uptake (Uptake I; Iversen, 1967) process in the membrane of newly formed axons.

Release of endogenous transmitter sufficient to alter the function of sinoatrial pacemaker cells and to ventricular muscle cells is first detected on the 16 th incubation day. Incubating cardiac tissues in NE did not change the time at which neuroeffector transmission could be detected (Higgins and Pappano, 1981b; Pappano and Loeffelholz, 1974). Because histochemical experiments indicated that incubation in NE or alpha-methyl NE enhanced axonal amine content, the delay between the appearance of axons and the detection of neuroeffector transmission cannot be attributed solely to a low transmitter concentration within budding axons.

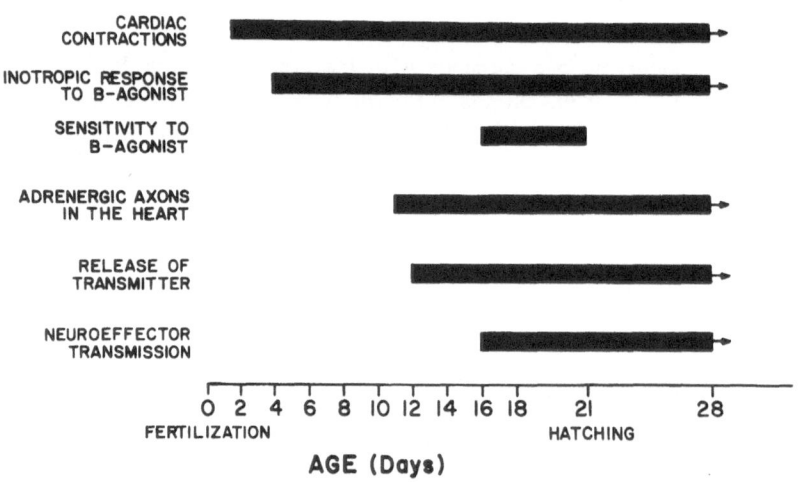

FIGURE 10 *Developmental changes that are pertinent to the formation of the cardiac adrenergic neuroeffector junction. Solid bars indicate the time a phenomenon is observed; the arrows indicate continuation beyond the 28th day (7 days after hatching).*

The delay between morphological and functional innervation seems to be the result of at least two factors: 1.) a poorly developed capacity to release transmitter and 2.) a great distance between axon and effector cell. Experiments with ^{3}H-NE showed that the retention of label in neuronal stores, as revealed by sensitivity to inhibition by cocaine or reserpine, was detectable on the 12th and 14th incubation days, respectively. The results with cocaine corroborate the conclusion from histochemical experiments concerning an early development of the neuronal uptake transport process (vide supra). It can be proposed that the reserpine-sensitive vesicular mechanism for intracellular storage of catecholamines develops between the 12th and 14th incubation days. There is some uncertainty in this proposition because of the observation that reserpine opposed ^{3}H-NE release by elevated K^+ from nerves on the 12th incubation day. This matter remains to be settled. Overall, the results of tracer experiments clearly indicate that adrenergic nerves are the principal source of ^{3}H-NE in the right ventricle. The increased retention of ^{3}H-NE with age paralleled the histochemical pattern for adrenergic axon development. Pharmacological evidence concerning retention (cocaine, reserpine, 6-hydroxydopamine) and release (Ca^{2+} deficiency, TTX, tyramine) of ^{3}H support the conclusion that adrenergic axons are the principal source of the label. The chromatographic analysis of products obtained during passive and stimulated overflow of ^{3}H as well as in the tissue indicate that ^{3}H-NE is stored in a protected position (intracellular granular vesicles) and released by stimuli from adrenergic axons.

The fact that ^{3}H-NE release by nerve impulse occurred by the 14th incubation day whereas neuroeffector transmission first appeared on the 16th incubation day indicates that stimulus-secretion coupling in the adrenergic axon was not the only limiting feature in the onset of transmission. (This conclusion assumes that the release of ^{3}H-NE occurred in the same manner as the release of endogenous NE.) The mechanisms for the delay between secretion and transmission can be accounted for by changes in 1.) the efficiency of stimulus-secretion coupling and 2.) in the number of axons within the myocardium. The results in Table III are consistent with the view that an increase in the efficiency of stimulus-secretion coupling occurs at about the time of the onset of transmission. Histochemical observations support the position that there are more axons within the myocardium. This factor is significant because the axons have moved closer to their effector cells (Higgins and Pappano, 1979).

We had previously observed a subsensitivity of the sinoatrial pacemaker to

ISO at the onset of adrenergic neuroeffector transmission (Loeffelholz and Pappano, 1974). The subsensitivity is also evident in the right ventricle (Table I; Higgins and Pappano, 1981a). Whereas administration of reserpine delayed the onset of adrenergic transmission in the right ventricle by at least 5 days, this treatment had no effect on the ontogenetic appearance of the subsensitivity to beta-adrenergic agonist or on the normal increase in heart weight (Higgins and Pappano, 1981a;cf. Deskin et al.,1980,for a different view). Although the subsensitivity coincides with functional cardiac innervation, these events are probably not causally related.

Adrenergic innervation begins at about the 11th incubation day in the embryonic avian heart. Tracer experiments indicate that at least some of the axons displayed uptake, intracellular storage and release of ^{3}H-NNE within 24 hours after being detected in the heart. Less than 48 hours later, the axons had incorporated TTX-sensitive Na channels and a Ca^{2+}- sensitive mechanism to permit impulse conduction that triggered exocytosis in a manner similar to that in adult animals. In the chick heart there is a relatively short delay between morphological and functional adrenergic innervation.

REFERENCES

Alexander, R.W., Galper, J.B., Neer, E.J. and Smith, T.W.: Development of beta-adrenergic receptors in embryonic heart. Circulation 57 and 58, Suppl. II-21, 1978.

Andrenyak, D., Higgins, D. and Pappano, A.: Detection of subpicomole amounts of ^{3}H-norepinephrine content and release from newly formed adrenergic nerves. Abstracts of New England Pharmacol. Soc., p. 22, 1980.

Bennett, T. and Malmfors, T.: The adrenergic nervous system of the domestic fowl (Gallus domesticus (L.)). Z. Zellforsch., 106: 22-50, 1970.

Claycomb, W.C.: Biochemical aspects of cardiac muscle differentiation. Possible control of deoxyribonucleic acid synthesis and cell differentiation by adrenergic innervation and cyclic adenosine 3':5'-monophosphate. J. Biol. Chem., 251: 6082-6089, 1976.

Culver, N.G. and Fischman, D.A.: A pharmacological analysis of sympathetic function in the embryonic chick heart. Am. J. Physiol., 232: R116-R123, 1977.

Deskin, R., Mills, E., Whitmore, W.L., Seidler, F.J. and Slotkin, T.A.: Maturation of sympathetic neurotransmission in the rat heart. VI. The effect of neonatal central catecholaminergic lesions. J. Pharmacol. Exp. Ther., 215: 342-347, 1980.

Epstein, M.L. and Gershon, M.D.: Development of monoaminergic neurons in the enteric nervous system of the chick embryo. Soc. for Neurosci., 4: 271 (Abs.), 1978.

Higgins, D.: The development of the adrenergic innervation of the chick embryo ventricle. Ph. D. Thesis, University of Connecticut, Storrs, 1980.

Higgins, D. and Pappano, A.: A histochemical study of the ontogeny of catecholamine-containing axons in the chick embryo heart. J. Mol. Cell. Cardiol., 11: 661-668, 1979.

Higgins, D. and Pappano, A.J.: Developmental changes in the sensitivity of the chick embryo ventricle to beta-adrenergic agonist during adrenergic innervation. Circ. Res., 48: 245-253, 1981a.

Higgins, D. and Pappano, A.J.: Development of transmitter secretory mechanisms by adrenergic neurons in the embryonic chick heart ventricle. Devel Biol. (in press), 1981b.

Ignarro, L.J. and Shideman, F.E.: The requirement of sympathetic innervation for the active transport of norepinephrine by the heart. J. Pharmacol. Exp. Ther., 159: 59-65, 1968.

Iversen, L.L.: The Uptake and Storage of Noradrenaline in Sympathetic Nerves, Cambridge University Press, London, 1967.

Kirby, M.L., Diab, I.M. and Mattio, T.F.: Development of adrenergic innervation of the iris and fluorescent ganglion cells in the choroid of the chick eye. Anat. Rec., 191: 311-320, 1978.

Kirby, M.L., McKenzie, J.W. and Weidman, T.A.: Developing innervation of the chick heart: A histofluorescence and light microscopic study of sympathetic innervation. Anat. Rec., 196: 333-340, 1980.

Kirshner, N.: Uptake of catecholamines by a particulate fraction of the adrenal medulla. J. Biol. Chem., 237: 2311-2317, 1962.

Lau, C. and Slotkin, T.A.: Accelerated development of rat sympathetic neurotransmission caused by neonatal triiodothyronine administration. J. Pharmacol. Exp. Ther., 208: 485-490, 1979.

Loeffelholz, K. and Pappano, A.J.: Increased sensitivity of sinoatrial pace-maker to acetylcholine and to catecholamines at the onset of autonomic neuroeffector transmission in chick embryo heart. J. Pharmacol. Exp. Ther., 191: 479-486, 1974.

MacKenzie, E. and Standen, N.B.: The postnatal development of adrenoceptor responses in isolated papillary muscles from rat. Pfluegers Arch., 383: 185-187, 1980.

Manasek, F.J.: Embryonic development of the heart. I. A light and electron microscopic study of myocardial development in the early chick embryo. J. Morph., 125: 329-366, 1968.

Markowitz, C.: Response of explanted embryonic cardiac tissue to epinephrine and acetylcholine. Am. J. Physiol., 97: 271-275, 1931.

McCarty, L.P., Lee, W.C. and Shideman, F.E.: Measurement of the inotropic effects of drugs on the innervated and noninnervated embryonic chick heart. J. Pharmac. Exp. Ther., 129: 315-321, 1960.

Pappano, A.J.: Onset of chronotropic effects of nicotinic drugs and tyramine on the sinoatrial pacemaker in chick embryo heart: Relationship to the development of autonomic neuroeffector transmission. J. Pharmacol. Exp. Ther., 196: 676-684, 1976.

Pappano, A.J.: Ontogenetic development of autonomic neuroeffector transmission and transmitter reactivity in embryonic and fetal hearts. Pharmacol. Rev., 29: 3-33, 1977.

Pappano, A.J. and Loeffelholz, K.: Ontogenesis of adrenergic and cholinergic neuroeffector transmission in chick embryo heart. J. Pharmacol. Exp. Ther., 191: 468-478, 1974.

Romanoff, A.L.: The Avian Embryo: Structural and Functional Development, The MacMillan Company, New York, 1960.

Seidler, F.J. and Slotkin, T.A.: Presynaptic and postsynaptic contributions to ontogeny of sympathetic control of heart rate in the pre-weanling rat. Br. J. Pharmac., 65: 431-434, 1979.

Shigenobu, K. and Sperelakis, N.: Failure of development of fast Na^+ channels during organ culture of young embryonic chick hearts. Devel. Biol., 39: 326-330, 1974.

Standen, N.B.: The postnatal development of adrenoceptor responses to agonists and electrical stimulation in rat isolated atria. Br. J. Pharmac., 64: 83-89, 1978.

REFERENCES

Abraham, R. and Robbin, J.: Transversal mapping and flows. Benjamin, New York, 1967.

Akwari, O.E., Kelly, K.A., Steinbach, J.H. and Code, C.F.: Electric pacing of intact and transected canine small-intestine and its computer model. Am. J. Physiol., 229: 1188-1197, 1975.

Albertini, D.F., Fawcett, D.W. and Olds, P.J.: Morphological variations in gap junctions of ovarian granulosa cells. Tissue and Cell, 7: 389-405, 1975.

Alcala, J., Lieska, N. and Maisel, H.: Protein composition of bovine lens cortical fiber cell membranes. Exp. Eye Res., 21: 581-595, 1975.

Alcala, J., Kuszak, J., Katar, M., Bradley, R.H. and Maisel, H.: Relationship of intrinsic and peripheral proteins to chicken lens gap junction morphology. J. Cell Biol., 83 (2, pt. 2): 269a, 1979.

Alexander, J.W.: On the doubtful validity of van der Pol's theory on relaxation oscillators. J. App. Sci. and Eng. Section A., 237-243, 1976.

Alexander, R.W., Galper, J.B., Neer, E.J. and Smith, T.W.: Development of beta-adrenergic receptors in embryonic heart. Circulation 57 and 58, Suppl. II-21, 1978.

Allessie, M.A. and Bonke, F.I.M.: Direct demonstration of sinus node reentry in the rabbit heart. Circ. Res., 44: 557-568, 1979.

Allessie, M.A., Bonke, F.I.M. and Schopman, F.J.G.: Circus movement in rabbit atrial muscle as a mechanism of tachycardia. Circ. Res., 33: 54-62, 1973.

Allessie, M.A., Bonke, F.I.M. and Schopman, F.J.G.: Circus movement in rabbit atrial muscle as a mechanism of tachycardia. II. The role of non-uniform recovery of excitability of the occurrence of uni-directional block, as studied with multiple microelectrodes. Circ. Res., 39: 168-177, 1976.

Allessie, M.A., Bonke, F.I.M. and Schopman, F.J.G.: Circus movement in rabbit atrial muscle as a mechanism of tachycardia: III. The "leading circle" concept: a new model of circus movement in cardiac tissue without the involvement of an anatomical obstacle. Circ. Res., 41: 9-18, 1977.

Almers, W.: Potassium conductance changes in skeletal muscle and the potassium concentration in the transverse tubules. J. Physiol. (London), 225: 33-56, 1972.

Altman, P.L.: Handbook of Circulation, Dittmer, D.S. and Grebe, R.M., eds., W.B. Saunders, Philadelphia, pp. 81-83, 1959.

Anderson, C.R. and Stevens, C.F.: Voltage clamp analysis of acetylcholine produced endplate current fluctuations at frog neuromuscular junction. J. Physiol. (London), 235: 655-691, 1973.

Anderson, E. and Albertini, D.F.: Gap junctions between the oocyte and companion follicle cells in the mammalian ovary. J. Cell Biol., 71: 680-686, 1976.

Anderson, R.H., Yen, H.S., Becker, A.E. and Gosling, J.A.: The development of the sinoatrial node. In: The Sinus Node. Structure, Function and Clinical Relevance, Bonke, F.I.M., ed., Martinus Nijhoff, The Hague, pp. 166-182, 1977.

Andrenyak, D., Higgins, D. and Pappano, A.: Detection of subpicomole amounts of ^{3}H-norepinephrine content and release from newly formed adrenergic nerves. Abstracts of New England Pharmacol. Soc., p. 22, 1980.

Angelakos, E.T., Maker, J.T. and Burlington, R.F.: Arrest of spontaneous atrial activity by cold at different potassium concentrations. Arch. Int. Physiol. Bioch., 79: 857-871, 1971.

Antzelevitch, C., Jalife, J. and Moe, G.K.: Characteristics of reflection as a mechanism of reentrant arrythmias and its relationship to parasystole. Circulation, 61: 182-191, 1980.

Anversa, P., Olivetti, G. and Loud, A.V.: Morphometric study of early postnatal development in the left and right ventricular myocardium of the rat. Circ. Res., 46: 495-502, 1980.

Asada, Y. and Bennett, M.V.L.: Experimental alteration of coupling resistance at an electrotonic synapse. J. Cell Biol., 49: 159-172, 1971.

Ashraf, M. and Halverson, C.: Ultrastructural modifications of nexuses (gap junctions) during early myocardial ischemia. J. Mol. Cell. Cardiol., 10: 263-269, 1978.

Attwell, D. and Cohen, I.: The voltage clamp of multicellular preparations. Prog. Biophys. Mol. Biol., 31: 201-245, 1977.

Attwell, D., Eisner, D.A. and Cohen, I.: Voltage-clamp and tracer flux data: effects of a restricted extracellular space. Q. Rev. Biophys., 12: 213-261, 1980.

Auerbach, A.A. and Bennett, M.V.L.: A rectifying synapse in the central nervous system of a vertebrate. J. Gen. Physiol., 53: 211-237, 1969.

Balakhovskii, I.S.: Several modes of excitation movement in ideal excitable tissue. Biophysics, 10: 1175-1179, 1965.

Baldwin, K.M.: The fine structure of healing over in mammalian cardiac muscle. J. Mol. Cell. Cardiol., 9: 959-966, 1977.

Baldwin, K.M.: Cardiac gap junction configuration after an uncoupling treatment as a function of time. J. Cell Biol., 82: 66-75, 1979.

Barr, L.: Electrical transmission between the cells of vertebrate cardiac muscle. In: Comparative Physiology of the Heart: Current Trends. McCann, F.V., ed., Birkhauser Verlag, Basel and Stuttgart, pp. 102-110, 1969.

Barr, L., Dewey, M.M. and Berger, W.: Propagation of action potentials and the structure of the nexus in cardiac muscle. J. Gen. Physiol., 48: 797-823, 1965.

Barr, L., Berger, W. and Dewey, M.M.: Electrical transmission at the nexus between smooth muscle cells. J. Gen. Physiol., 51: 347-368, 1968.

Barry, A.: The intrinsic pulsation rates of fragments of the embryonic chick heart. J. Exp. Zool., 91: 119-130, 1942.

Baumgarten, C.M. and Isenberg, G.: Depletion and accumulation of potassium in the extracellular clefts of cardiac Purkinje fibres during voltage-clamp hyperpolarization and depolarization. Pfluegers Arch., 368: 19-31, 1977.

Bayliss, W.M. and Starling, E.H.: On the electromotive phenomena of the mammalian heart. Monthly Internat. J. Anat. and Physiol., 9: 256-281, 1892.

Baylor, D.A., Fuortes, M.G.F. and O'Bryan, P.M.: Receptive fields of single cones in the retina of the turtle. J. Physiol. (London), 207: 77-92, 1971.

Beeler, G.W. and Reuter, H.: Reconstruction of the action potential of ventricular myocardial fibres. J. Physiol. (London), 268: 177-210, 1977.

Begenisich, T. and Stevens, C.F.: How many conductance states do potassium channels have? Biophys. J., 15: 843-846, 1975.

Benedetti, E.L. and Emmelot, P.: Hexagonal array of subunits in tight junctions seperated from isolated rat liver plasma membranes. J. Cell Biol., 38: 15-24, 1968.

Benedetti, E.L., Dunia, I. and Bloemendal, H.: Development of junctions during differentiation of lens fibres. Proc. Natl. Acad. Sci. USA, 71: 5073-5077, 1974.

Bennett, M.R.: Autonomic neuromuscular transmission. Cambridge University Press, Cambridge, (Monography of Physiological Society), 1972.

Bennett, M.V.L.: Function of electrotonic junctions in embryonic and adult tissue. Fed. Proc., 32: 65-75, 1973.

Bennett, M.V.L.: Electrical transmission: a functional analysis and comparison to chemical transmission. In: Handbook of Physiology. American Physiological Society, Bethesda, Maryland, 1977.

Bennett, M.V.L. and Goodenough, D.A.: Gap junctions, electrotonic coupling and intercellular communication. Neurosci. Res. Prog. Bull. 16: 373-486, 1978.

Bennett, M.V.LL., Dunham, B. and Pappas, G.D.: Ion fluxes through a "tight junction". J. Gen. Physiol., 50: 1094a. 1976.

Bennett, T. and Malmfors, T.: The adrenergic nervous system of the domestic fowl (Gallus domesticus (L.)). Z. Zellforsch., 106: 22-50, 1970.

Beress, L., Beress, R. and Wunderer, G.: Purification of three polypeptides with neuro and cardiotoxic activity from the sea anemone Anemonia sulcata. Toxicon, 13: 359-367, 1975.

Bergman, G., Dubois, J.M., Rojas, E. and Rathmayer, W.: Decreased rate of sodium conductance inactivation in the node of Ranvier induced by a polypeptide toxin from sea anemone. Biochem. Biophy. Acta., 455: 173-184, 1976.

Berkinblitt, M.B., Kovalev, S.A., Smolyaninov, S.S., Chilakhyan, L.M.: The electrical structure of myocardial tissue. Doklady Akademii Nauk SSSR, 163: 741-744, 1965.

Berkinblit, M.B., Kalinin, O., Kovalev, S.A. and Chilakhyan, L.M.: Study with the Noble model of synchronization of the spontaneously active myocardial cells bound by a highly permeable contact. Biofizika, 20: 121-125, 1975.

Bernard, C.: Establishment of ionic permeabilities of the myocardial membrane during embryonic development of the rat. In: Developmental and Physiological Correlates of Cardiac Muscle, Lieberman, M. and Sano, T., eds., Raven Press, New York, pp. 169-184, 1976.

Bernardini, G., Peracchia, C. and Venosa, A.: Uncoupling of lens fibers. J. Cell Biol., 87 (2, pt. 2): 207a, 1980.

Bernstein, J.: Ueber den Sitz der automatischen Erregung im froschherzen. Zentr. Med. Wiss. (Berlin), 14: 385-387, 1876.

Best, E.N.: Null space in the Hodgkin-Huxley equations. Biophys. J., 27: 87-104, 1979.

Birdsall, N.J.M., Burgen, A.S.V. and Hulme, E.C.: The binding of agonists to brain muscarinic receptors. Mol. Pharmacol., 14: 723-736, 1978.

Bleeker, W.K., Mackaay, A.J.C., Masson-Pevet, M., Bouman, L.N. and Becker, A.E.: Functional and morphological organization of the rabbit sinus node. Circ. Res., 46: 11-22, 1980.

Boethius, J. and Knutsson, E.: Resting membrane potential in chick muscle cells during ontogeny. J. Exp. Zool., 174: 281-286, 1970.

Bonke, F.I.M.: De Atrium Extrasystole. Thesis, Amsterdam, 1968.

Bonke, F.I.M.: Passive electrical properties of atrial fibers of the rabbit heart. Pfluegers Arch., 339: 1-15, 1973.

Bonke, F.I.M.: Electrotonic spread in the sinoatrial node of the rabbit heart. Pfluegers Arch., 339: 17-23, 1973.

Bonke, F.I.M.: A general introduction about the current status of the electrophysiology of the sinus node. In: The Sinus Node. Structure, Function and Clinical Relevance, Bonke, F.I.M., ed., Martinus Nijhoff, The Hague, pp. 225-232, 1977.

Bonke, F.I.M., Bouman, L.N. and van Rijn, H.E.: Change of cardiac rhythm in the rabbit after an atrial premature beat. Circ. Res., 24: 533-544, 1969.

Bonke, F.I.M., Bouman, L.N. and Schopman, F.J.G.: Effect of an early atrial premature beat on activity of the sinoatrial node and atrial rhythm in the rabbit. Circ. Res., 29: 704-715, 1971.

Boron, W.F. and De Weer, P.: Intracellular pH transients in squid giant axons caused by CO_2, NH_3 and metabolic inhibitors. J. Gen. Physiol., 67: 91-112, 1976.

Bouman, L.N., Gerlings, E.D., Biersteker, P.A. and Bonke, F.I.M.: Pacemaker shift in the sinoatrial node during vagal stimulation. Pfluegers Arch., 302: 225-267, 1968.

Bowditch, H.P.: Ueber die Eigenthuemlichkeiten der Reizbarkeit welche die Muskelfasern des Herzens zeigen. Arb. Physiol. Anstalt (Leipzig), pp. 139-176, 1871.

Bowditch, H.P.: Does the apex of the heart contract automatically. J. Physiol. (London), 1: 104-107,

1879.

Boyett, M.R. and Jewell, B.R.: Analysis of the effects of changes in rate and rhythm upon electrical activity in the heart. Prog. Biophys. Mol. Biol., 36: 1-52, 1980.

Branton, D.: Fracture faces of frozen membranes. Proc. Natl. Acad. Sci. U.S.A., 55: 1048-1056, 1966.

Bredikis, J.J., Bukauskas, F.F., Muckus, K.S. and Puodzius, S.S.: Ontogenetic pecularities of the electrical activity in cardiac fibres of human embryo. J. Evol. Biochem. Physiol. (Leningrad), 14: 43-48, 1978.

Brockes, J.P. and Hall, Z.W.: Acetylcholine receptors in normal and denervated rat diaphragm muscle II: comparison of junctional and extrajunctional receptors. Biochemistry, 14: 2100-2106, 1975.

Broekhuyse, R.M., Kuhlmann, E.D. and Stols, A.H.: Lens membrane. IV. Isolation and characterization of the main intrinsic polypeptide (MIP) of bovine lens fiber membranes. Exp. Eye Res., 23: 365, 1976.

Brooks, C.McC and Lu, H.H.: The sinoatrial pacemaker of the heart. Charles C. Thomas, Springfield, Illinois, 1972.

Brown, B.H., Duthie, H.L., Horn, A.R. and Smallwood, R.H.: A linked oscillator model of electrical activity of human small-intestine. Am. J. Physiol., 229: 384-388, 1975.

Brown, G.L. and Eccles, J.C.: The action of a single vagal volley on the rhythm of the heart beat. J. Physiol. (London), 82: 211-240, 1934.

Brown, G.L. and Eccles, J.C.: Further experiments on vagal inhibition of the heart beat. J. Physiol. (London), 82: 242-257, 1934.

Brown, H.F. and Noble, S.J.: Effects of adrenaline on membrane currents underlying pacemaker activity in frog atrial muscle. J. Physiol. (London), 238: 51P-53P, 1974.

Brown, H.F. and DiFrancesco, D.: Voltage clamp investigations of membrane currents underlying pacemaker activity in rabbit sino-atrial node. J. Physiol. (London), 308: 331-351, 1980.

Brown, H.F., Clark, A. and Noble, S.J.: Identification of the pacemaker current in frog atrium. J. Physiol. (London), 258: 521-545, 1976.

Brown, H.F., Giles, W. and Noble, S.J.: Membrane currents underlying activity in frog sinus venosus. J. Physiol. (London), 271: 783-816, 1977.

Brown, H.F., DiFrancesco, D. and Noble, S.J.: Cardiac pacemaker oscillation and its modulation by autonomic transmitters. J. Exp. Biol., 81: 175-204, 1979.

Brown, H.F., DiFrancesco, D. and Noble, S.J.: How does adrenaline accelerate the heart? Nature, 280: 235-236, 1979.

Brown, H.F., DiFrancesco, D. and Noble, S.J.: Adrenaline action on rabbit sinoatrial node. J. Physiol. (London), 290: 31P-32P, 1979.

Brown, H.F., DiFrancesco, D., Noble, D. and Noble, S.J.: The contribution of potassium accumulation to outward currents in frog atrium. J. Physiol. (London), 306: 127-149, 1980.

Brown, H.F., Kimura, J. and Noble S.J.: Evidence that the current i_f in sino-atrial node has a potassium component. J. Physiol. (London), 308: 33P, 1980.

Bruijne, J. de and Jongsma, H.J.: Membrane properties of aggregates of collagenase-dissociated rat heart cells. In: Advances in Myocardiology, Vol. I, Tajuddin, M., Das, P.K., Tariq, M. and Dhalla, N.S., eds., Baltimore, University Park Press, pp. 231-242, 1980.

Bukauskas, F.F. and Veteikis, R.P.: Passivve electrical properties of AV node region of rabbits heart. Biofizika, 22: 449-504, 1977.

Bukauskas, F.F., Kukushkin, N.I. and Saxon, M.E.: Model of two-dimensional anisotropic syncitium. Biofizika, 19: 712-716, 1974.

Bukauskas, F.F., Veteikis, R.P. and Gutman, A.M.: A model for passive three-dimensional anisotropic syncitium as continuous medium. Biofizika, 20: 1083-1086, 1975.

Bukauskas, F.F., Veteikis, R.P., Gutman, A.M. and Mutskus, K.S.: Intercellular coupling in the sinus node of the rabbit heart. Biofizika, 22: 108-112, 1977.

Burrows, M.T.: Rhythmical activity of isolated heart muscle cells in vitro. Science, 36: 90-92, 1912.

Cahn, R.D.: Developmental changes in embryonic enzyme patterns: the effect of oxidative substrates on lactic dehydrogenase in beating chick embryonic heart cell cultures. Devel. Biol., 9: 327-346, 1964.

Capelle, F.J.L. van, and Durrer, D.: Computer simulation of arrhythmias in a network of coupled excitable cells. Circ. Res., 47: 454-466, 1980.

Cardenas, J.M., Bandman, E. and Strohman, R.C.: Hybrid isozymes if pyruvate kinase appear during avian cardiac development. Biochem. and Biophys. Res. Comm., 80: 593-599, 1978.

Carmeliet, E.C. and Vereecke, J.: Electrogenesis of the action potential and automaticity. In: Handbook of Physiology, section 2: The Cardiovascular system, Vol 1: The Heart. Berne, R.M., Sperelakis, N. and Geiger, S.R., eds., Am. Physiol. Soc. Bethesda, Maryland, pp. 269-334, 1979.

Carmeliet, E., Horres, C.R., Lieberman, M. and Vereecke, J.S.: Potassium permeability in the chick heart: change with age external K, and valinomycin. In: Developmental and Physiological Correlates of Cardiac Muscle. Lieberman, M. and Sano, T., eds., Raven Press, New York, pp. 103-116, 1975.

Carmeliet, E., Horres, C.R., Lieberman, M. and Vereecke, J.S.: Developmental aspects of potassium flux and permeability of the embryonic chick heart. J. Physiol. (London), 254: 673-692, 1976.

Carrier, G.O. and Bishop, V.S.: The interaction of acetylcholine and norepinephrine on heart rate. J. Pharmacol. Exp. Ther., 180: 31-37, 1972.

Case, R.B., Nasser, M.G. and Crampton, R.S.: Biochemical aspects of early myocardial ischemia. Am. J. Cardiol., 24: 766-775, 1969.

Caspar, D.L.D., Goodenough, D.A., Makowski, L. and Phillips, W.C.: Gap junction structures. I. Correlated electron microscopy and X-ray diffraction. J. Cell Biol., 74: 605-628, 1977.

Castillo del, J. and Katz, B.: Production of membrane potential changes in the frog's heart by inhibitory nerve impulses. Nature, 175: 1035, 1955.

Cavanaugh, M.W.: Pulsation, migration and division in dissociated chick embryo heart cells in vitro. J. Exp. Zool., 128: 573-590, 1955.

Cavey, D., Vincent, J.P. and Lazdunski, M.: The muscarinic receptor of heart cell membranes: Association with agonists, antagonists and antiarrhythmic agents. FEBS Lett., 84: 110-114, 1977.

Chapman, R.A. and Fry, C.H.: An analysis of the cable properties of frog ventricular myocardium. J. Physiol. (London), 283: 263-282, 1978.

Chiba, S., Levy, M.N. and Zieske, H.: Chronotropic response to acetylcholine injected into the sinus node artery of the isolated atrium of the dog. Cardiovasc. Res., 9: 127-133, 1975.

Chicheportiche, R., Balerna, M. Lombet, A., Romey, G. and Lazdunksi, M.: Synthesis of new highly radioactive tetrodotoxin derivatives and their binding properties to the sodium channel. Eur. J. Biochem., 104: 617-625, 1980.

Clapham, D.E.: A whole tissue model of the heart cell aggregate: electrical coupling between cells, membrane impedance and the extracellular space. Doctoral dissertation, Emory University, Atlanta, Georgia USA, 1979.

Clapham, D.E., Shrier, A. and DeHaan, R.L.: Junctional resistance and action potential delay between embryonic heart cell aggregates. J. Gen. Physiol., 75: 633-654, 1980.

Clay, J.R. and DeHaan, R.L.: Fluctuations in interbeat interval in rhythmic heart cell clusters. Biophys. J., 28: 377-390, 1979.

Clay, J.R., DeFelice, L.J. and DeHaan, R.L.: Current noise parameters derived from voltage noise and impedance in embryonic heart cell preparations. Biophys. J., 28: 169-184, 1979.

Claycomb, W.C.: Biochemical aspects of cardiac muscle differentiation. Possible control of deoxyribonucleic acid synthesis and cell differentiation by adrenergic innervation and cyclic adenosine 3':5'-monophosphate. J. Biol. Chem., 251: 6082-6089, 1976.

Cobb, J.L.S.: Gap junctions in the heart of the teleost fish. Cell Tissue Res., 154: 131-134, 1974.

Cohen, I., Daut, J. and Noble, D.: The effects of potassium and temperature on the pacemaker current, i_{K_2}, in Purkinje fibres. J. Physiol. (London), 260: 55-74, 1976.

Cohen, I., Daut, J. and Noble, D.: An analysis of the actions of low concentrations of ouabain on membrane currents in Purkinje fibres. J. Physiol. (London), 260: 75-103, 1976.

Cohen, I., Eisner, D. and Noble, D.: The action of adrenaline on pacemaker activity in cardiac Purkinje fibres. J. Physiol. (London), 280: 155-168, 1978.

Cohen, I., Noble, D., Ohba, M. and Ojeda, C.: Actions of salicylate ions on the electrical properties of sheep cardiac Purkinje fibres. J. Physiol. (London), 297: 163-185, 1979.

Colquhoun, D. and Hawkes, A.G.: Relaxation and fluctuations of membrane currents that flow through drug-operated channels. Proc. R. Soc. Lond. B., 199: 231-262, 1977.

Cooley, J., Dodge, F. and Cohen, H.: Digital computer solutions for excitable membrane models. J. Cell. Comp. Physiol., 66, 99-108, 1965.

Copenhagen, D.R. and Owen, W.G.: Functional characteristics of lateral interactions between rods in the retina of snapping turtle. J. Physiol. (London), 259: 251-282, 1976.

Coraboeuf, E., LeDouarin, G. and Obrecht-Coutris, G.: Release of acetylcholine by chick embryo heart before innervation. J. Physiol. (London), 206: 383-395, 1970.

Coraboeuf, E., Obrecht-Coutris, G. and Le Douarin, G.: Acetylcholine and the embryonic heart. Am. J. Cardiol., 25: 285-291, 1970.

Couch, J.R., West, T.C. and Hoff, H.E.: Development of the action potential of the prenatal rat heart. Circ. Res., 24: 19-31, 1969.

Courtney, K.R., Jensen, R.A. and Davis, E.E.: Sodium ions affect adrenergic control of sinoatrial rate. J. Mol. Cell. Cardiol., 11: 237-244, 1979.

Cramer, M., Siegel, M., Bigger jr., J.Th. and Hoffman, B.F.: Characteristics of extracellular potentials recorded from the sinoatrial pacemaker of the rabbit. Circ. Res., 41: 292-300, 1979.

Cranefield, P.F.: The conduction of the cardiac impulse. The slow response and cardiac arrhythmias. Mount Kisco, N.Y., Futura, pp. 185, 1975.

Cranefield, P.F.: Action potentials, afterpotentials and arrhythmias. Circ. Res., 41: 415-423, 1977.

Cranefield, P.F.: Does spontaneous activity arise from phase 4 depolarization or from triggering? In: The Sinus Node. Structure, Function and Clinical Relevance, Bonke, F.I.M., ed., Martinus Nijhoff, The Hague, pp. 348-356, 1978.

Cranefield, P.F. and Greenspan, K.: The rate of oxygen uptake of quiescent cardiac muscle. J. Gen. Physiol., 44: 235-247, 1961.

Cranefield, P.F., Klein, H.O. and Hoffman, B.F.: Conduction of the cardiac impulse. I. Delay, block and one-way block in depressed Purkinje fibers. Circ. Res., 28: 199-219, 1971.

Culver, N.G. and Fischman, D.A.: A pharmacological analysis of sympathetic function in the embryonic chick heart. Am. J. Physiol., 232: R116-R123, 1977.

Dahl, G. and Isenberg, G.: Decoupling of heart muscle cells: correlation with increased cytoplasmic calcium and with changes of nexus ultrastructure. J. Memb. Biol., 53: 63-75, 1980.

Datardina, S.P. and Linkens, D.A.: Multimode oscillations in mutually coupled van der Pol type oscillators with fifth power non-linear characteristics. IEEE Trans. Cct. and Sys. CAS-25, 308-315, 1978.

Davis, C.L.: Development of the human heart from its first appearance to the stage found in embryos of 20 paired somites. Carnegie Inst. of Washington, Contr. to Embryology, 19: 245-284, 1927.

De Hemptinne, A.: Identification of ionic currents underlying the repolarization process in the frog auricle. European J. Cardiol., 7: Suppl. 5-15, 1978.

De la Fuente, D., Jedlicka, J. and Moe, G.K.: Time course of vagal effects on SA and AV nodes. Fed. Proc.,

28: 269, 1969.

De Mello, W.C.: Electrical uncoupling in heart fibres produced by intracellular injection of Na or Ca. The Physiologist, 17: 3, 1974.

De Mello, W.C.: Effect of intracellular injection of calcium and strontium on cell communication in heart. J. Physiol. (London), 250: 231-245, 1975.

De Mello, W.C.: Influence of the sodium pump on intercellular communication in heart fibres: effect of intracellular injection of sodium ion on electrical coupling. J. Physiol. (London), 263: 171-197, 1976.

De Mello, W.C.: Intercellular communication in heart muscle. In: Intercellular Communication, De Mello, W.C., ed., Plenum Press, New York, pp. 87-125, 1977.

De Mello, W.C.: Passive electrical properties of the atrioventricular node. Pfluegers Arch., 371: 135-139, 1977.

De Mello, W.C.: Effect of 2-4-dinitrophenol on intercellular communication in mammalian cardiac fibres. Pfluegers Arch., 380: 267-276, 1979.

De Mello, W.C.: On the decoupling action of ouabain. The Physiologist, 22: 4, 1979.

De Mello, W.C.: Effect of intracellular injection of La^{3+} and Mn^{2+} on electrical coupling of heart cells. Cell Biol. Intern. Rep., 3: 113-119, 1979.

De Mello, W.C.: Intercellular communication and junctional permeability. In: Membrane Structure and Function, Vol. 3, Bittar, E.E., ed., John Wiley and Sons, New York, pp. 127-170, 1980.

De Mello, W.C.: Influence of intracellular injection of H^{+} on the electrical coupling in cardiac Purkinje fibres. Cell Biol. Intern. Rep., 4: 51-55, 1980.

De Mello, W.C., Motta, G. and Chapeau, M.: A study on the healing over of myocardial cells of toads. Circ. Res., 24: 475-487, 1969.

Deck, K.A.: Dehnungseffekte am spontananschlagenden isolierten Sinusknoten. Pfluegers Arch., 280: 120-130, 1964.

Decker, R.S.: Hormonal regulation of gap junction differentiation. J. Cell Biol., 69: 669-686, 1976.

Decker, R.S.: Adrenocorticotropic hormone (ACTH) - induced formation of gap junctions between differentiating Y-1 tumor cells in vitro. J. Cell Biol., 70: 412a (Abstr.), 1976.

Decker, R.S. and Friend, D.S.: Assembly of gap junctions during amphibian neurulation. J. Cell Biol., 62: 32-47, 1974.

DeFelice, L.J. and Challice, C.E.: Anatomical and ultrastructural study of the electrophysiological atrioventricular node of the rabbit. Circ. Res., 24: 457-474, 1969.

DeHaan, R.L.: Cardia bifida and the development of pacemaker function in the early chick heart. Devel. Biol., 1: 586-602, 1959.

DeHaan, R.L.: Differentiation of the atrio-ventricular conducting system of the heart. Circulation, 24: 458-470, 1961.

DeHaan, R.L.: Regional organization of prepacemaker cells in the cardiac primordia of the early chick embryo. J. Embryol. Exp. Morphol., 11: 65-76, 1963.

DeHaan, R.L.: Avian embryo culture. In: Techniques for the Study of Development. Wilt, F.H. and Wessels, N.R., eds., Thomas Y. Crowell, New York, pp. 401-412, 1967.

DeHaan, R.L.: Regulation of spontaneous activity and growth of embryonic chick heart cells in tissue culture. Devel. Biol., 16: 216-249, 1967.

DeHaan, R.L.: The potassium sensitivity of isolated embryonic heart cells increases with development. Devel. Biol., 23: 226-240, 1970.

DeHaan, R.L.: Differentiation of excitable membranes. Cur. Topics Devel. Biol., 16: 117-164, 1980.

DeHaan, R.L. and Gottlieb, S.H.: The electrical activity of embryonic chick heart cells isolated in tissue culture singly or in interconnected cell sheets. J. Gen. Physiol., 52: 643-665, 1968.

DeHaan, R.L. and Hirakow, R.: Synchronization of pulsation rates in isolated cardiac myocytes. Exp. Cell Res., 70: 214-220, 1972.

DeHaan, R.L. and Sachs, H.G.: Cell coupling in developing systems: the heart-cell paradigm. Current Topics Devel. Biol., 7: 193-228, 1972.

DeHaan, R.L. and Fozzard, H.A.: Membrane responses to current pulses in spheroidal aggregates of embryonic heart cells. J. Gen. Physiol., 65: 207-222, 1975.

DeHaan, R.L. and DeFelice, L.J.: Oscillatory properties and excitability of the heart cell membrane. In: Theoretical Chemistry: Advances and Perspectives, Eyring, H., ed., Academic Press, New York, 4: 181-233, 1978.

DeHaan, R.L. and O'Rahilly, R.: Embryology of the heart. In: The Heart, Hurst, J.W., Logue, R.B., Schlant, R.C. and Wenger, N.K., eds., McGraw-Hill, New York, pp. 6-18, 1978.

DeHaan, R.L., McDonald, T.F. and Sachs, H.G.: Development of tetrodoxin sensitivity of embryonic chick heart cells in vitro. In: Developmental and Physiological Correlates of Cardiac Muscle, Lieberman, M. and Sano, T., eds., Raven Press, New York, pp. 155-168, 1975.

DeHaan, R.L., Williams, E.H., Ypey, D.L. and Clapham, D.E.: Intercellular coupling of embryonic heart cells. In: Mechanisms of Cardiac Morphogenesis and Teratogenesis: Perspectives in Cardiovascular Research, Pexieder, T., ed., Raven Press, New York, pp. 299-316, 1980.

Del Castillo, J. and Katz, B.: The membrane potential changes in frog's heart produced by inhibitory nerve impulses. Nature (London), 175: 1035, 1955.

Delaage, M., Roux, D. and Cailla, H.L.: Recent advances in cyclic nocleotide radioimmunoassay. In: Nato Advanced Study Institute on Cyclic Nucleotides, Paoletti, R., ed., Elsevier-North-Holland Biomedical Press, Amsterdam, 1977.

Deleze, J.: Possible reasons for drop of resting potential of mammalian heart preparations during hypothermia. Circ. Res., 8: 553-557, 1960.

Deleze, J.: Calcium ions and the healing over of heart fibers. In: Electrophysiology of the Heart, Taccardi B. and Marchetti, G., eds., Pergamon Press, Oxford, England, pp. 147-148, 1965.

Deleze, J.: The recovery of resting potential and input resistance in sheep heart injured by knife or laser. J. Physiol. (London), 208: 547-562, 1970.

Deskin, R., Mills, E., Whitmore, W.L., Seidler, F.J. and Slotkin, T.A.: Maturation of sympathetic neurotransmission in the rat heart. VI. The effect of neonatal central catecholaminergic lesions. J. Pharmacol. Exp. Ther., 215: 342-347, 1980.

Detwiler, P.B. and Hodgkin, A.L.: Electrical coupling between cones in the turtle retina. J. Physiol. (London), 291: 75-100, 1979.

Detwiler, P.B., Hodgkin, A.L. and McNaughton, P.M.: A surprising property of electrical spread in the network of rods in the turtle's retina. Nature, 274: 562-565, 1978.

Detwiler, P.B., Hodgkin, A.L. and McNaughton, P.A.: Temporal and spatial characteristics of the voltage response of rods in the retina of the snapping turtle. J. Physiol. (London), 300: 213-250, 1980.

Devreotis, P.N., and Fambrough, D.M.: Acetylcholine receptor turnover in membranes of developing muscle fibers. J. Cell Biol., 65: 335-358, 1975.

Dewey, M.M. and Barr, L.: Intercellular connection between smooth muscle cells: the Nexus. Science (Wash., D.C.), 137: 670-672, 1962.

DiFrancesco, D.: The pacemaker current "i_{K2}" in Purkinje fibres is carried by sodium and potassium. J. Physiol. (London), 308: 32P. 1980.

DiFrancesco, D.: A new interpretation of the pacemaker current i_{K2} in Purkinje fibres. J. Physiol. (London), 314: 359-376, 1981.

DiFrancesco, D.: A study of the ionic nature of the pacemaker current in Purkinje fibres. J. Physiol. (London), 314: 377-393, 1981.

DiFrancesco, D. and McNaughton, P.A.: The effects of calcium on outward membrane currents in the cardiac Purkinje fibre. J. Physiol. (London), 289: 347-373, 1979.

DiFrancesco, D. and Ojeda, C.: Properties of the pacemaker current i_f in the sinoatrial node of the rabbit: a comparison with the current i_{K2} in Purkinje fibres. J. Physiol. (London), 308: 353-367, 1980.

DiFrancesco, D. and Noble, D.: If "i_{K2}" is an inward current, how does it display potassium specificity? J. Physiol. (London), 305: 14-15P, 1980.

DiFrancesco, D. and Noble, D.: Reconstruction of Purkinje fibre currents in sodium-free solution. J. Physiol. (London), 308: 35P, 1980.

DiFrancesco, D., Ohba, M. and Ojeda, C.: Measurement and significance of the reversal potential for the pacemaker current (i_{K2}) in sheep Purkinje fibres. J. Physiol. (London), 297: 135-162, 1979.

DiFrancesco, D., Noma, A. and Trautwein, W.: Kinetics and magnitude of the time-dependent K current in the rabbit SA node: effect of external potassium. Pfluegers Arch., 381: 271-279, 1979.

DiFrancesco, D., Noma, A. and Trautwein, W.: Separation of current induced by potassium accumulation from acetylcholine induced relaxation current in the rabbit SA node. Pfluegers Arch., 387: 83-90, 1980.

Dong, E. and Reitz, B.A.: Effects of timing of vagal stimulation on heart rate in the dog. Circ. Res., 27: 635-646, 1970.

Dorticos, F.R. and Garcia-Barreto, D.: Electrophysiological effects of droperidol on sinoatrial nodal fibers. Arch. Int. Pharmacodyn, 240: 137-142, 1979.

Downar, E. and Waxman, M.B.: Depressed conduction and unidirectional block in Purkinje fibers. In: Conduction System of the Heart, Wellens, H.J.J., Lie, K.I. and Janse, M.J., eds., Stenfert Kroese, Leiden, pp. 393-409, 1976.

Draper, M.H. and Weidmann, S.: Cardiac resting and action potentials recorded with an intracellular electrode. J. Physiol. (London), 115: 74-94, 1951.

Dreifuss, J.J., Girardier, L. and Forssman, W.G.: Etude de la propagation de l'excitation dans le ventricule de rat au moyeu de solutions hypertoniques. Pfluegers Arch., 292: 13-33, 1966.

Dreyer, F., Peper, K. and Sterz, R.: Determination of dose-response curves by quantitative ionophoresis at the frog neuromuscular junction. J. Physiol. (London), 281: 395-419, 1978.

Dubois-Reymond, E.: Untersuchungen ueber thierische Electricitaet, Vol. 1, Verlag von G.Reimer, Berlin, 1848.

Dudel, J. and Trautwein, W.: Der Mechanismus der Automatischen Rhythmischen Impulsbildung der Herzmuskelfaser. Pfluegers Arch., 267: 553-565, 1958.

Duguid, J. and Revel, J.P.: The protein components of the gap junction. Cold Spring Harbor Symp. Quant. Biol., 40: 45-47, 1976.

Dunia, I., Sen Gosh, C., Benedetti, E.L., Zweers, A. and Bloemendal, H.: Isolation and protein pattern of eye fibres fiber junction. FEBS Lett., 45: 139-144, 1974.

Ebihara, L., Shigeto, N., Lieberman, M. and Johnson, E.A.: The initial inward current in spherical clusters of chick embryonic heart cells. J. Gen. Physiol., 75: 437-456, 1980.

Ehrhart, J.C. and Chauveau, J.: The protein component of mouse hepatocyte gap junctions. FEBS Letters, 78: 295-299, 1977.

Einthoven, W.: Ein neues Galvanometer. Annal. Physik. F. IV, 12: 1059, 1903.

Einthoven, W.: Weiteres ueber das Elektrocardiagramm. Arch. Ges. Physiol., 122: 517-584, 1908.

Eisner, D.A. and Lederer, W.J.: Characterisation of the electrogenic sodium pump in cardiac Purkinje fibres. J. Physiol. (London), 303, 441-474, 1980.

Elias, P.M. and Friend, D.S.: Vitamin-A-induced mucous metaplasia. An in vitro system for modulating tight and gap junction differentiation. J. Cell Biol., 68: 173-188, 1976.

Elsas, L.J., Wheeler, F.B., Danner, D.J. and DeHaan, R.L.: Amino acid transport by aggregates of cultured chicken heart cells (Effect of insulin), J. Biol. Chem., 250: 9381-9390, 1975.

Enemar, A., Flack, B. and Hakanson, R.: Observations on the appearance of norepinephrine in the sympathetic nervous system of the chick embryo. Devel. Biol., 11: 268-283, 1965.

Engelmann, Th. W.: Zur Physiologie des Ureter. Pfluegers Arch., 2: 243-293, 1869.

Engelmann, Th. W.: Ueber die Leitung der Erregung im Herzmuskel. Pfluegers Arch., 2: 465-480, 1875.

Engelmann, Th. W.: Ueber Degeneration von Nervenfasern. Pfluegers Arch., 13: 474-491, 1876.

Engelmann, Th. W.: Vergleichende Untersuchungen zur Lehre von der Muskel- und Nervenelektricitaet. Pfluegers Arch., 15: 116-148, 1877.

Epstein, M.L. and Gershon, M.D.: Development of monoaminergic neurons in the enteric nervous system of the chick embryo. Soc. for Neurosci., 4: 271 (Abs.), 1978.

Erlanger, J. and Blackman, J.R.: A study of relative rhythmicity and conductivity in various regions of the auricles of the mammalian heart. Amer. J. Physiol., 19: 125-174, 1907.

Evans, W.H. and Gurd, J.W.: Preparation and properties of nexuses and lipid enriched vesicles from mouse liver plasmamembranes. Biochem. J., 128: 691-700, 1972.

Eyster, J.A.E. and Meek, W.J.: The origin and conduction of the heart beat. Physiol. Rev., 1: 1-43, 1921.

Farquhar, M.G. and Palade, G.E.: Cell junctions in amphibian skin. J. Cell Biol., 25: 263-291, 1965.

Fawcett, D. and McNutt, N.S.: The ultrastructure of the cat myocardium I. Ventricular papillary muscle. J. Cell Biol., 42: 1-45, 1969.

Fayet, G., Couraud, F., Miranda, F. and Lissitzky, S.: Electro-optical system for monitoring activity of heart cells in culture: Application to the study of several drugs and scorpion toxin. Eur. J. Pharmac., 27: 165-174, 1974.

Field, R.J. and Troy, W.C.: The existence of solitary travelling wave solutions of a model of the Belousov-Zhabotinskii reaction. SIAM J. Appl. Math., 37: 561-581, 1979.

Fields, J.Z., Roeske, W.R., Morkin, E. and Yamamura, H.I.: Cardiac muscarinic cholinergic receptors: Biochemical identification and characterization. J. Biol. Chem., 253: 3251-3258, 1978.

Fine, I.H., Daplan, N.V. and Kuftinec, D.: Developmental changes of mammalian lactic dehydrogenases. Biochem., 4: 116-124, 1963.

Fischer, A.: The interaction of two fragments of pulsating heart tissue. J. Exp. Med., 39: 577-583, 1924.

Flagg-Newton, J.L., Simpson, I. and Loewenstein, W.R.: Permeability of the cell-to-cell membrane channels in mammalian cell junction. Science, 205: 404-407, 1979.

Forssmann, W.G. and Girardier, L.: A study of the T-system in rat heart. J. Cell Biol., 44: 1-19, 1970.

Fox, L.: In: Modern Computing Methods, Chapter 12. H.M.S.O. London, 1961.

Fozzard, H.A.: Conduction of the action potential. In: Handbook of Physiology: the Cardiovascular System. Sect. 2, Vol. 1. The Heart, Berne, R.M., ed., Am. Physiol. Soc. Bethesda, Md, pp. 335-356, 1979.

Fozzard, H.A. and Schoenberg, M.: Strength-duration curves in cardiac Purkinje fibers: effects of liminal length and charge distribution. J. Physiol. (London), 226: 593-618, 1972.

Frank, J.S., Beydler, S., Kreman, M. and Rau, E.E.: Structure of the freeze-fractured sarcolemma in the normal and anoxic rabbit myocardium. Circ. Res., 47: 131-143, 1980.

Freeman, S.E. and Turner, R.J.: Effects of temperature change and adrenaline on sinoatrial and atrioventricular nodal potentials. Cardiovasc. Res., 8: 443-450, 1974.

Freer, R.J., Pappano, A.J., Peach, M.J., Bing, K.T., McLean, M.J., Vogel, S. and Sperelakis, N.: Mechanism for the positive inotropic effect of angiotensin II on isolated cardiac muscle. Circ. Res., 39: 178-183, 1976.

Fujii, S., Hirota, A. and Kamino, K.: Optical signals from early embryonic chick heart stained with potential sensitive dyes: evidence for electrical activity. J. Physiol. (London), 304: 508-518, 1980.

Fujisawa, H. and Morioka, H.: A simple method for freeze-cleaving of cells grown on plastic culture dish. Cell Struct. Funct., 2: 361-365, 1977.

Fujisawa, H., Morioka, H., Nakamura, H. and Watanabe, K.: Gap junctions in the differentiated neural retinae of newly hatched chickens. J. Cell Sci., 22: 597-606, 1976.

Furshpan, E.G., Potter, D.D.: Transmission at the giant motor synapses of the crayfish. J. Physiol. (London), 145: 289-325, 1959.

Gabella, G.: Inpocketings of the cell membrane (caveolae) in the rat myocardium. J. Ultrastruct. Res., 65: 135-147, 1978.

Gadsby, D.C. and Cranefield, P.F.: Two levels of resting potential in cardiac Purkinje fibres. J. Gen. Physiol., 70: 725-746, 1977.

Gadsby, D.C., Wit, A.L. and Cranefield, P.F.: Overdrive suppression of triggered atrial tachycardia arising in the canine coronary sinus. (Abstr.) Am. J. Cardiol., 43: 374, 1979.

Galper, J.B. and Catteral, W.A.: Developmental changes in the sensitivity of embryonic heart cells to tetrodotoxin and D-600. Devel. Biol., 65: 216-227, 1978.

Galper, J.B., Klein, W. and Catterall, W.A.: Muscarinic acetylcholine receptors in developing chick heart. J. Biol. Chem., 23: 8692-8699, 1977.

Ganter, G. and Zahn, A.: Experimentelle Untersuchungen am Saugetierherzen ueber Reizbildung und Reizleitung in ihrer Beziehung zum spezifischen Muskelgewebe. Arch. Ges. Physiol., 144: 335-392, 1912.

Garnier, D., Nargeot, J., Ojeda, C. and Rougier, O.: The action of acetylcholine on background conductance in frog atrial trabeculae. J. Physiol. (London), 274: 381-396, 1978.

Garofolini, L.: Rhythmical contractions of single heart muscle cells in tissue culture in vitro. J. Physiol. (London), 63: V, 1927.

Garrey, W.E.: Nature of fibrillary contraction in the heart. Am. J. Physiol., 33: 397-414, 1914.

Gaskell, W.H.: On the tonicity of the heart and blood vessels. J. Physiol. (London), 3: 48-75, 1880.

Gaskell, W.H.: On the rhythm of the heart of the frog and on the nature of the action of the vagus nerve. Phil. Trans. Royal Soc., 3: 993-1033, 1882.

George, W.J., Polson, J.B., O'Toole, A.G. and Goldberg, N.D.: Elevation of guanosine 3', 5'-cyclic phosphate in rate heart after perfusion with acetylcholine. Proc. Natl. Acad. Sci. USA, 66: 398-403, 1970.

Gettes, L.S. and Reuter, H.: Slow recovery from inactivation of inward currents in mammalian myocardium. J. Physiol. (London), 240: 703-724, 1974.

Giles, W. and Tsien, R.W.: Effects of acetylcholine on membrane currents in frog atrial muscle. J. Physiol. (London), 246: 64P-66P, 1975.

Giles, W. and Noble, S.J.: Changes in membrane currents in bullfrog atrium produced by acetylcholine. J. Physiol. (London), 261: 103-123, 1976.

Gilula, N.B.: Gap junctions and cell communication. In: Int. Cell Biol., Brinkley, E. and Porter, K., eds., Rockefeller Univ. Press, New York, pp. 61-69, 1977.

Gilula, N.B., Reeves, O.R. and Steinbach, A.: Metabolic coupling, ionic coupling and cell contacts. Nature (Lond.), 235: 262-265, 1972.

Girard, H.: Arterial pressure in the chick embryo. Am. J. Physiol., 224: 454-460, 1973.

Glitsch, H.G.: An effect of the electrogenic sodium pump on the membrane potential in beating guinea-pig atria. Pfluegers Arch., 334: 169-180, 1973.

Glitsch, H.G. and Reuter, H.: The effect of internal sodium concentration on calcium fluxes in isolated guinea-pig auricles. J. Physiol. (London), 209: 25-43, 1970.

Glitsch, H.G. and Pott, L.: Effects of acetylcholine and parasympathetic nerve stimulation on membrane potential in quiescent guinea-pig atria. J. Physiol. (London), 279: 655-668, 1978.

Goodenough, D.A.: Methods for the isolation and structural characterization of hepatocyte gap junctions. In: Methods in Membrane Biology, Vol. 3, Korn, E.D., ed., Plenum Publishing Corp., New York, pp. 51-80, 1975.

Goodenough, D.A.: Lens gap junctions: A structural hypothesis for non-regulated low resistance intercellular pathways. Invest. Ophtalmol. Vis. Sci., 18: 1104-1122, 1979.

Goodenough, D.A. and Stoeckenius, W.: The isolation of mouse hepatocyte gap junctions. Preliminary chemical characterization and X-ray diffraction. J. Cell Biol., 54: 646-656, 1972.

Gorman, A.L.F. and Herman, A.: Internal effects of divalent cations on potassium permeability in molluscan neurons. J. Physiol. (London), 296: 393-410, 1979.

Goshima, K.: Synchronized beating of and electrotonic transmission between myocardial cell, mediated by heterotypic strain cells in monolayer culture. Exp. Cell Res., 58: 420-426, 1969.

Goshima, K.: Formation of nexuses and electrotonic transmission between myocardial and FL cells in monolayer culture. Exp. Cell Res., 63: 124-130, 1970.

Goshima, K.: Beating of myocardial cells in culture. In: Developmental and Physiological Correlates of Cardiac Muscle, Lieberman, M. and Sano, T., eds., Raven Press, New York, pp. 197-208, 1976.

Goshima, K. and Tonomura, Y.: Synchronized beating of mouse myocardial cells mediated by FL cells in monolayer culture. Exp. Cell Res., 56: 387-392, 1969.

Goss, C.M.: The first contractions of the heart in rat embryos. Anat. Rec., 70: 505-524, 1938.

Goto, J. and Irisawa, H.: Effects of lithium ions on rabbit sinoatrial node cell. Japan Circ. J., 41: 749, Abst., 1977.

Gough, W.B., Angelakos, E.T. and Morad, M.: Dependence of pacemaker activity on tissue epinephrine content and $(Ca^{2})_0$. Proc. Int. Union Physiol. Sci., vol XIII, 277, 1977.

Grattarola, M. and Torre, V.: Necessary and sufficient conditions for synchronization of non-linear oscillators with a given class of coupling. IEEE Trans., 24: 209-215, 1977.

Griepp, E.B. and Revel, J.P.: Gap junctions in development. In: Intercellular Communication, De Mello, W.C., ed., Plenum Publishing Corp., New York, pp. 1-14, 1977.

Griepp, E.B., Peacock, J.H., Bernfield, M.R. and Revel, J.P.: Morphological and functional correlates of synchronous beatng between embryonic heart cell aggregates and layers. Exp. Cell Res., 113: 273-282, 1978.

Gros, D., Mocquard, J.P., Challice, C.E. and Schrevel, J.: Formation and growth of gap junctions in mouse myocardium during ontogenesis. A freeze-cleave study. J. Cell Sci., 30: 45-61, 1978.

Gros, D., Mocquard, J.P., Challice, C.E., and Schrevel, J.: Formation and growth of gap junctions in mouse myocardium during ontogenesis. Quantitative data and their implications on the development of intercellular communication. J. Mol. Cell. Cardiol., 11: 543-554, 1979.

Gros, D., Mocquard, J.P., Schrevel, J. and Challice, C.E.: Assembly of gap junctions in developing mouse cardiac muscle. In: Perspectives in Cardiovascular Research, vol. 5, Pexieder, T., ed., Raven Press, New York, pp. 285-298, 1980.

Gros, D., Potreau, D. and Mocquard, J.P.: Myocardial plasma membrane during ontogenesis: Density and size of intramembranous particles. J. Cell Sci., 43: 301-317, 1980.

Gross, W.O.: Reizleitungsphaenomene zwischen Herzmuskelzellen in der Kultur (Film). Anat. Anz., 128: 303-310, 1971.

Guckenheimer, J., Oster, G. and Ipaktchi, A.: The dynamics of density dependent population models. J. Math. Biol., 4: 101-147, 1977.

Guidotti, G., Kanemeishi, D. and Foa, P.P.: Chick embryo heart as a tool for studying cell permeability and insulin action. Am. J. Physiol., 201: 863-868, 1961.

Guidotti, G., Loreti, L., Gaja, G. and Foa, P.P.: Glucose uptake in the developing chick embryo heart. Am. J. Physiol., 211: 981-987, 1966.

Gulko, F.B. and Petrov, A.A.: Mechanism of formation of closed pathways of conduction in excitable media. Biofizika, 17: 261-270, 1972.

Gumbel, E.J.: The statistics of extremes. New York, Columbia University Press, 1958.

Guttman, R., Lewis, S. and Rinzel, J.: Control of repetitive firing in squid axon membrane as a model for a neuron oscillator. J. Physiol. (London), 305: 377-395, 1980.

Hagiwara, S., Miyazaki, S., Moody, W. and Patlak, J.: Blocking effects of barium and hydrogen ions on the potassium current during anomalous rectification in the starfish egg. J. Physiol. (London), 279: 167-185, 1978.

Hama, K. and Saito, K.: Gap junctions between the supporting cells in some acoustico-vestibular receptors. J. Neurocytol., 6: 1-12, 1977.

Hamburger, V. and Hamilton, H.L.: A series of normal stages in the development of the chick embryo. J. Morphol., 88: 49-92, 1951.

Hanna, R.B., Keeter, J.S. and Pappas, G.D.: The fine structure of a rectifying electrotonic synapse. J. Cell Biol., 79: 764-773, 1978.

Harary, I. and Farley, B.: In vitro studies on single beating heart cells. II: Intercellular communication. Exp. Cell Res., 29: 466-474, 1963.

Harary, I., Seraydarian, M. and Gerschenson, L.E.: Effects of lipids on contractility of cultured heart cells. In: Factors Influencing Myocardial Contractility, Tanz, R.D., Kavaler, F. and Robers, J., eds., Academic Press, New York, pp. 231-243, 1967.

Harris, A.S.: Delayed development of ventricular ectopic rhythms following experimental coronary occlusion. Circulation, 1: 1318-1328, 1950.

Harris, A.S. and Rojas, A.G.: The initiation of ventricular fibrillation due to coronary occlusion. Exp. Med. and Surg., 1: 105, 1943.

Harris, E.J. and Hutter, O.F.: The action of acetylcholine on the movements of potassium ions in the sinus venosus of the heart. J. Physiol. (London), 133: 58P, 1956.

Harris, W., Days, R., Johnson, C., Finkelstein, I., Stallworth, J. and Hubert, C.: Studies on avian heart pyruvate kinase during development. Biochem. Biophys. Res. Commun., 75: 1117-1121, 1977.

Harsch, M. and Green, J.W.: Electrolyte analyses of chick embryonic fluids and heart tissues. J. Cell. Comp. Physiol., 62: 319-326, 1963.

Hart, G., Noble, D. and Shimoni, Y.: Adrenaline shifts the voltage dependence of the Na^+ and K^+ components of i_f in sheep Purkinje fibres. J. Physiol. (London), 308: 34P, 1980.

Hartree, E.F.: Determination of protein: a modification of the lowry method that gives a linear photometric response. Anal. Biochem., 48: 422-427, 1972.

Harvey, W.: De Motu Cordis. In: Classics of Cardiology (1941), Willius, F.A. and Keys, T.E., eds., Dover, New York, pp. 18-79, 1628.

Hashimoto, K., Suzuki, Y. and Chiba, S.: Influence of calcium and magnesium ions on the sinoatrial pacemaker of the canine heart. Tohuku J. Exp. Med., 113: 187-196, 1974.

Hauswirth, O., Noble, D. and Tsien, R.W.: Adrenaline: mechanism of action on the pacemaker potential in cardiac Purkinje fibres. Science, N.Y., 162: 916, 1968.

Hauswirth, O., Noble, D. and Tsien, R.W.: The mechanism of oscillatory activity at low membrane potentials in cardiac Purkinje fibres. J. Physiol. (London), 200: 255-265, 1969.

Hax, W., van Venrooij, G. and Vossenberg, J.: Cell communication: a cyclic-AMP mediated phenomenon. J. Memb. Biol., 19: 253-266, 1974.

Henderson, D., Eibl, H. and Weber, K.: Structure and biochemistry of mouse hepatic gap junctions. J. Mol. Biol., 132: 193-218, 1979.

Herbschleb, J.N., Heethaar, R.M., Van der Tweel, I., Zimmerman, A.N.E. and Meijler, F.L.: Signal analysis of ventricular fibrillation. Computers in Cardiology, 49-53, 1980.

Hermann, L.: Allgemeine Muskelphysiologie. In: Handbuch der Physiologie, Vol. I, Vogel, Leipzig, 1879.

Hermsmeyer, K.: Angiotensin II increases electrical coupling in mammalian ventricular myocardium. Circ. Res., 47: 524-529, 1980.

Hertzberg, E.L. and Gilula, N.B.: Isolation and characterization of gap junctions from rat liver. J. Biol. Chem., 254: 2138-2147, 1979.

Hess, P. and Weingart, R.: Intracellular free calcium modified by pH_i in sheep cardiac Purkinje fibres. J. Physiol. (London), 307, 60P, 1980.

Hibbs, R.G.: Electron microscopy of developing cardiac muscle in chick embryos. Am. J. Anat., 99: 17-52, 1956.

Higgings, C.B., Vatner, S.F. and Braunwald, E.: Parasympathetic control of the heart. Pharmacol. Rev., 25: 119-155, 1973.

Higgins, D.: The development of the adrenergic innervation of the chick embryo ventricle. Ph. D. Thesis, University of Connecticut, Storrs, 1980.

Higgins, D. and Pappano, A.: A histochemical study of the ontogeny of catecholamine-containing axons in the chick embryo heart. J. Mol. Cell. Cardiol., 11: 661-668, 1979.

Higgins, D. and Pappano, A.J.: Developmental changes in the sensitivity of the chick embryo ventricle to beta-adrenergic agonist during adrenergic innervation. Circ. Res., 48: 245-253, 1981.

Higgins, D. and Pappano, A.J.: Development of transmitter secretory mechanisms by adrenergic neurons in the embryonic chick heart ventricle. Devel. Biol. (in press), 1981.

Hill-Smith, I. and Purves, R.D.: Synaptic delay in the heart: an ionophoretic study. J. Physiol. (London), 279: 31-54, 1978.

Hino, N. and Ochi, R.: Effect of acetylcholine on membrane currents in guinea-pig papillary muscle. J. Physiol. (London), 307: 183-197, 1980.

Hodgkin, A.L. and Rushton, W.A.H.: The electrical constants of a crustacean nerve fibre. Proc. Roy. Soc. London, B133: 444-479, 1946.

Hodgkin, A.L. and Huxley, A.F.: A quantitative description of membrane current and its application to conduction and excitation in nerve. J. Physiol. (London), 117: 400-544, 1952.

Hodgkin, A.L. and Horowicz, P.: The influence of potassium and chloride ions on the membrane potentials of single muscle fibres. J. Physiol. (London), 148: 127-160, 1959.

Hoffman, B.F.: Atrioventricular conduction in mammalian hearts. Ann. N.Y. Acad. Sci., 127: 105-112, 1965.

Hoffman, B.F., Paes de Carvalho, A., DeMello, W.C. and Cranefield, P.: Electrical activity of single fibers of the atrioventricular node. Circ. Res., 2: 11-18, 1959.

Holden, A.V.: On the variability of pacemaker activity. Proceedings of the 5th European Meeting on Cybernetic and Systems Research, 1980.

Holman, M.E. and Hirst, G.D.S.: Junctional transmission in smooth muscle and the autonomic nervous system. In: Handbook of Physiology, American Physiological Society, Bethesda, Maryland, 1977.

Hunter, P.J., Mc Naughton, P.A. and Noble, D.: Analytical models of propagation in excitable cells. Progr. Biophys. Mol. Biol., 30: 99-144, 1975.

Hutter, O.F. and Trautwein, W.: Vagal and sympathetic effects on the pacemaker fibres in the sinus venosus of the heart. J. Gen. Physiol., 39: 715-733, 1956.

Hutter, O.F. and Noble, D.: Rectifying properties of heart muscle. Nature, 188: 495, 1960.

Hyde, A., Blondell, B., Matter, A., Cheneval, J.P., Filloux, B. and Girardier, L.: Homo and heterocellular junctions in cell cultures: an electrophysiological and morphological study. Prog. Brain Res., 31: 283-311, 1969.

Iano, T.L., Levy, M.N. and Lee, M.H.: An acceleratory component of the parasympathetic control of heart rate. Am. J. Physiol., 224: 997-1005, 1973.

Ignarro, L.J. and Shideman, F.E.: Catechol-o-methyl transferase and monoamine oxidase activities in the heart and liver of the embryonic and developing chick. J. Pharmacol. Exp. Ther., 159: 29-37, 1968.

Ignarro, L.J. and Shideman, F.E.: The requirement of sympathetic innervation for the active transport of norepinephrine by the heart. J. Pharmacol. Exp. Ther., 159: 59-65, 1968.

Ikemoto, Y. and Goto, M.: Nature of the negative inotropic effect of acetylcholine on the myocardium: an elucidation on the bullfrog atrium. Proc. Japan Acad., 51: 501-505, 1975.

Ikemoto, Y. and Goto, M.: Effects of ACh on slow inward current and tension components of the bullfrog atrium. J. Mol. Cell. Cardiol., 9: 313-326, 1977.

Imanaga, I.: Cell-to-cell diffusion of Procion Yellow in sheep and calf Purkinje fibers. J. Memb. Biol., 16: 381-388, 1974.

Irisawa, H.: Comparative physiology of the cardiac pacemaker mechanism. Physiol. Rev., 58: 461-498, 1978.

Irisawa, H.: Ionic currents underlying spontaneous rhythm of the cardiac primary pacemaker cells. In: The Sinus Node. Structure, Function and Clinical Relevance, Bonke, F.I.M., ed., Martinus Nijhoff, The Hague, pp. 368-375, 1978.

Irisawa, H. and Yanagihara, K.: The slow inward current of the rabbit sino-atrial nodal cells. In: The Slow Inward Current and Cardiac Arrhythmias, Zipes, D.P. and Bailey, J.C., eds., Martinus Nijhoff, The Hague, pp. 265-284, 1980.

Iriuchijima, J. and Kumada, M.: Efferent cardiac vagal discharge in response to electrical stimulation of sensory nerves. Jap. J. Physiol., 13: 599-605, 1963.

Isenberg, G.: Cardiac Purkinje fibres: Caesium as a tool to block inward rectifying potassium currents. Pfluegers Arch., 365: 99-106, 1976.

Isenberg, G.: Cardiac Purkinje fibers. Ca^{2+} controls steady state potassium conductance. Pfluegers Arch., 371: 71-76, 1977.

Isenberg, G. and Trautwein, W.: The effect of dihydroouabain and lithium ions on the outward current in cardiac Purkinje fibers: evidence for electrogenicity of active transport. Pfluegers Arch., 350: 41-54, 1974.

Isenberg, G. and Kloeckner, U.: Glycocalyx is not required for slow inward calcium current in isolated rat heart myocyte. Nature, 284: 358-360, 1980.

Ishima, Y.: The effect of tetrodoxotin and sodium substitution on the action potential in the course of development of the embryonic chicken heart. Proc. of Jap. Acad., 44: 170-175, 1978.

Ivanitskii, G.P., Krinskii, V.I. and Selkov, E.E.: The Mathematical Biophysics of Cells, Science Publishers, Moscow, 1978.

Iversen, L.L.: The Uptake and Storage of Noradrenaline in Sympathetic Nerves, Cambridge University Press, London, 1967.

Jack, J.J.B., Noble, D. and Tsien, R.W.: Electric current flow in excitable cells. Clarendon Press, Oxford, 1973.

Jalife, J. and Moe, G.K.: Effect of electrotonic potentials on pacemaker activity of canine Purkinje fibres in relation to parasystole. Circ.Res., 39: 801-808, 1976.

Jalife, J. and Antzelevitch, C.: Phase resetting and annihilation of pacemaker activity in cardiac tissue. Science, 206: 695-697, 1979.

Jalife, J. and Moe, G.K.: Phasic effects of vagal stimulation on pacemaker activity of the isolated sinus node of the young cat. Circ. Res., 45: 595-608, 1979.

Jalife, J. and Moe, G.K.: A biological model of parasystole. Am. J. Cardiol., 43: 761-772, 1979.

Jalife, J., Antzelevitch, C.: Pacemaker annihilation: diagnostic and therapeutic implications. Am. Heart J., 100: 128-130, 1980.

Jalife, J., Hamilton, A.J., Lamanna, V.R. and Moe, G.K.: Effects of current flow on pacemaker activity of the isolated kitten SA node. Am. J. Physiol., 238 (Heart Circ. Physiol. 7): H307-H316, 1980.

Jalife, J., Hamilton, A.J. and Moe, G.K.: Desensitization of the cholinergic receptor at the sinoatrial cell of the kitten. Am. J. Physiol., 238 (Heart Circ. Physiol. 7): H439-H448, 1980.

James, T.N.: Cardiac conduction system: fetal and postnatal development. Am. J. Cardiol., 25: 213-226,

1970.

James, T.N. and Sherf, L.: Ultrastructure of the human atrioventricular node. Circulation, 37: 1049-1070, 1968.

James, T.N., Sherf, L., Fine, G. and Morales, A.R.: Comparative ultrastructure of the sinus node in man and dog. Circulation, 34: 139-163, 1966.

Janse, M.J., Van Capelle, F.J., Morsink, H., Kleber, A.G., Wilms-Schopman, F., Cardinal, R., D'Almoncourt, C. and Durrer, D.: Flow of "injury" current and patterns of excitation during early ventricular arrhythmias in acute regional myocardial ischemia in isolated porcine and canine hearts. Circ. Res., 47: 151-165, 1980.

Jewett, J.D.: Activity of single efferent fibers in the cervical vagus nerve of the dog, with special reference to cardioinhibitory fibers. J. Physiol. (London), 175: 321-357, 1964.

Johnson, E.A. and Tille, J.: Investigations of the electrical properties of cardiac muscle fibres with the aid of intracellular double-barrelled electrodes. J. Gen. Physiol., 44: 443-467, 1961.

Johnson, E.A. and Lieberman, M.: Heart: excitation and contraction. Ann. Rev. Physiol., 33: 479-532, 1971.

Johnson, R.G., Hammer, M., Sheridan, J. and Revel, J.P.: Gap junctions between reaggregated Novikoff hepatoma cells. Proc. Natl. Acad. Sci. USA, 71: 4536-4540, 1974.

Johnstone, P.N.: Studies on the physiological anatomy of the embryonic heart. I. Bull. Johns Hopkins Hosp., 35: 87-90, 1924.

Johnstone, P.N.: Studies on the physiological anatomy of the embryonic heart. II: An inquiry into the development of the heart beat in chick embryos. Bull. Johns Hopkins Hosp., 36: 299-311, 1925.

Jongsma, H.J., Masson-Pevet, M., Hollander, C.C. and DeBruyne, J.: Synchronization of the beating frequency of cultured rat heart cells. In: Developmental and Physiological Correlates of Cardiac Muscle, Lieberman, M. and Sano T., eds., Raven Press, New York, pp. 185-196, 1975.

Jongsma, H.J. and Van Rijn, H.E.: Electrotonic spread of current in monolayer cultures of neonatal rat heart cells. J. Memb. Biol., 9: 341-360, 1972.

Jose, A.D. and Collison, D.: The normal range and determinants of the intrinsic heart rate in man. Cardiovasc. Res., 4: 160-167, 1970.

Josephson, I., Renaud, J-F., Vogel, S., McLean, M. and Sperelakis, N.: Mechanism of the histamine-induced positive inotropic action in cardiac muscle. Europ. J. Pharmacol., 35: 393-398, 1967.

Joyner, R.W., Westerfield, M. and Moore, J.W.: Effects of cellular geometry on current flow during a propagated action potential. Biophysical J., 31: 183-194, 1980.

Kamiyama, A. and Matsuda, K.: Electrophysiological properties of the canine ventricular fiber. Jap. J. Physiol., 16: 407-420, 1966.

Kaneko, A.: Electrical connexions between horizontal cells in the dogfish retina. J. Physiol. (London), 213: 95-105, 1976.

Karfunkel, H.R.: Zur Theorie der Anregbarkeit und Ausbreitung von Erregungswellen in chemischen Reaktionssystemen. Dissertation, Universitaet zu Tubingen, 1975.

Karrer, H.E.: Cell interconnections in normal human cervical epithelium. J. Biophys. Biochem. Cytol., 7: 181-183, 1960.

Karrer, H.E.: The striated musculature of blood vessels. II. Cell interconnections and cell surface. J. Biophys. Biochem. Cytol., 8: 135-150, 1960.

Kass, R.S. and Tsien, R.W.: Multiple effects of calcium antagonists on plateau currents in cardiac Purkinje fibers. J. Gen. Physiol., 66: 169-192, 1975.

Kasuya, Y., Matsuki, N. and Shigenobu, K.: Changes in sensitivity to anoxia of the cardiac action potential plateau during chick embryonic development. Devel. Biol., 58: 124-133, 1977.

Katona, P.G., Poitras, J.W., Barnett, G.O. and Terry, B.S.: Cardiac vagal efferent activity and heart period in the carotid sinus reflex. Am. J. Physiol., 218: 1030-1037, 1970.

Katz, B.: Les constantes électriques de la membrane du muscle. Archs. Sci. Physiol., 3: 285-300, 1949.

Katz, B. and Miledi, R.: The statistical nature of the acetylcholine potentials and its molecular components. J. Physiol. (London), 224: 665-699, 1972.

Katzung, B.G.: Electrically induced automaticity in ventricular myocardium. Life Sci., 14: 1133-1140, 1974.

Katzung, B.G.: Effects of extracellular calcium and sodium on depolarization-induced automaticity in guinea pig papillary muscle. Circ. Res., 37: 118-127, 1975.

Kaufman, R. and Theophile, U.: Automatie-foerdernde Dehnungseffekte an Purkinje Faeden, Papillarmuskeln und Vorhoftrabekeln von Rhesus-Affen. Pluegers Arch., 297: 174-189, 1967.

Kawamura, K. and Konishi, T.: Ultrastructure of the cell junction of heart muscle with special reference to its functional significance in excitation conduction and in the concept of "disease of intercalated discs". Japan. Circ. J., 31: 1533-1543, 1967.

Keeter, J.S., Deschenes, M., Pappas, G.D. and Bennett, M.V.L.: Fine structure and permeability studies of a rectifying electrotonic synapse. Biol. Bull., 147: 485, 1974.

Keith, A. and Flack, M.W.: The auriculo-ventricular bundle of the human heart. Lancet, 2: 359-364, 1906.

Kelly, K.A. and Laforce, R.C.: Pacing the canine stomach with electric stimulation. Am. J. Physiol., 222: 588-594, 1972.

Kensler, R.W. and Goodenough, D.A.: Isolation of mouse myocardial gap junctions. J. Cell Biol., 86: 755-764, 1980.

Kensler, R.W., Brink, P. and Dewey, M.M.: Nexus of frog ventricle. J. Cell Biol., 73: 768-781, 1977.

Khodorov, B.I. and Timin, E.N.: Nerve impulse propagation along nonuniform fibers. Progr. Biophys. Mol. Biol., 30: 145-184, 1975.

Kim, S. and Baba, N.: Atrioventricular node and Purkinje fibers of the guinea pig heart, Am. J. Anat.,

132: 339-353, 1971.

Kirby, M.L., Diab, I.M. and Mattio, T.F.: Development of adrenergic innervation of the iris and fluorescent ganglión cells in the choroid of the chick eye. Anat. Rec., 191: 311-320, 1978.

Kirby, M.L., McKenzie, J.W. and Weidman, T.A.: Developing innervation of the chick heart: A histofluorescence and light microscopic study of sympathetic innervation. Anat. Rec., 196: 333-340, 1980.

Kirshner, N.: Uptake of catecholamines by a particulate fraction of the adrenal medulla. J. Biol. Chem., 237: 2311-2317, 1962.

Kistler, J. and Bullivant, S.: Lens gap junctions and orthogonal arrays are unrelated. FEBS Lett., 111: 73-78, 1980.

Kistler, J. and Bullivant, S.: The connexon order in isolated lens gap junctions. J. Ultrastruct. Res., 72: 27-38, 1980.

Kleber, A.G., Janse, M.J., van Capelle, F.J.L. and Durrer, D.: Mechanisms and time course of S-T and T-Q segment changes during acute regional myocardial ischemia in the pig heart determined by extracellular and intracellular recordings. Circ. Res., 42: 603-613, 1978.

Kline, R. and Morad, M.: Potassium efflux and accumulation in heart muscle. Evidence from K^+ electrode experiments. Biophys. J., 16: 367-372, 1976.

Kodama, J., Goto, J., Ando, S., Toyama, J. and Yamada, K.: Effects of rapid stimulation on the transmembrane action potentials of rabbit sinus node pacemaker cells. Circ. Res., 46: 90-99, 1980.

Koelliker, A. and Mueller, H.: Nachweis der negativen Schwankung des Muskelstroms am naturlich sich contrahierende Muskel. Verhandl. J. Physiol. Med. Gessellsch. in Wurzberg, 6: 528-533, 1855.

Kohlhardt, M., Bauer, B., Krause, H. and Fleckenstein, A.: Differentiation of the transmembrane Na and Ca channels in mammalian cardiac fibers by use of specific inhibitors. Pfluegers Arch., 335: 309-322, 1972.

Kohlhardt, M., Figulla, H.R. and Tripathi, O.: The slow membrane channel as the predominant mediator of the excitation process of the sinoatrial pacemaker cell. Basic Res. Cardiol., 71: 17-26, 1976.

Korn, H. and Faber, D.S.: An electrically mediated inhibition in goldfish medulla. J. Neurophysiol., 38: 430-451, 1975.

Kreitner, D.: Effect of polarization and of inhibitors of ionic conductances on the action potentials of nodal and perinodal fibers in rabbit sinoatrial node. In: The Sinus Node. Structure, Function and Clinical Relevance, Bonke, F.I.M., eds., Martinus Nijhoff, The Hague, pp. 270-278, 1978.

Krinskii, V.I.: Spread of excitation in an inhomogeneous medium. Biofizika, 11: 676-683, 1966.

Krinskii, V.I.: Fibrillation in excitable media. Prob. Kibernetiki, 20: 59-80, 1968.

Krinskii, V.I.: Mathematical models of cardiac arrhythmias (spiral waves). Pharmac. Ther. B., 3: 539-555, 1978.

Kronhaus, K.D., Spear, J.F., Moore, E.N. and Kline, R.P.: Sinus node extracellular potassium transients following vagal stimulation. Nature, 275: 322-324, 1978.

Kukushkin, N.I., Bukauskas, F.F. and Saxon, M.E.: II. Model of two-dimensional anisotropic syncitium. Biofizika, 19: 888-893, 1974.

Kunze, D.L.: Reflex discharge patterns of cardiac vagal efferent fibres. J. Physiol. (London), 222: 1-15, 1972.

Kuramoto Y.: Diffusion-induced chaos in reaction system. Prog. Theor. Phys., 64: (supplement), 346-367, 1978.

Kutchai, H., King, S.L., Martin, M. and Daves, E.D.: Glucose uptake by chicken embryo hearts at various stages of development. Devel. Biol., 55: 92-102, 1977.

Lamb, T.D. and Simon, E.J.: The relation between intercellular coupling and electrical noise in turtle photoreceptors. J. Physiol. (London), 263: 257-286, 1976.

Lane, M.A., Sastre, A., Law, M. and Salpeter, M.M.: Cholinergic and adrenergic receptors on mouse cardiocytes in vitro. Devel. Biol., 57: 254-269, 1977.

Lange, G.: Action of driving stimuli from intrinsic and extrinsic sources on in situ cardiac pacemaker tissues. Circ. Res., 17: 449-459, 1965.

Langendorff, O.: Studien ueber Rhythmik und Automatie des Froschherzens. Arch. Physiol. (Leipzig), 1: 133, 1884.

Langer, G.A., Frank, J.S. and Nudd, L.M.: Correlation of calcium exchange, structure and function in myocardial tissue culture. Am. J. Physiol., 237: H239-H246, 1979.

Lapicque, L.: Recherches quantitatives sur l'excitation électrique des nerfs traitée comme une polarisation. J. Physiol. (Paris), 9: 620-635, 1907.

Larsen, W.J.: Gap junctions and hormone action. In: Transport of Ions and Water in Epithelia, Walls, B.J., Oschman, J.L., Moreton, D. and Gupta, B., eds., Academic Press, London, pp. 333-363, 1977.

Larsen, W.J.: Structural diversity of gap junctions. Tissue and Cell, 9: 373-394, 1977.

Lasansky, A. and Vallerga, S.: Horizontal cell responses in the retina of the larval tiger salamander. J. Physiol. (London), 236: 171-191, 1975.

Lau, C. and Slotkin, T.A.: Accelerated development of rat sympathetic neurotransmission caused by neonatal triiodothyronine administration. J. Pharmacol. Exp. Ther., 208: 485-490, 1979.

Lavallee, M. and Webb, J.L.: Mesure directe de l'acidose cellulaire sur le muscle cardiaque au cours de l'anoxie (abstr.). Memorias del IV Congreso Mundial de Cardiologia, Mexico, 5: 249, 1963.

Lawrence, T.S., Beers, W.H. and Gilula, N.B.: Transmission of hormonal stimulation by cell-to-cell communication. Nature (Lond.) 272: 501-506, 1978.

Le Douarin, G., Obrecht, G. and Coraboeuf, E.: Détermination régionales dans l'aire cardiaque présomptive mises en evidence chez l'embryon de poulet par la méthode microélectrophysiologique. J. Embryol. Exp. Morphol., 15: 153-167, 1966.

Le Douarin, G., Renaud, J.D., Renaud, D. and Coraboeuf, E.: Influence of insulin on sensitivity to tetroto-
    doxin of isolated chick embryo heart cells in culture. J. Mol. Cell. Cardiol., 6: 523-529, 1974.
Lea, T.J. and Ashley, C.C.: Increase in free Ca^{2+} in muscle after exposure to CO_2, Nature, 275:   236,
    1978.
Ledbetter, M.L. and Lubin, M.: Transfer of potassium. A new measure of cell-cell coupling. J. Cell Biol.,
    80: 150-165, 1979.
Lee, I. and Challice, C.E.: A freeze-cleave study of the influence of cyclohexamide on the development of
    gap junctions in vitro. IRCS Medical Sci., 8: 49-50, 1980.
Lee, J.P., Kuo, J.F. and Greengard, P.: Role of muscarinic cholinergic receptors in regulation of guanosine
    3', 5'. Monophosphate content in mammalian brain, heart muscle and intestinal smooth muscle. Proc.
    Natl. Acad. Sci. USA, 69: 3287-3291, 1972.
Lehmkuhl, D. and Sperelakis, N.: Electrotonic spread of current in cultured chick heart cells.   J. Cell.
    Comp. Physiol., 66: 119-133, 1965.
Lehninger, A.L.: Dynamics and mechanism of active ion transport across the mitochondria membrane.   N.   Y.
    Acad. Sci., 137 (2): 700-707, 1966.
Lenfant, J.: Analyse des propriétés de la membrane myocardique sino-auriculaire: génèse de l'activité spon-
    tanée. Theses, Poitiers, 1972.
Levin, K.R. and Page, E.: Quantitative studies on plasmalemmal folds and caveolae of rabbit ventricular myo-
    cardial cells. Circ. Res.: 46: 244-255, 1980.
Levy, M.N. and Zieske, H.: Synchronization of the cardiac pacemaker with repetitive stimulation of the caro-
    tid sinus nerve in the dog. Circ. Res., 30: 634-641, 1972.
Levy, M.N., Martin, P.J., Iano, T. and Zieske, H.: Paradoxical effect of vagus nerve stimulation on heart
    rate in dogs. Circ. Res., 25: 303-314, 1969.
Levy, M.N., Marti, P.J., Iano, T. and Zieske, H.: Effects of single vagal stimulus on heart rate and atrio-
    ventricular conduction. Am. J. Physiol., 218: 1256-1262, 1970.
Levy, M.N., Iano, T. and Zieske, H.: Effects of repetitive bursts of vagal activity on heart rate.   Circ.
    Res., 30: 186-195, 1972.
Levy, M.N., Wexberg, S., Eckel, C. and Zieske, H.: The effect of changing interpulse intervals on the nega-
    tive chronotropic response to repetitive bursts of vagal stimuli in the dog. Circ. Res., 43: 570-576,
    1978.
Lewis, M.R.: Muscular contractions in tissue culture. Contr. to Embryol., Carnegie Inst. of Washington, 9:
    191-209, 1920.
Lewis, T.: Galvanometric curves yielded by cardiac beats generated in various areas of the auricular muscula-
    ture. The pacemaker heart. Heart, 2: 23-46, 1910.
Lewis, T.: The Mechanism and Graphic Registration of the Heart Beat. Shaw and Sons, London, 452 pp., 1920.
Lewis, T., Oppenheimer, A. and Oppenheimer, B.S.: The site of origin of the mammalian heart beat: the pace-
    maker in the dog. Heart, 2: 147-169, 1910.
Lewis, W.H.: The influence of temperature on the rhythm of the isolated heart of the young chick embryo.
    Bull. Johns Hopkins Hosp., 35: 253, 1924.
Lieberman, M., Kootsey, J.M., Johnson, E.A. and Sawanobori, T.: Slow conduction in cardiac muscle: a bio-
    physical model. Biophys. J. 13: 37-55, 1973.
Lieberman, M., Sawanobori, T., Kootsey, J.M. and Johnson, E.A.: A synthetic strand of cardiac muscle.   Its
    passive electrical properties. J. Gen. Physiol., 65: 527-550, 1975.
Lieberman, M., Horres, C.R., Aiton, J.F. and Johnson, E.A.: Active transport and electrogenicity of cardiac
    muscle in tissue culture. XXVIIth Proc. of Internat. Cong. of Physiol. Sci. (Paris), 13: 446,
    1977.
Linkens, D.A.: The stability of entrainment conditions for RLC coupled van der Pol oscillators. Bull. Math.
    Biol., 39: 359-372, 1977.
Linkens, D.A.: Theoretical analysis of beating and modulation phenomena in weakly inter-coupled van der Pol
    oscillator systems for biological modeling. J. Theor. Biol., 79: 31-54, 1979.
Linkens, D.A.: Canine colonic pacing and coupled oscillator synchronisation. J. Physiol. (London), 278:
    26P, 1978.
Linkens, D.A. and Datardina, S.: Frequency entrainment of coupled Hodgkin-Huxley type oscillators for model-
    ing gastrointestinal electrical activity. IEEE Trans. Biom.. Eng., BME 24: 362-365, 1977.
Linkens, D.A., Taylor, I. and Duthie, H.L.: Mathematical Modelling of the colorectal myoelectrical activity
    in humans. IEEE Trans. Bio. Med. Eng., BME 23, 101-110, 1976.
Lipsius, S.L. and Vassalle, M.: Dual excitatory channels in the sinus node. J. Mol. Cell. Cardiol., 10:
    753-767, 1978.
Lipsius, S.L. and Vassalle, M.: Characterization of a two-component upstroke in the sinus node subsidiary
    pacemakers.   In: The Sinus Node. Structure, Function and Clinical Relevance, Bonke, F.I.M., ed., Mar-
    tinus Nijhoff, The Hague, pp. 2330244, 1978.
Loeffelholz, K. and Pappano, A.J.: Increased sensitivity of sinoatrial pacemaker to acetylcholine and to ca-
    techolamines at the onset of autonomic neuroeffector transmission in chick embryo heart. J. Pharmacol.
    Exp. Ther., 191: 479-486, 1974.
Loeffelholz, K. and Pappano, A.J.: Ontogenetic changes in the pacemaker activity in the chick heart.   Life
    Sci., 14: 1755-1763, 1974.
Loewenstein, W.R.: Permeability of membrane junctions. Ann. N.Y. Acad. Sci., 137: 441-472, 1966.
Loewenstein, W.R.: Permeable junctions. Cold Spring Harbor Symp. Quant. Biol., 40: 49-63, 1975.
Loewenstein, W.R.: The cell-to-cell membrane channel in development and growth. In: Differentiation and De-
    velopment, Ahmad, F., Russell, T.R., Schultz, J. and Werner, R., eds., Academic Press, New York, pp.

399-409, 1978.

Loewenstein, W.R., Nakas, M. and Socolar, S.J.: Junctional membrane uncoupling: permeability transforma-
    tions at a cell membrane junction. J. Gen. Physiol., 50: 1865-1981, 1967.

Loewenstein, W.R., Kanno, Y. and Socolar, S.J.: The cell-to-cell channel. Fed. Proc., 37: 2645-2650,
    1978.

Loewenstein, W.R., Kanno, Y. and Socolar, S.J.: Quantum jumps of conductance during formation of membrane
    channels at cell-to-cell junction. Nature (London), 274: 133-136, 1978.

Lombet, A., Renaud, J.F., Chicheportiche, R. and Lazdunski, M.: A cardiac tetrodotoxin-binding component:
    biochemical identification, characterization and properties. Biochemistry, 20: 1279-1285, 1981.

Lompre, A.M., Poggioli, J. and Vassort, G.: Maintenance of fast sodium channels during primary culture of
    embryonic chick heart cells. J. Mol. Cell. Cardiol., 11: 813-825, 1979.

Lorber, V. and Bertaud, W.S.: Cellular surfaces of amphibian atrial muscle. J. Cell. Sci., 9:   427-433,
    1971.

Lowe, D.A., Bush, B.M.H. and Ripley, S.H.: Pharmacological evidence for "fast" sodium channels in nonspiking
    neurones. Nature, 274: 289-290, 1978.

Lu, H., Lange, G. and Brooks, C.C.: Factors controlling pacemaker action in cells of the sinoatrial node.
    Circ. Res., 17: 460-471, 1965.

Lu, H.H.: Shifts in pacemaker dominance within the sinoatrial region of cat and rabbit hearts resulting from
    increase of extracellular potassium. Circ. Res., 26: 339-345, 1970.

MacGregor, D.C., Wilson, D.J., Tanaka, S., Holness, D.E., Lixfeld, W., Silver, M.D., Rubis, L.J., Goldstein,
    W. and Gunstensen, J.: Ischemic contracture of the left ventricle. J. Thor. Cardiovasc. Surg., 70:
    945-954, 1975.

Mackaay, A.J.C., Bleeker, W.K., Op 't Hof, T. and Bouman, L.N.: Temperature dependence of the chronotropic
    action of Ca. J. Mol. Cell. Cardiol., 12: 433-443, 1980.

Mackaay, A.J.C., Op 't Hof, T., Bleeker, W.K., Jongsma, H.J. and Bouman, L.N.: Interaction of adrenaline and
    acetylcholine on cardiac pacemaker function. Functional inhomogeneity of the rabbit sinus node. J.
    Pharmacol. Exp. Ther., 214: 417-422, 1980.

MacKenzie, E. and Standen, N.B.: The postnatal development of adrenoceptor responses in isolated papillary
    muscles from rat. Pfluegers Arch., 383: 185-187, 1980.

Makowski, L., Caspar, D.L.D., Phillips, W.C. and Goodenough, D.A.: Gap junction structures. II. Analysis
    of the X-ray diffraction data. J. Cell Biol., 74: 629-645, 1977.

Mallart, A. and Trautmann, A.: Ionic properties of the neuromuscular junction of the frog; effects of den-
    ervation and pH. J. Physiol. (London), 234: 553-567, 1973.

Manasek, F.J.: Embryonic development of the heart. I. A light and electron microscopic study of myocardial
    development in the early chick embryo. J. Morph., 125: 329-366, 1968.

Mann, J.E. and Sperelakis, N.: Further development of a model for electrical transmission between myocardial
    cells not connected by low-resistance pathways. J. Electrocardiol., 12: 23-33, 1979.

Markowitz, C.: Response of explanted embryonic cardiac tissue to epinephrine and acetylcholine. Am. J.
    Physiol., 97: 271-275, 1931.

Martin, P.J.: Dynamic vagal control of atrial-ventricular conduction: theoretical and experimental studies.
    Ann. Biomed. Eng., 3: 275-295, 1975.

Martin, P.J.: Paradoxical dynamic interaction of heart period and vagal activity on atrioventricular conduc-
    tion in the dog. Circ. Res., 40: 81-89, 1977.

Martins-Ferreira, H., de Oliveiro Castro, G., Struchinea, C.J. and Rodriques, P.S.: Circling spreading de-
    pression in isolated chicken retina. J. Neurophys., 37: 773-784, 1974.

Masson-Pevet, M.A.: The fine structure of cardiac pacemaker cells in the sinus node and in tissue culture.
    (Doct. Thesis), Rodopi, Amsterdam, 1979.

Masson-Pevet, M.A., Jongsma, H.J. and De Bruijne, J.: Collagenase and trypsin-dissociated heart cells: A
    comparative ultrastructural study. J. Mol. Cell. Cardiol., 8: 747-757, 1976.

Masson-Pevet, M., Bleeker, W.K., Mackaay, A.J.C., Gros, D. and Bouman, L.N.: Ultrastructural and functional
    aspects of the rabbit sinoatrial node. In: The Sinus Node. Structure, Function and Clinical Relevance,
    Bonke, F.I.M., ed., Martinus Nijhoff, The Hague, pp. 195-211, 1978.

Masson-Pevet, M., Bleeker, W.K. and Gros, D.: The plasma membrane of leading pacemaker cells in the rabbit
    sinus node. Circ. Res., 45: 621-629, 1979.

Masson-Pevet, M., Bleeker, W.K., Mackaay, A.J.C., Bouman, L.N. and Houtkoper, J.M.: Sinus node and atrium
    cells from the rabbit heart: a quantitative electron microscope description after electrophysiological
    localization. J. Mol. Cell. Cardiol., 11: 555-568, 1979.

Masson-Pevet, M., Gros, D. and Besselsen, E.: The caveolae in rabbit sinus node and atrium. Cell Tissue
    Res., 208: 183-196, 1980.

Masuda, M.O. and Paes de Carvalho, A.: Sinoatrial transmission and atrial invasion during normal rhythm in
    the rabbit heart. Circ. Res., 37: 414-421, 1975.

Matter, A.: A morphometric study on the nexus of rat cardiac muscle. J. Cell Biol., 56: 690-696, 1973.

Maughan, D.N.: Some effect of prolonged depolarization on membrane currents in bullfrog atrial muscle. J.
    Memb. Biol., 11: 331-352, 1973.

May, R.: Simple mathematical models with very complicated dynamics. Nature, 261: 459, (erratum: Nature,
    262: 236), 1978.

Mayer, A.G.: Rhythmical pulsation in scyphomedusae. Papers of the Tortugas Lab. of the Carnegie Inst. of
    Wash., 1: 115-131, 1908.

Mayer, A.G.: The relation between degree of concentration of one electrolytes of seawater and rate of nerve
    conduction in Cassiope. Papers of the Tortugas Lab. of Carnegie Inst. of Wash. 6: 25-54, 1914.

Mayer, A.G.: Rhythmical pulsation in Scyphomedusae: II. In: Papers from the Tortugas Laboratory of the Carnegie Institution of Washington. I: 113-131 (Carnegie Institution of Washington, Publication No. 102, part VII), 1908.

Mazet, F.: Mise en évidence et étude des variations morphologiques des gap-junctions dans les tissues électriquement couplés. Applications aux tissus cardiaques. These de Doctorat d'Etat, University of Paris XI (Orsay), France, 1977.

Mazet, F.: Freeze-fracure studies of gap junctions in the developing and adult amphibian cardiac muscle. Devel. Biol., 60: 139-152, 1977.

Mazet, F. and Cartaud, J.: Freeze-fracture studies of frog atrial fibres. J. Cell Sci., 22: 427-434, 1976.

Mazet, F.: Etude ultrastructurale des jonctions présentes dans le myocarde de poulet. Biol. Cell. (Paris), 29: 27a, 1977.

McAllister, R.E. and Noble, D.: The time and voltage dependence of the slow outward current in cardiac Purkinje fibres. J. Physiol. (London), 186: 632-662, 1966.

McAllister, R.E., Noble, D. and Tsien, W.: Reconstruction of the electrical activity of cardiac Purkinje fibres. J. Physiol. (London), 251: 1-59, 1975.

McCall, D.: Effect of quinidine and temperature on sodium uptake and contraction frequency of cultured rat myocardial cells. Circ. Res., 39: 730-735, 1976.

McCarty, L.P., Lee, W.C. and Shideman, F.E.: Measurement of the inotropic effects of drugs on the innervated and noninnervated embryonic chick heart. J. Pharmac. Exp. Ther., 129: 315-321, 1960.

McDonald, T.F. and DeHaan, R.L.: Ion levels and membrane potential in chick heart tissue and cultured cells. J. Gen. Physiol., 61: 89-109, 1973.

McDonald, T.F. and Sachs, H.G.: Electrical activity in embryonic heart cell aggregates (Developmental aspects). Pfluegers Arch., 354: 151-164, 1975.

McDonald, T.F. and Trautwein, W.: The potassium current underlying delayed rectification in cat ventricular muscle. J. Physiol. (London), 274: 217-246, 1978.

McDonald, T.F., Sachs, H.G. and DeHaan, R.L.: Development of sensitivity to tetrodotoxin in beating chick embryo hearts, single cells, and aggregates. Science, L76: 1248-1250, 1972.

McGuigan, J.A.S.: Some limitations of the double sucrose gap and its use in a study of the slow outward current in mammalian ventricular muscle. J. Physiol. (London), 240: 775-806, 1974.

McLean, M.J. and Sperelakis, N.: Rapid loss of sensitivity to tetrodotoxin of chick ventricular myocardial cells after separation from the heart. Exp. Cell Res., 86: 351-364, 1974.

McLean, M.J. and Sperelakis, N.: Retention of fully differentiated electrophysiological properties of chick embryonic heart cells in culture. Devel. Biol., 50: 134-142, 1976.

McLean, M.J. and Sperelakis, N.: Differences in degree of electrotonic interaction between highly differentiated and reverted cultured heart cell reaggregates. J. Memb. Biol., (in press), 1980.

McLean, M.J., Lapsley, R.A., Shigenobu, K., Murad, R. and Sperelakis, N.: High cyclic AMP levels in young chick embryonic hearts. Devel. Biol., 42: 196-201, 1975.

McLean, M.J., Renaud, J.F., Sperelakis, N. and Nio, M.C.: RNA induction of fast Na^+ channels in cultured cardiac myoblasts. Science, 191: 297-299, 1976.

McLean, M.J., Renaud, J-F., Niu, M.C. and Sperelakis, N.: Membrane differentiation of cardiac myoblasts induced in vitro by an RNA-enriched fraction from adult heart. Exp. Cell Res.,110: 1-14, 1977.

McLean, M.J., Renaud, J.F. and Sperelakis, N.: Cardiac-like action potentials recorded from spontaneously-contracting structures induced in post-nodal pieces of chick blastoderm exposed to an RNA-enriched fraction from adult heart. Differentiation, 11: 13-17, 1978.

McLean, M.J., Pelleg, A. and Sperelakis, N.: Electrophysiological recordings from spontaneously contracting reaggregates of cultured smooth muscle cells from guinea pig vas deferens. J. Cell Biol., 80: 539-552, 1979.

McNutt, N.S.: Ultrastructure of intercellular junctions in adult and developing cardiac muscle. Am. J. Cardiol., 25: 169-182, 1970.

McNutt, N.S. and Weinstein, R.S.: The ultrastructure of the nexus. A correlated thin-section and freeze-cleave study. J. Cell Biol., 47: 666-688, 1970.

McNutt, N.S. and Weinstein, R.S.: Membrane ultrastructure at mammalian intercellular junctions. Progr. Biophys. Mol. Biol., 26: 45-101, 1973.

Meda, M. and Ferroni, A.: Early functional differentiation of heart muscle cells. Experientia, 15: 427-428, 1959.

Meda, P., Perrelet, A. and Orci, L.: Gap junctions and beta-cell function. Horm. Metab. Res. Suppl., (in press), 1980.

Meech, R.H. and Thomas, R.C.: The effect of calcium injection on the intracellular sodium and pH of snail neurones. J. Physiol. (London), 265: 867-879, 1977.

Mela, L.: Interactions of La^{3+} and local anesthetic drugs with mitochondria, Ca^{++} and Mn^{++} uptake. Archiv. Biochim. Biophys., 123: 286-293, 1968.

Mendez, C. and Moe, G.K.: Some characteristics of transmembrane potentials of AV nodal cells during propagation of premature beats. Circ. Res., 19: 993-1010, 1966.

Mendez, C., Mueller, W.J., Meredith, J. and Moe, G.K.: Interaction of transmembrane potentials in canine Purkinje fiber-muscle junctions. Circ. Res., 24: 361-372, 1969.

Meves, H. and Voelkner, K.G.: Die Wirkung von CO_2 auf das Ruhemembranpotential und die elektrischen Konstanten der quergestreiften Muskelfaser. Pfluegers Arch., 265: 457-476, 1959.

Mines, G.R.: On circulating excitations on heart muscles and their possible relation to tachycardia and fibrillation. Trans. R. Soc. Can., 4: 43-53, 1914.

Mobley, B.A. and Page, E.: The surface area of sheep cardiac Purkinje fibers. J. Physiol. (London), 220: 547-563, 1972.

Moe, G.K.: On the multiple wavelet hypothesis of atrial fibrillation. Arch. Int. Pharmacodyn., 140: 183-188, 1962.

Moe, G.K. and Abildskov, J.A.: Atrial fibrillation as a selfsustaining arrhythmia independent of focal discharge. Am. Heart J., 58: 59-70, 1959.

Moe, G.K., Rheinboldt, W.C. and Abildskov, J.A.: A computer model of atrial fibrillation. Am. Heart J., 67: 200-220, 1964.

Moore, G.P., Perkel, D.H. and Segundo, J.P.: Stability patterns in interneuronal pacemaker regulation. In: Proc. San Diego Symp. Biomed. Eng., Paul A., ed., La Jolla, California, 1963.

Moscona, A.A.: Rotation-mediated histogenetic aggregation of dissociated cells. Exp. Cell Res., 22: 455-475, 1961.

Myerburg, R.J., Conde, C.A., Sung, R.J., Mayorga-Cortes, A., Mallon, S.M., Sheps, D.A., Appel, R.A. and Castellanos, A.: Clinical, electrophysiologic and hemodynamic profile of patients resuscitated from prehospital cardiac arrest. Am. J. Med., 68: 568-576, 1980.

Nagumo, J., Suzuki R. and Sato, S.: Electrochemical Active Network. Notes of Professional Group on Nonlinear Theory of IECE (Japan), Feb. 26, 1963.

Nakas, M., Higashino, S. and Loewenstein, W.R.: Uncoupling of an epithelial cell membrane junction by calcium-ion removal. Science (Wash., D.C.), 151: 89-91, 1966.

Nathan, R.D., and DeHaan, R.L.: In vitro differentiation of a fast sodium conductance in embryonic heart cell aggregates. Proc. Natl. Acad. Sci. USA, 75: 2776-2780, 1978.

Nathan, R.D. and DeHaan, R.L.: Voltage clamp analysis of embryonic heart cell aggregates. J. Gen. Physiol., 73: 175-198, 1979.

Nawrath, H., TenEick, R.E., McDonald, T.F. and Trautwein, W.: On the mechanism underlying the action of D 600 on slow inward current and tension in mammalian myocardium. Circ. Res., 40: 408-414, 1977.

Nayler, W. and Seabra-Gomes, R.: Effect of methylprednisolone sodium succinate on hypoxic heart muscle. Cardiovasc. Res., 10: 349-358, 1976.

Nayler, W.G., Poole-Wilson, P.A. and Williams, A.: Hypoxia and calcium. J. Mol. Cell. Cardiol., 11: 683-706, 1979.

New, D.A.T.: A new technique for the cultivation of the chick embryo in vitro. J. Embryol. Exp. Morphol., 3: 320-331, 1955.

Nishi, K., Yoshikawa, Y., Sugahara, K. and Monoka, T.: Changes in electrical activity and ultrastructure of sinoatrial nodal cells of the rabbit's heart exposed to hypoxic solution. Circ. Res., 46: 201-213, 1980.

Nishiye, H.: The mechanism of Ca^{2+} action on the healing-over process in mammalian cardiac muscles: a kinetic analysis. Jap. J. Physiol., 27: 451-466, 1977.

Niu, M.C. and Deshpande, A.K.: The development of tubular heart in RNA-treated post-nodal pieces of chick blastoderm. J. Embryol. Exp. Morphol., 29: 485-501, 1973.

Noble, D.: Electrical properties of cardiac muscle attributable to inward-going (anomalous) rectification. J. Cell. Comp. Physiol., 66: 127-136, 1965.

Noble, D.: Conductance mechanisms in excitable cells. Biomembranes 3, Kreuzer, F. and Slegers, J.F.G., eds., Plenum Press, New York, pp. 427-447, 1972.

Noble, D.: The Initiation of the Heart Beat, Clarendon Press, Oxford, 1979.

Noble, D. and Stein, R.B.: The threshold conditions for initiation of action potentials by excitable cells. J. Physiol. (London), 187: 129-162, 1966.

Noble, D. and Tsien, R.W.: The kinetic and rectifier properties of the slow potassium current in cardiac Purkinje fibres. J. Physiol. (London), 195: 185-214, 1968.

Noble, D. and Tsien, R.W.: Outward membrane currents activated in the plateau range of potentials in cardiac Purkinje fibres. J. Physiol. (London), 200, 205-231, 1969.

Noble, D. and Tsien, R.W.: The repolarization process of heart cells. In: Electrical phenomena in the heart, De Mello, W.C., ed., Academic Press, New York, pp. 133-161, 1972.

Noble, S.J.: Potassium accumulation and depletion in frog atrial muscle. J. Physiol. (London), 258: 579-613, 1976.

Noble, S.J. and Shimoni, Y.: The calcium and frequency dependence of the slow inward current "staircase" in frog atrium. J. Physiol. (London), 310: 57-75, 1981.

Noma, A.: Mechanisms underlying cessation of rabbit sinoatrial node pacemaker activity in high potassium solution. Jap. J. Physiol., 26: 619-630, 1976.

Noma, A. and Irisawa, H.: The effect of sodium ion on the initial phase of the sinoatrial pacemaker action potentials in rabbits. Jap. J. Physiol., 24: 617-632, 1974.

Noma, A. and Irisawa, H.: Contribution of an electrogenic sodium pump to the membrane potential in rabbit sinoatrial node cells. Pfluegers Arch., 358: 289-301, 1975.

Noma, A. and Irisawa, H.: Effects of Na^+ and K^+ on the resting membrane potential of the rabbit sinoatrial node cell. Jap. J. Physiol., 25: 287-302, 1975.

Noma, A. and Irisawa, H.: Effects of calcium ion on rising phase of the action potential in rabbit sinoatrial node cells. Jap. J. Physiol., 26: 93-99, 1976.

Noma, A. and Irisawa, H.: Membrane currents in the rabbit sinoatrial node cell as studied by the double microelectrode method. Pfluegers Arch., 364: 45-52, 1976.

Noma, A. and Irisawa, H.: A time- and voltage-dependent potassium current in the rabbit sinoatrial node cell. Pfluegers Arch., 366: 251-258, 1976.

Noma, A. and Trautwein, W.: Relaxation of the ACh-induced potassium current in the rabbit sinoatrial node

cell. Pfluegers Arch., 377: 193-200, 1978.
Noma, A., Yanagihara, K. and Irisawa, H.: Inward current of the rabbit sinoatrial node cell. Pfluegers Arch., 372: 43-51, 1977.
Noma, A., Peper, K. and Trautwein, W.: Acetylcholine-induced potassium current fluctuations in the rabbit sino-atrial node. Pfluegers Arch., 381: 255-262, 1979.
Noma, A., Osterrieder, W. and Trautwein, W.: The effect of external potassium on the elementary conductance of the ACh-induced potassium channel in the sino-atrial node. Pfluegers Arch., 381: 263-269, 1979.
Noma, A., Kotake, H. and Irisawa, H.: Slow inward current and its role mediating chronotropic effect of epinephrine. Pfluegers Arch., 388: 1-9, 1980.
Norwood, C.R., Castaneda, A.R. and Norwood, W.I.: Heterogeneity of rat cardiac cells of defined origin in single cell culture. J. Mol. Cell. Cardiol., 12: 201-210, 1980.
Ohta, M., Naharashi, T. and Keeler, R.F.: Effects of veratrum alkaloids on membrane potential and conductance of squid and crayfish giant axons. J. Pharmacol. Exp. Ther., 184: 143-154, 1973.
Op 't Hof, T., Mackaay, A.J.C., Bleeker, W.K., Jongsma, H.J. and Bouman, L.N.: Dependence of the chronotropic effects of adrenaline and acetylcholine and of the site of the dominant pacemaker on cycle length in the rabbit sinus node. J. Pharmacol. Exp. Ther., submitted, 1981.
Op 't Hof, T., Mackaay, A.J.C., Bleeker, W.K., Jongsma, H.J. and Bouman, L.N.: Magnesium and sinus node function. Magnesium Bulletin, accepted, 1981.
Opie, L.H., Nathan, D. and Lubbe, W.: Biochemical aspects of arrhythmogenesis and ventricular fibrillation. Am. J. Cardiol., 143: 131-147, 1979.
Osterhout, W.J.V. and Hill, S.E.: Salt bridges and negative variations. J. Gen. Physiol., 13: 547-552, 1930.
Osterrieder, W., Noma, A. and Trautwein, W.: On the kinetics of the potassium channel activated by acetylcholine in the SA node of the rabbit heart. Pfluegers Arch., 386: 101-109, 1980.
Osterrieder, W., Yang, Q.-f. and Trautwein, W.: The time course of the muscarinic response to ionophoretic acetylcholine application to the SA node of the rabbit heart. Pfluegers Arch., 389: 283-291, 1981.
Paes de Carvalho, A., De Mello, W.C. and Hoffman, B.F.: Electrophysiological evidence for specialized fibertypes in rabbit atrium. Am. J. Physiol., 196: 483-488, 1959.
Paff, G.H.: Transplantation of sinoatrium to conus in the embryonic heart in vitro. Am. J. Physiol., 117: 313-317, 1936.
Page, E. and Storm, S.R.: Cat heart muscle in vitro. Active transport of sodium in papillary muscles. J. Gen. Physiol., 48: 957-972, 1965.
Pappano, A.J.: Calcium-dependent action potentials produced by catecholamines in guinea pig atrial muscle fibers. Circ. Res., 27: 379-390, 1970.
Pappano, A.J.: Sodium-dependent depolarization of non-innervated embryonic chick heart by acetylcholine. J. Pharmacol. Exp. Ther., 180: 340-350, 1972.
Pappano, A.J.: Development of autonomic neuroeffector transmission in the chick embryo heart. In: Developmental and Physiological Correlates of Cardiac Muscle, Lieberman, M. and Sano, T., eds., Raven Press, New York, pp. 235-248, 1976.
Pappano, A.J.: Onset of chronotropic effects of nicotinic drugs and tyramine on the sinoatrial pacemaker in chick embryo heart: Relationship to the development of autonomic neuroeffector transmission. J. Pharmacol. Exp. Ther., 196: 676-684, 1976.
Pappano, A.J.: Ontogenetic development of autonomic neuroeffector transmission and transmitter reactivity in embryonic and fetal hearts. Pharmacol. Rev., 29: 3-33, 1977.
Pappano, A.J. and Sperelakis, N.: Low K^+ conductance and low resting potentials of isolated single cultured heart cells. Am. J. Physiol., 217: 1076-1082, 1969.
Pappano, A.J. and Loeffelholz, K.: Ontogenesis of adrenergic and cholinergic neuroeffector transmission in chick embryo heart. J. Pharmacol. Exp. Ther., 191: 468-478, 1974.
Pappas, G.D., Asada, Y. and Bennett, M.V.L.: Morphological correlates of increased coupling resistance at an electrotonic synapse. J. Cell Biol., 49: 173-188, 1971.
Patten, B.M.: Initiation and early changes in the character of the heart beat in vertebrate embryos. Physiol. Rev., 29: 31-47, 1949.
Patten, B.M. and Kramer, T.C.: The initiation of contraction in the embryonic heart. Am. J. Anat., 53: 349-375, 1933.
Patton, R.J. and Linkens, D.A.: Hodgkin-Huxley type electronic modelling of gastrointestinal electrical activity. Med. and Biol. Eng. and Comp., 16: 195-202, 1978.
Pavlidis, T.: Biological Oscillators: Their mathematical analysis. Academic Press, New York and London, 1973.
Pavlidis, T.: Qualitative similarities between the behavior of coupled oscillators and circadian rhythms. Bull. Math. Biol., 40: 675-692, 1978.
Payton, B.W., Bennett, M.V.L. and Pappas, G.D.: Temperature-dependence of resistance at an electrotonic synapse. Science (Wash., D.C.), 165: 594-597, 1969.
Payton, B.W., Bennett, M.V.L. and Pappas, G.D.: Permeability and structure of junctional membranes at an electrotonic synapse. Science (Wash., D.C.), 166: 1641-1643, 1969.
Pearson, O.H., Hastings, A.B. and Bunting, H.: Metabolism of cardiac muscle: utilization of C^{14} labelled pyruvate and acetate by heart slices. Am. J. Physiol., 158: 251-260, 1949.
Pelleg, A., Vogel, S., Belardinelli, L. and Sperelakis, N.: Overdrive suppression of automaticity in cultured chick myocardial cells. Am. J. Physiol., 238: H24-H30, 1980.
Peper, K. and Trautwein, W.: A note on the pacemaker current in Purkinje fibres. Pfluegers Arch., 309: 356-361, 1969.

Peracchia, C.: Low resistance junctions in crayfish. I. Two arrays of globules in junctional membranes. J. Cell Biol., 57: 54-65, 1973.

Peracchia, C.: Low resistance junctions in crayfish. II. Structural details and further evidence for intercellular channels by freeze-fracture and negative staining. J. Cell Biol., 57: 66-76, 1973.

Peracchia, C.: A structure-function correlation in gap junctions of crayfish. Proc. Int. Cong. Electron Microsc., 8th Canberra, II, 226-227, 1974.

Peracchia, C.: Gap junctions: structural changes after uncoupling procedures. J. Cell Biol., 72: 628-641, 1977.

Peracchia, C.: Calcium effects on gap junction structure and cell coupling. Nature (Lond.), 271: 669-671, 1978.

Peracchia, C.: Structural correlates of gap junction permeation. Int. Rev. Cytol., 66: 81-146, 1980.

Peracchia, C. and Dulhunty, A.F.: Gap junctions: structural changes associated with changes in permeability. J. Cell Biol., 63: (2, pt. 2): 263a, 1974.

Peracchia, C. and Dulhunty, A.F.: Low resistance junctions in crayfish: structural changes with functional uncoupling. J. Cell Biol., 70: 419-439, 1976.

Peracchia, C. and Peracchia, L.L.: Gap junction dynamics: reversible effects of divalent cations. J. Cell Biol., 87: 708-718, 1980.

Peracchia, C. and Peracchia, L.L.: Gap junction dynamics: reversible effects of hydrogen ions. J. Cell Biol., 87: 719-727, 1980.

Peracchia, C., Bernardini, G. and Peracchia, L.L.: Uncoupling mechanism: a hypothesis. J. Cell Biol., 83: (2, pt. 2): 86a, 1979.

Perkel, D.H., Schulman, J.H., Bullock, T.H., Moore, G.P. and Segundo, J.P.: Pacemaker neurons: Effects of regularly spaced synaptic input. Science, 145: 61-63, 1964.

Petersen, O.H., Findlay, I., Meda, P., Laugier, R. and Iwatsuki, N.: Control of cell-to-cell communication in exocrine glands by the intracellular hydrogen ion concentration. In: Hydrogen Ion Transport in Epithelia, Schulz, I., ed., Elsevier (North Holland Press), pp. 227-234, 1980.

Pickering, J.W.: Observations on the physiology of the embryonic heart. J. Physiol. (London), 14: 383-466, 1893.

Pinsker, H.M.: Aplysia bursting neurons as endogenous oscillators. II. Synchronization and entrainment by pulsed inhibitory synaptic input. J. Neurophysiol., 40: 544-556, 1976.

Pinto da Silva, P. and Gilula, N.B.: Gap junctions in normal and transformed fibroblasts in culture. Exp. Cell Res., 71: 393-401, 1972.

Pittendrigh, C.A.: On the mechanism of entrainment of a circadian rhythm by light cycles. In: Circadian Clocks, Aschoff, J., ed., Amsterdam, North Holland, pp. 277-297, 1965.

Pitts, J.D.: Molecular exchange and growth control in tissue culture. In: Growth Control in Cultures, Wolstenholme, G.E.W. and Knight, J., eds. Churchill Livingstone, London, pp. 89-105, 1971.

Pitts, J.D.: Direct communication between animal cells. In: International Cell Biology, Brinkley, B.R. and Porter, K.R., eds., The Rockefeller University Press, New York, pp. 43-49, 1977.

Politoff, A. and Pappas, G.D.: Mechanism of increase in coupling resistance at electrotonic synapses of the crayfish septate axon. Anat. Record, 172: 384-385, 1972.

Politoff, A., Pappas, G.D. and Bennett, M.V.L.: Cobalt ions cross an electrotonic synapse if cytoplasmic concentration is low. Brain Res., 76: 343-346, 1974.

Pollack, G.H.: Intercellular coupling in the atrioventricular node and other tissues of the rabbit heart. J. Physiol. (London), 255: 275-298, 1976.

Pott, L.: On the time course of the acetylcholine-induced hyperpolarization in quiescent guinea-pig atria. Pfluegers Arch., 380: 71-77, 1979.

Pott, L. and Pusch, H.: A kinetic model for the muscarinic action of acetylcholine. Pfluegers Arch., 383: 75-77, 1979.

Prystowsky, E.N., Grant, A.O., Wallace, A.G. and Strauss, H.C.: An analysis of the effects of acetylcholine on conduction and refractoriness in the rabbit sinus node. Circ. Res., 44: 112-120, 1979.

Purdy, J.E., Lieberman, M., Roggeveen, A.E. and Kirk, R.G.: Synthetic strands of cardiac muscle; formation and ultrastructure. J. Cell Biol., 55: 563-578, 1972.

Purves, R.D.: Current flow and potential in a three-dimensional syncitium. J. Theor. Biol., 60: 147-163, 1976.

Purves, R.D.: Function of muscarinic and nicotinic acetylcholine receptors. Nature, 261: 149-151, 1976.

Purves, R.D.: The time course of cellular response to ionophoretically applied drugs. J. Theor. Biol., 65: 327-344, 1977.

Rae, J.L.: The movement of procion dye in the crystalline lens. Invest. Ophtalmol. Vis. Sci., 13: 147-150, 1974.

Ramon, F. and Moore, J.W.: Propagation of action potentials in squid giant axons. Repetitive firing at regions of membrane inhomogeneities. J. Gen. Physiol., 73: 595-603, 1979.

Rathamayer, W. and Beress, L.: The effect of toxins from Anemonia sulcata (coelenterata) on neuromuscular transmission and nerve action potentials in the crayfish (Astacus Leptodactylus). J. Comp. Physiol., 109: 373-382, 1976.

Raviola, E., Goodenough, D.A. and Raviola, G.: The native structure of gap junctions rapidly frozen at 4°K. J. Cell Biol., 79 (2, pt. 2): 229a, 1978.

Raviola, E., Goodenough, D.A. and Raviola, G.: Structure of rapidly frozen gap junctions. J. Cell Biol., 87: 273-279, 1980.

Reid, J.V.O.: The cardiac pacemaker: effects of regularly spaced nervous input. Am. Heart J., 78: 58-64, 1969.

Renaud, D.: Etude électrophysiologique de la différentiation cardiaque chez l'embryon de poulet. Thesis Univ. of Nantes, 1973.

Renaud, J-F.: Use of cell cultures as tool to elucidate physiological, pharmacological and biochemical membrane properties of the embryonic heart. Biol. Cellulaire, 37: 97-104, 1980.

Renaud, J-F. and Sperelakis, N.: Electrophysiological properties of chick embryonic hearts grafted and organ cultured in vitro. J. Mol. Cell. Cardiol., 8: 889-900, 1976.

Renaud, J-F., Sperelakis, N. and LeDouarin, G.: Increase of cyclic AMP levels induced by isoproterenol in cultured and non-cultured chick embryonic hearts. J. Mol. Cell. Cardiol., 10: 281-286, 1978.

Renaud, J.F., Barhanin, J., Cavey, D., Fosset, M. and Lazdunski, M.: Comparative properties of in ovo and in vitro differentiation of the muscarinic cholinergic receptor in embryonic heart cells. Devel. Biol., 78: 184-200, 1980.

Reshodko, L.V. and Bures, J.: Computer simulation of reverberating spreading depression in a network of cell automata. Biol. Cyb., 18: 181-189, 1975.

Reuter, H.: Ueber die Wirkung von Adrenalin auf den cellulaeren Ca-Umsatz des Meerschweinchen-vorhofs. Naunyn-Schmiedebergs Arch. Pharmakol., 251: 401, 1965.

Reuter, H.: Divalent cations as charge carriers in excitable membranes. Prog. Biophys. Mol. Biol., 26: 1-43, 1973.

Reuter, H. and Seitz, H.: The dependence of calcium efflux from cardiac muscle on temperature and external ion composition. J. Physiol. (London), 195: 451-470, 1968.

Reuter, H. and Scholz, H.: A study on the ion selectivity and the kinetic properties of the calcium dependent slow inward current in mammalian cardiac muscle. J. Physiol. (London), 264: 17-47, 1977.

Revel, J.P.: Contacts and junctions between cells. SEM Symp., 28: 447-461, 1974.

Revel, J.P. and Karnovsky, M.J.: Hexagonal array of subunits in intercellular junctions of the mouse heart and liver. J. Cell Biol., 33: C7-C12, 1967.

Revel, J.P., Griepp, E.B., Finbow, M. and Johnson, R.: Possible steps in gap junction formation. Zoon, 6: 139-144 (Proc. Symp. "Formshaping Movements in Neurogenesis", Uppsala, Sept. 1977), 1978.

Roberts, L.A. and Hughs, M.J.: Chronotropic response of spontaneously beating rabbit atria to hyperosmotic media. Am. J. Physiol., 233: H228-H233, 1977.

Robertson, J.D.: The occurrence of a subunit pattern in the unit membranes of club endings in Mauthner cell synapses in Goldfish brains. J. Cell Biol., 19: 201-222, 1963.

Robertson-Dunn, B. and Linkens, D.A.: A mathematical model of the slow-wave electrical activity of the human small-intestine. Med. and Biol. Eng., 750-758, 1974.

Romanoff, A.: The Avian Embryo, Structure and Functional Development, Macmillan Press, New York, 1960.

Romey, G. and Lazdunski, M.: Scorpion and sea anemone neurotoxins actions on axonal membrane. 5th International Biophysics Congress, Copenhagen, 503, 1975.

Romey, G., Abita, J.P., Schweitz, H., Wunderer, G. and Lazdunski, M.: Sea anemone toxin: a tool to study molecular mechanisms of nerve conduction and excitation-secretion coupling. Proc. Natl. Acad. Sci. USA, 73: 4055-4059, 1976.

Romey, G., Jacques, Y., Schweitz, H., Fosset, M. and Lazdunksi, M.: The sodium channel in non-impulsive cells. Interaction with specific neurotoxins. Biochim. Biophys. Acta, 556: 344-353, 1979.

Romey, G., Renaud, J.F., Fosset, M. and Lazdunksi, M.: Pharmacological properties of the interaction of a sea anemone polypeptide toxin with cardiac cells in culture. J. Pharmacol. Exp. Ther., 213: 607-615, 1980.

Rose, B. and Loewenstein, W.R.: Permeability of cell junction depends on local cytoplasmic calcium activity. Nature (London), 254: 250, 1975.

Rose, B. and Loewenstein, W.R.: Permeability of a cell junction and the local cytoplasmic free ionized calcium concentration: a study with aequorin. J. Memb. Biol., 28: 87-119, 1976.

Rose, B. and Rick, R.: Intracellular pH, intracellular free Ca and junctional cell-cell coupling. J. Memb. Biol., 44: 337-415, 1978.

Rossler, O.E.: Chemical turbulence; chaos in a simple reaction-diffusion system. Zeit. Naturforsch., 31a: 1168-1172, 1976.

Rossler, O.E.: Chemical turbulence - a synopsis. In Synergetics, H. Haken, Ed. Lecture Notes in Physics, Springer-Verlag, Berlin, 1978.

Rossler, O.E. and Kahlert, C.: Winfree meandering in a 2-dimensional 2-variable excitable medium. Z. Naturforsch., 34a: 565-570, 1979.

Rothschuh, K.E.: Ueber den funktionellen Aufbau des Herzens aus elektrophysiologischen Elementen und ueber den Mechanismus der Erregungsleitung im Herzen. Pfluegers Arch., 253: 238-251, 1951.

Rothschuh, K.E.: Geschichte der Physiologie, Springer, Berlin, Goettingen, Heidelberg, 1953.

Rougier, O., Vassort, G. and Stampfi, R.: Voltage-clamp experiments frog atrial heart muscle fibers with the sucrose-gap technique. Pfluegers Arch., 301: 91-108, 1968.

Rovetto, M.J., Whitmer, J.T. and Neely, J.R.: Comparison of the effects of anoxia and whole heart ischemia on carbohydrate utilization in isolated working rat heart. Circ. Res., 32: 669-711, 1973.

Rozenshtraukh, L.V., Kholopov, A.V. and Yushmanova, A.V.: Vagus inhibition-cause of formation of closed pathways of conduction of excitation in the auricles. Biofizika, 15: 690-700, 1970.

Sachs, F.: Electrophysiological properties of tissue cultured heart cells grown in linear array. J. Memb. Biol., 28: 373-399, 1976.

Sachs, H.G. and DeHaan, R.L.: Embryonic myocardial cell aggregates; volume and pulsation rate. Devel. Biol., 30: 233-240, 1973.

Sachs, H.G., Mc Donald, T.F. and DeHaan, R.L.: Tetrodotoxin sensitivity of cultured embryonic heart cells depends on cell interactions. J. Cell Biol., 56: 255-258, 1973.

Sakson, M.E., Bukauskas, F.F., Kukushkin, N.I. and Nasonova, V.V.: Study of electrotonic distribution on the surface of cardiac structures. Biofizika, 19: 1045–1049, 1974.

Sanderson, J.B. and Page, F.J.M.: On the time-relations of the excitatory process in the ventricle of the heart of the frog. J. Physiol. (London), 2: 384–435, 1880.

Sano, T. and Yamagishi, S.: Spread of excitation from the sinus node. Circ. Res., 16: 423–430, 1965.

Sano, T. and Iida, Y.: Sinoatrial connection and wandering pacemaker. J. Electrocardiol., 1: 147–153, 1968.

Sano, T., Yamagishi, S. and Iida, Y.: Several aspects on the spontaneous activity of the sinus node and its spread. Jap. Circ. J., 30: 134–138, 1966.

Sano, T., Sawanobori, T. and Adaniya, H.: Mechanism of rhythm determination among pacemaker cells of the mammalian sinus node. Am. J. Physiol., 235: H379–H384, 1978.

Sarna, S.K. and Daniel, E.E.: Electrical stimulation of gastric electrical control activity. Am. J. Physiol., 225: 125–131, 1973.

Sarna, S.K. and Daniel, E.E.: Electrical stimulation of small intestinal electrical control activity. Gastroenterol., 69: 660–667, 1975.

Sarna, S.K., Daniel, E.E. and Kingma, Y.J.: Simulation of slow-wave electrical activity of small-intestine. Am. J. Physiol., 221: 166–175, 1971.

Sarna, S.K., Daniel, E.E. and Kingma, Y.J.: Simulation of the electrical control activity of the stomach by an array of relaxation oscillators. Am. J. Dig. Dis., 17: 299–310, 1972.

Sastre, A., Gray, D.B. and Lane, M.A.: Muscarinic cholinergic binding sites in the developing avian heart. Devel. Biol., 55: 201–205, 1977.

Schaer, H.: Antagonistische Wirkungen von Magnesium-, Calcium- und Natriumionen auf die Impulsbildung im Sinusknoten des Meerschweinchenherzens. Pfluegers Arch., 298: 359–371, 1968.

Schanne, O.F.: Measurement of cytoplasmic resistivity by means of the glass microelectrodes. In: Glass microelectrodes, Lavallee, M., Schanne, O.F. and Herbert, N.C., eds., Wiley Sons, New York-London-Sydney-Toronto, pp. 299–321, 1969.

Schanne, O.F., Ruiz-Ceretti, E., Payet, M.D. and Deslauriers, Y.: Influence of varied Ca^{2+}_o and Na^+_o on electrical activity of clusters of cultured cardiac cells from neonatal rats. J. Mol. Cell. Cardiol., 11: 477–484, 1979.

Schmitt, F.O. and Erlanger, J.: Directional differences in the conduction of the impulse through heart muscle and their possible relation to extrasystolic and fibrillary contractions. Am. J. Physiol., 87: 326–347, 1928.

Schreurs, W., van Leeuwen, J.R. and Jongsma, H.J.: An optically clear heating plate for tissue culture experiments. Submitted, 1981.

Scott, S.: Stimulation simulations of young yet cultured beating hearts. Ph. D. Thesis, State University of New York, Buffalo, 1979.

Seidler, F.J. and Slotkin, T.A.: Presynaptic and postsynaptic contributions to ontogeny of sympathetic control of heart rate in the pre-weanling rat. Br. J. Pharmac., 65: 431–434, 1979.

Seltzer, J.L. and McDougal, D.B.: Enzyme levels in chick embryo heart and brain from 1 to 21 days of development. Devel. Biol., 42: 95–105, 1975.

Senges, J., Mizutani, T., Pelzer, D., Brachmann, J., Sonnhof, U. and Kuebler, W.: Effect of hypoxia on the sinoatrial node, atrium and atrioventricular node in the rabbit heart. Circ. Res., 44: 856–863, 1979.

Senges, J., Hennig, E., Brachmann, J., Pelzer, D., Mizutani, T. and Kuebler, W.: Effects of orciprenaline on the sinoatrial and atrioventricular nodes in presence of hypoxia. J. Mol. Cell. Cardiol., 12:135–147, 1980.

Seyama, I.: Characteristics of the rectifying properties of the sinoatrial node cell of the rabbit. J. Physiol. (London), 255: 379–397, 1976.

Seyama, I.: Effect of grayanotoxine I on SA node and right atrial myocardia of the rabbit. Am. J. Physiol., 235: C136–C142, 1978.

Seyama, I.: Characteristics of the anion channel in the sinoatrial node cell of the rabbit. J. Physiol. (London), 294: 447–460, 1979.

Shcherbunov, A.I., Kukushkin, N.I. and Saxon, M.E.: Reverberator in a system of interrelated fibers described by the Noble equation. Biofizika, 18: 519–525, 1973.

Shearin, N.L., Bowes, K.L., Kingma, Y.J. and Koles, Z.T.: Frequency analysis of electrical activity in dog colon. 6th Inst. Symp. on G.I. Motility, Edinburgh, 1977.

Sheridan, J.D.: Cell coupling and cell communication during embryogenesis. In: The Cell Surface in Animal Embryogenesis and Development. Poste, G. and Nicolson, G.L., eds., Elsevier/North-Holland Biomedical Press, Amsterdam, pp. 409–447, 1976.

Shibata, M. and Bures, J.: Reverberation of cortical spreading depression along closed-loop pathways in rat cerebral cortex. J. Neurophys., 35: 381–388, 1973.

Shibata, M. and Bures, J.: Optimum topographical conditions for reverberating cortical spreading depression in rats. J. Neurobiol., 5: 107–118, 1974.

Shibata, Y.: Comparative ultrastructure of cell membrane specializations in vertebrate cardiac muscles. Arch. Histol. Jap., 40: 391–406, 1977.

Shibata, Y. and Yamamoto, T.: Gap junctions in the cardiac muscle cells of the lamprey. Cell Tissue Res., 178: 477–482, 1977.

Shibata, Y. and Yamamoto, T.: Freeze-fracture studies of gap junctions in vertebrate cardiac muscle cells. J. Ultrastructure Res., 67: 79–88, 1979.

Shigenobu, K. and Sperelakis, N.: Development of sensitivity to tetrodotoxin of chick embryonic hearts with age. J. Mol. Cell. Cardiol., 3: 271–286, 1971.

Shigenobu, K. and Sperelakis, N.: Ca^{++} current channels induced by catecholamines in chick embryonic hearts whose fast Na$^+$ channels are blocked by tetrodotoxin or elevated K$^+$. Circ. Res., 31: 932-952, 1972.

Shigenobu, K. and Sperelakis, N.: Failure of development of fast Na$^+$ channels during organ culture of young embryonic chick hearts. Devel. Biol., 39: 326-330, 1974.

Shigenobu, K., Schneider, J.A. and Sperelakis, N.: Blockade of slow Na$^+$ and Ca^{++} currents in myocardial cells by verapamil. J. Pharmacol. Exp. Ther., 190: 280-288, 1974.

Shimada, Y., Moscona, A.A. and Fischman, D.A.: Scanning electron microscopy of cell aggregation: cardiac and mixed retina-cardiac cell suspensions. Devel. Biol., 36: 428-446, 1974.

Shimamoto, K. and Toda, N.: Modifications by propranolol of the response of isolated rabbit atria to endogeneous and exogeneous noradrenaline. Br. J. Pharmacol. Chemo. Ther., 32: 539-545, 1968.

Shimizu, Y. and Tasaki, K.: Electrical excitability of developing cardiac muscle in chick embryos. Tohoku J. Exp. Med., 88: 49-56, 1966.

Shrier, A. and Clay, J.R.: Low K$^+$ conductance and low resting potentials of isolated single cultured heart cells. Nature, 283: 670-671, 1980.

Simon, E.J.: Two types of luminosity horizontal cells in the retina of the turtle. J. Physiol. (London), 230: 199-211, 1973.

Sjöstrand, F.S. and Andersson, E.: Electron microscopy of the intercalated discs of cardiac muscle tissue. Experimentia, 10: 369-370, 1954.

Sjöstrand, F.S., Andersson-Cedergren, E. and Dewey, M.M.: The ultrastructure of the intercalated discs of frog, mouse and guinea pig cardiac muscle. J. Ultrastruct. Res., 1: 271-287, 1958.

Smith, E.E. and Guyton, A.C.: An iron heart model for study of cardiac impulse transmission. Physiologist, 4: 112, 1961.

Smolyaninov, V.V.: Mathematical models of biological tissues (in Russian), Nauka, Moscow, 1980.

Somjen, G.G. and Baskerville, E.N.: Effect of excess magnesium on vagal inhibition and acetylcholine sensitivity of the mammalian heart in situ and in vitro. Nature, 217: 679-680, 1968.

Spear, J.F. and Moore, E.N.: Influence of brief vagal and stellate nerve stimulation on pacemaker activity and conduction within the atrioventricular conducting system of the dog. Circ. Res., 32: 27-41, 1973.

Spear, J.F., Kronhaus, K.D., Moore, E.N. and Kline, R.P.: The effect of brief vagal stimulation on the isolated rabbit sinus node. Circ. Res., 44: 75-88, 1979.

Speicher, D.W. and Mc Carl, R.L.: Evaluation of a proteolytic enzyme mixture isolated from crude trypsin in tissue desaggregation. In Vitro, 14: 849-853, 1978.

Sperelakis, N.: Electrophysiology of cultured chick heart cells. In: Electrophysiology and Ultrastructure of the Heart, Sano, T., Mizuhira, V. and Matsuda, K., eds., Bunkodo Co., Ltd., Tokyo, pp. 81-108, 1967.

Sperelakis, N.: Na$^+$, K$^+$-ATPase activity of embryonic chick heart and skeletal muscles as a function of age. Biochim. Biophys. Acta, 266: 230-237, 1972.

Sperelakis, N.: Electrical properties of embryonic heart cells. In: Electrical Phenomena in the Heart, De Mello, W.C., ed., Academic Press, New York, pp. 1-61, 1972.

Sperelakis, N.: Origin of the cardiac resting potential. In: Handbook of Physiology, the Cardiovascular System, Vol. 1, Berne, R.M. and Sperelakis, N., eds., Am. Physiol. Soc., Bethesda, pp. 187-267, 1979.

Sperelakis, N. and Lehmkuhl, D.: Effect of current on transmembrane potentials in cultured chick heart cells. J. Gen. Physiol., 47: 895-927, 1964.

Sperelakis, N. and Lehmkuhl, D.: Insensitivity of cultured chick heart cells to autonomic agents and tetrodotoxin. Am. J. Physiol., 209: 693-698, 1965.

Sperelakis, N. and Lehmkuhl, D.: Ionic interconversion of pacemaker and nonpacemaker cultured chick heart cells. J. Gen. Physiol., 49: 867-895, 1966.

Sperelakis, N. and Lehmkuhl, D.: Effects of temperature and metabolic poisons on membrane potentials of cultured heart cells. Am. J. Physiol., 213: 719-724, 1967.

Sperelakis, N. and Pappano, A.J.: Depolarization of cultured heart cells by a lipid soluble acetylcholine analogue. Am. J. Physiol., 217: 625-629, 1969.

Sperelakis, N. and Lee, E.E.: Characterization of (Na$^+$, K$^+$)-ATPase isolated from embryonic chick hearts and cultured chick heart cells. Biochim. Biophys. Acta, 233: 562-579, 1971.

Sperelakis, N. and Shigenobu, K.: Changes in membrane properties of chick embryonic hearts during development. J. Gen. Physiol., 60: 430-453, 1972.

Sperelakis, N. and Macdonald, R.L.: Ratio of transverse to longitudinal resistivities of isolated cardiac muscle fiber bundle. J. Electrocardiol., 7: 301-314, 1974.

Sperelakis, N. and Shigenobu, K.: Organ-cultured embryonic hearts of various ages. Part I: Electrophysiology, J. Mol. Cell. Cardiol., 5: 449-471, 1974.

Sperelakis, N. and McLean, M.J.: The electrical properties of embryonic chick cardiac cells. In: Fetal and Newborn Cardiovascular Physiology. Vol. 1, Longo, L.D. and Renaud, D.D., eds., Garland Press, New York, pp. 191-236, 1978.

Sperelakis, N., Hoshiko, T. and Berne, R.M.: Non-syncytial nature of cardiac muscle: membrane resistance of single cells. Am. J. Physiol., 198: 531-536, 1960.

Sperelakis, N., Schneider, M.F. and Harris, E.J.: Decreased K$^+$ conductance produced by Ba^{++} in frog sartorius fibers. J. Gen. Physiol., 50: 1565-1583, 1967.

Sperelakis, N., Forbes, M. and Rubio, R.: The tubular systems of myocardial cells: ultrastructure and possible function. In: Recent Advances in Studies on Cardiac Structure and Metabolism, Vol. 4, Dhalla, N.S. and Rona, G., eds., University Park Press, Baltimore, pp. 163-194, 1974.

Sperelakis, N., Shigenobu, K. and McLean, M.J.: Membrane cation channels: changes in developing hearts, in cell culture and in organ culture. In: Developmental and Physiological Correlates of Cardiac Muscle, Lieberman, M. and Sano, T., eds., Raven Press, New York, pp. 209-234, 1976.

Spray, D.C., Harris, A.L. and Bennett, M.V.L.: Voltage dependence of junctional conductance in early amphibian embryos. Science, 204: 432-434, 1979.

Staehelin, L.A.: Structure and function of intercellular junctions. Int. Rev. Cytol., 39: 191-283, 1974.

Standen, N.B.: The postnatal development of adrenoceptor responses to agonists and electrical stimulation in rat isolated atria. Br. J. Pharmac., 64: 83-89, 1978.

Standen, N.B. and Stanfield, P.R.: A potential- and time-dependent blockade of inward rectification in frog skeletal muscle fibres by barium and strontium ions. J. Physiol. (London), 280: 169-181, 1978.

Stannius, H.F.: Zwei Reihen Physiologischer Versuche. I. Versuche am Froschherzen. Arch. f. Anat. und Physiol., pp. 85, 1852.

Steinbeck, G., Allessie, M.A., Bonke, F.I.M. and Lammers, W.J.E.P.: Sinus-node response to premature atrial stimulation in the rabbit studied with multiple microelectrode impalements. Circ. Res., 43: 695-704, 1978.

Steinbeck, G., Bonke, F.I.M., Allessie, M.A. and Lammers, W.J.E.P.: The effect of ouabain on the isolated sinus node preparation of the rabbit studied with microelectrodes. Circ. Res., 46: 404-414, 1980.

Stibitz, G.R. and Rytand, D.A.: On the path of the excitationwave in atrial flutter. Circulation, 37: 75-81, 1968.

Strauss, H.C. and Bigger jr., J.Th.: Electrophysiological properties of the rabbit sinoatrial perinodal fibers. Circ. Res., 31: 490-506, 1972.

Stuesse, S.L., Levy, M.N. and Zieske, H.: Phase-related sensitivity of the sinoatrial node to vagal stimuli in the isolated rat atrium. Circ. Res., 43: 217-224, 1978.

Suga, H. and Oshima, M.: Modulation-characteristics of heart rate by vagal stimulation. Japan J. Med. Electron. Biol. Eng., 6: 465-471, 1968.

Suga, H. and Oshima, M.: Periodic variation of heart rate caused by repetitive electric stimulation of cardiac vagus nerve. J. Physiol. Soc. Japan, 31: 33-34, 1969.

Suzuki, R.: Electrochemical neuron model. Adv. Biophys., 9: 115-156, 1976.

Tanaka, I. and Sasaki, Y.: On the electrotonic spread in cardiac muscle of the mouse. J. Gen. Physiol., 49: 1089-1110, 1966.

Taniguchi, T., Fujiwara, M., Ja Lee, J. and Hidaka, H.: Effect of acetylcholine on the norepinephrine induced positive chronotropy and increase in cyclic nucleotides of isolated rabbit sinoatrial node. Circ. Res., 45: 493-504, 1979.

Taylor, J.J., d'Agrosa, L.S. and Burns, E.M.: The pacemaker cell of the sinoatrial node of the rabbit. Am. J. Physiol., 235: H407-H412, 1978.

TenEick, R., Nawrath, H., McDonald, T.F. and Trautwein, W.: On the mechanism of the negative inotropic effect of acetylcholine. Pfluegers Arch., 361: 207-213, 1976.

TenEick, R.E., Singer, D.H. and Solberg, L.E.: Coronary occlusion effect on cellular electrical activity of the heart. Med. Clin. North Am., 60: 49-67, 1976.

Toda, N.: Influence of sodium ions on the membrane potential of the sino-atrial node in response to sympathetic nerve stimulation. J. Physiol. (London), 196: 677-691, 1968.

Toda, N.: Electrophysiological effects of potassium and calcium ions in the si noatrial node in response to sympathetic nerve stimulation. Pfluegers Arch., 310: 45-63, 1969.

Toda, N. and West, T.C.: Changes in sinoatrial node transmembrane potentials on vagal stimulation of the isolated rabbit atrium. Nature, 205: 808-809, 1965.

Toda, N. and West, Th.: Interactions of K, Na and vagal stimulation in the sinoatrial node of the rabbit. Am. J. Physiol., 212, 416-423, 1967.

Toda, N. and West, Th.: Interaction between Na, Ca, Mg and vagal stimulation in the sinoatrial node of the rabbit. Am. J. Physiol., 212: 424-430, 1967.

Toda, N. and Shimamoto, K.: The influence of sympathetic stimulation on transmembrane potentials in the s-a node. J. Pharmacol. Exp. Ther., 159: 298-305, 1968.

Toda, N., Fu, W.L.H. and Osumi, Y.: Age-dependence of the chronotropic response to noradrenaline, acetylcholine and transmural stimulation in isolated rabbit atria. Jap. J. Pharmacol., 26: 359-366, 1976.

Torre, V.: A theory of synchronization of heart pacemaker cells. J. Theor. Biol., 61: 55-71, 1976.

Tranum-Jensen, J.: The fine structure of the sinus node. A survey. In: The Sinus Node. Structure, Function and Clinical Relevance, Bonke, F.I.M., ed., Martinus Nijhoff, The Hague, pp. 149-165, 1978.

Trautwein, W.: Membrane currents in cardiac muscle fibers. Physiol. Rev., 53: 793-835, 1973.

Trautwein, W. and Zink, K.: Ueber Membran und Aktionspotentials einzelner Myokardfasern des Kalt und Warmblueterherzens. Pfluegers Arch., 256: 68-84, 1952.

Trautwein, W. and Dudel, J.: Zum Mechanismus der Membranwirkung des Acetylcholin an der Herzmuskelfaser. Pfluegers Arch., 266: 324-334, 1958.

Trautwein, W. and Uchizono, K.: Electron microscopic and electrophysiologic study of the pacemaker in the sinoatrial node of the rabbit heart. Z. Zellforsch., 61: 96-109, 1963.

Troy, W.C.: Mathematical modeling of excitable media in neurobiology and chemistry. Theoretical Chemistry, 4, Eyring, H. and Henderson, D., eds., Academis Press, New York, pp. 133-157, 1978.

Truex, R.C.: The sinoatrial node and its connections with the atrial tissue. In: The Conduction System of the Heart, Wellens, H.J.J., Lie, K.I. and Janse, M.J., eds., Stenfert Kroese, B.V., Leiden, pp. 209-227, 1976.

Tsien, R.W. and Weingart, R.: Cyclic-AMP: cell-to-cell movement and inotropic effect in ventricular muscle, studied by a cut-end method. J. Physiol. (London), 242: 95P-96P, 1974.

Tsien, R.W. and Weingart, R.: Inotropic effect of cyclic AMP in calf ventricular muscle studied by a cut end method. J. Physiol. (London), 260: 117-141, 1976.

Turin, L. and Warner, A.E.: Carbon dioxide reversibly abolishes ionic communication between cells of early amphibian embryo. Nature, 270: 56, 1977.

Turin, L. and Warner, A.E.: Intracellular pH in early Xenopus embryos: its effect on current flow between blastomeres. J. Physiol. (London), 300: 489-504, 1980.

Turlapaty, P.D.M.V. and Carrier sr., O.: Influence of magnesium on calcium induced responses of atrial and vascular muscle. J. Pharmacol. Exp. Ther., 187: 86-98, 1973.

Tyson, J.J.: The Belousov-Zhabotinskii Reaction, Lecture Notes in Biomathematics, vol. 10, Leven, S., ed., Springer-Verlag, Berlin, 1976.

Ulbricht, W.: The effect of veratridine on excitable membranes of nerve and muscle. Ergeb. Physiol. Biol. Chem. Exp. Pharm., 61: 18-71, 1969.

Unwin, P.N.T. and Zampighi, G.: Structure of the junction between communicating cells. Nature (Lond.), 283: 545-549, 1980.

Van Mierop, L.H.S.: Location of pacemaker in chick embryo heart at the time of initiation of heart beat. Am. J. Physiol., 212: 407-415, 1967.

Vassalle, M.: Cardiac pacemaker potentials at different extra- and intracellular K concentrations. Am. J. Physiol., 208: 770-775, 1965.

Vassalle, M.: Analysis of cardiac pacemaker potential using a "voltage clamp" technique. Am. J. Physiol., 210: 1335-1341, 1966.

Vassalle, M.: Automaticity and automatic rhythms. Am. J. Cardiol., 28: 245-252, 1971.

Vassalle, M., Cummins, M., Castro, C. and Stuckey, J.H.: The relationship between overdrive suppression and overdrive excitation in ventricular pacemakers in dogs. Circ. Res., 38: 367-374, 1975.

Vassalle, M., Knob, R.E., Cummins, M., Lara, G.A., Castro, C. and Stuckeu, J.H.: An analysis of fast idioventricular rhythm in the dog. Circ. Res., 41: 218-226, 1977.

Vassort, G., Rougier, O., Garnier, D., Sauviat, M.P., Coraboeuf, E., Gargouil, Y.-M.: Effects of adrenaline on membrane inward currents during the cardiac action potential. Pfluegers Arch., 309: 70, 1969.

Vincenzi, F.F. and West, T.C.: Release of autonomic mediators in cardiac tissue by direct subthreshold electrical stimulation. J. Pharmacol. Exp. Ther., 141: 185-194, 1963.

Vincenzi, F.F. and West, T.C.: Modification by calcium of the release of autonomic mediators in the isolated sinoatrial node. J. Pharmacol. Exp. Ther., 150: 349-360, 1965.

Viragh, S. and Porte, A.: The fine structure of the conducting system of the monkey heart (Macaca mulatta). I. The sinoatrial node and the internodal connections. Zeitschrift fuer Zellforschung, 145: 191-211, 1973.

Von Holst, E.: Entwurf eines systems der lokomotorischen Periodenbildungen bei Fischen. Zeitschr. f. Vergl. Physiologie, 26: 481-528, 1939.

Wallick, D.W., Levy, M.N., Felder, D.S. and Zieske, H.: Effects of repetitive bursts of vagal activity on atrioventricular junctional rate in dogs. Am. J. Physiol., 237: H275-H281, 1979.

Weidmann, S.: Effect of current flow on the membrane potential of cardiac muscle. J. Physiol. (London), 115: 227-236, 1951.

Weidmann, S.: The electrical constants of Purkinje fibres. J. Physiol. (London), 118: 348-360, 1952.

Weidmann, S.: Electrophysiologie der Herzmuskelfaser. Huber, Bern, 1956.

Weidmann, S.: Shortening of the cardiac action potential due to a brief injection of KCl following the onset of activity. J. Physiol. (London), 132: 157-163, 1956.

Weidmann, S.: The diffusion of radiopotassium across intercalated disks of mammalian cardiac muscle. J. Physiol. (London), 187: 323-342, 1966.

Weidmann, S.: Electrical constants of trabecular muscle from mammalian heart. J. Physiol. (London), 210: 1041-1054, 1970.

Weingart, R.: The permeability to tetraethylammonium ions of the surface membrane and intercalated disks of sheep and calf myocardium. J. Physiol. (London), 240: 741-762, 1974.

Weingart, R.: The action of ouabain on intercellular coupling and conduction velocity in mammalian ventricular muscle. J. Physiol. (London), 264: 341-365, 1977.

Weingart, R. and Reber, W.: Influence of internal pH on r_i of Purkinje fibres from mammalian heart. Experientia, 35: 929, 1979.

West, T.C: Ultramicroelectrode recording from the cardiac pacemaker. J. Pharmacol. Exp. Ther., 115: 283-290, 1955.

West, T.C.: Effects of chronotropic influences on subthreshold oscillations in the sino-atrial node. In: The Specialized Tissues of the Heart, Paes de Carvalho, A., de Mello, W.C. and Hoffman, B.F., eds., Amsterdam, Elsevier, pp. 81-94, 1961.

West, T.C. and Toda, N.: Response of the AV node of the rabbit to stimulation of the intracardiac cholinergic nerves. Circ. Res., 20: 18-31, 1967.

West, T.C., Falk, G. and Cervoni, P.: Drug alteration of transmembrane potentials in atrial pacemaker cells. J. Pharmacol. Exp. Ther., 117: 245-252, 1956.

Wever, R.: Virtual synchronization towards the limits of the range of entrainment. J. Theor. Biol., 36: 119-132, 1972.

Wiener, N. and Rosenblueth, A.: The mathematical formulation of the problem of conduction of impulses in a network of connected excitable elements, specifically in cardiac muscle. Arch. Inst. Cardiologia de Mexico, 16: 205-265, 1946.

Wier, W.G.: Calcium transients during excitation-contraction coupling in mammalian heart: aequorin signals of canine Purkinje fibers. Science, 207: 1085-1087, 1980.

Williams, E.H. and DeHaan, R.L.: Electrical coupling among heart cells in the absence of ultrastructurally defined gap junctions. J. Memb. Biol., 60: 237-248, 1981.

Winfree, A.T.: Integrated view of resetting a circadian clock. J. Theor. Biol., 28: 327-374, 1970.

Winfree, A.T.: Oscillatory glycolysis in yeast: the pattern of phase resetting by oxygen. Arch. Biochem. Biophys., 149: 388-401, 1972.

Winfree, A.T.: Spiral waves of chemical activity. Science, 175: 634-636, 1972.

Winfree, A.T.: Wavelike activity in biological and biochemical media. In: Lecture Notes in Biomathematics, 2, Van den Driessche, P., ed., Springer-Verlag, Berlin, pp. 243-260, 1974.

Winfree, A.T.: Phase control of neural pacemakers. Science, 197: 761-762, 1977.

Winfree, A.T.: Stable rotating patterns of reaction and diffusion. In: Theoretical Chemistry, 4, Eyring, H. and Henderson, D., eds., Academic Press, New York, pp. 1-51, 1978.

Winfree, A.T.: The Geometry of Biological Time. Springer-Verlag, N.Y., 1980.

Winfree, A.T.: Peculiarities in the impulse response of pacemaker neurons. In: Mathematical Aspects of Physiology, Lectures in Applied Mathematics 19, Hoppensteadt, F., ed., Am. Math. Soc., Providence, pp. 265-279, 1981.

Wit, A.L. and Cranefield, P.F.: Effect of verapamil on the sinoatrial and atrioventricular nodes of the rabbit and the mechanism by which it arrests reentrant atrioventricular nodal tachycardia. Circ. Res., 35: 413-425, 1974.

Wit, A.L. and Cranefield, P.F.: Triggered activity in cardiac muscle fibers of the simian mitral valve. Circ. Res., 38: 85-98, 1976.

Wit, A.L. and Cranefield, P.F.: Triggered and automatic activity in the canine coronary sinus. Circ. Res., 41: 435-455, 1977.

Wit, A.L. and Cranefield, P.F.: Reentrant excitation as a cause of cardiac arrhythmias. Am. J. Physiol., 235: H1-H17, 1978.

Wit, A.L., Hoffman, B.F. and Cranefield, P.F.: Slow conduction and re-entry in the ventricular conducting system. I. Return extrasystole in canine Purkinje fibers. Circ. Res., 30: 1-10, 1972.

Wojtczak, J.: Contractures and increase in internal longitudinal resistance of cow ventricular muscle induced by hypoxia. Circ. Res., 44: 88-95, 1979.

Wunderer, G., Fritz, H., Wachter, E. and Machleidt, W.: Amoni-acid sequence of a coelenterate toxin: Toxin II from anemonia sulcata. Eur. J. Biochem., 68: 193-198, 1976.

Wybauw, M.R.: Sur le point d'origine de la systole cardiaque dans l'oreillette droite. Arch. Int. Physiol., 10: 78-89, 1910.

Yamaguchi, I., Obayashi, K. and Mandel, W.J.: Electrophysiological effects of verapamil. Cardiovasc. Res., 12: 597-608, 1978.

Yamaguchi, I., Singh, B. and Mandel, W.J.: Electrophysiological actions of mexiletine on isolated rabbit atria and canine ventricular muscle and Purkinje fibers. Cardiovasc. Res., 13: 288-296, 1979.

Yamasaki, J., Fujiwana, M. and Toda, N.: Effects of intracellularly applied cyclic 3', 5''-adenosine monophosphate and dibutyryl cyclic 3', 5'-adenosine monophosphate on the electrical activity of the sinoatrial nodal cells of the rabbit. J. Pharmac. Exp. Ther., 190: 15-20, 1974.

Yanagihara, K. and Irisawa, H.: Inward current activated during hyperpolarization in the rabbit sinoatrial node cell. Pfluegers Arch., 385: 11-19, 1980.

Yanagihara, K. and Irisawa, H.: Potassium current during the pacemaker depolarization in rabbit sinoatrial node cell. Pfluegers Arch., 388: 255-260, 1980.

Yancey, B.S., Easter, D. and Revel, J.P.: Cytological changes in gap junctions during liver regeneration. J. Ultrastructure Res., 67: 229-242, 1979.

Yee, A.G. and Revel, J.P.: Loss and reappearance of gap junctions in regenerating liver. J. Cell Biol., 78: 554-564, 1978.

Young, J.M.: Desensitization and agonist binding to cholinergic receptors in intestinal smooth muscle. FEBS Lett., 46: 354-356, 1974.

Ypey, D.L., Clapham, D.E., DeHaan, R.L.: Development of electrical coupling and action potential synchrony between paired aggregates of embryonic heart cells. J. Memb. Biol., 51: 75-96, 1979.

Ypey, D.L., VanMeerwijk, W.P.M., Ince, C. and Groos, G.: Mutual entrainment of two pacemaker cells. A study with an electronic parallel conductance model. J. Theor. Biol., 86: 731-755, 1980.

Zaikin, A.N. and Zhabotinsky, A.M.: Concentration wave propagation in two-dimensional liquid-phase self-oscillating systems. Nature, 225: 535-537, 1970.

Zampighi, G. and Unwin, P.N.T.: Two forms of isolated gap junctions. J. Mol. Biol., 135: 451-464, 1979.

Zampighi, G., Corless, J.M. and Robertson, J.D.: On gap junction structure. J. Cell Biol., 86: 190-198, 1980.

INDEX